Neurology

FOR THE

Non-Neurologist
Fourth Edition

Neurology

FOR THE

Non-Neurologist

Fourth Edition

Edited by

William J. Weiner, M.D.

Professor of Neurology
Director of the Parkinson's Disease
and Movement Disorders Center
Department of Neurology
University of Miami
School of Medicine
Miami, Florida

and

Christopher G. Goetz, M.D.

Professor of Neurological Sciences
and Associate Chairperson
Department of Neurological Sciences
Rush Medical College
Rush Presbyterian-St. Luke's Medical Center
Chicago, Illinois

With 35 additional contributors

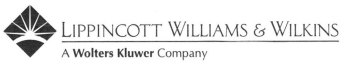

LIPPINCOTT WILLIAMS & WILKINS
A **Wolters Kluwer** Company
Philadelphia · Baltimore · New York · London
Buenos Aires · Hong Kong · Sydney · Tokyo

Acquisitions Editor: Anne M. Sydor
Developmental Editor: Sonya L. Seigafuse
Manufacturing Manager: Chuck Wagner
Production Manager: Robert Pancotti
Production Editor: Aureliano Vázquez, Jr.
Cover Designer: David Levy
Indexer: Nancy Newman
Compositor: Circle Graphics
Printer: R. R. Donnelly, Crawfordsville

Printed in the United States of America

9 8 7 6 5 4 3 2

Library of Congress Cataloging-in-Publication Data

Neurology for the non-neurologist / edited by William J. Weiner and
    Christopher G. Goetz ; with 35 additional contributors. — 4th ed.
        p.   cm.
    Includes bibliographical references and index.
    ISBN 0-7817-1707-8
    1. Neurology.   2. Nervous system—Diseases.   I. Weiner, William
J. II. Goetz, Christopher G.
    [DNLM: 1. Nervous System Diseases.   WL 140 N4928 1999]
    RC346.N453   1999
    616.8—dc21
    DNLM/DLC
    for Library of Congress   99-11318
                                                                  CIP

To our families

Contents

Contributing Authors

David A. Bennett, M.D.
Associate Professor
Department of Neurological Sciences
Rush Medical College
Director
Rush Alzheimer's Disease Center
Rush-Presbyterian-St. Luke's Medical Center
710 South Paulina Street
8 North J.R. Bowman
Chicago, Illinois 60612

Donna C. Bergen, M.D.
Associate Professor
Department of Neurological Sciences
Rush Medical College
Associate Attending Physician
Rush-Presbyterian-St. Luke's Medical Center
1725 West Harrison Street, Suite 755
Chicago, Illinois 60612

Joseph R. Berger, M.D.
Professor and Chairman
Department of Neurology
University of Kentucky
Kentucky Clinic, Room L445
Lexington, Kentucky 40536-0284

Thomas P. Bleck, M.D.
Professor of Neurology, Neurosurgery, and Medicine
University of Virginia
Director
Department of Neurocritical Care
University of Virginia
Neurology, Box 394
Charlottesville, Virginia 22908

Brian Bowen, M.D.
Associate Professor
Department of Radiology
MRI Center
University of Miami School of Medicine
1501 NW 9th Avenue
Miami, Florida 33136

Richard W. Byrne, M.D.
Assistant Professor
Department of Neurosurgery
1653 West Congress Parkway, Suite 1491
Chicago, Illinois 60612

Cynthia L. Comella, M.D.
Associate Professor
Department of Neurological Sciences
Rush Medical College
Associate Attending Physician
Rush-Presbyterian-St. Luke's Medical Center
1725 West Harrison Street, Suite 1106
Chicago, Illinois 60612

Charles M. D'Angelo, M.D.
Associates in Neurological Surgery, SC
Associate Professor
Rush-Presbyterian-St. Luke's Medical Center
1725 West Harrison Street, Suite 1117
Chicago, Illinois 60612

Larry E. Davis, M.D.
Chief, Neurology Services
VA Medical Center
1501 San Pedro Avenue
Alburquerque, New Mexico 87108
Professor
Department of Neurology
University of New Mexico School of Medicine

Stewart A. Factor, D.O.
Associate Professor and Riley
Family Chair in Parkinson's Disease
  at the Department of Neurology
Albany Medical College
and Parkinson's Disease and Movement Disorders Center
Albany Medical Center
215 Washington Avenue
Albany, New York 12203

Morris A. Fisher, M.D.
Professor
Department of Neurology
Loyola University Stritch School of Medicine
Attending Neurologist
Department of Neurology (127)
Hines VA Hospital
Hines, Illinois 60141

Russell H. Glantz, M.D.
Parkview Musculoskeletal Institute
7600 West College Drive
Palos Heights, Illinois 60463

Christopher G. Goetz, M.D.
Professor and Associate Chairperson
Department of Neurological Sciences
Rush Medical College
Senior Attending Physician
Rush-Presbyterian-St. Luke's Medical Center
1725 West Harrison Street, Suite 1106
Chicago, Illinois 60612

James A. Goodwin, M.D.
Associate Professor
Department of Ophthalmology and Neurology
The University of Illinois at Chicago
Director of Neuro-Ophthalmology
Department of Ophthalmology
University of Illinois Eye and Ear Infirmary
1855 West Taylor Street
Chicago, Illinois 60612

Deborah Olin Heros, M.D.
Clinical Neuro-oncologist
Department of Neurology
Mount Sinai Comprehensive Cancer Center
4306 Alton Road
Miami Beach, Florida 33140

Lawrence S. Honig, M.D.
Assistant Professor of Neurology
University of Texas South Western Medical Center
5323 Harry Hines Boulevard
Dallas, Texas 75235-9036

Judd M. Jensen, M.D.
Assistant Professor
Penobscot Bay Medical Center
4 Glen Cove Drive, Suite 105
Rockport, Maine 04856

Roger E. Kelley, M.D.
Professor and Chairman
Department of Neurology
Louisiana State University Medical Center-Shreveport
1501 Kings Highway
Shreveport, Louisiana 71130

William C. Koller, M.D., PH.D.
Professor
Department of Neurology
University of Kansas Medical Center
3901 Rainbow Boulevard
Kansas City, Kansas 66160

Ružica Kovačević-Ristanović, M.D.
Associate Professor
Department of Neurological Sciences
Rush Medical College
Associate Attending Physician
Rush-Presbyterian-St. Luke's Medical Center
1725 West Harrison Street, Suite 755
Chicago, Illinois 60612

David S. Kushner, M.D.
Assistant Clinical Professor
Department of Neurology
University of Miami School of Medicine
Medical Director
University Neurorehabilitation Institute
Health South Rehabilitation Hospital
20601 Old Cutler Road
Miami, Florida 33189

Steven L. Lewis, M.D.
Assistant Professor
Rush Medical College
Associate Attending Physician
Rush Presbyterian-St. Luke's Medical Center
1725 West Harrison Street, Suite 1106
Chicago, Illinois 60612

Sundeep M. Nayak, M.D.
Assistant Clinical Professor
Department of Radiology
University of California at San Francisco
Staff Neuroradiologist
Department of Imaging
University of California at San Francisco
Fresno VA Medical Center
2615 East Clinton Avenue
Fresno, California 93703-2286

Hans E. Neville, M.D.
Professor
Department of Neurology
University of Colorado
Staff Neurologist
Neurology Services
Denver VA Medical Center
9th & Clarmont
Denver, Colorado 90220

Lois Margaret Nora, M.D., J.D.
Associate Professor
Department of Neurology
University of Kentucky
Associate Dean, Academic Affairs and Administration
Office of Academic Affairs
University of Kentucky
Chandler Medical Center
800 Rose Street
Lexington, Kentucky 40536

Robert E. Nora
Attorney-at-Law
Oak Park, Illinois

Peter Portegies, PH.D.
Lecturer
Department of Neurology
University of Amsterdam
Neurologist
Department of Neurology
Academic Medical Centre H2-222
Meibergdreef 9
1105 AZ Amsterdam, The Netherlands

Priscilla F. Potter, M.D., PH.D.
Assistant Professor
Department of Neurology
University of Miami
1501 NW 9th Avenue
Miami, Florida 33136

Ruth G. Ramsey, M.D.
Professor of Radiology
and Chief, Section of Neuroradiology
Department of Radiology, MC 2026
The University of Chicago Hospital
5841 South Maryland Avenue
Chicago, Illinois 60637-1470

Steven P. Ringel, M.D.
Professor
Department of Neurology
University of Colorado School of Medicine
Director, Office of Clinical Practice and Quality
Management
and Director, Neuromuscular Section
University Hospital
4200 East 9th Avenue
Denver, Colorado 80262

José G. Romano, M.D.
Assistant Professor
Department of Neurology
University of Miami School of Medicine
Attending Physician
Department of Neurology
Jackson Memorial Hospital
1611 NW 12th Avenue
Miami, Florida 33136

Joel R. Saper, M.D., F.A.C.P, F.A.A.N
Clinical Professor of Neurology
Michigan State University
Founder and Director
Michigan Head-Pain and Neurological Institute
3120 Professional Drive
Ann Arbor, Michigan 48104

Kathleen M. Shannon, M.D.
Associate Professor
Department of Neurological Sciences
Rush Medical College
Associate Attending Physician
Rush-Presbyterian-St. Luke's Medical Center
1725 West Harrison Street, Suite 1106
Chicago, Illinois 60612

William A. Sheremata, M.D., F.R.C.P.C.
Professor of Clinical Neurology
Department of Neurology
University of Miami School of Medicine
1501 NW 9th Avenue
Miami, Florida 33136

Lisa M. Shulman, M.D.
Assistant Professor
Department of Neurology
University of Miami School of Medicine
1501 NW 9th Avenue
Miami, Florida 33136

Jordan L. Topel, M.D.
Associate Professor
Department of Neurological Sciences
Rush-Presbyterian-St. Luke's Medical Center
1725 Harrison Street, Suite 1106
Chicago, Illinois 60612

William J. Weiner, M.D.
Director of the Parkinson's Disease and Movement
  Disorder Center
and Professor
Department of Neurology
University of Miami School of Medicine
1501 NW 9th Avenue
Miami, Florida 33136

Robert S. Wilson, PH.D.
Professor
Department of Neurological Sciences
Director, Section of Cognitive Neuroscience
Rush-Presbyterian-St. Luke's Medical Center
1645 West Jackson, Suite 675
Chicago, Illinois 60612

Preface

The life, career, and words of William Osler are pertinent anchors for a discussion of neurology among non-neurologists. A Canadian by birth, Osler worked at McGill University early in his career, then at the University of Pennsylvania before becoming the first chairman of the Department of Medicine at the newly formed Johns Hopkins Medical School. Always a proud internist who opposed the risk of isolation found in medical specialization, Osler showed an enormous breadth in his medical, scientific, and philosophical contributions. Of note to this discussion, throughout his life Osler found that neurological issues related to the general practice of medicine, and his works on cerebrovascular disease, infections, chorea, and pediatric disabilities remain pillars in the medical literature. To honor Osler as the archetype of the non-neurologist who used neurology at its highest level, we cite several of his words as we introduce this text.

The fourth edition of *Neurology for the Non-Neurologist* maintains its focus on educating health care professionals who deal with nervous system disease regularly but who have not committed their careers to neuroscience. This group of colleagues includes internists, family practitioners, psychiatrists, geriatricians, rehabilitation specialists, and advanced nurses. As neurology has broadened its scope and depth over the past years, we have not only updated the third edition of this book but also expanded it to encompass new areas of interest and clinical concern. We have prepared this book not as a comprehensive text but rather as a series of focused and concise essays on major topics in neurology. As such, the book may be read in its entirety to give an overview of contemporary clinical neurology as it relates to medicine; or it can be used as a reference source on individual topics. The book's size is purposefully moderate, manageable for carrying on hospital rounds and being used in a busy office practice. Although each chapter is composed by different authors, the editors have placed an overall discipline on the work to maintain a homogeneity for readers who search for a consistent level and manner of presentation:

> *To the physician particularly a scientific discipline is an incalculable gift, which leavens his whole life, giving exactness to habits of thought and tempering the mind with that judicious faculty of distrust, which can alone, amid the uncertainty of practice, make him wise.*
> *Osler, 1893*

The initial chapters of this edition deal with topics of general pertinence, such as the basic neurological examination and the ordering of neurological tests. To this section we have added a new chapter on several commonly encountered neurological syndromes, with an emphasis on key information in the patient's history that will guide the diagnostic evaluation. The repertoire of diagnostic tests has increased recently, as has their expense, and an overview of the usefulness and expected yield of various examinations helps to guide the treating physician in a logical evaluation sequence. Furthermore, a common and difficult decision is "When should a neurologist be consulted?" Although there is no simple textbook answer, these early chapters are written to help frontline physicians capture the core principles of neurology. With this information, they can place their individual patients into a clinical context and maximally utilize the neurological examination and testing opportunities to arrive at diagnostic, treatment, and referral decisions. Equally important, these first chapters are designed to dispel biases that neurological topics are obscure, overly complicated, and rarely linked to practical solutions.

The very first step towards success in any occupation is to become interested in it.

Osler, 1903

Subsequent chapters guide the reader through the frequently encountered neurological problems of medically ill patients. Some of these chapters are based on contributions from the third edition but have been revised to incorporate comments and feedback that we received in using this book in various educational contexts. As with the prior editions, the authors are primarily faculty of national reputation from our two institutions, with added experts from several other university and practice centers. We have selected our authors based not only on their teaching experience, but also on their keen abilities to distill information and prioritize the most important elements for a non-neurologist's practice.

It is often harder to boil down than to write.

Osler, 1903

The topics covered in this book range from primary neurology, such as cerebrovascular diseases, headaches, multiple sclerosis, and neuropathies, to chapters on neurological dilemmas consequent to medical illnesses or their treatment. The chapters on infections and AIDS are up-to-date discussions of how these disorders impact the nervous system, especially in the instances of initial disease presentation. The chapter on neurological complications of pregnancy addresses the alarmingly frequent abnormalities affecting childbearing women, and stresses the prompt recognition of these problems and the issues related to a decision on treatment or observation. We have added a new chapter on neurorehabilitation because many medical disorders of both acute or chronic nature have neurological manifestations that are clearly associated with significant functional gains after rehabilitative efforts. In hospital practice as well as outpatient care, a clear perspective on the role of neurorehabilitation provides the health care practioner with resources on therapies, devices, and educational opportunities that can be pivotal for patients in their reintegration into the community. Whereas the emphasis of each chapter is necessarily neurological, the authors have attempted to place these features always in a comprehensive context that maintains a respectful view of total patient care.

Care more particularly for the individual patient than for the special features of the disease.

Osler, 1894

We consider this fourth edition of *Neurology for the Non-Neurologist* our best and most comprehensive effort in the long-standing commitment to continuing medical education. As with the other editions, this revision and expansion has offered us the opportunity to continue working towards an admittedly unattainable goal. Like Osler, however, we have proudly found the process of trying to achieve a perfect project nourishing and of continued interest. We look to our readers to provide us with the necessary feedback to maintain an agile and critical eye for the future of this book.

The artistic sense of perfection in work is another much-to-be-desired quality to be cultivated. No matter how trifling the matter on hand, do it with feeling that it demands the best that is in you, and when done, look it over with a critical eye, not sparing a strict judgement of yourself.

Osler, 1903.

William J. Weiner, M.D.
Christopher G. Goetz, M.D.

Citations derived from: RB Bean, *Sir William Osler: Aphorisms from his bedside teachings and writings.* CC Thomas, Springfield, 1961.

Preface

to the First Edition

Neurology for the Non-Neurologist is an outgrowth of over 20 years of continued participation in the education and training of undergraduate neuroscience students, postgraduate residents, and practicing physicians. Our experience has been that despite the diverse backgrounds and interests of these groups, there is a common point at which they begin to acquire their working knowledge of neurology. Based on this assumption, this text has been designed to be valuable to both pre- and postgraduate physicians, as well as to students, and concisely covers the implications of neurologic disease for clinical medicine and neuroscience.

Most neurology texts are organized by anatomy (diseases of the hemispheres, brain stem, peripheral nerves, and muscles) or etiology (genetic, infectious, autoimmune neurologic diseases). Some entities are more easily and clearly discussed from the former vantage and others are better understood when approached from the latter. This text integrates both approaches, emphasizing the anatomic method of organization in some chapters (peripheral neuropathy, muscle disorder, neuroophthalmology, and so forth) and the etiologic organization in others (epilepsy, infections, and tumors). Other chapters are descriptive and aim to guide the physician in a reasonable and satisfying therapeutic approach to common neurologic dilemmas: trauma, behavioral neurology, minimal brain dysfunction, sleep disorders, and so forth.

We have not attempted to write a comprehensive neurologic textbook, but instead to collect a series of concise essays concerning areas of current clinical relevance to neurology. Each chapter includes a description of a clinical disorder with emphasis on signs, symptomatology, pathophysiology, clinical therapeutics, and an overall view of research trends in that particular field. At the conclusion of each chapter there are several self-study questions with appropriate discussion provided for the reader. The book may be read in its entirety to give an overview of clinical neurology to medical students and beginning neurology residents, psychiatrists, students in related fields or neurosciences, and practicing physicians in internal medicine or family practice. *Neurology for the Non-Neurologist* may also be used as a selective reference work, since each chapter can stand entirely by itself.

William J. Weiner, M.D.
Christopher G. Goetz, M.D.

Acknowledgments

We thank Maynard M. Cohen, M.D., Ph.D., for his enthusiasm, dedication, and interest in this book when the first edition was being prepared. His guidance was instrumental in the publication of this series. We also thank Maria Macias, Rebeca Barquero, and Marilynn Payton, who provided invaluable help in the preparation of this manuscript.

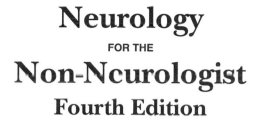

Neurology
FOR THE
Non-Neurologist
Fourth Edition

Neurology for the Non-Neurologist, Fourth Edition,
edited by William J. Weiner and
Christopher G. Goetz. Lippincott
Williams & Wilkins, Philadelphia © 1999.

C H A P T E R   1

The Neurologic Examination

Priscilla F. Potter

William J. Weiner

The neurologic examination is the foundation of the practice of neurology. It includes the patient interview and the physical examination. Unlike other medical disciplines that place much weight on ancillary studies, the neurologic investigations are wholly guided by the information gleaned from the neurologic interview and examination. The neurologic exam itself is guided by the information obtained in the interview. Every patient does not require a complete neurologic examination. The information obtained in the interview directs the examiner to the relevant parts of the examination.

The examination starts when the examiner enters the room of the patient. Observation is key. The examiner needs to observe who is in the room besides the patient, who is telling the history of the patient, the language used in the history, and the body movements of the patient during the interview. All of this information is potentially relevant to the neurologic examination and diagnosis. The information obtained in the history should be used to formulate a hypothesis and direct the neurologic evaluation.

The neurologic interview/history should be obtained with great care. The nature of the problem, its tempo, onset, duration, acuity, progression, frequency, associated symptoms, and exacerbating and alleviating circumstances should be elicited. Anatomic regions that are affected should be defined.

In some instances, the history has to be obtained from others. The patient who has a generalized seizure or an episode of impairment of consciousness will not be able to provide a complete history of the event. The patient with cognitive deficits or speech difficulties will also be unable to provide adequate historical information. It is important to question the spouse, a relative, or witnesses to a specific event to obtain a more complete and often more accurate story.

The neurologic examination in divided into several components. These include examination of the mental status, cranial nerves, sensory system, motor system, coordination, gait, and reflexes. Each of these components has several parts that will be addressed in this chapter. The depth of the examination of these components is directed by the information obtained in the history of the problem. If the patient is complaining of numbness and weakness of the hands, the examination concentrates on the peripheral nervous system. If, however, the patient is complaining of dysarthria and hemibody paresis, the examination is directed at the central nervous system. The tempo of these neurologic changes also becomes important. If the speech and hemibody paresis were sudden in onset, a vascular event is suspected, whereas a slowly progressive tempo would suggest a space-occupying lesion such as a tumor. The following description of the neurologic examination is written for the use by non-neurologists.

Certain neurologic conditions are commonly associated with a normal neurologic examination [e.g., primary generalized epilepsies, transient ischemic attacks (TIAs), migraine, and other headaches]. In these and other disorders, initial diagnostic considerations depend on obtaining a complete history. If the neurologic examination detects abnormalities, additional diagnostic alternatives may be raised. For example, a positive Babinski sign days after a grand mal seizure suggests that the seizure may have been of focal onset, so that a search for a structural brain lesion has to be considered. The finding of mild hand clumsiness after an acute event points to a stroke rather than a TIA. Therapeutic choices may differ depending on whether the patient had a TIA or a completed cerebrovascular accident (CVA).

Since the neurologic examination is often crucial in establishing the correct diagnosis, it is important for all physicians to be able to perform a complete, albeit often brief, evaluation of the nervous system. The often-written chart note for the neurologic examination found on non-neurology services (neuro-WNL, meaning within normal limits) should be avoided; most often, WNL is interpreted as "We never looked." The neurologic examination should be conducted with a consistent routine so that portions of the evaluation are not forgotten.

MENTAL STATUS

The examination for mental status begins with the interview. The examiner notes whether information is provided by the patient or by the person accompanying the patient. Is the patient capable of giving the information, or does he/she have a depressed level of consciousness or perhaps a psychiatric condition that interferes with the information-giving process? The examiner observes the patient's behavior, mood, and affect. Furthermore, the examiner looks for signs of illusions, delusions, hallucinations, and misinterpretations in the patient's answers. If the patient has significant signs of psychiatric problems, an examination by a psychiatrist is in order.

The goal of the mental status examination is to determine the level of consciousness; orientation to person, place, and time; attention span; concentration; memory; insight; judgment; and ability to calculate. This assessment is useful in determining the global cortical functioning of the patient as well as more localized functioning of such areas as the hippocampus, which is concerned with memory. Questions used to assess these functions should be woven into the interview so that the patient does not feel that

he/she is being examined. It should be recognized that a patient who fully participates in the history taking and provides a coherent accurate history interspersed with accurate references to current social or political events, and who follows instructions during the examination, may not require a formal evaluation of mental status, memory, and language functions. A withdrawn, nonparticipating patient may have cognitive dysfunction (with or without dementia) or may be depressed. A patient with significant cognitive deficits in memory or language will not be able to provide adequate information even while trying hard to communicate. The physician should also note other aspects of behavior. Avoidance of eye contact and a depressed face suggest depression. Irritability, distractibility, aimless picking on clothing or surrounding objects, and indifference to serious symptoms being discussed suggest cognitive impairment. A clear indication that a formal mental evaluation should be conducted is the clinical situation in which the spouse or caregiver asks to give the history and then proceeds to do so. In such instances, the patient often sits quietly, not speaking spontaneously, while an entire discussion ensues of how his personality and behavior have changed.

When the history suggests memory dysfunction or changes in behavior, historical information from relatives, friends, coworkers, and employers may be required. Often patients with early, mild dementing processes may still be smarter than their evaluators, and they often use various tricks of social grace and convention to evade specific questions. Patients may become belligerent if deficits are revealed, and this should be done cautiously. For example, specific mental status testing may be performed by telling patients in a nonthreatening manner that silly questions have to be asked, and by requesting them to please cooperate.

The formal examination of mental status starts with questions related to orientation to time, place, and person. Orientation to time should progress from year through season, month, and date to day of the week. Orientation to space starts with the current actual location (e.g., Dr. Smith's office) and city, then goes to county, state, and country. The patient should be asked to state his full name and try to identify any person accompanying him. Memory evaluation should be divided into tests of immediate and recent recall. Immediate recall is tested by asking the patient to immediately repeat a random sequence of numbers (digit span). Digits can be presented in groups of increasing numbers (from three to six). Normal adults can readily repeat sequences of five to six numbers without error. Most adults are able to reverse the number sequence successfully, and great difficulty in reversing the sequence may be a subtle sign of cognitive impairment. Many patients with early to moderate dementing illness can successfully perform digit spans. Recent recall is tested by presenting the patients with three to four unrelated words, asking the patient to remember them, and then proceeding with other elements of the mental status evaluation. After 3 to 5 minutes, the patient should be asked to repeat the previously given words. Unimpaired patients will be able to recall at least two to three of the words. Impairment of recent recall is often affected early in dementing processes and may reflect the frequent historical complaint that the patient has to be repeatedly told things and does not seem to remember events.

Concentration and calculating ability are evaluated by the use of serial 7s. The patient is asked to subtract 7 in a sequential manner from 100 (100, 93, 86, 79, 72, 65). Finger gnosis, right–left orientation, and ability to perform three-step commands can be assessed by asking the patient to take his right index finger and touch his right ear and close his eyes.

Language can be quickly assessed by evaluating spontaneous speech, repetition, comprehension of spoken and written material, and the ability to write. Speech may be fluent or nonfluent, and this observation may be very useful in localizing a potential cortical lesion. Nonfluent speech (Broca's aphasia) is localized to the dominant posterior inferior frontal region and is often associated with a hemiparesis, whereas fluent aphasic speech (Wernicke's aphasia), which sounds normal in delivery but makes little or no sense, is localized to the posterior temporal area and is not associated with a marked paresis. The presence of aphasia may prevent adequate memory and other cognitive testing.

Apraxia (difficulty in performance of motor acts independent of motor or primary sensory impairment) can be evaluated by asking the patient to demonstrate how he would comb his hair, salute, or use a screwdriver. The apractic patient may use his hand as a tool instead of pretending to hold the object or may simply be unable to demonstrate the essential movement involved in the act. Apraxia can also be suspected if the patient displays difficulties in the execution of motor tasks such as finger tapping or hand pronation or supination that appear to be more than mere slowness, clumsiness, or weakness. Language disturbances (aphasia), calculation difficulties (dyscalculia), and the apraxias may each represent involvement of the dominant hemisphere, or

they may be a sign of more widespread cognitive impairment (dementia).

The ability to draw a clock and to copy a three-dimensional representation of a cube can be interpreted as a function of visual spatial orientation. This ability may be impaired as a result of focal disease (nondominant hemisphere) or a dementing illness. Clock drawing may also detect a visual field deficit when the patient repeatedly draws only a half or a quarter of the clock.

In the office, it is useful to have a quantifiable standardized tool to screen for dementing process. The Folstein Mini-Mental Status evaluation is widely used and provides not only scores that can be compared with normals but also a baseline by which to judge patient's future performance.

CRANIAL NERVES

There are twelve pairs of cranial nerves, each of which serves specific functions as illustrated in Table 1-1. A systematic examination of each pair of the cranial nerves is an essential part of the neurologic exam as it provides information on the integrity of the medulla, pons, midbrain, and limbic and visual systems. A superficial examination of the cranial nerves should be incorporated into any neurologic examination and can be done in just a few minutes. Of course, if any abnormality is found on the cursory exam, a more detailed study of that area is necessary.

OLFACTORY NERVE

Loss of smell is most frequently due to trauma, but it may result from a lesion in the anterior fossa of the cranium. The olfactory nerve (cranial nerve I) is usually not tested unless the patient is complaining of loss of smell. The olfactory nerves can be tested with aromatic coffee grounds, cloves, or flavorings. A small vial of the aromatic substance is held under the nostril while the other nostril is occluded. The patient is asked to breathe through the unobstructed nostril and identify the odor. The exercise is repeated on the other side with a different aromatic substance.

OPTIC NERVE

Evaluation of the optic nerve (cranial nerve II) includes examination of visual acuity, visual fields, and color vision. It further includes examination of

TABLE 1-1. Cranial Nerves and Their Functions

CRANIAL NERVE	NAME OF CRANIAL NERVE	FUNCTION
I	Olfactory	Smell
II	Optic	Vision
III	Oculomotor	Elevate, depress and adduct the eye, pupillary constriction
IV	Trochlear	Depression, adduction, and intorsion of the eye
V	Trigeminal	Sensation of the face and motor control of the muscles of mastication
VI	Abducens	Abduction of the eye
VII	Facial	Muscles of facial expression, taste for anterior ⅔ of tongue, sensation from ear
VIII	Vestibulocochlear	Hearing and balance
IX	Glossopharyngeal	Taste posterior ⅓ of tongue, sensation from ear, gag reflex, contraction of stylopharyngius muscle
X	Vagus	Gag reflex motor to soft palate, pharynx, larynx; autonomic fibers to esophagus, stomach, small intestine, heart, trachea; sensation from ear; viscera
XI	Spinal accessory	Motor control of the sternocleidomastoid and trapezius muscles
XII	Hypoglossal	Motor control of the tongue

the retina of the eye. The optic nerve is the connection between the retina, the optic chiasm, optic radiation, and the occipital cortex. Central vision is tested by examination of visual acuity. The patient is asked to read printed material from a book or newspaper, or the examiner can use the Snellen card for a more accurate test of near vision. The eyes are tested individually. The patient may use corrective lenses if necessary. If the patient cannot see the printed letters, then the ability to count fingers, distinguish movement of hands, or detect light can be used to assess impairment of central vision.

Visual fields are tested by confrontation. The examiner faces the patient, points to his own nose, and asks him to concentrate on it. The examiner then holds up some of his own fingers briefly in each of the four quadrants of the visual field and asks the patient to count them. If an abnormality was seen on the initial screening, the visual fields of both eyes are examined separately (by covering the other eye). Visual field defects of one eye suggest that the lesion is localized to that globe or in the prechaismatic optic nerve. A defect in both eyes suggests lesions involving the optic chiasm, tract, radiations, or visual cortex. Defects involving the temporal half of one eye and the nasal portion of the other eye (homonymous hemianopsia) suggests a lesion of the optic radiation or occipital cortex, whereas a bi-temporal field defect is found in a lesion of the optic chiasm.

The optic nerve head is evaluated during the funduscopic examination. Items to be evaluated include the optic disc, the retinal vessels that traverse the center of the optic nerve head, and the retina. The optic disc is evaluated for clarity and depth. Papilledema is associated with swelling of the optic disc and is visualized as indeterminate disc margins and loss of venous pulsations in the optic veins. It is bilateral and associated with preserved visual acuity except for extremely advanced cases. The presence of papilledema suggests increased intracranial pressure and can be seen with brain tumors, occlusions of the cerebral venous drainage, and benign intracranial hypertension. Glaucoma is associated with a deep optic disc, but all deep optic discs do not denote glaucoma. Optic neuritis is a common neurologic condition associated with some eye pain, decreased visual acuity that is not corrected by lenses, and an afferent pupillary defect (Marcus–Gunn pupil). Light shown into the affected pupil causes minimal or no pupillary restriction because the inflamed optic nerve is unable to transmit the light stimulus fully or at all. This results in the seeming paradox of the affected pupil dilating in response to a light stimulus. Light shown in the nonaffected eye does cause pupillary constriction in the opposite eye because of the consensual pupillary reflex (see later). Optic neuritis may be bilateral and in that case the patient would have bilateral pupillary defects.

OCULOMOTOR, TROCHLEAR, AND ABDUCENS NERVES

The oculomotor (cranial nerve III), trochlear (cranial nerve IV), and abducens (cranial nerve VI) primarily control the movements of the extraocular eye muscles, which are yoked in their actions. Contraction of the right lateral rectus and the left medial rectus causes the eyes to move toward the right, while contraction of the superior rectus muscles causes the eyes to deviate superiorly. The oculomotor nerve supplies the superior, inferior, and medial rectus and inferior oblique muscles. These muscles elevate, depress, and adduct the eye. The levator palpebrae muscle is also innervated by this cranial nerve. Denervation of this muscle would result in ptosis of the superior eyelid. The oculomotor nerve also carries parasympathetic fibers to the pupilloconstrictor and ciliary muscles, which cause constriction of the pupil to light and thickening of the lens during accommodation, respectively.

The trochlear nerve supplies the superior oblique muscle. Contraction of this muscle results in depression, adduction, and intorsion of the eye. The abducens nerve supplies the lateral rectus muscle. Contraction of this muscle results in abduction of the eye.

These three cranial nerves are tested together. The examiner first notes the position of the eyes in primary gaze. Are both eyes looking forward, or is one (or are both) deviated from the primary gaze position? The examiner asks the patient to follow his finger as he moves it in the four peripheral quadrants. He notes whether each eye is able to move in all four quadrants of gaze, and whether the eye movements are symmetrical (conjugate) or dysconjugate. If the eye movements are dysconjugate, each eye's movements are tested individually. Nystagmus may be noted during this exam.

Pupillary function is under the control of the parasympathetic and sympathetic nerves. The parasympathetic fibers are carried on the oculomotor nerve while the sympathetic fibers are carried on the carotid and intracranial blood vessels. Pupillary size and equality should be observed during the examination of the eyes and extraocular muscles. A difference of up to 1 mm in the size of the pupils is considered normal. Pupillary reaction to light and accommodation is tested. A bright light is shone into first one eye and the pupillary response is observed in both eyes. The direct response is the response of the pupil that had the light shone in it. The constriction of the opposite pupil when light stimulates only one eye is called the consensual light reflex. These responses are usually equal. Pupils that are not reac-

tive to light stimulus but that do constrict with accommodation are seen in light-near dissociation. These pupils, called Argyll Robertson pupils, are seen in conditions such as neurosyphilis, diabetes, and autonomic neuropathies. Lesions of the sympathetic pathway, either central or peripheral, result in miosis and ptosis of the affected eye (Horner's syndrome).

Involvement of cranial nerves III, IV, and VI, or of the muscles they serve, is almost invariably accompanied by diplopia except in long-standing squints and progressive external ophthalmoplegia (a rare muscular disorder). Involvement of cranial nerve III distal to its nucleus may present with unilateral ptosis and deficits of adduction, depression, or elevation of the eye with or without associated mydriasis. Bilateral asymmetrical extraocular movement deficits without pupillary involvement may represent disease of the ocular muscles (Graves' disease) or the neuromuscular junction (myasthenia gravis). A lesion of cranial nerve VI will result in a deficit of abduction of the eye on straight-ahead gaze. A lesion of cranial nerve IV will result in a deficit of intorsion (internal rotation) of the eye (superior oblique weakness) when the affected eye is attempting to look down and in.

Impairment of conjugate eye movements implies pathology of the cerebral centers controlling eye movements. This may be seen in cerebral hemisphere strokes or basal ganglia degenerative diseases (e.g., progressive supranuclear palsy). These disorders are not accompanied by diplopia.

TRIGEMINAL NERVE

The trigeminal nerve (cranial nerve V) has two components: One conveys sensory information from the face, and the motor component controls the muscles of mastication (temporalis, masseter, and pterygoid) and the tensor vali palatini. The sensory portion of the trigeminal nerve is composed of three divisions, ophthalmic, maxillary and mandibular. Figure 1-1 shows the distribution of these divisions. Sensation of crude touch, pinprick, and temperature on the face can be tested in three separate divisions by cotton whisp, pin, or cold and warm test tubes. The examiner should note the presence of symmetry of the sensation. The corneal reflex is also evaluated during the sensory examination of the face. A whisp of cotton is touched to the cornea while the patient is looking away from the examiner. The normal response is a blink of both eyes. The strength of the masticator muscles is checked by examining jaw-opening strength, palpating jaw muscles while the teeth are being clenched, and evaluating side-to-side jaw movements. Unilateral

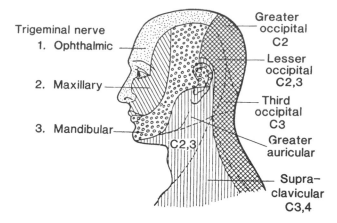

Trigeminal nerve
1. Ophthalmic
2. Maxillary
3. Mandibular

Greater occipital C2
Lesser occipital C2,3
Third occipital C3
Greater auricular
Supra-clavicular C3,4
C2,3

FIG. 1-1. Distribution of the three divisions of the trigeminal nerve. The sensory portion of the trigeminal nerve has three divisions: I, ophthalmic; II, maxillary; and III, mandibular. Their approximate locations are illustrated. *(From Members of the Department of Neurology, Mayo Clinic and Mayo Foundation for Medical Education and Research, Clinical Examinations in Neurology, 6th Ed., St. Louis: Mosby Year Book, 1991, p. 270.)*

weakness will cause the jaw to deviate to that side upon jaw opening. The jaw jerk is a jaw closure movement elicited by tapping the partially opened jaw at its midline. This reflex may become hyperactive, affecting connections between cortex and the cranial nerves subserving mastication, speech, and deglutition (e.g., bilateral hemispheral CVAs).

FACIAL NERVE

The facial nerve (cranial nerve VII) is a compound nerve carrying motor, general sensory, special sensory, and parasympathetic fibers. It supplies motor innervation to the muscles of facial expression, sensory fibers to the external ear, and special sensory fibers for taste reception from the anterior two thirds of the tongue. Parasympathetic fibers from the salivatory nucleus that mediate vasodilatation and secretion of the submandibular and sublingual glands travel along the facial nerve.

Examination of the facial nerve begins with observation of the patient's facial movements while he/she is speaking, frowning, smiling. The muscles of facial expression are examined by having him wrinkle his forehead, close his eyes tightly against resistance, smile, grimace, puff out his cheeks, and whistle. Symmetry is noted during these various movements. Having him protrude his tongue and then placing sugar, salt, or similar substances gently on one side of the tongue tests taste. The patient should identify the substance before withdrawing his tongue into his mouth, as the test substance can diffuse in the mouth to the posterior or the opposite side of the tongue.

The ability to wrinkle the forehead is often used to distinguish between upper and lower motor neuron involvement of the facial nerve. The forehead being spared when the lower face is paralyzed is suggestive of upper motor neuron involvement such as is seen in cortical lesions (CVA). If the forehead is involved in the paralytic process, the lesion is likely to be lower motor neuron (the nucleus or the nerve itself) as in Bell's palsy. The sense of taste may be involved in lower motor neuron type of facial paralysis if the lesion is proximal to the chordi tympani nerve.

ACOUSTIC NERVE

The acoustic nerve (cranial nerve VIII) is a compound nerve that has two divisions: The cochlear division is involved in hearing, and the vestibular division is involved in balance. Hearing ability is assessed by whispering in each ear with the other ear blocked, or by holding a ticking wristwatch to the ear so that the patient can hear the ticktock. A tuning fork (256 vibrations per second) is used to assess air conduction in Rinne's test. The vibrating tuning fork is held against the mastoid bone and the patient is instructed to tell the examiner when he can no longer hear the noise. The head of the fork is then placed beside the patient's ear. The test result is normal when the patient can hear the vibrating tuning fork much longer when it is placed beside the ear (air conduction is greater than bone conduction). An abnormal Rinne's test, when bone conduction is greater than air conduction, could be the result of a blockage in the external canal or a lesion in the ossicles of the middle ear.

In Weber's test for hearing, a vibrating tuning fork is placed on the mid frontal area of the head. Normally, sound is perceived in both ears. If there is a conduction block of the ear, the sound will lateralize to that ear. If there is a sensorineural defect blocking sound perception, the sound will localize to the opposite ear with the intact nerve. Dysfunction of the vestibular component of the acoustic nerve is suggested by complaints of vertigo and findings of nystagmus on examination of extraocular eye movements.

GLOSSOPHARYNGEAL NERVE

The glossopharyngeal nerve (cranial nerve IX) carries special sensory fibers transmitting taste sensation from the posterior one third of the tongue and general sensation from the auditory tube and middle ear. This nerve also contains motor fibers that control secretion from the parotid gland and contraction of the stylopharynglius muscle. Testing of this nerve involves placing a tongue depressor on the posterior wall of the pharynx. The normal response is a contraction of these muscles, the gag reflex. It is difficult to attribute this response to cranial nerve IX alone, since there is also innervation to the pharynx from the vagus nerve (cranial nerve X).

VAGUS NERVE

The vagus nerve (cranial nerve X) is a mixed nerve that carries somatic fibers to the soft palate, pharynx, and larynx; autonomic fibers to muscles of the esophagus, stomach, small intestine, heart, and trachea; and sensory fibers from the viscera and external ear. It is difficult to test all portions of the vagus nerve. The usual exam consists of observing the movement of the soft palate while asking the patient to say Ahh. A normal response is for the palate to elevate symmetrically. Weakness on one side of the palate will cause deviation in the direction of the intact side. A unilateral lesion of the vagus does not normally result in swallowing difficulties, while bilateral lesions result in regurgitation and dysphagia. Lesion of the recurrent laryngeal nerve causes unilateral paralysis of vocal cords in the abducted position, resulting in hoarseness of the voice.

The gag reflex need not be performed in every patient. There exists a wide range of responses to this test, and many normal people are hypersensitive to it. Some patients will start to gag as soon as they see the tongue blade. The gag reflex may also be almost absent in a normal patient. A history of swallowing difficulties and speech changes and assorted neurologic abnormalities need to be present before the gag reflex assumes meaning. Isolated reports that the gag reflex is hypersensitive or absent are usually meaningless.

SPINAL ACCESSORY NERVE

The spinal accessory nerve (cranial nerve XI) arises from the upper five cervical segments of the spinal cord. It ascends through the foramen magnum and exits through the jugular foramen. The spinal accessory nerve innervates the sternocleidomastoid and trapezius muscles. Having the patient turn his head to the right tests the left sternocleidomastoid muscle. The trapezius is examined by having him shrug his shoulders while the examiner pushes down on them.

HYPOGLOSSAL NERVE

The hypoglossal nerve (cranial nerve XII) provides innervation to the tongue. Examination of the tongue includes looking for bulk of the muscle, midline protrusion, and rapid movements from side to side and in and out of the mouth. Unilateral lower motor neuron lesions will cause ipsilateral wasting of the tongue and protrusion toward the stronger side. Bilateral lower motor neuron lesions result in bilateral atrophy of the tongue, poor protusion, and poor lingual sounds such as "La la la." Bilateral upper motor lesions cause a decrease in the rapidity of tongue movements while unilateral upper motor neuron lesions have little effect since the hypoglossal nuclei have some bilateral innervation.

SENSORY SYSTEM

The sensory examination is very dependent on the subjective responses of the patient. If the patient is confused, demented, aphasic, or has an altered state of consciousness, the responses will be invalid and this portion of the neurologic exam can be omitted. On the other hand, if the patient is anxious, seems to have limited tolerance to testing or a limited but not totally impaired attention span, and the history suggests that the sensory examination will be important in reaching a diagnosis, the examination should begin with sensory testing. The patient does not need to undress for the exam, but the legs below the knees and the arms below the elbows should be exposed. If a spinal cord problem is suspected, the trunk should be accessible.

The sensory exam is divided into primary sensations and cortical sensations. The primary sensations, including pain, light touch, temperature, vibration, and joint position, are carried on two different tracts. The sensations of pain and temperature are transmitted to the ventroposterior lateral nucleus of the thalamus by the crossed spinothalamic tract. Vibration, joint position, and two-point discrimination are transmitted via the uncrossed posterior columns to the same thalamic nucleus. Both the spinothalamic and posterior columns transmit light touch. The combined sensations are then transmitted to the primary sensory cortex via the fibers of the posterior limb of the internal capsule. Cortical sensations include double simultaneous stimulation, stereognosis, and graphesthesia. These sensations can be evaluated only in the presence of intact primary sensory modalities.

The sensory system should be evaluated in an organized manner. Side-to-side and proximal-to-distal comparisons should be made. Hemibody loss of all primary sensory modalities is due to lesions in the contralateral sensory pathways of the brainstem or cerebral hemispheres. A useful examination technique is to quickly compare the patient's appreciation of pinprick from proximal to distal and from side to side. If a particular area of decreased sensation to pinprick is identified in a part of a limb, careful attention to its boundaries will suggest root (dermotomal), plexus, or peripheral nerve involvement (Fig. 1-2). Temperature can be tested by comparing the touch of a cool tuning fork and a warm finger on the skin, or by using cold and warm test tubes. A cursory survey of temperature discrimination involves touching the three divisions of the trigeminal nerve with the warm and cool objects, followed by testing the dorsum of the hands and feet. If the patient lacks temperature discrimination in any of these areas, a more detailed examination of that area is required. If any loss of temperature sensation is found, it should be determined if there is a corresponding loss of pinprick sensation, as these are carried on the same spinothalamic pathway. The pinprick test includes discrimination between sharp and dull sensations. The patient's response should be immediate, either "sharp" or "dull." A delayed response could suggest either inattention to the activity or that the sensation is traveling along the more diffuse polysynaptic pathway through the reticular formation. Testing of pain and temperature is quite useful, especially when looking for a spinal cord level, since spinothalamic fibers cross within a few segments of entering the spinal cord. The examination should be conducted with disposable pins so that they are not used from patient to patient.

Vibratory sense and joint position are sensations carried in the dorsal columns that do not cross until the cervicomedullary junction. Vibratory sense is tested by placing a vibrating tuning fork (either 128 or 256 Hz) on the nail or knuckle of the fingers and toes while the examiner places his or her finger under the patient's digit. In this way the examiner can tell when the vibration has ceased. The patient is asked to tell the examiner if the vibration is felt and when it stops. In this way, a difference in sensory discrimination can be noted if present. The examiner should also use a null stimulus such as a nonvibrating tuning fork for an accurate assessment of this sensory modality.

Gripping the digit by the sides and moving it up, down, or into the neutral position tests joint proprioception. The digits on either side of the digit to be tested should be spread apart so that they do not touch the digit being tested. Using three choices for the answer lessens the possibility of guessing and thus is more reliable. A normal test of joint position would have no incorrect responses. If there is evidence of loss of joint-position sensation in the digits, then testing of the more proximal joints of wrist and ankle is indicated.

Testing higher sensory functions (graphesthesia, stereoagnosia, two-point discrimination, and simultaneous sensation) can reveal information about cortical sensory association areas. It is essential that the primary modality of sensation be present prior to testing these higher cortical functions. Graphesthesia is the patient's ability to recognize written numbers or letters. With the patient's eyes closed, the examiner traces numbers or letters on the patient's palm using a blunt object. A normal test in an educated patient has few errors. Stereoagnosia is the patient's ability to recognize forms. Various objects such as safety pins, keys, coins, or pencils are placed in the patient's hand after the patient closes his eyes. He is allowed to move the object around in his hand to fully appreciate the form. A normal exam has few errors.

Two-point discrimination is the patient's ability to recognize two distinct pressure points. This ability changes with areas of the face and hand far more sensitive and the back less sensitive. This sensory test is dependent on the patient having a mental image of body parts. Double simultaneous stimulation is a useful test in patients where inattention to body parts is suspected such as those with right parietal lesions. The examiner alternately touches body parts either on one side or on both sides at the same time. The patient identifies what body parts have been touched. Patients with inattention due to parietal lesions will not attend to double stimuli. If the hand is paretic, stereognosis can still be evaluated by moving the object around in the patient's palm.

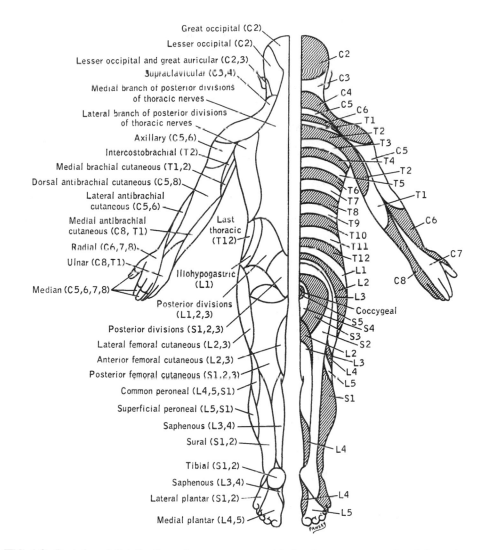

FIG. 1-2. Peripheral distribution of sensory nerves with the dermatomes on the right and cutaneous nerves on the left. *(From House EL, Pansky B: A Functional Approach to Neuroanatomy. New York: McGraw-Hill, 1960, p. 286.)*

MOTOR EXAMINATION

Dysfunction of the motor system can occur at any level, at the muscle, neuromuscular junction, peripheral nerve, or central nervous system. Careful and systematic examination of the motor system will give clues to the site of the dysfunction. The motor exam-

ination assesses muscle tone, bulk, and strength. It also assesses rapidity of movements, the presence of abnormal movements, and reflexes. First, the patient's muscles are observed for bulk (looking for evidence of atrophy or hypertrophy), fasciculations, and abnormal movements such as tremors. Next, *tone,* operationally defined as the resistance offered by the limb or other body segment when it is passively mobilized, is assessed as the examiner moves the limb through a full range of flexion and extension movements at the elbow, wrist, knee, ankle, and neck. Tone may be normal, decreased (in lower motor neuron or cerebellar lesions), or increased (in upper motor neuron and extrapyramidal disorders). The increase in tone may be perceived as a ratchety feeling of intermittent tone releases like cogwheels (cogwheel rigidity), or as an increase in tone that suddenly gives way, reminiscent of a razor blade (spastic), or as a more diffuse feeling of resistance to movement without any "give" to it (lead-pipe rigidity, as seen occasionally in dystonias and akinetic rigid syndromes or the gegenhalten of the demented patient). To examine tone, the examiner asks the patient to relax. Then the upper extremities are examined by holding the arm above the elbow and at the hand, and moving the arm through full extension and flexion. For examination of the lower extremities, the patient is placed in the supine position and again asked to relax. The leg is grasped at the level of the knee and quickly raised into the air. The heel of patients with normal or flaccid tone will stay on the bed, but it will elevate off the bed in patients with hypertonicity.

The muscle groups should be examined side to side and proximal to distal, allowing comparisons of strength to be made. Weakness of all muscle groups on one side would suggest a hemiparesis. Proximal muscle weakness would suggest a primary muscle problem (myopathy), while distal muscle weakness is suggestive of a neuropathic process. There are also patterns of weakness that suggest cervical or lumber spinal root involvement. In general, C5 innervates deltoids and biceps; C6, wrist extensions; C7, wrist flexors; C8, finger flexion; and T1, finger abduction and adduction. L1, L2, and L3 innervate the iliopsoas muscle (hip flexion); L2, L3, and L4 control knee extension; L5 controls dorsiflexion, version, and inversion of the foot; and S1 controls plantar flexion. Muscle strength is graded on a scale from 0 to 5: 0 = absence of movement, 1 = a flicker of movement, 2 = movement on the horizontal plane with gravity removed, 3 = movement against gravity but with no resistance, 4 = movement against gravity with resistance that can be overcome, and 5 = movement against gravity with resistance that cannot be overcome.

To test rhythm of movement (after assessing for strength), the patient is asked to open and close the hand rapidly, to alternate movements between pronation and supination, or to tap the toes. The examiner is looking for the speed, amplitude, and regularity of these movements. Impairment is suggestive of dysfunction of either the basal ganglia or cerebellum if the strength has been preserved.

Abnormal movements are observed while the patient is at rest and while he has his hands outstretched. These abnormal movements will be discussed in Chapter 11 on movement disorders.

REFLEXES

The deep tendon reflexes (DTRs) also known as muscle stretch reflexes (MSRs) are responses of muscle spindles to rapid stretch. The stretch causes rapid firing of muscle spindles. Information from the stretched muscle spindle fibers is transmitted via afferent fibers to the spinal cord where they synapse on anterior horn cells. Efferent fibers from the anterior horn cells synapse with muscle fibers at the neuromuscular junction. Stimulation of the neuromuscular junction results in muscle contraction. Although there are numerous DTRs, only some of them are used in a routine neurologic examination. These reflexes are the biceps, brachioradialis, and triceps reflexes of the upper extremities, and the patellar and ankle responses of the lower extremities. To test a reflex, the examiner places the patient in either the supine or sitting position and asks him to relax. The examiner then strikes the tendon of the muscle to be tested with a light but firm tap of the reflex hammer. The examiner observes the reflex contraction of the muscle and grades the response as normal, hypo-, or hyperreflexic. Asymmetrical decrease or loss of a particular reflex is seen with radiculopathies, plexopathies, or mononeuropathies. Examples include ipsilateral loss of biceps and brachioradialis reflexes in pathology of the sixth cervical root, and the loss of the knee reflex in femoral neuropathy. Decrease or loss of reflexes in the upper extremities with hyperreflexia in the lower extremities suggests spinal cord pathology at the cervical level or amyotropic lateral sclerosis. Bilateral decrease or absence of distal DTRs suggests peripheral neuropathy.

Hyperreflexia is seen in diseases affecting the upper motor neuron (motor cortex or corticospinal tract) and is associated with increase in tone (spasticity) and a positive Babinski reflex. It is seen with degenerative, neoplastic, inflammatory, vascular, and posttraumatic disease affecting the brain, brain stem, or spinal cord.

The plantar response is obtained most commonly by stroking the lateral surface of the sole of the foot from heel to toe. The great toe flexes in a normal response and extends in an abnormal response (Babinski sign).

CEREBELLAR FUNCTION EXAM

The cerebellum is an integrating way station for the control of volitional muscular movements. It integrates information from the various sensory and motor systems that result in fluid movements and postures. Dysfunction of this system is manifest in disorders of gait, abnormal speech and eye movements, hypotonia, tremors, and clumsiness of movements. Cerebellar syndromes may consist of four components, including ataxia, dysarthria, hypotonia, and nystagmus.

The clinical manifestations of these disorders can be evaluated by listening to the patient's speech; using examination techniques to demonstrate incoordination, kinetic tremor, and decomposition of movement; and observing the gait. The presence of weakness in the limbs, involuntary movements, or any other concomitant neurologic deficit will affect the cerebellar examination. In evaluating specific motor functions, the patient's ability to judge the speed, power, and distance to carry out an act should be noted. If these are faulty, dysmetria is present. If the patient has difficulty in carrying out repetitive successive acts or in stopping one motor maneuver and immediately starting an opposite motor act, dysdiadochokinesia is present.

Appendicular movements test coordination of movements of the extremities. The cerebellar hemispheres modulate these movements. The finger-to-nose-to-finger test and the heel-to-shin maneuver test appendicular movements. In the former, the patient is asked to touch his finger to the examiner's finger and then to touch his finger to his own nose. The patient's eyes are open during this testing. The examiner positions his finger at a distance such that the patient must fully extend the arm to touch it. In this way, any tremor at the extreme of arm extension can be seen. This tremor, the intention tremor, is a side-to-side pendular tremor as the patient tries to touch the examiner's finger or his own nose. An intention or kinetic tremor can also be observed in the lower extremity when the patient is asked to put his heel on his knee and then to run his heel down his shin. This is performed with the patient supine.

Midline cerebellar dysfunction is characterized by ataxia of the trunk. The patient is observed sitting upright or walking to determine the ability to hold the trunk and head still. Patients with midline cerebellar lesions are unable to hold the head and trunk in position and have a swaying movement.

GAIT EXAMINATION

Like the mental examination, the gait examination starts the moment the physician greets the patient. The gait exam is best interpreted after the symptoms and signs have been gathered and diagnostic hypotheses have been framed.

The patient is asked to arise from a chair with his arms crossed. Mild difficulties are present if the patient performs this task slowly, flexing the knees while bringing the upper body forward, or sliding the buttocks forward over the seating surface before trying to stand up. A measure of more difficulty in rising is the need for repeated attempts before accomplishing the task or the need to use the hands to push the body up. More severe degrees of impairment are indicated by the need for assistance. Difficulties in this area can be the result of proximal muscle weakness, basal ganglia disease, or pain in the low back or proximal lower extremities.

The patient's posture is observed. Patients with Parkinson's disease exhibit a stooping (simian) posture, which may be associated with thoracic kyphosis and additional lateral bending. Patients with progressive supranuclear palsy—another extrapyramidal disorder causing bradykinesia and rigidity—frequently display an erect or hypererect posture. An exaggerated lumbar lordosis may be seen in patients with proximal lower extremity weakness, as seen in muscular dystrophies and other myopathies.

The patient's ambulation is analyzed for speed, stride length, turning, and associated movements. Diseases affecting the pyramidal tract or the extrapyramidal system may shorten the stride length, slow ambulation, decrease the vertical displacement of the advancing foot, and be associated with a decrease or absence of the associated arm movement on the same side. It is sometimes impossible to distinguish, on gait exam alone, a patient who has only partially recovered from a stroke from a patient with early Parkinson's disease. Patients with cerebellar disease, progressive supranuclear palsy, or labyrinthine disease may exhibit a cautious, wide-based stance with consequent slowing of ambulation. The festinating gait of the parkinsonian patient is characterized by rapid, increasingly accelerating short steps, and the patient may have difficulty coming to an immediate halt at will.

Weakness of the tibialis anterior muscle results in inability to adequately dorsiflex the foot as the foot is being advanced, and in a resultant compensatory marked elevation of the leg in what is called a steppage gait (seen in common peroneal neuropathy or L5 radiculopathy). Weakness of the same muscle may be manifested by an inability to heel walk (also seen in pyramidal tract disease). Toe walking difficulty is indicative of gastrocnemius weakness (seen in posterior tibial neuropathy or S1–S2 radiculopathies).

Efficient turning is accomplished by an act of sequential pivoting of both legs. The leg opposite the desired direction of turn is the one making the final advance prior to the turning moment, and the posteriorly placed leg is the first to pivot. Difficulties in this area are manifested by the substitution of multiple steps or the appearance of sudden interruptions of the movement (freezing). It is at this juncture that falls are more likely to occur, and the examiner should be reasonably close to the patient to prevent this. Adequate turning or pivoting may be affected in disorders of basal ganglia, cerebellar disease, or labyrinthine disease. Freezing is viewed exclusively as an extrapyramidal (basal ganglion) dysfunction.

The patient is then asked to stand with one foot next to the other. Patients with cerebellar disease, advanced basal ganglia disease, or acute labyrinthine disease may be unable to successfully accomplish this task and may find it necessary to separate the distance between their feet. Only after a standing stance has been successfully accomplished can the clinician proceed to perform the Romberg test. The patient is asked to close his eyes while trying to stand still. Oscillations in the lateral or anteroposterior direction may normally appear, but the feet will not move. Wider oscillations culminating in a loss of equilibrium suggest proprioceptive difficulties in the lower extremities, implying dysfunction in the posterior columns, although it can also be seen with severe sensory neuropathies.

Postural stability can be checked in the anteroposterior direction by having the clinician place him- or herself behind the standing patient and firmly push the patient on the midsternal area or the anterior aspect of both shoulders. A normal response results in quick return of the displaced upper body to its preperturbation position. At times, a normal subject may have to take one or two steps back to avoid a fall. Abnormal responses are variable, ranging from the need for multiple steps, to the failure of multiple steps to avoid the fall, to the loss of generation of these multiple steps with a tendency to fall *en bloc*, sometimes without the compensatory forward elevation of the upper extremities. The most severely affected patients are those who need to be held while standing or walking. Basal ganglia and cerebellar disease are the most frequent causes of problems in this area.

Postural stability is checked in the lateral direction by asking the patient to walk in tandem. Difficulties in this area include cerebellar disease, labyrinthine disease, proprioceptive difficulties in the lower extremities, and basal ganglia disease.

QUESTIONS AND DISCUSSION

1. A 62-year-old man has had a feeling of generalized weakness for the preceding 3 weeks, associated with difficulty in chewing and swallowing and a change in the quality of speech. Further questioning reveals that he has been suffering from intermittent diplopia and droopiness of one eyelid for the preceding year. The examination reveals ptosis of the left eye associated with deficit of abduction. There is weakness of jaw opening and nasality of speech. Gag reflexes are present. The soft palate shows decreased symmetrical excursion to both reflex and command. Weakness is generalized, affecting both proximal and distal muscles. There are no cognitive findings (including no emotional lability) and no sensory findings. Reflexes are symmetrical and normoreactive, there are no Babinski responses, and the tone is normal. The likely site of the lesion is:

A. Both cerebral hemispheres.
B. The neuromuscular junction.
C. The brain stem affecting cranial nerves III, V, VI, IX, and X.
D. The peripheral nerves in a diffuse fashion as seen in Guillain–Barré syndrome.

The answer is not (A). Bilateral hemisphere dysfunction capable of causing difficulty in chewing, swallowing, and speaking is known as a pseudobulbar state. It implies bilateral involvement of corticobulbar fibers (i.e., a dysfunction of those connections between the cerebral hemispheres and the brain-stem nuclei). This may be seen in individuals who have suffered multiple strokes. This patient had diplopia, a symptom that cannot be explained by lesions proximal to the brain-stem nuclei. He also lacked cranial hyperreflexia (hyperactive jaw jerk and gag reflexes), limb hyperreflexia, Babinski responses, limb spasticity, and cognitive changes (slowness of mental function, emotional lability).

The answer is (B). Myasthenia gravis is the most commonly seen disease of the neuromuscular junction. It can affect eye movements in an asymmetrical fashion, with diplopia being a frequent early complaint. This patient had difficulty in chewing because of jaw muscle weakness but no evidence of direct cranial nerve V involvement (no sensory findings over the face). The patient's difficulty in swallowing and his nasality of voice were expressive of involvement of the soft palate musculature. The fact that gag reflexes and jaw jerk were not hyperactive spoke against the involvement of corticobulbar fibers. The fact that the generalized weakness was not accompanied by reflex, tone, or sensory abnormalities spoke against involvement of central (corticospinal tracts at brain, brainstem, or spinal cord level) or peripheral motor fibers.

The answer is not (C). A brain-stem event may in fact be associated with diplopia by affecting cranial nerve nuclei or fibers connecting them (medial longitudinal fasciculus). Ptosis of the one eye in such a context could be due to Horner's syndrome, but the ipsilateral pupil was not miotic. It could also be caused by involvement of cranial nerve III or its fibers before they emerge from the brain stem, but cranial nerve III–dependent functions were not affected (no deficit of eye adduction, elevation, or depression; no pupillary dilatation). A brain-stem event could also be associated with dysphagia. Dysarthria (deficit in articulation) or anarthria (absence of articulation) rather than nasality of voice is a more likely speech difficulty. An acute brain-stem event (e.g., CVA) may be associated with quadriparesis but would also be associated with flaccidity of tone and hyporeflexia. As the patient recovers, spasticity and hyperreflexia will appear. Neither feature was present in this case.

The answer is not (D). An acute inflammatory polyradiculoneuropathy (Guillain–Barré syndrome) can be associated with rapid onset of generalized weakness, including bulbar dysfunction (dysphagia, difficulty with mastication, voice nasality) but is not likely to be preceded by diplopia for months, as was the case for this patient. Areflexia is a very important feature of this condition. Sensory findings may also be present, such as distal loss or decrease of sensation to light touch, pinprick, temperature, vibration, or position.

2. A 55-year-old woman has noticed gradual loss of dexterity of her left hand and increasing difficulty with ambulation. Examination discloses a wasted left hand and bilateral lower extremity spasticity. The left lower extremity is weaker than the right, while pinprick is better perceived on that same side. The decrease in sensation to pinprick on the right side extends to the mid trunk. There are no cranial nerve findings, and cognitive functions are intact. The likely site of the lesion is:

A. An asymmetrical polyneuropathy affecting the left median nerve and both sciatic nerves.
B. A cervical cord–compressive syndrome.
C. A diffuse motor neuron disorder (amyotrophic lateral sclerosis).

The answer is not (A). Polyneuropathy does not cause lower extremity spasticity, which is a sign of upper motor neuron dysfunction.

The answer is (B). An asymmetrical spasticity with the weaker lower extremity on the left and decreased sensation to pinprick on the opposite side places the site of pathology in the spinal cord, predominantly on the left side. The reason pinprick is diminished on the right is that the sensory fibers cross to the opposite side shortly after entering the spinal cord. Thus, a lesion that affects the pathways for pain sensation (spinothalamic tracts) on one side of the cord will be experienced as decreased sensation to pinprick on the opposite side. The precise location of the lesion is given by the wasting of the left hand, a lower motor neuron lesion that suggests involvement of the lower motor neurons at the C8 segment. The sensory level in this case falsely localizes the process to the mid thoracic area.

The answer is not (C). Motor neuron disease can present with a combination of upper and motor neuron signs such as in this case, but there is no sensory involvement.

3. A 35-year-old woman presents with complaints of painful burning feet and difficulty with ambulation. The examination discloses severe loss of position and vibration sense in the lower extremities—distal more than proximal—associated with spasticity, hyperreflexia, and Babinski responses. The upper extremities disclose a similar sensory deficit but to a milder degree. There are no cranial nerve or cognitive deficits. The likely site of the lesion is:

A. The posterior columns and corticospinal tracts at the level of the spinal cord.
B. The peripheral nerves, particularly the large myelinated fibers that conduct proprioceptive information.
C. The brain stem, affecting the proprioceptive fibers (medial lemnisci) and corticospinal tracts.

The answer is (A). The loss of proprioceptive information can be caused by a peripheral neuropathy affecting large myelinated fibers, or to disease affecting the posterior columns in the spinal cord. The concurrent presence of upper motor neuron signs (spasticity, hyperreflexia, and Babinski responses) points to the spinal cord as the site of pathology.

The answer is not (B). A peripheral neuropathy could be associated with selective or preferential involvement of those fibers conducting proprioceptive information, but it would not be the cause of the associated upper motor neuron syndrome.

The answer is not (C). The patient does not have evidence of involvement of other brain-stem structures such as cranial nerves, gaze centers, or other sensory modalities.

4. A 25-year-old myopic woman presents with the complaint of blurred vision of the left eye associated with eye pain for the preceding 7 days. Past history reveals that she has been experiencing amenorrhea for the preceding 6 months. There is a very strongly positive history of glaucoma in the family. The extra-ocular movements are intact, and there is no ptosis. The eye examination discloses no overt abnormalities of the cornea, iris, or lens. Visual acuity of the left eye is 20/80, uncorrected by glasses, while it is 20/25 in the right eye with glasses. The left pupil dilates as a light is directed from the right to the left eye. Fundoscopic exam reveals blurred margins of the left disk. There are no other findings on neurologic exam. The likely site of the lesion is:

A. The optic chiasm as a result of compression by a pituitary gland tumor.
B. The right occipital lobe or right optic radiations.
C. This represents an acute attack of glaucoma.
D. The left optic nerve

The answer is not (A). Although the patient's amenorrhea warrants investigation, it is unlikely to explain her symptoms and signs because a lesion at the level of the optic chiasm would cause loss of both temporal fields of vision and not a uniocular decrease in visual acuity.

The answer is not (B). A lesion of the right occipital lobe or the optic radiations would cause a loss of vision in the nasal field of the right eye and the temporal field of the left eye (left homonymous hemianopia).

The answer is not (C). Sudden loss of vision due to an acute attack of glaucoma can be associated with eye pain and even with an unreactive pupil. It is not associated with swelling of the optic disc. The patient's positive family history for glaucoma proves to be a red herring rather than a clue in this particular case.

The answer is (D). The patient's picture is very characteristic of an acute optic neuritis with a decrease of central vision in one eye, associated with an afferent pupillary defect and swelling of the optic disc. Sometimes the swelling of the optic nerve may occur more posteriorly and the disc may appear normal (retrobulbar neuritis). Approximately 30% of patients who suffer optic neuritis will eventually develop multiple sclerosis

SUGGESTED READING

Adams RD, Victor M: Principles of Neurology, 5th ed., pp. 5–9. New York: McGraw-Hill, 1993

De Myer WE: Technique of the Neurological Examination, A Programmed Text, 4th ed. New York: McGraw-Hill, 1994

Glaser JS. Neuro-Ophthalmology, 2nd ed., pp. 37–60. Philadelphia: JB Lippincott, 1990

Haerer AF: DeJong's The Neurologic Examination, 5th ed. Philadelphia: JB Lippincott, 1992

Medical Research Council: Aids to the Examination of the Peripheral Nervous System. London: HMSO, 1976

Members of the Department of Neurology, Mayo Clinic and Mayo Foundation for Medical Education and Research: Clinical Examinations in Neurology, 6th ed. St. Louis: Mosby, 1991

Neurology for the Non-Neurologist, Fourth Edition, edited by William J. Weiner and Christopher G. Goetz. Lippincott Williams & Wilkins, Philadelphia © 1999.

C H A P T E R 2

An Approach to Neurologic Symptoms

Steven L. Lewis

In neurologic diagnosis, individual symptoms and constellations of symptoms can be of telling diagnostic importance both anatomically and etiologically. Thus, a detailed neurologic history that puts together various symptoms and their temporal development helps to define neurologic entities, often with as much precision as an isolated examination.

COMMON NEUROLOGIC TERMS

Before proceeding with a discussion of specific neurologic symptoms, it is worthwhile to define some terms that can be useful in characterizing neurologic symptom complexes. These words are used to indicate certain *localizations* of pathology.

Encephalopathy means disease of the brain. Although theoretically the term *encephalopathy* could refer to any process involving any part of the brain, it is generally used to connote dysfunction that involves the entirety of both cerebral hemispheres. Thus, the terms *encephalopathy* and *diffuse encephalopathy,* in common usage, are essentially synonymous. A common type of encephalopathy is metabolic encephalopathy, caused by uremic, hepatic, or other metabolic dysfunction.

Myelopathy means disease of the spinal cord. A patient with any symptoms or signs that are caused by spinal cord dysfunction has a myelopathy. A common type of myelopathy is *compressive* myelopathy caused by a tumor compressing the spinal cord, causing weakness, sensory loss, and spasticity below the level of the compression.

Radiculopathy, disease of the nerve roots (*radix* is Latin for root; a radish is a root vegetable), is the term used for any process involving single or multiple nerve roots in the cervical, thoracic, or lumbar spine. For example, a herniated lumbar disc between the fourth and fifth lumbar spine might cause an L5 radiculopathy; Guillain-Barré syndrome would cause a *polyradiculopathy* due to dysfunction of multiple nerve roots.

Neuropathy means disease of a nerve. The term connotes dysfunction of one (*mononeuropathy*), several (*mononeuropathy multiplex*), or many/diffuse (*polyneuropathy*) peripheral nerves. Dysfunction of a cranial nerve would be called a *cranial neuropathy. Myopathy* refers to any disease of muscle.

These generic terms are very helpful to the clinician in categorizing sites of pathology or dysfunction. A specific causative lesion, or causative process, is not conveyed by any of these terms. Unless there is a preceding adjective (e.g., *compressive* myelopathy, or *demyelinative* polyneuropathy), a cause or mechanism is not implied. Likewise, substitution of the suffix *-itis* for *-pathy* (e.g., myositis instead of myopathy) implies, specifically, an inflammatory process, rather than an as-yet-unknown process affecting that region of the nervous system.

AN APPROACH TO SPECIFIC NEUROLOGIC SYMPTOM COMPLEXES

The essential elements of the neurologic diagnostic process are an accurate and detailed history, followed by a neurologic examination. Imaging and laboratory studies follow, as appropriate. The goal is to determine *where* in the nervous system the problem lies, as well as *how* the dysfunction occurred. This section discusses the *where* part of the neurologic formulation using the history and examination. Using the history of the evolution of symptoms to help determine the *mechanism* of dysfunction will be discussed later in this chapter. Now, several specific symptom complexes are discussed: mental status changes, weakness, sensory symptoms, and gait disorders.

MENTAL STATUS CHANGES

When confronted with a patient who has had a mental status change, the clinician should try to determine whether there is an alteration in the *level* of consciousness or an alteration of the *content* of consciousness.

Alterations in the *level* of consciousness manifest in the continuum between drowsiness and coma. They are due either to dysfunction of both cerebral hemispheres, or to dysfunction of the upper brainstem (mid pons or above), or to a combination of hemispheric and upper brainstem dysfunction. The clinical approach to the patient who presents with an alteration in level of consciousness is discussed in more detail in Chapter 5. A major goal of the neurologic exam of these patients is to determine whether there is focal brainstem dysfunction. If brainstem function is intact, the cause of the problem is unlikely to be due to a focal structural brainstem process, and more likely due to a diffuse encephalopathic process (involving both cerebral hemispheres, or the hemispheres and the brainstem). The actual processes that may affect the level of consciousness are vast and are discussed in more detail in Chapter 5.

Neurologic processes can affect the mental status of patients, however, by affecting the *content* of consciousness without necessarily altering the level of consciousness (see Chapters 15 and 16). Alterations in the content of consciousness are exemplified by psychiatric disorders, or by neurologic processes that affect memory, language, awareness, or global intellectual functioning. Patients with *chronic dementing illnesses* (Chapter 16) usually have normal alertness despite the deterioration in cognitive functioning.

Aphasic patients—particularly those with fluent aphasias (Chapter 15)—often appear to be confused. More careful attention to the patient's speech pattern to determine the presence of paraphasic errors and neologisms will often help the clinician determine that the "confused" patient is actually aphasic; the presence of aphasia is usually a clue to focal dysfunction in the dominant (usually left) hemisphere. Patients with lesions affecting the right hemisphere may also appear to be "confused," neglectful, and unaware, whereas they actually have neglect of the left side of space and may be oblivious of their deficit (anosagnosia) because of the nondominant hemisphere dysfunction.

WEAKNESS

"Weakness" as a patient complaint may have several possible meanings, besides the usually presumed meaning of a decrease in motor function in one or several extremities. The clinician should keep in mind that some patients might use the term *weakness* to describe generalized fatigue, malaise, or asthenia. Some patients might describe as weakness a symptom such as the generalized bradykinesia of parkinsonism (Chapter 10). As in all neurologic diagnosis, an accurate history and examination should suffice for clarification. Muscular *fatigue*, although very nonspecific, suggests the possibility of a disorder of the neuromuscular junction such as myasthenia gravis (see Chapter 19), or a disease of muscle (myopathy), in addition to primarily non-neurologic processes causing generalized malaise and fatigue.

The following are definitions of some common terms used to describe decreases in motor function. *Paresis* refers to muscular weakness but not complete paralysis. *Plegia* is the term used to describe complete paralysis. *Monoparesis* and *monoplegia* are terms sometimes used to describe weakness or paralysis in one extremity. *Hemiparesis* and *hemiplegia* refer to weakness or paralysis in the arm and leg on one side of the body. *Paraparesis* and *paraplegia* describe weakness or paralysis in both legs, and *quadriparesis* and *quadriplegia* denote weakness or paralysis in all four extremities.

Muscular weakness can occur as a result of dysfunction at any level of the central or peripheral nervous system. To illustrate this, it is worth considering the neuroanatomic pathway for muscle movement.

The pathway for muscle movement begins in nerve cells that are located on the precentral gyrus of each frontal lobe. The axons from these nerve cells comprise the *corticospinal tract*. The corticospinal tracts travel through the white matter of each cerebral hemisphere, through the internal capsule, and further downward into the brainstem, where each corticospinal tract crosses to the opposite side in the low medulla. From the medulla, the corticospinal tracts travel downward through each side of the spinal cord.

Within the spinal cord, the corticospinal tract on each side synapses with nerve cells in the anterior horns located in the spinal cord gray matter. Axons from these second-order neurons become the cervical, thoracic, and lumbosacral nerve roots. The cervical nerve roots then form the brachial plexus, and the nerves that are formed in the brachial plexus travel into the upper extremities and innervate the muscles of the upper extremities. The lumbar nerve roots travel downward within the lumbar spinal canal as the cauda equina, before exiting and forming the lumbosacral plexus and ultimately the nerves that innervate the lower extremity musculature.

A lesion at any level of the above pathway, from the cerebral cortex to the muscles themselves, can cause weakness. The location of this lesion causing weakness, or a history of weakness, is not always immediately obvious, even to an experienced clinician who has performed an accurate history and examination. However, there are typical, or classic, patterns of muscle weakness that lesions at various levels of the pathway for motor function will usually produce. Recognition of these typical patterns can be very helpful in attempting to decide on possible localizations of pathology in patients who present with motor weakness.

UPPER MOTOR NEURON SYNDROMES

Lesions that cause dysfunction of the corticospinal tracts are called *upper motor neuron* lesions; their distinctive features, in addition to weakness, include increased or pathologic reflexes, and increased tone and spasticity in chronic lesions. It should also be recognized that these classic findings of upper motor neuron dysfunction might not always be evident. Upper motor neuron syndromes can result from lesions of the corticospinal tract at various levels of the central nervous system. Further clinical details—described later—help to specify whether the lesion is cortical, subcortical, or in the spinal cord. When symptoms of *transient* motor dysfunction occur, no abnormalities would be expected on the examination, and the site of the lesion must be inferred by the patient's description of the areas of transient weakness and associated symptoms.

Hemispheric motor cortex lesions involving the cortical motor neurons of the *lateral* surface of one hemisphere usually cause upper motor neuron weakness of the contralateral face (see Chapter 1) and arm, with less weakness of the leg. A lesion in this region, like all corticospinal tract lesions, will often cause predominant weakness in the extensors of the arm and flexors of the leg, with relative preservation of strength in arm flexors and leg extensors. As such, the affected arm is held mildly flexed while walking and the leg is overextended, causing it to drag stiffly, sometimes catching the toe. Hemispheric motor cortex lesions involving the *medial* aspect of one frontal lobe will predominantly cause contralateral leg weakness. Weakness due to lesions affecting cortical motor neurons is often accompanied by other signs of cortical dysfunction, giving a clue to the localization of the problem. For example, left hemisphere cortical lesions are often accompanied by abnormalities of language function (see Chapter 15). Right hemisphere cortical lesions are often accompanied by denial of the left-sided weakness or even unawareness of the presence of the left extremities (asomatagnosia). Any complex behavioral change of these types suggests that the upper motor neuron lesion is cortical. Cortical lesions causing weakness are often also accompanied by some contralateral sensory disturbance because of the proximity of the cortical sensory neurons to the motor cortex.

Deep hemispheric or *internal capsule* lesions will also cause weakness of the contralateral body but without accompanying signs of cortical dysfunction. Lesions affecting the corticospinal tract fibers in the posterior limb of the internal capsule may produce a characteristic *pure motor hemiparesis* (or hemiplegia) involving the contralateral face, arm, and leg (Chapter 6). This is characterized by significant weakness of one side of the body without sensory disturbance or signs of cortical dysfunction such as aphasia. This distinctive form of isolated weakness occurs because the corticospinal fibers from a large area of the motor cortex all lie close together in the internal capsule, segregated from the sensory fibers, and deep to the cortical structures. In contrast, a hemispheric lesion that would be large enough to cause significant weakness of an entire side of the body would most likely also involve sensory signs or symptoms, and signs of cortical dysfunction.

Brainstem lesions that involve the corticospinal tract on one side will also cause weakness of the contralateral side of the body. Some unilateral ventral pontine lesions—affecting only the corticospinal tract but no other brainstem pathways—may even produce an isolated pure motor hemiparesis clinically indistinguishable from an internal capsular lesion. However, many brainstem processes producing weakness also produce *brainstem signs* or *brainstem symptoms* such as diplopia, vertigo, nausea, and vomiting, or cranial nerve palsies, which are clues to the brainstem localization of the process (Chapter 6). One of the pillars of neurologic localization is that a brainstem lesion can cause weakness of the contralateral body (as a result of involvement of the corticospinal tract) and dysfunction of an ipsilateral cranial nerve (as a result of involvement of a cranial nerve nucleus, or the cranial nerve itself, before it exits the brainstem). An example would be a right peripheral facial palsy and left body weakness due to a right pontine lesion. In addition, because both the right and the left corticospinal tracts are relatively close together in the brainstem, bilateral extremity weakness can be seen in brainstem disease.

Lesions of the corticospinal tracts in the *spinal cord* cause weakness below the level of the spinal cord lesion. Although it is possible to have unilateral weakness resulting from a spinal cord lesion, many lesions affecting the spinal cord cause bilateral weakness because of involvement of the corticospinal tracts on both sides of the cord. The level of the spinal cord lesion causing the weakness is not always immediately obvious to the examiner, however. The corticospinal fibers destined for arm function end in the lower cervical/first thoracic portion of the spinal cord. The corticospinal tract fibers for leg function need to pass through the cervical and thoracic portions of the spinal cord before ending in the lumbosacral cord. Therefore, weakness of the upper *and* lower extremities, when due to a single lesion, must be due to a lesion at least as high as the cervical spinal cord. However, weakness of the legs without weakness of the arms is not necessarily due to a lesion below the neck. A partial or early process affecting the high (e.g., cervical) spinal cord could potentially cause clinical dysfunction primarily affecting that portion of the corticospinal tract destined for lower extremity function, without obviously affecting those fibers involved in upper extremity function. This has important implications in the imaging of patients with suspected spinal cord lesions.

LOWER MOTOR NEURON LESIONS

Lower motor neuron dysfunction occurs when there is dysfunction at the level of the anterior horn cell, motor nerve root, plexus, peripheral nerve, or neuromuscular junction (see Chapters 13 and 19). Lesions of the lower motor neuron may cause, in addition to weakness, decreased reflexes in the involved limb (if a clinically testable reflex is subserved by the nerve in question). In chronic lesions, lower motor neuron dysfunction may lead to clinically evident atrophy and fasciculations of muscle due to the trophic influence the lower motor neuron plays in muscle maintenance. In these cases, patients may complain that their muscles are shrinking and have small, visible twitches. Lower motor neuron weakness may be due to either a *focal* or *diffuse* process.

Clinical localization of the source of a patient's weakness to a particular *focal* lower motor neuron lesion mainly rests in the finding of muscle dysfunction that appears to fit the territory of a specific nerve root (*radiculopathy*), region of plexus (*plexopathy*), or peripheral nerve distribution (*neuropathy*)—see Chapter 13. In addition, when such a lesion is also affecting sensory fibers (as do most lower motor neuron lesions that are distal to the anterior horn cell), the concomitant sensory dysfunction can also be an important clue to the localization of the problem.

Examples of common *diffuse* lower motor neuron processes include processes that simultaneously affect multiple peripheral nerves (*polyneuropathies*) or multiple nerve roots (*polyradiculopathies*). Diffuse polyneuropathies (Chapter 13) typically predominantly affect the most distal extremities, causing weakness that is often limited to the distal fingers and foot muscles. Distal reflexes are usually diminished or lost, fairly symmetrically. In most diffuse polyneuropathies, such as diabetic neuropathies, the sensory symptoms are more prominent than the distal motor findings, at least initially. *Multifocal,* rather than diffuse polyneuropathies are characterized as a *mononeuropathy multiplex.* This would be seen clinically by dysfunction in the territories of two or more peripheral nerves. Polyradiculopathic processes clinically resemble (and may be difficult to initially distinguish from) the diffuse polyneuropathies but are suggested by the presence of motor dysfunction that appears to involve multiple motor nerve *root* territories. Concomitant sensory symptoms such as *radicular* pain (see later), when present, are helpful diagnostic clues to the presence of a radicular or polyradicular localization.

Disease of muscle (*myopathy*) is suggested when a patient presents with weakness that is predominantly proximal in distribution. However, proximal weakness is not pathognomonic for myopathy and can be also be seen, for example, in some myelopathic and radiculopathic processes. It should also be noted that some myopathies cause unusual patterns of weakness (e.g., inclusion body myositis) or even predominantly distal weakness (e.g., myotonic dystrophy)—see Chapter 19. Often, myopathies cause pain and tenderness in the involved muscles, especially in inflammatory conditions.

PAIN AND SENSORY SYNDROMES

One can arguably consider all pain to be neurologic in origin, since all pain must be transmitted through sensory fibers and perceived in central nervous system structures. However, in this section, primary *neurologic* pain and other neurologic abnormalities of sensation are discussed and can be defined as pain and other sensory symptoms that are directly due to dysfunction of nervous system structures. Back pain is discussed in Chapter 21 and headache in Chapter 7—these topics will therefore not be specifically addressed in this section.

Patients often report "numbness" as a neurologic symptom. However, this term has many potential meanings, including the expected sensory symptoms (also described in Chapter 13) of decreased sensation (*hypoesthesia* or *anesthesia*), a tingling/pins and needles sensation (*paresthesias*), or very uncomfortable/burning sensations (*dysesthesias*). Patients, however, sometimes use the word *numbness* to describe weakness or other nonsensory symptoms. A careful history, specifically asking the patient to explain the symptom of numbness in more detail, will usually suffice for clarification.

The pathways for cutaneous sensation will be grossly described here. Sensation starts in the peripheral nerve endings, and it travels up the sensory nerves to the dorsal nerve roots and into the spinal cord. In the spinal cord, the sensory pathways ascend as the *spinothalamic tract* (mainly subserving pain and temperature sensation), and the *posterior columns* (mainly subserving vibration and proprioceptive sensation). These ascending sensory tracts in the spinal cord synapse in the thalamus. From the thalamus, thalamocortical projections send impulses to the cerebral cortex.

Abnormalities at any level of the sensory pathway—peripheral sensory nerve, nerve root, spinal cord, thalamus, or sensory cortex—may produce sensory symptoms. Lesions at some of these levels, particularly the sensory nerve, nerve root, or thalamus, may also produce pain.

The sensory symptoms of peripheral nerve lesions (see Chapter 13) generally consist of hypoesthesia, paresthesias, or dysesthesias conforming to the territory of the nerve. When this occurs *focally*, as a result of a focal peripheral nerve process, the area of numbness is usually well circumscribed, corresponding to a particular peripheral nerve distribution. When the peripheral nerve process is *diffuse and symmetrical*, such as in a distal polyneuropathy, the area of sensory disturbance characteristically occurs in a *stocking* or *stocking-glove* pattern. The fact that these symptoms are likely due to a neurologic process is usually evident from the history and exam.

Like peripheral neuropathic lesions, *radiculopathies* may cause paresthesias or hypoesthesia in the territory of a nerve root. However, these nerve root lesions often cause characteristic *radiculopathic* pain, characterized by sharp shooting pain, *radiating* proximally to distally in the distribution of the root (see Chapter 21). Radicular pain due to cervical or lumbar root processes can occur even in the absence of obvious neck or back pain. The possibility of a cervical or lumbar radiculopathic localization of a patient's symptoms is often apparent given the characteristic symptoms. However, *thoracic* radiculopathies are less common and may produce radiating pain, paresthesias, or severe dysesthesias in the territory of one or several thoracic nerve roots. Causes of thoracic radiculopathies include herpes zoster, diabetic thoracic radiculopathies, or structural lesions. Thoracic radiculopathies may mimic serious systemic processes such as intra-abdominal or cardiac pathology. A clue to the primary neurologic, radicular cause of the patient's symptoms would be the presence of clearcut *cutaneous* hypoesthesia or dysesthesia on the surface of the skin, conforming to a thoracic dermatomal distribution.

Spinal cord lesions (*myelopathies*) that affect the ascending sensory tracts cause sensory symptoms (hypoesthesia and paresthesias) below the level of the lesion. Total interruption of these sensory fibers at any level of the cord would cause complete anesthesia below that level. Myelopathies may cause *Lhermitte's sign,* which is an uncomfortable feeling of electricity, vibration, or tingling that radiates down the neck and/or back and sometimes into the extremities, occurring upon neck flexion (Chapter 9). Lhermitte's sign is caused by dysfunction of nerve fibers in the posterior columns. Although it can be seen in multiple sclerosis, it can occur as a result of any process affecting the cord, including compressive lesions. Therefore, when a patient reports a Lhermitte's sign, it can be a helpful clue to a myelopathic localization of pathology.

Thalamic lesions may cause decreased sensation and paresthesias over the contralateral body. This may be quite marked, and some patients with thalamic strokes, for example, may have severe sensory dysfunction over an entire half of the body up to the midline. Thalamic lesions, particularly chronic ones, may sometimes also cause severe dysesthesias (*thalamic pain*) in addition to the cutaneous sensory loss. *Cortical* lesions involving the sensory cortex will cause paresthesias or hypoesthesia in the regions of the contralateral body corresponding to the cortical territory involved. Such sensory cortical lesions may also be associated with motor abnormalities or other signs of cortical dysfunction.

GAIT DISORDERS

Disorders of gait and balance may be due to non-neurologic or neurologic causes. Non-neurologic causes of gait dysfunction are primarily the result of orthopedic problems, such as spine, pelvic, hip, or knee problems. Gait dysfunction due to pain in a lower extremity is termed an *antalgic* gait. It is usually, although not always, evident from the history and examination that a disorder of gait is related to an orthopedic, as opposed to a primary neurologic, process.

The neurologic structures that control gait and balance include the frontal lobes, basal ganglia, cerebellum, and pathways for motor and sensory function. Gait problems can occur as a result of dysfunction in any of these regions, and they cause characteristic abnormalities evident on history and examination.

Frontal lobe disorders, as can be seen resulting from hydrocephalus or bifrontal mass lesions, or as an accompaniment of aging or dementia in some patients, cause a characteristic difficulty with initiation of gait. Patients may complain that their feet are "glued" to the floor. The resulting gait disorder is very similar to a parkinsonian gait, with very short steps, although the way the feet appear to be nearly stuck to the floor and the absence of other parkinsonian features help in distinguishing this from parkinsonism. Patients with a frontal lobe gait disorder may or may not have other symptoms of frontal lobe dysfunction, such as incontinence or dementia.

When the *basal ganglia* dysfunction of *Parkinson's disease* affects walking, it causes a characteristic flexed posture and a slow, *bradykinetic* gait, with multiple steps needed for turns, which may be accompanied by impairment of *postural reflexes*. Patients may complain that they have a difficult time stopping their forward progress while walking, termed the *festination* of gait. Parkinson's disease is discussed in more detail in Chapter 10.

Disorders of the *cerebellum* or cerebellar pathways (e.g., in the brainstem) produce an *ataxic* gait, a wide-based, unsteady gait indistinguishable from the gait disorder of acute alcohol intoxication.

Unilateral *corticospinal tract* disease will produce a *hemiparetic* gait, often with characteristic circumduction of the stiff, overextended, hemiparetic leg, pivoting around the axis of the strong leg. Bilateral corticospinal tract disease, such as can occur as a result of *myelopathies,* causes both legs to be stiff, and the resulting *spastic* gait may include a scissoring motion of each leg around the other while moving forward.

Disorders of the *lower motor neuron* (or *muscle*) of the lower extremities can also affect the gait. The resulting gait abnormality depends on the muscles that are weakened. When there is weakness of extension at the knee joint, the patient may lose the ability to lock the knee, and this may cause buckling and falling. This may be most bothersome in maneuvers that require the knee to lock for stabilization, and patients may therefore note buckling of a leg particularly when walking down stairs. Weakness of foot dorsiflexion may cause the patients to complain of tripping over their toes. Severe foot dorsiflexion weakness will therefore produce a *steppage* gait, with the leg lifted higher than normal to avoid tripping over the toes of the weak foot.

Patients with severely impaired sensation in the lower extremities may also complain of difficulty with gait, even in the absence of motor impairment. Examples include severe peripheral neuropathies or other disorders affecting proprioceptive sensory function in the legs, as can be seen, for example, as a result of vitamin B_{12} deficiency. Often, these patients present to the physician because of the gait disorder; usually, they do not realize that there is an underlying disorder of extremity sensation that is the cause, especially when paresthesias or dysesthesias are not prominent. When patients have such a severe loss of proprioceptive sensation in the feet, the resulting wide-based gait disorder is a *sensory ataxia.* These patients need to look at their feet while walking, and they often describe a particular tendency to fall in the dark, where visual cues are lost (Romberg's sign).

THE ROLE OF THE TEMPORAL COURSE OF NEUROLOGIC ILLNESS IN NEUROLOGIC DIAGNOSIS

An accurate and detailed neurologic history is the cornerstone of neurologic diagnosis. One of the most telling parts of the history is the *temporal pattern* of the neurologic symptomatology. This time course of neurologic symptoms can give the clinician important clues as to the probable *mechanism* of central nervous system dysfunction. In neurologic diagnosis, it is usually most helpful to try to decide which *general mechanism* of disease is most likely to be present, before proceeding further diagnostically. Neurologic disease processes can be categorized as producing their dysfunction through one of these general mechanisms: *compressive, degenerative, epileptic, hemorrhagic, infectious, inflammatory* (including *demyelinative*), *ischemic, migrainous, metabolic* (including *toxic*), or *traumatic*. (Some congenital neurologic processes may also produce disease that results from the *congenital absence* of certain normal structures or tissues—whether on a subcellular or macroscopic level—thereby leading to abnormal neurologic function.)

These mechanisms of acquired neurologic disease are generic; for example, the *compressive* mechanism would include such diverse disease processes as a subdural hematoma causing mass effect on the brain, a benign or malignant tumor (with or without associated edema) compressing or infiltrating brain tissue, or a cervical disc compressing the spinal cord. In addition, single pathologic processes can produce clinical symptoms via different potential mechanisms; for example, an intracerebral aneurysm may produce disease because of hemorrhage, or because of compression of important structures (e.g., a posterior communicating artery aneurysm causing a compressive oculomotor nerve palsy).

Consideration of the temporal pattern, although not specific for a single mechanism, can be most helpful in including or excluding some of these mechanisms; other clues from the history and examination can then be incorporated to narrow the choices of mechanism and specific disease process. The following discussion presents some common temporal patterns of symptomatology and the disease mechanisms they particularly suggest.

Transient focal neurologic symptoms, which may or may not be recurrent, are usually seen due to *ischemia, migraine,* or *seizure.* Although these three mechanisms may seem to be quite different from each other, they are not always easy to distinguish. *Ischemic* symptoms, when transient, can produce focal neurologic dysfunction lasting from seconds to hours. *Migrainous* brain dysfunction (see Chapter 7) can produce a variety of focal neurologic manifestations (even without headache). In addition to the visual scintillations of classic migraine, other neurologic symptoms can be seen as migrainous phenomena, including weakness, paresthesias, and aphasia. These migrainous symptoms typically progress and spread over a period of minutes (e.g., 15 to 30 minutes) before resolving. In contrast, the focal neurologic symptoms of *seizures* tend to spread somewhat more quickly (Chapter 8). The patient's age, associated medical conditions, and other clues from history and examination may assist in the delineation of the likely mechanism of transient focal neurologic dysfunction. It should be noted that *demyelinating disease* (e.g., multiple sclerosis—see Chapter 9) causes focal neurologic dysfunction that can resolve and then recur in a different region of the central nervous system. However, the symptoms of an acute attack of multiple sclerosis usually last at least days to weeks before improving, unlike the more transient symptoms of ischemia, migraine, or epilepsy. As noted in Chapter 9, some patients with multiple sclerosis do experience very brief (as short as seconds), repetitive *paroxysmal* neurologic symptoms. This is presumably due to "short circuits" between adjacent demyelinated axons in a multiple sclerosis plaque, and the resulting very brief paroxysmal event can be simply considered as a white matter electrical (seizure-like) event.

Sudden-onset neurologic symptoms suggest ischemia or hemorrhage. A *progressive focal neurologic symptom* primarily suggests a compressive lesion, but ischemic, inflammatory, or focal infectious processes can progress gradually as well. Degenerative diseases may also produce progressive focal neurologic dysfunction, but the dysfunction is usually more diffuse, even if not symmetric. Ischemic or compressive lesions can also cause *waxing and waning* focal neurologic symptoms. More *diffuse waxing and waning* symptoms would also be expected in some toxic or metabolic processes.

Progressive diffuse neurologic symptoms are most suggestive of degenerative processes, infectious or inflammatory processes, or metabolic abnormalities. The specific time course in question can be quite helpful. For example diffuse neurologic dysfunction that has been progressing over days would more likely be ascribed to a metabolic or infectious process, whereas the same kind of symptoms progressing over years would be more likely caused by a degenerative disease.

QUESTIONS AND DISCUSSION

1. A 35-year-old man presents to the emergency room with a 3-day history of numbness and tingling from his mid chest down to his legs, and mild weakness in both legs. He also describes an unusual electric-shock-like sensation whenever he flexes his neck forward. He also has some urinary urgency. Examination shows normal mental status and cranial nerves. There is mild weakness in both legs (4/5). Sensory examination shows that pinprick is felt differently (it feels less sharp, although somewhat tingly) below the level of the nipples, including the lower chest, abdomen, and legs, than above that level. Reflexes are normal in the

arms but are brisk in the legs. Toes are upgoing to plantar stimulation.

Which of the following terms best describes the localization of this patient's clinical syndrome?

A. Encephalopathy
B. Myelopathy
C. Radiculopathy
D. Neuropathy
E. Plexopathy
F. Myopathy

The answer is (B). This patient has symptoms of spinal cord (*myelopathic*) dysfunction. Clues to a spinal cord localization of his symptoms include the bilateral motor dysfunction in the legs, as well as the bilateral sensory dysfunction with a sensory level over the trunk. There are also brisk reflexes in both legs and bilateral *Babinski signs,* suggestive of bilateral upper motor neuron (corticospinal tract) dysfunction as the cause of the leg weakness. Although brainstem lesions can similarly cause bilateral motor and sensory symptoms, the absence of cranial nerve abnormalities is evidence that the lesion is below the level of the brainstem. Urinary symptoms, including urgency, are not uncommon in spinal cord processes. This patient also describes *Lhermitte's sign,* the electric-like sensation upon neck flexion, a finding suggestive of a spinal cord process affecting the posterior columns.

Although the cause of this patient's spinal cord dysfunction is not yet clear, the clinical realization that his symptoms are *myelopathic* is important and will guide the clinician to the appropriate choice of imaging and other studies. Whether his myelopathy is *compressive,* or due to a *demyelinative* or *inflammatory* (*myelitis*) cause, or other process, will need to be determined by additional investigations. The next step in workup of this patient would include magnetic resonance imaging (MRI) to look for a structural lesion outside the spinal cord (e.g., a compressive process) or within the spinal cord (e.g., an inflammatory process). Despite the fact that the level of the lesion appears most likely to be thoracic, imaging of both the thoracic and cervical spinal cord would be appropriate, as a cervical cord lesion could also cause these symptoms.

This patient's clinical symptoms and signs are not suggestive of pathology in the brain (*encephalopathy*), nerve root (*radiculopathy*), nerve (*neuropathy*), cervical or lumbosacral plexus (*plexopathy*), or muscle (*myopathy*).

2. A 72-year-old woman with a 2-year history of diabetes mellitus presents to your office because of severe pain under her right breast and right scapula.

The pain has been present for 4 weeks and has been excruciating and unremitting. She describes the pain as a burning feeling. There is an occasional severe, sharp, shooting sensation from her right mid/upper back to beneath her right breast. The pain is not worse with breathing, but she notes that the skin in this area is very uncomfortable for her to touch. It bothers her when clothes touch this region. Her only medication is an oral hypoglycemic agent. She has seen multiple physicians for this pain, and she has undergone extensive gastrointestinal and cardiac evaluations for it, which were unrevealing.

The patient's general physical examination is normal and there is no skin rash. Neurologic examination shows normal mental status and cranial nerves. Motor strength is normal. Sensory testing shows that she has severe discomfort when the skin under the right breast and below the right scapula is touched with either a cotton swab or the point of a pin. This area of sensory abnormality is a strip about 2 cm in height but extending from the right mid/upper thoracic spine posteriorly to the lower sternum anteriorly. Reflexes are 1+ and symmetric, and toes are downgoing to plantar stimulation.

Which of the following terms best describes the localization of this patient's pain syndrome?

A. Encephalopathy
B. Myelopathy
C. Radiculopathy
D. Neuropathy
E. Plexopathy
F. Myopathy

The best answer is (C). This patient has characteristic symptoms and signs of a *thoracic radiculopathy.* (Answer (D)—*neuropathy*—is not entirely incorrect, as it would be difficult at the bedside to be certain that her lesion is not of a thoracic *nerve* rather than *root.*) The major clue to a probable *nerve root* localization of her disease process is the distribution of her sensory symptoms and sensory findings to the cutaneous territory of a particular nerve root. In this case, her findings map out the territory of either the right T5 or T6 root. Another clue to this *radicular* localization of her symptoms is the occasional proximal-to-distal shooting pains in the territory of a right thoracic nerve root.

The generic diagnosis of a thoracic radiculopathy does not in itself give a specific clinical diagnosis for this patient. However, the clinical realization that this is the likely syndrome allows the physician to narrow the causative possibilities, and to reasonably exclude many possibilities, prior to further investigation. Realization that this patient's cutaneous sensory symptoms and signs are most compatible with a thoracic radicular process, and not a visceral process, would probably have saved her from some unnecessary investigation. One caveat is that visceral disease can cause *referred* pain syndromes suggestive of neurologic or spinal processes, such as thoracic or lumbar spine pain from deep chest, abdominal, or retroperitoneal processes.

In this patient, the most likely cause of her thoracic radicular syndrome is a *diabetic thoracic radiculopathy*. Herpes zoster (shingles) in this distribution would cause similar symptoms, but it is less likely given the absence of herpetic skin lesions. The clinical diagnosis of a diabetic thoracic radiculopathy can probably be made in this case without the necessity of much further investigation. However, the clinician could elect to order an MRI scan of the thoracic spine to exclude the unlikely possibility of a structural cause (e.g., a *compressive radiculopathy*) of her symptoms.

3. Your office nurse tells you that your next patient is complaining of intermittent episodes of dizziness that have been occurring for the last 2 months. The patient is a 54-year-old woman whom you have been following for several years for routine general medical care. She has no significant illnesses other than hypertension. Prior to coming to your office today, the patient had a few tests done, including an MRI scan of the brain and a 24-hour ambulatory heart monitor test. (The patient works in a hospital, and the technicians did these tests for her as a favor.)

Which of the following choices would be the most appropriate *next step* in your evaluation of this patient?

A. Review the results of the previous workup.
B. Take a history from the patient.
C. Perform a general physical examination.
D. Perform a neurologic examination, including testing for positional vertigo.

The answer is (B). Although all of the choices can be very important and helpful, the first step in any neurologic evaluation should be the taking of a neurologic history. Once the neurologic history is obtained, the clinician should usually have enough clues to determine the likely locations of the lesion (the *where* part of the neurologic diagnostic process) and the possible disease mechanisms involved (the *how* part of the diagnostic process). The neurologic examination can be a very helpful adjunct to the neurologic history, and in some cases it may help exclude or include certain processes that are under consideration. The role of the neurologic history and examination in the evaluation of patients with dizziness is discussed in Chapter 14.

The results of ancillary laboratory tests, although often very important in excluding or confirming specific diagnostic considerations, should be ordered and interpreted in light of the clinical history (first) and the neurologic exam (second). Clinical interpretation of a patient's diagnostic studies without regard to the findings of history and examination is fraught with potential hazard. Just as incidental abnormalities may be overinterpreted for clinical importance (red herrings), the clinician might also get false reassurance from the results of normal studies that do not answer the appropriate clinical question at hand.

4. A 25-year-old woman presents to your office because of a 5-year history of intermittent episodes of face and arm numbness and difficulty with vision and speech. The attacks are all very similar, and she has had about two attacks per year, the last one being several days ago. Most of the episodes have involved the right side of vision, and the right face and arm, and are described as follows. They begin with the visual disturbance, which she describes as difficulty seeing the right side of people's faces, or the right side of a page, "as if they are obscured by heat waves." This is then followed, within a few minutes, by numbness and tingling in the right cheek. This numb sensation then gradually descends over the next 15 minutes to involve the right arm and hand. During the attacks, she has had difficulty with speech, which she describes as a feeling that "I know what I want to say, but I can't get the words out." These symptoms last a total of about 30 minutes, then resolve, and are usually followed by a moderately severe throbbing headache over the left temporal region. Although the majority of her episodes have involved her right vision and body, she recalls having had a few episodes that involved only the left side of her vision, face, and arm, but without the speech disturbance. She has no significant past medical history, except for additional occasional headaches that occur (about once a month) without neurologic or visual symptoms, located over either or both temples, relieved by over-the-counter analgesics. She is on no other medications and is not on birth control pills. Her neurologic examination is normal when she is seen in your office.

Which of the following general mechanisms of neurologic dysfunction is the most likely cause of this patient's presenting symptoms?

A. Ischemia
B. Migraine
C. Epilepsy
D. Demyelinative

The answer is (B). This patient has recurrent episodes of transient focal neurologic dysfunction, most likely of *migrainous* etiology. Recurrent transient focal neurologic symptoms are usually due to *ischemia, epilepsy,* or *migraine.* In this case, migraine is the most likely cause of her visual symptoms, which sound typical of migraine auras. Her other neurologic symptoms, which occur subsequent to the onset of her visual symptom, suggest the focal neurologic symptomatology that migraine can sometimes produce (see Chapter 7), and they progress with a typical migrainous tempo. The subsequent headache after the neurologic disturbance is also suggestive of migraine, although migrainous neurologic symptoms can sometimes occur without headache, and headache can occur with other neurologic processes, including ischemia and epilepsy. Ischemia is less likely to be the cause of this patient's symptoms, because of the number of episodes (stereotypic, but sometimes affecting either side of the brain) she has had over many years without obvious sequelae. Her age would also make ischemia less likely, although the clinician could consider the possibility of a hypercoagulable state such as the antiphospholipid antibody syndrome. A focal seizure is also possible, but less likely because of the slow tempo of progression and the fact that her symptoms have occurred on either side. *Demyelinating disease* is an unlikely cause of this patient's symptoms.

Despite the clinical diagnosis of a likely migrainous cause of this patient's episodes, however, further workup is indicated. This would include blood tests, as well as MRI of the brain to exclude focal structural pathology (for example, an arteriovenous malformation or mass) that could serve as a nidus for focal neurologic symptoms such as migraine or seizure.

5. A 72-year-old right-handed woman with a 10-year history of diabetes mellitus and hypertension presents to the emergency room because of right face, arm, and leg weakness. She is very alert and conversant, and upon taking her history, she tells you that she was well until this morning, when after she awakened she realized that her right arm and leg were very weak and she was unable to move them at all. She also noted that the right side of her mouth was droopy. She called the paramedics herself, who brought her to the hospital. Her weakness has not improved. Although she notes that her right arm and leg are completely paralyzed, she also tells you that when the paramedics touched her on her right side, the sensation of her right arm and leg seemed normal. She is taking an oral hypoglycemic agent and an angiotensin convert-

ing enzyme inhibitor. Her blood pressure is 140/90 and her heart rate is 68/minute and regular.

Even prior to your examination of this patient, you attempt to hypothesize the most likely location of her neurologic lesion. Of the following choices, which is the most likely localization of her lesion?

A. Cerebral cortex
B. Subcortical white matter
C. Cervical spinal cord
D. Nerve root

The answer is (B). This patient's history alone suggests that she most likely has the clinical syndrome of a *pure motor hemiplegia.* She describes severe weakness of her right arm and leg, without obvious sensory symptoms. In addition, her ability to give such a detailed history without obvious language impairment suggests intact left hemisphere *cortical* function. This combination of pure motor weakness with intact sensory and cortical function is most consistent with a *subcortical* stroke. The syndrome of a pure motor hemiparesis can occur as a result of a small lesion in either the posterior limb of the internal capsule or on one side of the base of the pons. In either of these subcortical locations, the corticospinal fibers are segregated from sensory fibers and are deep to the cortex; therefore a lesion in these locations will cause motor weakness without cortical or sensory dysfunction. The most likely cause of a lesion in this region would be a *lacunar* stroke (see Chapter 6), although a small *hypertensive hemorrhage* can cause lesions in the same locations and result in a similar clinical picture.

This patient's symptoms would not likely be from a *cortical* stroke, because of the intact right hemisphere cortical function. In addition, a cortical stroke large enough to cause paralysis of an entire side of the body would be expected to cause some concomitant sensory dysfunction. A *cervical spinal cord* localization of her lesion would be unlikely because of the facial droop, and because of the unilateral nature of her severe deficit—without the patient's description of any motor or sensory symptoms on the other side. This patient's symptoms are not suggestive of a *nerve root* localization.

Therefore, the most likely localizations and etiology of this patient's problem can be surmised by a simple, but careful, history. The results of the subsequent neurologic examination—in particular, testing motor strength, sensory function, and assessing for left hemisphere cortical function—would then help support or refute the probable diagnosis of the syndrome of a pure motor hemiplegia. Imaging studies are then helpful in excluding a hemorrhagic, as opposed to an ischemic, lesion in the internal capsule or pons causing this patient's stroke syndrome.

SUGGESTED READING

Brazis PW, Masdeu JC, Biller J: Localization in Clinical Neurology, 3rd ed. Boston, Little, Brown, 1996

Gelb DJ: Introduction to Clinical Neurology. Boston, Butterworth-Heinemann, 1995

Gilman S, Newman SW: Manter & Gatz's Essentials of Clinical Neuroanatomy and Neurophysiology, 9th ed. Philadelphia, FA Davis, 1996

Haerer AF: DeJong's The Neurologic Examination, 5th ed. Philadelphia, JB Lippincott, 1992

Patten JP: Neurological Differential Diagnosis, 2nd ed. London, Springer-Verlag, 1996

Neurology for the Non-Neurologist, Fourth Edition,
edited by William J. Weiner and
Christopher G. Goetz. Lippincott
Williams & Wilkins, Philadelphia © 1999.

| C H A P T E R | 3 |

Clinical Use of Neurologic Diagnostic Tests

Thomas P. Bleck

The diagnostic tests used in neurologic practice are most effectively employed as adjuncts to the history and physical examination. Prior to the advent of computerized imaging studies, the noninvasive electrodiagnostic tests were often ordered as a battery to determine whether invasive radiologic studies or diagnostic cranial exploration was indicated. As computed tomography (CT) and magnetic resonance imaging (MRI) have advanced, the electrophysiologic studies are less important anatomically; however, as pathophysiologic studies they remain unchallenged. Similarly, cerebrospinal fluid (CSF) examination is less often indicated in the work-up of mass lesions but is prominent in the study of neuroimmunologic disorders. Hence, diagnostic studies can now be more appropriately tailored, with a considerable decrease in risk, time, and expense. However, if these tests are used indiscriminately, rather than to include or exclude specific clinical hypotheses, they can increase costs and delay diagnosis and treatment.

Cerebrospinal fluid examination and electrodiagnostic procedures are considered in this chapter. Neuroradiologic studies, discussed in Chapter 4, are mentioned here only as an alternative means of acquiring data.

CEREBROSPINAL FLUID EXAMINATION

Since Quincke introduced the diagnostic lumbar puncture (LP) at the end of the 19th century, CSF evaluation has been applied to most neurologic disorders. As other diagnostic tests have become more sophisticated, CSF examination is no longer a standard part of the analysis of all central nervous system (CNS) disorders. This procedure is most commonly indicated for the diagnosis of CNS infection, neoplastic invasion of the subarachnoid space, multiple sclerosis (MS), acute inflammatory demyelinating polyneuropathy (Guillain–Barré syndrome), other neuroimmunologic disorders, and pseudotumor cerebri.

TECHNIQUE

An LP is usually performed with the patient lying on his side, with the knees flexed as close to the chest as possible. The patient should be informed about each stage of the procedure and he should be positioned with his back as close to the edge of the bed as possible. The location of the intended puncture should be determined before cleansing the skin. A line connecting the posterior iliac crests crosses the L3–L4 interspace, which is usually the most rostral space employed. The caudal end of the spinal cord is at L2 in most adults. After palpating the spinous processes, the examiner can mark the L4–L5 and L5–S1 interspaces with thumbnail pressure prior to gloving. The skin is cleansed with iodine followed by alcohol, and sterile drapes are positioned around the area to be punctured. The skin is anesthetized with 1% lidocaine, using a 25-gauge needle, which is then exchanged for a 22-gauge needle. This longer, stiffer needle is used to anesthetize the deeper tissue down to the epidural space. As the needle is advanced, the syringe is aspirated to avoid intravascular or subarachnoid injection. The epidural space is recognized by the sudden loss of resistance to injection.

A 20- or 22-gauge spinal needle is adequate for most LPs; smaller-caliber needles make pressure measurements difficult. The needle should always be advanced with the stylet in place (to avoid subarachnoid introduction of epidermal tissue). Although some experts replace the stylet when withdrawing the needle to avoid entrapping a spinal nerve root, the rare incidence of this complication does not appear to differ between these two techniques. The needle should be advanced with the bevel up, to separate the fibers of the ligamentum flavum. The needle is angled 15 degrees cephalad to avoid the spinous processes. Dural puncture produces a "pop"; the stylet is then withdrawn. If free CSF flow does not occur, rotating the bevel toward the head is often useful. (With all movements of the needle, the stylet should be replaced). Should it be necessary to redirect the needle, it must be withdrawn almost to the skin. Newer spinal needles, which have a conical tip and a side port rather than a beveled tip, may produce less of a dural tear and therefore fewer, less severe postprocedural headaches.

When free flow has been established, the CSF pressure is measured with a manometer attached to the needle by means of a stopcock. The patient's legs should be extended to prevent a falsely increased reading. The respiration and pulse should both fluctuate.

For accurate pressure readings, patients on ventilators (especially those receiving positive end-expiratory pressure) should, if possible, be transiently disconnected to lower the transmitted intrathoracic pressure. The Queckenstedt jugular compression test is unreliable and dangerous. Following pressure measurement, four tubes of CSF are withdrawn and processed for cell counts (at the start and end), bio-chemical and immunologic studies, and microbiologic analysis. The usefulness of closing pressure measurement is uncertain.

Following the withdrawal of the needle, pressure should be applied to the site of entry and the patient should be placed in the prone position. Although the evidence is inconclusive, many experts feel that 1 to 3 hours prone is the most effective method of preventing a post-LP headache, which is the major complication of the procedure.

If the physician is unable to enter the subarachnoid space with this technique, the patient should be placed in a sitting position. With the patient leaning forward on a support, the spinous processes will be palpable in the midline. When the needle is in the subarachnoid space, the patient should be returned to the recumbent position for a pressure measurement.

When lumbar spine disease or the question of an intraspinal mass prevents the lumbar approach, a lateral cervical approach can be performed by a physician trained in this technique. Fluoroscopic guidance can be employed with either approach.

CONTRAINDICATIONS

Prior to LP, the physician must be certain that the patient does not have an intracranial or intraspinous mass. A CSF examination is rarely useful in this situation, and the withdrawal of CSF may alter the CNS pressure dynamics sufficiently to cause herniation.

The absence of papilledema does not exclude an intracranial mass, although its presence mandates a CT scan prior to LP (as does an asymmetry on neurologic examination). It is *not* necessary that all patients be scanned before an LP is performed, especially if acute bacterial meningitis is suspected. If LP is delayed for CT scanning when bacterial meningitis is suspected, one should consider a single dose of empirically chosen antibiotics prior to the CT scan (after blood cultures have been obtained).

Coagulopathy is a relative contraindication to LP, because epidural hematomas can arise at the puncture site. Infusions of fresh frozen plasma or platelets, as appropriate, should be given prior to the procedure if possible. If the coagulopathy is discovered after the LP, therapy should still be given because bleeding may occur for many hours. The patient should be examined frequently for signs of cauda equina dysfunction, which may necessitate surgical extirpation of the extravasated blood.

Cutaneous infection at the intended puncture site requires that a different approach (e.g., lateral cervical) be used.

INTERPRETATION OF RESULTS

Normal lumbar CSF is under a pressure of no more than 180 mm (of CSF) with the patient in a recumbent position. An elevated pressure suggests the presence of infection, a mass lesion, or increased CSF production or its diminished resorption. Normal pressure does not exclude an infection or a mass.

The glucose concentration in CSF is normally at least two thirds of the serum glucose; as glucose takes time to equilibrate in the subarachnoid space, the CSF value tends to lag behind the serum by about 30 minutes. Low CSF glucose concentrations are seen with meningeal inflammatory processes (e.g., infection or meningeal spread of neoplasms). The protein concentration primarily reflects albumin derived from the serum; in the lumbar space, it is usually 15 to 45 mg/dl. Elevation usually reflects an increased transudation of albumin, generally as a consequence of inflammation. The protein concentration may be low or low-normal in pseudotumor cerebri.

High-resolution electrophoretic studies of CSF proteins reveal the presence of *oligoclonal antibodies* in over 90% of patients with MS. This finding is also seen in other settings in which immunoglobulins are produced in the subarachnoid space (e.g., infections), and rarely in the presence of primary brain tumors. They are also frequently present in the Guillain–Barré syndrome.

A cytologic examination of normal CSF should reveal no more than 5 lymphocytes per mL, and no polymorphonuclear leukocytes (PMNs). The presence of PMNs indicates an acute inflammatory process; lymphocytes predominate generally in aseptic, chronic, or resolving conditions.

Cultures and stains for microbial agents should be obtained if any possibility of infection arises. These include Gram stains, India ink preparations, stains for acid-fast bacilli (AFB), routine bacterial cultures, fungal cultures, and AFB cultures. Various newer studies are available for the analysis of bacterial infective agents; these studies include counterimmunoelectrophoresis (CIE) for specific bacterial antigens and the limulus test for endotoxin. Routine viral cultures of CSF seldom reveal the etiology of aseptic meningitis or encephalitis except for human immunodeficiency virus-1 (HIV-1), but antibody titers in the CSF and serum may be helpful. Serologic testing for syphilis is increasingly important.

Although subarachnoid hemorrhage is usually diagnosed by CT, an LP may be necessary to confirm the diagnosis. The scan may not detect small amounts of subarachnoid blood in patients without atrophy; in this case, LP is required. The procedure may also be used to reduce CSF pressure, and thus symptoms, if there is no intraparenchymal extension of bleeding.

Tables 3-1 and 3-2 summarize the expected CSF findings associated with the more common indications for LP.

ELECTROENCEPHALOGRAPHY

Indications for electroencephalography (EEG) have varied during the 60-year history of this technique. Imaging studies have supplanted it as a method for localizing anatomic pathology. This has freed EEG to develop as a pathophysiologic tool, detecting abnormal cerebral *function* that cannot be visualized radiographically or magnetically. Thus, the use of EEG is greatest in the evaluation of transient states (e.g., seizures), evolving conditions (e.g., herpes simplex encephalitis), global disorders (e.g., dementia), and neonates. As with the other procedures considered in this chapter, the usefulness of EEG data depends on the clinical hypothesis being tested. Only a few EEG patterns are diagnostic of particular diseases, but the test is helpful in deciding among diagnostic alternatives.

TECHNIQUE

The quality of EEG recording and interpretation varies dramatically among laboratories. In evaluating the standards of practice used, the physician should expect the following:

1. The technologists are trained specifically in EEG and are either eligible for, or have obtained, certification by the American Board of Registration in Electrodiagnostic Technology.
2. The technologists participate in regular continuing education activities, both locally and nationally.
3. The electroencephalographers are neurologists certified by both the American Board of Psychiatry and Neurology and the American Board of Clinical Neurophysiology.
4. The laboratory meets the accreditation standards of the American Electroencephalographic Society.
5. The patient's head is always measured prior to the application of electrodes, according to the International 10–20 System.
6. The equipment employed has at least 16 channels and is calibrated prior to each use.

(*text continues on page 32*)

TABLE 3-1. Cerebrospinal Fluid Abnormalities in Common Meningitides

	ACUTE BACTERIAL MENINGITIS	ASEPTIC MENINGITIS	TUBERCULOUS MENINGITIS	CRYPTOCOCCAL MENINGITIS	PARTIALLY TREATED BACTERIAL MENINGITIS	NEOPLASTIC MENINGITIS	ACUTE HIV-1 INFECTION
Pressure (mm CSF)	Up to 1000	Up to 350	300–500	300–500	Up to 500	Up to 500	Up to 350
Glucose (mg/dl)	0–40 (<35% of serum)	10–40	1–40	5–40	May be low	5–40	Usually normal
Protein (mg/dl)	Up to 1000	Up to 200	Up to 1000	Up to 500	May be elevated	Up to 500	Up to 200
WBCs (per mL)	500–50,000	15–200	100–500	100–500	Often elevated	20–500	Up to 500
Polys (%)	>90	May predominate early	5–15	5–15	Up to 30%	Occasional	Rare
Lymphs (%)	10	Predominant later	85–95	85–95	Predominant	Predominant	Predominant
Microbiologic studies	Gram stain culture	Culture (rarely)	AFB smear culture	India ink culture	Gram stain culture		Culture
Immunologic studies	CIE; limulus test	Antibodies; VDRL		Cryptococcal antigen	CIE; limulus test	β-2 microglobulin	Antigen, antibody studies
Other						Cytology	

AFB = acid-fast bacilli; CSF = cerebrospinal fluid; CIE = counterimmunoelectrophoresis; VDRL = Venereal Disease Research Laboratory test; WBC = white blood cell count.

TABLE 3-2. Cerebrospinal Fluid Abnormalities in Other Disorders

	HERPES SIMPLEX ENCEPHALITIS	SUBACUTE SCLEROSING PANENCEPHALITIS	ACUTE INFLAMMATORY DEMYELINATING POLYNEUROPATHY	CYSTICERCOSIS	ACUTE TOXOPLASMOSIS	MULTIPLE SCLEROSIS	SUBARACHNOID HEMORRHAGE
Pressure (mm CSF)	Up to 450	Normal	Normal	Up to 250	Normal	Normal	Up to 500 (may be normal)
Glucose (mg/dl)	30–70	Normal	Normal	Normal	Normal	Normal	Usually normal
Protein (mg/dl)	Up to 200	Up to 100	Up to 100 (rarely, to 1000)	Up to 50	Up to 100	Up to 60	Often elevated
WBCs (per mL)	Up to 1000	6–500	0–5	Up to 300	10–50	Up to 20	Acutely, proportional to blood entry; later, elevated
Polys (%) Lymphs (%)	Up to 30 Predominant	Rare Predominant	Rare Up to 100	Rare Predominant	Rare Predominant	Rare Predominant	Acutely Predominate later
Immunologic studies	Viral antibodies (late)	Measles and oligoclonal antibodies	Oligoclonal antibodies	Antibody titers	Antibody titers	Oligoclonal antibodies	
Other					Occasional eosinophils		Gross blood within 1–2 hours; xanthochromia

CSF = cerebrospinal fluid; WBC = white blood cell count.

7. Each record performed includes both wakefulness and sleep (and states this clearly).
8. Hyperventilation and photic stimulation are used routinely as activation procedures unless contraindicated.
9. Extra electrodes (e.g., sphenoidal) are employed when indicated.
10. The EEG report includes both a technical description and a clinical interpretation. This interpretation attempts to correlate the EEG with the patient's history. Although it may contain suggestions for further evaluation (e.g., a sleep-deprived EEG), management recommendations beyond the scope of an EEG (e.g., the suggestion of specific medications) are inappropriate.

TOPOGRAPHIC MAPPING

Many manufacturers have adapted computer interpolation techniques to produce colorful "brain maps" of EEG (and evoked potential) data. Although these maps have a great deal of emotional appeal and may eventually be found to aid in EEG interpretation, they currently require expert technologists and electroencephalographers to be certain that the data entered are free of artifacts. The statistical analysis of these maps is in its initial stage. At present, they cannot substitute for a standard EEG.

INTERPRETATION

The interpretation of an EEG is an attempt to answer clinical questions about the cerebrum in light of the electrophysiologic data; thus, the interpretation is most useful when the questions are well defined and are appropriate for the examination. An EEG is one of the most useful studies in the evaluation of suspected seizures, for example, but is seldom valuable in the analysis of headaches or dizziness. The most commonly encountered EEG abnormalities are epileptiform events, slowing of normal rhythms, and disorders of age-specific patterns.

EPILEPTIFORM EVENTS

The term *epileptiform* is used because spikes and other sharp activity on the EEG rarely represent actual seizures. The usual EEG signature of a seizure disorder is the *interictal spike*. Such irritative events do occur (albeit rarely) in individuals without seizures, and their presence does not diagnose a seizure disorder (unless the actual seizure is recorded). Similarly, the absence of epileptiform abnormalities never

excludes the diagnosis of a seizure disorder: this is a clinical decision.

Epileptiform activity may be divided broadly into *focal*, *multifocal*, and *generalized* events. In complex partial seizures of temporal lobe origin, for example, the abnormality is often localized over one anterior temporal region. In absence epilepsy, the 3-Hz discharges are typically widespread and bilaterally synchronous. This distinction is most crucial in the patient with a generalized convulsion, for whom the work-up, treatment, and prognosis depend on an accurate distinction between *primary generalized epilepsy* and *partial epilepsy with secondary generalization*. Other syndromes with specific EEG patterns, such as benign Rolandic epilepsy of childhood, have predictable courses and seldom require imaging studies or further work-up.

Several special EEG techniques are helpful in the diagnosis of epilepsy. Partial sleep deprivation may bring out otherwise undetected epileptiform abnormalities and should be performed whenever the routine EEG is unrevealing. Various extra electrodes have been developed and are most useful when a focal EEG abnormality is detected but is not definitely epileptiform. The most commonly employed are nasopharyngeal electrodes; however, studies have shown that extra true temporal (T1 and T2) electrodes are just as valuable and are less noxious. Sphenoidal electrodes or double-density electrode arrays may be suggested by the electroencephalographer in particular clinical situations, but they are not indicated routinely. Ambulatory 24-hour EEG technology is improving and can contribute to the differential diagnosis of intermittent behavioral episodes. Prolonged inpatient recordings, sometimes employing intracranial electrodes, are occasionally necessary for a definitive diagnosis.

The normal EEG contains several benign variants that may be confused with truly epileptiform activity. Small sharp spikes, positive occipital sharp transients of sleep, 14- and 6-Hz–positive spikes, "phantom" spikes, and "psychomotor variant" are embedded in the older literature but are of dubious significance. EEG reports that stress their association with epilepsy or "neurovegetative disorders" should prompt the clinician to find another electroencephalographer.

SLOW WAVE ABNORMALITIES

As with epileptiform activity, the crucial distinction is among focal, multifocal, and diffuse abnormalities. A focal abnormality may result from gray or white matter dysfunction in that area; this distinction is based on other EEG characteristics. Recall here that the

EEG is a physiologic test; postictal slowing from a recent seizure and the constant slowing emitted by cerebral tissue adjacent to a brain tumor may be indistinguishable on a single EEG. Imaging and electrophysiology are thus complementary, and unexplained focal slowing should prompt a radiologic or magnetic investigation.

Diffuse abnormalities are commonly a consequence of a toxic (e.g., drug), metabolic (e.g., hepatic), degenerative (e.g., Alzheimer's disease), infectious (e.g., encephalitis), or postictal condition. Pure diffuse slowing has few characteristics that distinguish among these possibilities; EEGs are most useful when acquired serially to monitor change in the patient's condition. Specific patterns, such as triphasic waves that exhibit temporospatial lags in hepatic encephalopathy, may suggest an etiology but are rarely diagnostic of a particular metabolic cause. Some forms of dementia (e.g., subacute spongiform encephalopathy) have specific EEG signatures that are usually diagnostic of that particular disorder. A paucity of EEG abnormality in an apparently demented patient raises the possibility of depressive pseudodementia.

The combination of focal and diffuse disturbances is often a useful finding. In herpes simplex encephalitis, the EEG is the earliest diagnostically useful test to become abnormal and is often used to determine the site of brain biopsy before radiologic studies are abnormal. Multifocal abnormalities, especially if intermixed with epileptiform discharges, may suggest the embolic origin of a stroke.

Electrocerebral silence ("flat EEG") is the most extreme diffuse abnormality. If hypothermia and hypnosedative drug intoxication are excluded, this finding may be used to diagnose cerebral cortical inactivity. As the EEG does not reflect brain-stem activity, the EEG is not a substitute for a physical examination in the diagnosis of "brain death." The American Electroencephalographic Society has strict published criteria for these recordings. Such a study is only supportive, however, and is subject to false-negative interpretation because of artifacts. Studies that image intracranial blood flow are more useful in this setting.

AGE-SPECIFIC PATTERNS

Neonatal EEG recordings provide the clinician with the opportunity to assess cerebral development, as well as to detect the abnormalities previously described. The more subtle manifestations of seizures in newborns may be detected only by EEG.

A modest degree of focal slowing in the temporal regions commonly accompanies normal aging and may be overread by inexperienced interpreters.

EVOKED POTENTIALS

The role of evoked potential studies (EPs) has been in flux during the past decade. Prior to the wide availability of MR and CSF oligoclonal antibody studies, EPs were often essential in the diagnosis of MS because of their ability to detect subclinical lesions. Although they still play an ancillary role here, they are being applied increasingly to other areas.

Several sensory modalities can be investigated by evoked potentials; the most commonly studied are the visual, auditory, and somatosensory systems. "Cognitive" potentials and the cerebral events associated with motor output are areas of current research interest that may find a clinical application in the next several years.

TECHNIQUE

Evoked potentials rely on computer averaging to eliminate signals that are not related temporally to the stimulus used. Many reliable commercial systems for acquiring and displaying EP data are now available; problems arise because of variability in stimulus parameters, data manipulation, and interpretation. Standardization of techniques and interpretation is currently poor. At a minimum, the clinician should expect that the laboratory performing EPs have validated its technique and normative data by testing at least 20 normal subjects. Since the definitions of abnormality in EPs are based on numerical differences of latency and amplitude from a control population, the criteria of abnormality employed must be clearly stated. The number of falsely positive and negative studies depends on how these criteria are defined, rather than on a qualitatively abnormal measurement. To reduce false-positive results, most laboratories now use three standard deviations from the control mean as the definition of abnormality.

VISUAL EVOKED RESPONSES

Visual evoked responses (VERs) can be elicited with various stimuli: the most commonly employed are reversing checkerboard patterns, sinusoidal gratings, and repetitive flashes. The size of checks (or the spatial frequency of the grating), the luminance of the pattern, the ambient light, and the repetition rate of the stimuli are all important variables. Thus, norms derived in one laboratory may not apply to another.

The response is recorded over the occipital region. Each eye is tested separately to examine for prechiasmal lesions; stimulation of individual fields may also be performed if postchiasmal dysfunction is suspected.

Visual acuity is an important determinant of the response; if the patient wears glasses, they should be used during pattern testing.

For pattern reversal and sinusoidal gratings, the major potential of interest is a surface positive wave occurring about 100 msec after the stimulus (termed P100). Flash responses elicit a surface negative wave approximately 80 msec after the stimulus (N3).

BRAIN-STEM AUDITORY EVOKED RESPONSES

Although the auditory evoked response can be followed up to the cortex, the major use of this test on brain-stem auditory evoked responses (BAERs) is the evaluation of brain-stem structures. The stimuli are clicks, delivered monaurally through headphones. The frequency spectra of the clicks, their intensity, their duration, and their repetition rate influence the latency and amplitude of the responses.

Five waves are routinely recorded. Wave I originates from the eighth nerve, wave II from the cochlear nucleus, wave III from the superior olivary complex, wave IV from the lateral lemniscus, and wave V from the inferior colliculus. All of these responses normally occur within 6 msec of the stimulus.

SOMATOSENSORY EVOKED RESPONSES

Upper extremity somatosensory evoked responses (SSERs) are recorded following stimulation of the median nerve, and lower extremity SSERs from the posterior tibial nerve. The stimulus intensity is adjusted according to the motor response. These stimuli travel in the posterior column/medial lemniscal system, so that digit movement, rather than discomfort, is used to determine the stimulation level. Repetition rate and stimulus intensity affect the latency and amplitude of the responses.

From the upper extremity, responses are recorded over the brachial plexus, at the dorsal root entry zone, and over the contralateral primary sensory cortex. Lower extremity responses are measured at the popliteal fossa, the dorsal root entry zone, and the midline scalp over the somatosensory cortex (the foot area being located in the interhemispheric fissure).

INTERPRETATION

The major use of EPs is in the detection of subclinical lesions. Within the visual system, asymptomatic optic neuritis is easily detected; its presence may aid in the diagnosis of MS. Abnormalities of the optic nerves are poorly visualized by MRI, making VERs an important adjunct when the diagnosis of demyelinat-ing disease is in doubt. Similarly, BAERs and SSERs can detect physiologic lesions below the limit of resolution of imaging techniques. This is especially true for MS plaques in the spinal cord, another area where MRI has been disappointing.

In infants, VERs have been used to assess the integrity of the visual system when blindness is suspected. Paradigms to determine refractive error are under investigation.

In addition to detecting asymptomatic brain-stem lesions in MS, auditory evoked responses are an excellent screening procedure when tumors of the eighth nerve are suspected. The sensitivity of BAERs in the setting is over 90%. BAERs are often employed in the operating room to help protect the eighth nerve during resection of posterior fossa lesions. The test is also useful when neuromuscular junction blockade or large doses of hypnosedative drugs have abolished the clinically testable brain-stem reflexes. The presence of BAERs (beyond wave I) confirms the activity of the brain stem and can also help to localize brain-stem lesions producing coma.

Analysis of BAER wave latencies as a function of intensity serves as a useful marker of auditory acuity in infants. This technique allows the early selection of hearing-impaired children for hearing aids and helps prevent their misdiagnosis as autistic or mentally retarded.

Somatosensory evoked responses are also useful in suspected MS, because they allow the documentation of unsuspected or poorly defined sensory dysfunction. As the technique evolves, dermatomal SSERs may allow better definition of nerve root compression (e.g., by a herniated disc). SSERs also have a place in the operating room, guiding the degree of tension on distracting rods during scoliosis surgery.

ELECTROMYOGRAPHY AND NERVE CONDUCTION STUDIES

These procedures are valuable primarily in the analysis of peripheral nerve and muscular disorders. They serve as adjuncts to the patient's history and physical examination and must be tailored to a specific clinical question.

TECHNIQUE

Electromyography (EMG) demands a high degree of clinical and technical skill from the physician performing the study. The laboratory should be directed by a member of the American Association of Electromyography and Electrodiagnosis. Many variables influence the interpretation of results, including anatomic variations and the cooperation of the patient.

The usual EMG study involves recording spontaneous, voluntary, and electrically stimulated muscle activity by way of small intramuscular needle electrodes. Since the voluntary contraction of muscles is crucial for some parts of the study, the procedures should be clearly explained to the patient. Some discomfort is unavoidable during the test. Patients can be premedicated with codeine or anxiolytic agents without altering the data obtained; this often results in better cooperation and tolerance.

Some conditions indicate special studies. Myasthenia gravis and the myasthenic (Eaton–Lambert) syndrome exhibit characteristic responses to repetitive stimulation; the requesting physician must communicate such suspicions to the electromyographer.

Nerve conduction velocity (NCV) studies can be performed by trained technologists under the electromyographer's supervision. These tests involve electrical stimulation of a peripheral nerve, measuring the rate of transmission and the amplitude of the response along the nerve. These results are compared to statistically derived normal ranges. Careful attention to variables such as limb temperature and length is required for a valid interpretation.

INTERPRETATION

Abnormalities of the EMG can be produced by disease anywhere in the motor unit, from the lower motor neuron cell body to the muscle fiber. Characteristic patterns have emerged that allow the electromyographer to suspect diagnoses, but the test results are only meaningful with reference to a particular clinical problem. The analysis of the EMG and NCV data best illuminates questions of primary motor neuron or muscle disease, demyelinative versus axonal neuropathy, nerve root versus plexus disorders, and the localization of a mononeuropathy.

Motor neuron disease (e.g., amyotrophic lateral sclerosis) results in abnormal spontaneous activity of motor units and individual muscle fibers. This activity is seen throughout the body. Muscle disorders (e.g., myotonic dystrophy) produce characteristically different patterns of spontaneous activity.

Polyneuropathies cause EMG and NCV abnormalities according to their pathophysiology. Demyelinative neuropathies produce slowed conduction with preserved amplitude, whereas axonal neuropathies reduce amplitude with little effect on NCV. Chronic axonal neuropathy produces diffuse denervation responses in muscle (similar in nature to those seen focally in mononeuropathies). These tests can thus narrow the diagnostic spectrum in polyneuropathy and should be performed early to help plan the subsequent work-up. In acute demyelinative neuropathies (e.g., the Guillain–Barré syndrome), special studies of conduction through the nerve roots (F responses and H reflexes) are often confirmatory when the routine NCV studies are normal.

The correct localization of a lesion along the course of a peripheral nerve (root, plexus, or at distal sites) is usually required for diagnosis and therapy. Root lesions produce denervation in paraspinal muscles in addition to distal changes; thus, a herniated disc can be separated from other pathologic lesions. Denervation changes require from 1 to 6 weeks to appear following an injury; thus, these studies are rarely indicated acutely. Such a study is important when multiple sites of pathology are detected along the course of a nerve. Some surgeons require EMG confirmation of focal lesions prior to removing a disc or transposing a peripheral nerve.

Entrapment syndromes are often diagnosed best by EMG and nerve conduction studies. The most common disorder is the carpal tunnel syndrome; this is also a situation in which clinical judgment in interpretation is crucial. Asymptomatic median nerve compression in the carpal tunnel is common; if the electrical studies are limited only to the wrist, pathology in the neck may be overlooked and the wrong therapy may be undertaken.

The routine use of EMG and NCV studies in the evaluation of neck, shoulder, or low back pain in the absence of neurologic deficits is costly and time consuming, and it seldom benefits the patient. The test is best used to confirm and define abnormalities seen on examination. Only if the clinical suspicion of a discrete lesion is high, or confirmation of equivocal imaging studies is required, should these tests be performed in such a situation.

SUMMARY

Neurodiagnostic studies can provide critical data for the evaluation of diagnostic alternatives. It is hoped that the preceding discussion has served to place these tests in their proper clinical perspective. One must use the information obtained as an extension of the history and physical examination, or incorrect diagnosis and improper therapy are likely.

The future of electrophysiologic studies is bright; improvements in automated data analysis and artificial intelligence will elicit more data from the available tests. As the power of these techniques increases, however, so does their potential for error. As the clinician becomes more dependent on other people's interpretation of data, it becomes increasingly important to be certain that the clinical laboratories used are appropriately certified.

QUESTIONS AND DISCUSSION

1. A patient presents with paraparesis and a history of optic neuritis in the left eye. An MRI study reveals no cerebral lesions and no evidence of spinal cord pathology. Which of the following tests is most likely to help confirm or refute the diagnosis of multiple sclerosis?

A. NCV studies
B. CSF evaluation for oligoclonal antibodies
C. Contrast myelography
D. BAERs
E. EEG

The answer is (B). Oligoclonal antibodies are present in over 90% of MS patients. Nerve conduction velocity is not affected in multiple sclerosis. Contrast myelography is unnecessary if the MR is normal. BAERs might be abnormal but would be superfluous if oligoclonal antibodies are present. The EEG is not helpful in diagnosing MS.

2. A patient with suspected complex partial seizures has a normal routine EEG. Which of these procedures would be most useful diagnostically?

A. VERs
B. LP
C. Repeat EEG with sleep deprivation and extra electrodes
D. 24-hour EEG monitoring
E. EMG studies

The answer is (C). Sleep deprivation and extra electrodes often demonstrate epileptiform activity when the routine EEG is unrevealing. Evoked response studies are not specifically abnormal in epilepsy. Twenty-four-hour EEG monitoring is helpful in special circumstances but is seldom necessary in routine practice. An EMG would not shed light on possible epilepsy.

3. Which of the following is *not* a contraindication to LP?

A. Papilledema, stiff neck, and fever
B. Cutaneous infection of the lower back
C. Suspected intraspinal mass
D. Posterior fossa tumor
E. Coagulopathy

The answer is (A). Papilledema is seen in states of increased intracranial pressure but does not necessarily imply a risk of herniation. In the setting of fever and stiff neck, papilledema is suggestive of meningitis so that a lumbar puncture is necessary. Patients with pseudotumor cerebri usually benefit symptomatically from an LP, and the test is necessary for the diagnosis. A CT scan, however, should precede an LP in the presence of papilledema. The other situations are all contraindications to an LP.

4. Which of the following tests is the most useful screening procedure for cerebellopontine angle tumors?

A. Skull films
B. EEG
C. VERs
D. BAERs
E. SSERs

The answer is (D). Although MRI is probably the most sensitive diagnostic test for cerebellopontine angle tumors, its expense is prohibitive for screening. BAERs are sensitive and are relatively inexpensive. Skull films and EEGs may be abnormal if the tumor is large, but not early in the course. VERs and SSERs are not characteristically affected by these lesions.

5. Nerve conduction studies in axonal neuropathies are characterized by:

A. Slow conduction and normal amplitude
B. No changes in either conduction velocity or amplitude
C. Loss of amplitude, with relative sparing of velocity
D. Increased conduction velocity
E. High-amplitude responses

The answer is (C). The amplitude reflects the number of nerve impulses that arrive at the neuromuscular junction; axonal neuropathies primarily reduce this number. Those impulses that are transmitted have a relatively normal conduction velocity. Demyelinative neuropathy slows conduction but does not reduce the number of fibers carrying impulses.

SUGGESTED READING

American Electroencephalographic Society: Guidelines in EEG and evoked potentials. J Clin Neurophysiol 3 (Suppl 1), 1986

Aminoff MJ (ed): Electrodiagnosis in Clinical Neurology, 3rd ed. New York, Churchill Livingstone, 1992

Chiappa K (ed): Evoked Potentials in Clinical Medicine, 3rd ed. New York, Raven Press, 1990

Cracco RQ, Bodis-Wollner I (eds): Evoked Potentials. New York, Alan R. Liss, 1986

Daly DD, Pedley TA: Current Practice of Clinical EEG. New York, Raven Press, 1990

Fishman RA: Cerebrospinal Fluid in Diseases of the Nervous System, 3rd ed. Philadelphia, WB Saunders, 1992

Liveson JA: Peripheral Neurology: Case Studies in Electrodiagnosis, 2nd ed. Philadelphia, FA Davis, 1991

Niedermeyer E, Lopes da Silva F (eds): Electroencephalography, 3rd ed. Baltimore, Urban and Schwarzenberg, 1992

Schaumburg HH, Spencer PS, Thomas PK: Disorders of Peripheral Nerves, 2nd ed. Philadelphia, FA Davis, 1991

Scheld WM, Whittley RJ, Durach DT (eds): Infections of the Central Nervous System, 2nd ed. New York, Raven Press, 1997

Neurology for the Non-Neurologist, Fourth Edition, edited by William J. Weiner and Christopher G. Goetz. Lippincott Williams & Wilkins, Philadelphia © 1999.

C H A P T E R   4

Neuroradiology—Which Tests to Order?

Sundeep M. Nayak

Ruth G. Ramsey

Magnetic resonance imaging (MRI) is a young modality in neuroradiology. Its birth and evolution resulted from a need to image the skull and its contents to superior anatomic advantage. Non-central nervous system (CNS) neurologic and body imaging applications were later extensions of this important technology. MRI exploits latent magnetic domains contained within native hydrogen atoms (protons) that are ubiquitous in various tissues but occur in different proportions. Each proton and its environment affect the magnetic field generated by the MR equipment: This property undergoes computerized manipulation to generate data that may be presented as a qualitative gray-scale image (MR image, or MRI), a spectrum of relative frequencies (MR spectroscopy, or MRS), or a quantitative evaluation of mobile protons (MR flow studies, or MRF, and diffusion MR). Besides the obvious advantage of not using any form of irradiation, the technique is noninvasive and displays the field of view with excellent contrast resolution. Innumerable MR sequences have been developed in the quest for diagnostic perfection and anatomic detail. The most commonly used spin-echo sequences are available as standard software on most MR scanners. Briefly put, short TR (also known as T1-weighted) sequences outline anatomy well, whereas long TR (either balanced or T2-weighted) sequences highlight pathology.

Computed tomography (CT), which revolutionized our understanding of sectional anatomy, was initially developed expressly for neuroimaging applications. Very simply, it utilizes the absorption of photons (generated from thinly collimated sources) by tissues to generate data that, after computerized postprocessing, are presented in a familiar gray-scale format. While there are no absolute contraindications, some factors cause significant image degradation. Recent advances in this technology include rapid helical (also known as spiral) CT scanning, which is particularly useful when imaging unstable patients and when there is limited time to arrive at an accurate diagnosis. Other noninvasive methods commonly used in central neuraxis imaging include isotope studies (typically utilizing gamma rays and positron emission tomography) and sonography (using gray-scale, spectral Doppler, Doppler color, and power/energy imaging).

Invasive neuroimaging includes myelography (imaging of the subarachnoid space and its contents) and angiography (imaging of vascular luminal anatomy). The role of angiography has now been expanded to encompass interventional (or therapeutic) neuroradiology to attack acquired and developmental neurovascular pathology.

Intravascular contrast agents currently being used have improved in availability, chemical composition, and packaging. Iodinated contrast agents are available in high osmolar and low osmolar forms. Low osmolar contrast media are associated with improved safety profiles. For contrast-enhanced MRI, gadolinium-diethylenetriamine pentaacetic acid (Gd-DTPA, a chelated compound) may be safely used in almost all cases. Intravascular contrast agents for improved sonographic quantification in low flow states are being developed; their exact role in neuroimaging is yet to be fully realized.

STROKE

Stroke, or a "brain attack," is one of the commonest clinical conundrums faced by the neurologist and the neuroradiologist. Cranial CT is the preferred initial study. Although it is not uncommon for the cranial CT to be unremarkable shortly after the event, its value is its ability to identify the presence of a subarachnoid hemorrhage, a hemorrhagic infarction (especially when immediate anticoagulation is a consideration), or other entities that can mimic the presentation of a stroke. Up to 70% of infarctions will be visible as cortex-based, wedge-shaped areas of hypoattenuation within a week of the ictus. While conventional MRI will doubtlessly reveal more parenchymal and vascular detail, it is not as accurate as CT in the detection of fresh blood in the parenchymal (axial) or extraxial spaces within the cranium. Mimics of the stroke presentation include subdural collections of blood, neoplasms, parenchymal hemorrhages (such as from hypertension), vascular anomalies (such as aneurysms and arteriovenous malformations), and subarachnoid hemorrhage.

A typical infarction is limited to a singular vascular territory and, because of flow dynamics, often favors the middle cerebral artery distribution. Lacunar (*lacuna* = lake) infarctions occur in the basal motor nuclei, and "watershed" infarctions usually are found at the junction of the anterior and middle cerebral arterial territories. Hyperacute infarctions (under 6 hours) may sometimes be barely visible as non-space-occupying lesions in varying shades of gray ("smudging"). Maximal cytotoxic edema occurs within 24 to 72 hours, and significant mass effect ensues; this might even result in ipsilateral ventricular compression, vascular compromise, or herniation (under the falx cerebri or through the tentorium cerebelli) (Fig. 4-1). Transtentorial herniation leading to brainstem compression may cause slit-like Duret hemorrhages that may be preterminal CT findings.

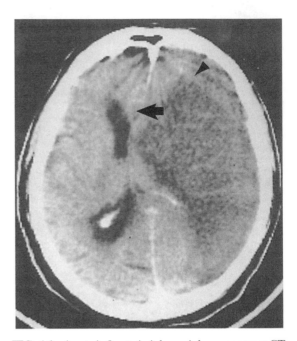

FIG. 4-1. Acute infarct. Axial cranial noncontrast CT (NCCT) image at the level of the ventricular trigone shows a cortex-based cone of hypoattenuation ("dark volume") involving nearly the entire left cerebral hemisphere (*arrowhead*) with marked mass effect and shift (*arrow*) to the contralateral side. An infarct with this degree of mass effect is approximately 24 to 48 hours old and may occasionally mimic the appearance of a chronic subdural hemorrhage.

Chronic infarctions are associated with regional parenchymal volume loss; as a result of progressive necrosis and tissue loss, there is increasing focal prominence of the ventricles and subarachnoid spaces as well as postinfarction leukomalacia (white matter gliosis). Leukomalacia will appear to follow the CT attenuation or MR signal intensity of cerebrospinal fluid (CSF) (Fig. 4-2).

Compared to CT imaging, MRI far more sensitively identifies infarctions as hyperintense (high-signal) areas on long TR images and will thus demonstrate them earlier. Additionally, many smaller infarctions will be identified only on MRI, which increases diagnostic confidence. This is especially true of small-vessel end-artery infarcts seen in the deep white matter. Advanced or long-standing small-vessel disease (leukoaraiosis) is manifest as periventricular white

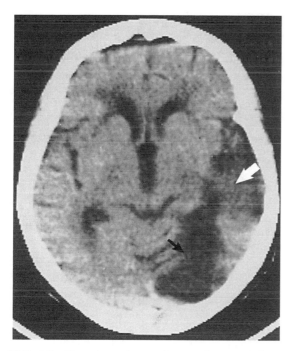

FIG. 4-2. Chronic and superimposed acute infarction. Axial cranial NCCT image at the level of the anterior pillars of the fornix shows the left occipital cortical infarction has progressed to an area of leukomalacia (*black arrow*) containing material of CSF attenuation. There is a new infarction in the left middle cerebral artery that is hypoattenuating (*white arrow*) but not quite the attenuation of CSF.

matter changes of CT hypoattenuation or MR hyperintensity on long TR images (Fig. 4-3).

Because of the physics of CT imaging, the evaluation of many structures in the posterior fossa (or infratentorial space) is limited by beam hardening streak artifacts generated at the interface of the heavily ossified petrous pyramids. MR is thus more sensitive for examining infratentorial structures for infarctions, which is especially important in the midbrain and pons as lesions located there often have devastating clinical consequences. Gd-DTPA highlights varying patterns of enhancement, which may aid in estimating the age of the infarction and thus in determining the prognosis, as patients with enhancing infarcts may do less well clinically. Typically, however, intravenous contrast infusion is not critical in diagnosing a classic infarction.

Whereas the focus of stroke imaging has traditionally centered around the stroke ictus, the current focus is on preventive imaging in the setting of transient ischemic attacks (TIA), as well as secondary prevention (using direct intraarterial infusion thrombolysis, an algorithm still being tested). TIA imaging, which earlier comprised carotid sonography and MR angiography (MRA), now also incorporates helical CT angiography using a three-dimensional (3D) technique of data presentation.

MAGNETIC RESONANCE ANGIOGRAPHY

Magnetic resonance angiography is a reliable noninvasive method of evaluating vascular structures without intravascular contrast infusion, utilizing instead the physical properties intrinsic to streaming red blood cells in the vascular tree. Different techniques ("bright blood," "dark blood"), primary effects responsible (phase-contrast, time-of-flight), and acquisition parameters (2D, 3D) are used depending on the region of interest. Each method has advantages and limitations as an angiographic technique, and these are reflected in their respective applications. At the Fresno VA Medical Center and the University of Chicago, every patient being worked up for cerebrovascular disorders is studied with a routine MRI study as well as with *conventional MRA* of the vessels in the neck (Fig. 4-4) or about the circle of Willis (Fig. 4-5), all technical parameters being individually tailored for maximal benefit. With conventional MRA, it is occasionally possible to demonstrate an aneurysm that was not seen by conventional catheter angiography.

Artifacts arising from respiration or patient motion, difficulties in the depiction of slow or turbulent flow, and in-plane saturation have impaired image quality and limited the popularity of conventional MRA as a diagnostic imaging tool. Many of these limitations may be overcome with *contrast-enhanced MRA* (CEMRA) using Gd-DTPA, a technique that permits the coverage of large volumes of interest in short acquisition times. The 3D data sets obtained may be reconstructed as maximum intensity projection (MIP) images, which resemble conventional catheter angiograms; shaded surface images, which resemble volumetric display; or even virtual intraluminal endoscopic (VIE) images, which provide angioscopic views of the vessel of interest. With high-performance gradient echo systems in use, imaging time is further reduced, making single-breath-hold acquisitions feasible. CEMRA is being

(*text continues on page 44*)

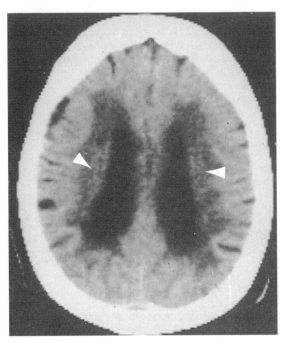

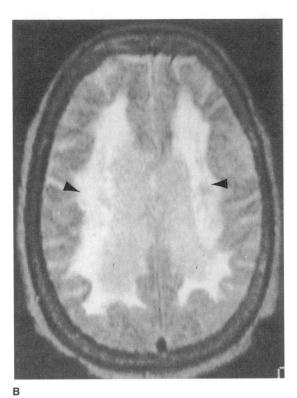

A   B

FIG. 4-3. Multiple deep white matter infarctions. **A.** Axial cranial NCCT image at the level of the centrum semiovale shows the typical bat-wing distribution of periventricular white matter changes (*white arrowheads*). **B.** Axial long TR/TE MR image shows corresponding hyperintense (high-signal) areas (*black arrowheads*).

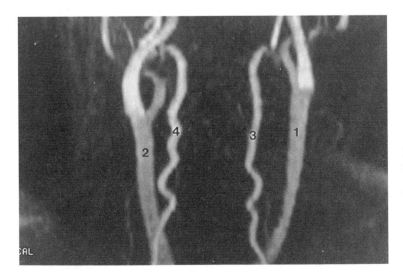

FIG. 4-4. Normal MRA of the neck. Photographic reconstructions from a two-dimensional (2D) phase-contrast study of normal neck vessels. 1: Left common carotid artery. 2: Left vertebral artery. 3: Right external carotid artery. 4: Right carotid bifurcation. 5: Right internal carotid artery.

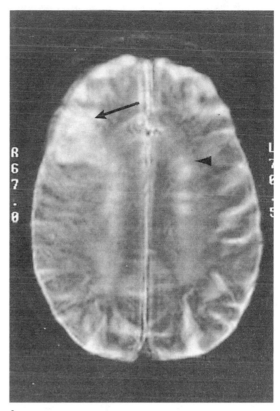

FIG. 4-5. Infarct with occluded right common carotid artery. **A.** Axial long TR image of the brain at the level of the corona radiata shows a cortex-based cone of hyperintensity (high signal) in the right frontal region, consistent with an infarction (*arrow*). Other scattered hyperintense areas (*arrowhead*) are consistent with scattered areas of ischemic-gliotic change from small foci of infarction.

A

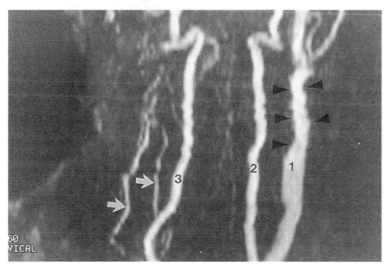

B. Photographic reconstruction from a 2D phase-contrast MRA of the neck vessels reveals complete occlusion of the right common carotid artery. Only the left carotid (1), left vertebral (2), and right vertebral (3) arteries are demonstrated. The left common carotid artery is diffusely irregular (*arrowheads*) secondary to atherosclerotic plaques when compared to Figure 4-4. The smaller vessels identified on the right side (small arrows) are attempts at collateral vessel system formation.

B

evaluated as a safe, sensitive, noninvasive, and rapid alternative to conventional catheter angiography used for routine diagnostic purposes.

INTRACRANIAL NEOPLASMS

Intracranial neoplasms are readily diagnosed by CT or MRI. While noncontrast cranial CT (NCCT) is the initial study of choice to evaluate for the presence of calcium and blood, contrast-enhanced MRI (CEMRI) using Gd-DTPA is the next step in imaging as it is more sensitive in determining the multiplanar extent and anatomic characteristics of the process that are so crucial in neurosurgical and radiotherapeutic planning. This is especially true in evaluating the infratentorial space.

GLIOBLASTOMA MULTIFORME

The glioblastoma is a malignant neoplasm seen most frequently in the third through fifth decades of life. Often large when first seen (Fig. 4-6), these tumors have variable presentations, ranging from innocuous headaches to dramatic symptoms such as seizures, hemiparesis, and paralysis. Cross-sectional imaging using CT (or MRI) typically reveals a large hypoattenuation (or complex) mass lesion primarily involving the white matter with frequent postcontrast enhancement of an irregular rim of tissue. These tumors are notorious for transcallosal extension to the contralateral hemisphere, fancifully referred to as butterfly glioma. Significant vasogenic edema is seen around the mass and extends along the neighboring white matter pathways.

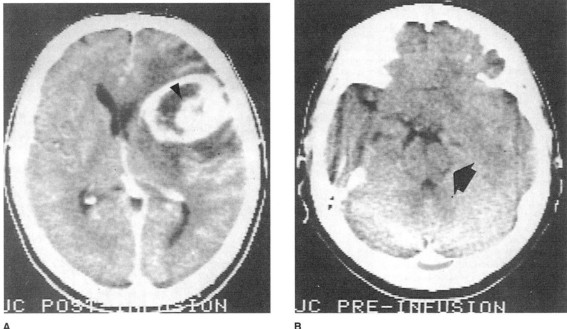

A   B

FIG. 4-6. Glioblastoma multiforme. **A.** Axial cranial contrast-enhanced CT (CECT) at the level of the third ventricle shows the tumor as a ring of intense enhancement (*arrow*) with a mural nodule (*arrowhead*) of enhancement, a hypoattenuating ("dark") central core, and surrounding vasogenic edema. **B.** Axial cranial CECT at the level of the midbrain in the same patient shows marked shift to the contralateral side with transtentorial herniation of the medial portion of the left temporal lobe and compression of the midbrain (*arrowhead*). Although the appearance is typical of the glioblastoma multiforme, metastatic disease or abscesses may have a similar appearance.

Computed tomographic imaging is critical to determine areas of amorphous calcification, which are difficult to identify on conventional MRI sequences. Often, massive infarctions and other space-occupying nonneoplastic lesions may appear tumefactive; in puzzling cases, a thorough clinical history will help the interpreting radiologist make exact determinations and recommendations, including a problem solving follow-up study. The histology or grading of the tumor type based on attenuation, intensity, or enhancement characteristics is not possible as significant overlap is seen.

MENINGIOMAS

Meningiomas arise from arachnoid "cap" cells embedded in the dura mater and are thus found in proportion to the concentration of these cells. They are most commonly encountered in the frontal high lateral convexities and less frequently at the skull base. Because of their high cellularity and microscopic calcium content, they are typically hyperattenuating ("bright") on CT and isointense (slightly low signal) on both short and long TR sequences in MRI. Intense and fairly uniform postcontrast enhancement is seen because meningiomas lack a blood–brain barrier. The digital CT tomogram often demonstrates enlargement of the groove of the middle meningeal artery (this vessel usually supplies the tumor). Mass effect upon, and white matter edema in, the neighboring parenchymal structures are variable findings that depend on the size and location of the meningioma. MR studies are invaluable in defining the patency of neighboring dural venous sinuses (using conventional MRI or MR venograms) in those cases where surgery is contemplated.

METASTASES

Intracranial metastatic deposits are equally likely to appear as singular or multifocal tumors, often having originated from breast and lung malignancies. Malignant melanoma commonly metastasizes to the brain parenchyma and, because of its high vascularity and blood product content, presents on CT as hyperattenuating enhancing masses, often multiple (Fig. 4-7). Blood products of varying signal intensities appear on different MR sequences because of temporal differences in their magnetic properties. Metastatic lesions typically have disproportionately significant perilesional edema, which may mask the underlying small tumors, acting instead as sentinels of their presence.

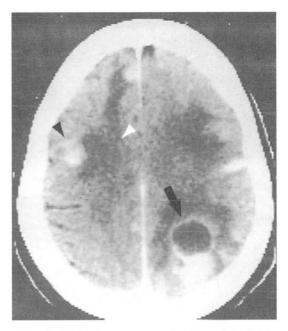

FIG. 4-7. Multiple metastases. Axial cranial CECT at the level of the corona radiata shows multiple nodules (*black arrowhead*) of enhancement, with one cystic area of enhancement (*arrow*) in the left posterior parietal lobe, probably reflecting a necrotic center. There is marked surrounding vasogenic edema (*white arrowhead*). This appearance is typical of metastatic disease.

As metastases are known to masquerade clinically as TIAs, CEMRI is always necessary to evaluate atypical cases. Occasionally, multiplicity and multifocality of intracranial neoplasms (such as metastatic deposits) may be displayed to advantage by using a higher dose of Gd-DTPA. Unexpected findings in the resulting images often dramatically alter treatment decisions.

ACQUIRED IMMUNE DEFICIENCY SYNDROME AND THE CENTRAL NERVOUS SYSTEM

Acquired immune deficiency syndrome (AIDS) is a systemic disorder caused by the human immunodeficiency virus (HIV), and a CNS affliction (CNS-HIV)

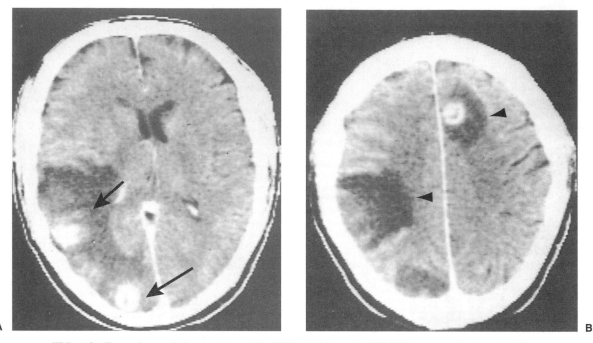

FIG. 4-8. Toxoplasmosis in a patient with AIDS. Axial cranial CECT images at the level of the trigone (**A.**) and corona radiata (**B.**) show multiple ring enhancing lesions (*arrows*) with marked surrounding edema (*arrowheads*). Multiple metastases will have a similar appearance.

may often be the AIDS-defining illness. NCCT may be unremarkable, or it may show significant atrophy for the patient's age, a result of the direct neurotropic effects of HIV often associated with the AIDS dementia complex (ADC). Opportunistic infections, unusual neoplasms, and white matter disorders are seen with alarming frequency using CEMRI. Unfortunately, the multifocal enhancing lesions seen in both toxoplasmosis (a protozoan opportunistic infection) (Fig. 4-8) and AIDS-related CNS lymphoma are known to mimic one another; in these cases, an empirical treatment plan followed by a repeat study will sometimes preclude a brain biopsy. A common preterminal event is progressive multifocal leukoencephalopathy (PML), which is best evaluated on CEMR.

TRAUMA

Computed tomography is the absolute standard for urgent care because of its ability to evaluate acute cases of blunt and penetrating cranial trauma and their life-threatening complications. Epidural and subdural collections of blood, if undiagnosed, may cause unnecessary morbidity and avoidable mortality. Subdural hemorrhages are more common in the young and the elderly, while epidural hemorrhages are frequent in middle-aged people.

Subdural hemorrhages occur from the tearing of bridging veins that traverse the subdural space. They are typically crescentic hyperattenuating collections. Usually unilateral, they vary in size: Large ones are capable of significant subfalcine or transtentorial herniation of underlying compressed, but otherwise normal, brain parenchyma. Bilateral ("balanced") subdural hemorrhages may show no shift of the structures of the midline. Subacute subdural hemorrhages display a hematocrit effect (Fig. 4-9) or have a mottled appearance. Chronic subdural collections are hypoattenuating ("dark"), but because of their higher protein content they display higher CT attenuation than CSF. Caution must be exercised in cases of isoattenuating subdural hemorrhages,

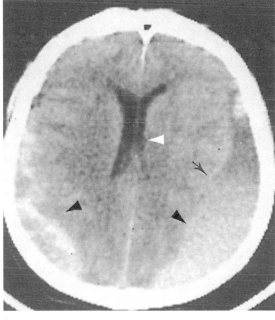

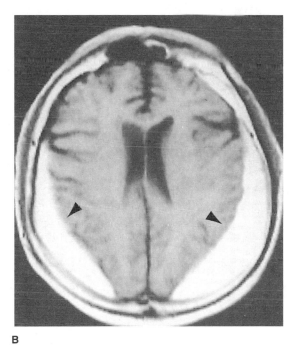

A   B

FIG. 4-9. Bilateral subdural hemorrhages. **A.** Axial cranial NCCT at the level of the body of the lateral ventricle shows bilateral mottled extracerebral collections (*black arrowheads*). There is a hematocrit effect on the left (*arrow*), secondary to settling of blood products. The lateral ventricles (*white arrowhead*) are compressed toward the midline and are elongated, reflecting the bilateral nature of the process. **B.** Axial short TR cranial MR image at the corresponding level better demonstrates the hyperintense ("bright") extracerebral collections (*black arrowheads*), as a result of the formation of methemoglobin, which is present only after the initial 48 hours.

which are known to efface prominent cortical sulci in the elderly, giving rise to a deceptively normal-appearing study. A combination of high clinical suspicion, thin-section follow-up imaging, contrast infusion, and MRI will help resolve the issue.

Epidural hemorrhages are usually secondary to arterial bleeding and are frequently associated with those calvarial fractures that violate the groove for the middle meningeal artery. The outer layer of the dura mater forms the periosteum of the inner calvarial table, from which attachment it is peeled away by the dissecting presence of an epidural fluid collection, resulting in the classic lentiform (lens-shaped) configuration. These hemorrhages are life threatening and warrant urgent intervention.

Other posttraumatic lesions seen include cerebral contusions and hemorrhages, subarachnoid and ven-tricular hemorrhages, diffuse cerebral edema, and shearing injuries. While CT is unchallenged in its role in determining the acute presence of blood, MRI is excellent in evaluating patients after the initial crucial 48 hours—in the subacute and chronic phases—to assess the extent of injury, evaluate its evolution, and recognize prognostic indicators.

DEGENERATIVE, TOXIC, AND METABOLIC DISORDERS

Multiple sclerosis (MS) is a common acquired myelinoclastic affliction that results in the demyelination of the nerves of the central neuraxis while sparing the peripheral nerves. Because of its superior sensitivity

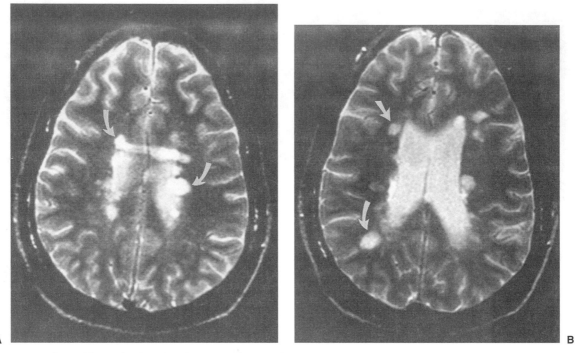

FIG. 4-10. Multiple sclerosis. **A.** Axial cranial MR image in the plane of the centrum semiovale shows demyelinating plaques in the anterior reflected portion of the corpus callosum (*anterior curved arrow*) and perpendicular to the periventricular white line (*posterior curved arrow*). **B.** Axial cranial MR image in the plane of the body of the cerebral ventricle shows demyelinating plaques in the subcortical white matter (*anterior curved arrow*) and the subcortical U-type fibers (*posterior curved arrow*). The diagnosis is based on the topographic distribution of the lesions rather than on the morphology of individual lesions.

and improved specificity, MRI using balanced (or intermediate) sequences (Fig. 4-10) is the imaging modality of choice. Classic plaques of demyelination are seen perpendicular to the periventricular zones, in the subcortical U-type fibers and in the middle cerebellar peduncles (Fig. 4-11). Callosal involvement is frequent and variably manifests as edema, irregularity, or atrophy.

Carbon monoxide poisoning results in necrosis of the globus pallidus in a bilateral and symmetric manner, appearing as hypoattenuating areas on CT, and as high-signal intensity foci on long TR images using MRI.

Adrenoleukodystrophy, a hereditary disease, is one of several disorders of the myelin sheath characterized by defective myelin generation and poor myelin maintenance. Adrenal insufficiency is the presenting symptom in some boys, and occipital cortical involvement is associated with blindness. MRI reveals corresponding hyperintense (high-signal) areas on long TR images. Other demyelinating and dysmyelinating disorders are also similarly best evaluated with MRI. MRS is helpful in the diagnosis of various degenerative, toxic, and metabolic disorders.

VASCULAR LESIONS

Arteriovenous malformations (AVMs) are commonly encountered developmental vascular anomalies. Other lesions include cryptic (not demonstrated arteriographically) vascular malformations, develop-

Subarachnoid hemorrhage (SAH) may result from a bleeding AVM but is more commonly a result of trauma or the rupture of an aneurysm. CT is the diagnostic study of choice as it demonstrates hyperattenuating subarachnoid cisterns in up to 95% of cases of SAH (Fig. 4-12), while not actually displaying the culprit aneurysm itself. A complete vascular study (Fig. 4-13) of the carotid and basilar systems is always recommended to define the anatomy of the aneurysm (for neurosurgical planning) and multiplicity (as high as 20%). While traditional approaches have included conventional catheter arteriography (CCA), both MRA and CT angiography (with 3D reconstruction and virtual imaging techniques) are being revisited, reserving CCA (Fig. 4-14) for equivocal cases or those patients who would require neurointerventional techniques such as percutaneous transcatheter ablation, particulate embolization, or microcatheter balloon occlusion.

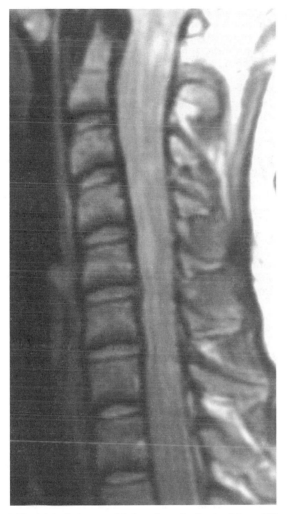

FIG. 4-11. Spine multiple sclerosis. Sagittal long TR cervical spine MR image shows multiple oval hyperintense (high-signal) foci parallel to the long axis of the spinal cord. They represent MS plaques.

mental venous anomalies (formerly known as venous angiomas in the mistaken belief that they represented true neoplasms), and vein of Galen varices. The latter is a manifestation of the draining dilated venous channel of an upstream AVM or, unusually, a fistulous connection to the posterior cerebral artery. MRI is a very efficient noninvasive modality in diagnosing these abnormalities.

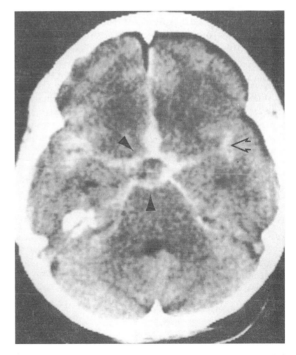

FIG. 4-12. Subarachnoid hemorrhage. Axial cranial NCCT at the level of the suprasellar cistern shows significant hyperattenuation ("brightness") in the basal cisterns (*arrowheads*) and outlining the great Sylvian fissures (*arrow*) bilaterally.

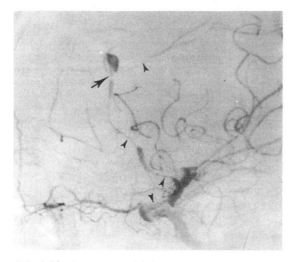

FIG. 4-13. Aneurysm with hemorrhage. Lateral view from injection of the left internal carotid artery in the arterial phase of a conventional catheter angiogram shows a typical berry aneurysm (arrow) at the bifurcation of the pericallosal and callosomarginal arteries. Blood in the subarachnoid space is irritative and causes vascular spasm (*arrowheads*).

While conventional MRA is useful in the diagnosis of vascular malformations (especially AVMs), MR venography (MRV) is being increasingly performed for the evaluation of such venous flow disorders as superior sagittal sinus thrombosis.

SPINE

Its multiplanar architecture makes the vertebral column and its content ideal for a thorough evaluation by MRI, which is the primary modality of choice in spinal imaging. MRI effectively analyzes disorders such as discogenic disease (Fig. 4-15), spinal stenosis, spinal metastases, congenital disorders (such as the Chiari type I malformation (Fig. 4-16), tethered

cord, meningomyelocele), syringohydromyelia, discospondylitis, intraspinal lipomas, and vertebral column tumors (Fig. 4-17).

Tears in the annulus fibrosus of the intervertebral discs permit herniation of portions of the central nucleus pulposus, which may compress the thecal sac, nerve rootlets, or nerve root sheath complex. Planning for spinal surgery demands the evaluation of lumbar intervertebral discs and facet hypertrophic changes using postmyelographic follow-through CT performed after instillation of nonionic iodinated contrast material into the subarachnoid space under fluoroscopic guidance. At the University of Chicago, a follow-through CT study is always performed after a conventional contrast myelogram for optimal evaluation. Postprocessing techniques can display the source data at soft tissue and bone "settings," as well as photographic reconstructions in the coronal and sagittal planes, which help substantially in presurgical planning.

Traditionally examined by myelography, spinal tumors may be classified into three major classes, each with a typical myelographic appearance (Table 4-1). *Medullary* lesions cause a diffuse expansion of the cord volume or shadow. *Intradural* processes displace the cord to the contralateral side, compressing the cord shadow; "capping" of the lesion by the contrast material forms a meniscus effect. *Extradural* pathology causes compression of the cord shadow in one plane while simultaneously causing apparent widening in the orthogonal plane. MRI has now entirely replaced myelography by more completely defining the anatomy and extent of spinal tumors using the intrinsic high-intensity (signal) of CSF to evaluate the subarachnoid space in detail. Recent advances focus on using the myelographic effect of CSF in the subarachnoid space using newer MRI sequences as a noninvasive alternative imaging modality; extraosseous anatomic definition on MRI is quite superior to that of CT while being an entirely noninvasive, outpatient, and cost-effective procedure.

In spinal surveys for metastatic disease, MRI is the modality of choice. Fat-suppressed short TR sequences and Gd-DTPA infusion have increased both the sensi-

TABLE 4-1. Spinal Tumors Classified by Spinal Column Compartments[a]

INTRADURAL	INTRAMEDULLARY	EXTRADURAL
Neurofibroma/schwannoma	Hemangioblastoma	Metastases
Meningioma	Astrocytoma/ependymoma	Herniated disc
Metastases	Metastases	Epidural hemorrhage

[a] Note that metastases may occur in any spinal column compartment.

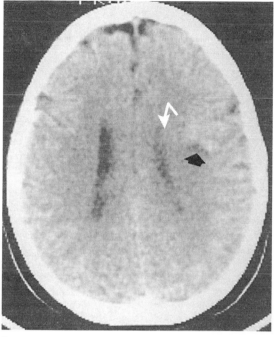

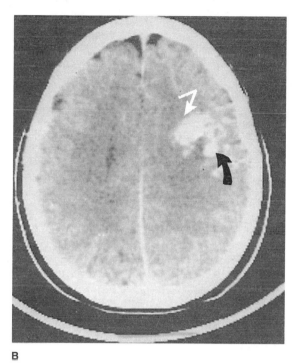

A   B

FIG. 4-14. Arteriovenous malformation. **A.** Cranial NCCT at the level of the body of the lateral ventricle shows an ill-defined area of hyperattenuation (*black arrow*) with a smaller posterior area of hypoattenuation. Slight mass effect causes compression of the body of the left lateral ventricle (*white arrow*). **B.** CECT at the corresponding level shows dense serpentine enhancement of the lesion, outlining the enlarged feeding arteries (*black arrow*) and draining veins (*white arrow*).

tivity and specificity of MRI in the diagnosis of osseous metastases. After irradiation therapy, a relative increase in marrow fat content causes uniform hyperintensity in the marrow space included in the radiation port (Fig. 4-18). Thus, MRI may also be used to follow the response to therapy. CEMRI is also very helpful in detecting leptomeningeal or dural carcinomatosis, which appears as nodules or sheets of abnormal post-contrast enhancement (Fig. 4-19).

ORBIT

Computed tomography is ideal for the evaluation of the osseous orbital pyramid and its contents, including the globe. Orbital pathology detected includes maxillofacial fractures, thyroid ophthalmopathy, orbital

hemangiomas, lacrimal apparatus neoplasms, optic nerve sheath complex neoplasms (gliomas, meningiomas), and orbital pseudotumor. CT permits a rapid diagnosis of sinusitis and orbital or periorbital (facial) cellulitis. It not only defines the aggressive osteolytic changes often seen in neoplastic processes but also readily evaluates the invasion of adjacent vital structures, particularly by violation of the epidural space.

MAGNETIC RESONANCE SPECTROSCOPY

Magnetic resonance spectroscopy enables neuroradiologists to make routine direct clinical diagnoses that were previously unavailable by radiologic or clinical tests. It is one of the many spectroscopic tools used to

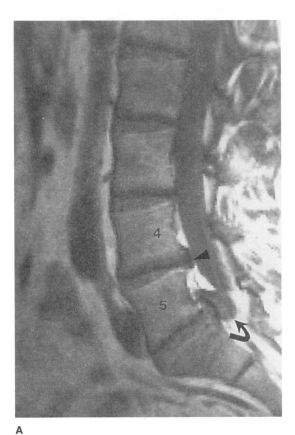

A

FIG. 4-15. Herniated disc. **A.** Sagittal short TR lumbar spine MR image shows a herniated disc (*arrow*) at the L5-S1 level and a bulging disc (*arrowhead*) at the L4-5 level. (L = lumbar; S = sacral.)

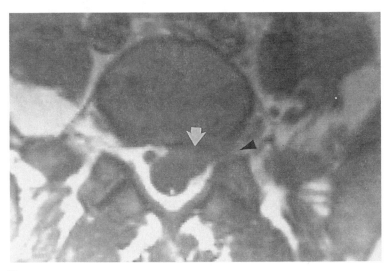

B

B. Axial short TR lumbar spine MR image shows the disc (*arrow*) to be left sided. There is interruption of the hyperintense (high signal) epidural fat and encroachment on the left intervertebral neural foramen (*arrowhead*).

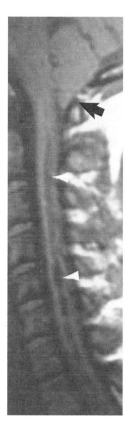

FIG. 4-16. Chiari malformation. Sagittal short TR cervical spine MR image shows peglike cerebellar tonsils (*black arrow*) extending inferiorly below the level of the foramen magnum. There is a multiloculated syringohydromyelia (*arrowheads*) in the cervical spinal cord.

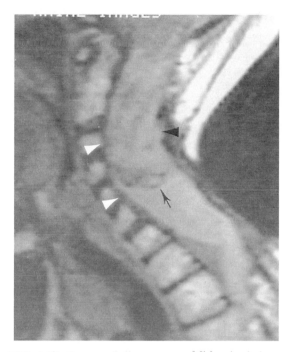

FIG. 4-17. Intramedullary tumor. Midsagittal short TR cervical spine MR image shows marked expansion (*black arrowhead*) of the cervical cord volume by a mixed-signal-intensity tumor. The lower margin of this tumor appears to end in a curvilinear fashion (*arrow*), although the cord volume is expanded and kinked below this level. As a result of the long-standing nature of this tumor, there is pressure erosion (*white arrowheads*) of the posterior margin of the cervical vertebral bodies.

determine the molecular structure of a compound or to determine the compound's presence. MRS is based on the phenomenon that the nuclei of certain atoms have characteristic magnetic properties; as a result, signals can be received and displayed as an image plot of water concentration (MRI) or as a spectrum of other biochemical compounds (MRS). The MR signal detectable from a representative volume element (a voxel), which is carefully chosen by the neuroradiologist, is directly proportional to the concentration of biochemicals within it (Fig. 4-20). This helps differentiate, for example, strokes from neoplasms. MRS is also used in problem-solving when recurrent tumor, irradiation-induced neoplasia, and necrosis cannot be

readily differentiated on the basis of MRI. MRS is currently seen as having a complementary role when standard clinical and radiologic tests are too invasive or fail to indicate a definitive diagnosis. Besides achieving clinical utility in monitoring the evolution of disease and associated therapies, MRS has been shown to be of diagnostic value for the evaluation and monitoring of the progression of stroke, asphyxiation or ischemic injury, intracranial tumors and tumor-like lesions, multiple sclerosis, encephalopathies, leukodystrophies (especially adrenoleukodystrophy), dementias, and CNS-HIV disease.

Like any tool, MRS cannot answer every clinical question, but if properly utilized in conjunction with MRI,

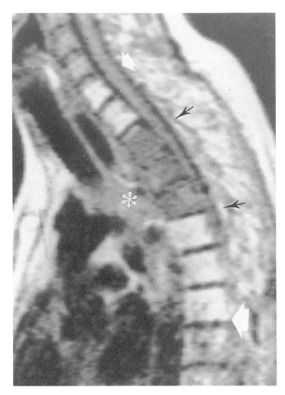

FIG. 4-18. Metastatic disease with radiation therapy effect. Midsagittal short TR thoracic spine MR image shows hypointense (*low-signal*) tumor (*black arrows*) replacing three vertebral bodies and hyperintensity (high signal) involving the two vertebrae above and three vertebrae below because of a relative increase in the marrow fat content (*white arrow*) following irradiation. A prevertebral mass (*asterisk*) from anterior tumor extension is seen.

it will assist clinicians to better manage their patients. At the Fresno VA Medical Center and the University of Chicago, every case demonstrating an intracranial neoplasm or a white matter disorder on conventional MRI is further analyzed by tailored MRS, a sequence that requires under 10 minutes of scanner time but vastly improves our understanding of biochemical composition.

SUMMARY

The work-up of patients with neurologic disease often includes several neurodiagnostic imaging tests that

TABLE 4-2. Neurologic Indications for CT

Acute cerebrovascular disease
Acute head trauma
Extracerebral tumors (especially meningiomas)
Intracranial calcifications or osseous lesions
Lumbar spine presurgical planning (postmyelogram follow-though CT)
Osseous trauma
Subarachnoid hemorrhage

have been developed over the last several years. In general, noninvasive, noncontrast CT imaging is the initial study of choice in the diagnosis of subarachnoid hemorrhage and acute stroke, both in a posttraumatic setting and in situations where MRI is contraindicated (for example, because of longer scanner times when patient cooperation drops steeply, although this will soon change with the availability of improved techniques such as echoplanar and modified gradient echo imaging) (Table 4-2). In all other clinical settings, particularly in spinal and neurodegenerative brain imaging, MRI has a firmly established role (Table 4-3).

Plain radiographs have been relegated to a limited role in preliminary spinal imaging and pre-MR screening for intraorbital foreign body exclusion. While CT angiography and MRA are the initial tests in the evaluation of vascular pathology, conventional catheter angiography has a new role in neurointerventional techniques. MRS is being increasingly used in problem-solving cases and is rapidly gaining wide acceptance with standardization in technique and a greater understanding of its biochemical and physical principles. MR diffusion imaging and functional MRI (f-MRI) are under intense scrutiny for validation by the imaging community and for outcomes analysis before their presentation as acceptable clinical technologies for everyday use.

TABLE 4-3. Neurologic Indications for MRI

Acute stroke[a]
Cervical spine
Demyelinating disorders
Head trauma (after the acute phase)
Inflammatory disorders
Intracranial tumors (axial)
Osseous vetebral column metastases
Posterior fossa and craniovertebral junction lesions
Seizures
Spinal cord lesions

[a] Future emergency role for functional MRI (f-MRI), such as diffusion imaging, blood volume maps, and oxygen consumption plots.

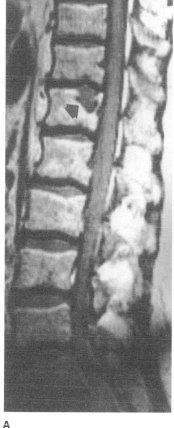
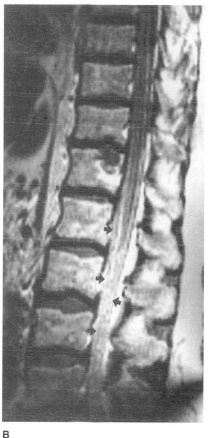

A   **B**

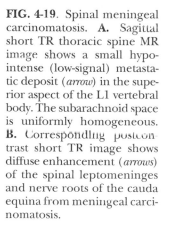

FIG. 4-19. Spinal meningeal carcinomatosis. **A.** Sagittal short TR thoracic spine MR image shows a small hypointense (low-signal) metastatic deposit (*arrow*) in the superior aspect of the L1 vertebral body. The subarachnoid space is uniformly homogeneous. **B.** Corresponding postcontrast short TR image shows diffuse enhancement (*arrows*) of the spinal leptomeninges and nerve roots of the cauda equina from meningeal carcinomatosis.

QUESTIONS AND DISCUSSION

1. Magnetic resonance angiography (MRA) is a new technique that (choose one or more):

A. Requires the infusion of intravascular contrast material such as Gd-DTPA.
B. Is useful for the detection of extracranial carotid artery stenosis.
C. While useful for arterial abnormalities, is not useful for venous system evaluation.
D. Cannot as yet be used in the diagnosis of aneurysms.
E. Is frequently used independent of conventional MR imaging (MRI).

The answer is (B) only. MRA depends on the intrinsic properties of normal blood flow, and routine Gd-DTPA infusion is not necessary. MRA can be used for the diagnosis of both arterial and venous system disorders. It is a good screening tool in aneurysm detection. It is always used in conjunction with routine MRI.

2. For the evaluation of acute stroke, which of the following is (are) true?

A. MRI is more sensitive than CT for the diagnosis of acute subarachnoid hemorrhage (SAH).
B. A noncontrast CT (NCCT) is the initial study of choice.
C. A contrast-enhanced CT (CECT) should be immediately performed.
D. MRI is more sensitive than NCCT and often reveals infarctions earlier and in addition to those seen on CECT.
E. CECT is more sensitive than MRI in the evaluation of the midbrain and brain stem.

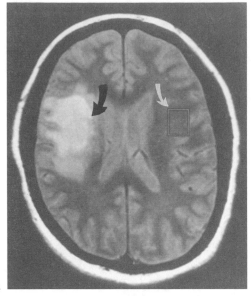

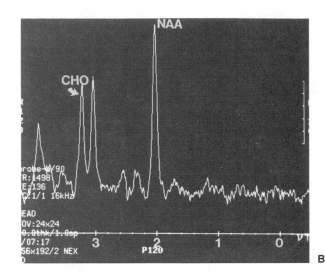

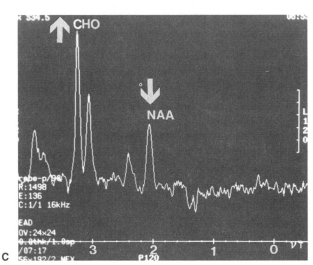

FIG. 4-20. MR spectroscopy. **A.** Proton spectrum acquired at 1.5 tesla from a normal-appearing (control-volume) left anterior parietal subcortex using 12 × 12 × 12 mm representative voxel (*curved white arrow*) with PRESS software using the SV-PROBE (TR/TE = 1,498/136 msec) acquisition method (General Electric Medical Systems, Milwaukee, WI). **B.** Spectrum shows dominant N-acetyl aspartate (NAA) peak and normal choline (CHO) peak height. This is the normal adult white matter spectral profile. **C.** Spectral analysis of lesion voxel in right anterior parietal subcortex (*curved black arrow*) shows depression of the NAA peak and elevation of the CHO peak. The CHO peak height is twice that of NAA. This is the characteristic tumor profile.

The answers are (B) and (D). NCCT is more accurate than MRI for the evaluation of acute SAH as well as hemorrhage in other locations. MRI is useful after hemorrhage has been ruled out, as it is more accurate in evaluating the presence of hyperacute and acute infarctions and is more sensitive in identifying additional areas of infarction. CECT studies are not recommended in the acute setting; enhancing infarctions are apparent after 1 week and may persist for a variable period of time from 6 weeks to years after the stroke ictus.

3. For the diagnosis of primary and secondary intracranial neoplasms, which of the following is true?

A. A contrast-enhanced study is not necessary with MRI as metastases are apparent on long TR images as hyperintense (bright) areas.

B. CECT is the modality of choice.

C. Conventional MRI is much more sensitive than NCCT for the diagnosis of areas of calcification.

D. MRI reveals a different enhancement pattern than CECT and may result in inaccurate tumor localization.

E. NCCT is more accurate than conventional MRI in the diagnosis of osseous metastases.

The answer is (E). Bone is poorly demonstrated on conventional MRI studies, making NCCT more accurate in the diagnosis of osseous metastases. Although metastases are frequently demonstrated on long TR images, preinfusion and contrast-enhanced short TR images must always be performed for complete evaluation. Contrast-enhanced MRI (CEMR) is a more sensitive technique and the modality of choice in the diagnosis of intracranial tumors. Although the patterns of enhancement in CECT and CEMR are essentially similar, CEMR is more sensitive and may reveal more intense enhancement as well as additional areas not visualized on the CECT. Calcification is much more accurately diagnosed by NCCT than by MR.

4. MR of the spine has become the diagnostic procedure of choice for all lesions of the spine. Regarding spinal MR, which of the following is or are true?

A. Approximately half of all spinal cord tumors exhibit postcontrast enhancement.

B. Plaques of multiple sclerosis (MS) are not visible by MRI, as they are usually too small to be demonstrated.

C. Herniated disc material is visible on the sagittal MR images; however, the lateralization of these discs is more accurately evaluated by NCCT.

D. MRI is the procedure of choice in the diagnosis of osseous metastatic disease.

E. MRI, even with contrast infusion, cannot diagnose spinal meningeal carcinomatosis.

The answer is (D). MRI is the modality of choice in imaging osseous metastases, readily demonstrating the level of involvement, the amount and extent of soft tissue abnormality, and the degree of spinal cord compression. CEMR is the most accurate method of imaging spinal meningeal carcinomatosis. Nearly all spinal cord tumors enhance on CEMR. MS plaques are uncommon in the spinal cord but may be identified by MRI as hyperintense (bright) areas on balanced (proton-weighted or intermediate) images. Herniated disc material is accurately demonstrated

on MRI in both the sagittal and axial planes. Surgery is being increasingly performed based on the MRI findings alone.

5. Regarding the use of MRI in the diagnosis of various abnormalities of the brain and spine, which of the following is or are true?

A. MRI uses a slightly greater amount of ionizing radiation than CT and less than conventional radiographic techniques.

B. Contrast material such as Gd-DTPA in the subarachnoid space enhances on long TR images.

C. The use of MRI and MRA will result in a decrease in the number of conventional catheter arteriograms (CCA) needed to diagnose many vascular abnormalities.

D. MRI is useful in the diagnosis of superior longitudinal (sagittal) sinus thrombosis.

The answers are (C) and (D). MRI and MRA will definitely result in a decrease in the routine diagnostic use of CCA. An unequivocally normal carotid sonogram or MRA of the extracranial carotid arteries precludes the need for CCA. MRA provides adequate evaluation of the vessels about the circle of Willis in the screening for aneurysms. MRI and MRA are very accurate for the evaluation of superior longitudinal (sagittal) sinus thrombosis. At this time, no contrast material has been granted FDA approval in the continental United States for instillation in the subarachnoid space. MRI does not use ionizing radiation.

SUGGESTED READING

Barkovich AJ: Neuroimaging of pediatric brain tumors. Neurosurg Clin N Am 3:739, 1992

Castillo M, Kwock L, Mukherji SK: Clinical applications of proton MR spectroscopy. Am J Neuroradiol 17:1, 1996

Chua SL, Goh PS, Tan LK: Magnetic resonance imaging of leptomeningeal metastases to the spine. Singapore Med J 34:253, 1993

Cousins JP: Clinical MR spectroscopy: Fundamentals, current applications, and future potential. AJR 164:1337, 1995

Curnes JT, Shogry ME, Clark DC, et al: MR angiographic demonstration of an intracranial aneurysm not seen by conventional angiography. AJNR 14:971, 1993

Davis CP, Hany TF, Wildermuth S et al: Postprocessing techniques for gadolinium-enhanced three-dimensional MR angiography. RadioGraphics 17:1061, 1997

Engelbrecht V, Rassek M, Gartner J et al: The value of new MRI techniques in adrenoleukodystrophy. Pediatr Radiol 27:207, 1997

Fischer G, Brotchi J: Intramedullary spinal cord tumors. New York: Thieme, 1996

Graves MJ: Magnetic resonance angiography. Br J Radiol 70:6, 1997

Heinz ER: Aneurysms and MR angiography. AJNR 14:974, 1993

Marks MP: Computed tomography angiography. Neuroimaging Clin N Am 6:899, 1996

Mayr NA, Yuh WT, Muhonen MG et al: Cost-effectiveness of high-dose MR contrast studies in the evaluation of brain metastases. Am J Neuroradiol 15:1053, 1994

Ramsey RG, Gean AD: Neuroimaging of AIDS. I. Central nervous system toxoplasmosis. Neuroimaging Clin N Am 7:171, 1997

Rosovsky MA, Litt AW, Krinsky G: Magnetic resonance carotid angiography of the neck. Clinical Implications. Neuroimaging Clin N Am 6:863, 1996

Selman WR, Tarr R, Landis DM: Brain attack: Emergency treatment of ischemic stroke. Am Fam Physician 55:2655, 1997

Simeone A, Carriero A, Armillotta M et al: Spiral CT angiography in the study of the carotid stenoses. J Neuroradiol 24:18, 1997

Sklar EM, Quencer RM, Bowen BC et al: Magnetic resonance applications in cerebral injury. Radiol Clin North Am 30:353, 1992

Thurnher MM, Thurnher SA, Schindler E: CNS involvement in AIDS: Spectrum of CT and MR findings. Eur Radiol 7:1091, 1997

Van Dijk P, Sijens PE, Schmitz PL et al: Gd-enhanced MR imaging of brain metastases: Contrast as a function of dose and lesion size. Magn Reson Imaging 15:535, 1997

Yussen PS, Swartz JD: The acute lumbar disc herniation: Imaging diagnosis. Semin Ultrasound CT MR 14:389, 1993

Neurology for the Non-Neurologist, Fourth Edition,
edited by William J. Weiner and
Christopher G. Goetz. Lippincott
Williams & Wilkins, Philadelphia © 1999.

| C | H | A | P | T | E | R | 5 |

Examination of the Comatose Patient

Jordan L. Topel

Steven L. Lewis

DEFINITIONS AND CLINICAL SYNDROMES

A discussion of the evaluation and treatment of the comatose patient necessitates the definition of certain terms regarding different states and levels of consciousness and unconsciousness. Although the examination and diagnostic studies must be carried out in a rather organized and systematic manner, the definitions of different levels of consciousness are, by themselves, confusing and often contradictory. When one physician's understanding of terms (e.g., lethargy, stupor, or obtundation) differs from that of his colleagues, he may think that a patient's condition has deteriorated, although only the terminology has changed between observers. It is better to describe specifically a patient's spontaneous movements, respiratory patterns, and reactions to external stimuli, for example, than to categorize the patient as being lethargic, semicomatose, or stuporous.

Consciousness is the awareness of one's self and the environment. This is a poor definition, because one can argue that a sleeping person is unconscious, that is, unaware of himself and his environment. Clinically, however, no one regards a sleeping person as unconscious: he can be aroused to appropriate physical and mental activity with appropriate, non-noxious stimuli.

Consciousness comprises a continuum from full alertness to deep coma, or total unresponsiveness. Drowsiness or lethargy is characterized by easy arousability with light stimuli. There may be a verbal response or appropriate limb movements to pain. Stupor reflects arousability by persistent or vigorous stimuli only, and the arousal is incomplete. There is little verbal response, but limb movements may still be appropriate to the stimulus. Mental and physical activity are reduced to a minimum. Coma reflects the state in which the patient cannot be aroused to make purposeful responses. This is subgrouped into light coma, in which there may be reflex, primitive, or disorganized responses to noxious stimuli (e.g., decorticate and decerebrate responses), and deep coma, in which there is no response to painful stimuli.

Hysterical coma is a psychiatric phenomenon in which the patient appears unresponsive but is physiologically awake. The heart and respiratory rates are usually normal. The patient lies with the eyes closed, and the eyelids are frequently difficult to separate. Muscle tone is normal. Although there may be little resistance to passive movement, suspending the patient's hand over his face usually results in its falling to the side instead of directly downward. Pupils are equal and reactive unless certain eyedrops have been used. Ice water caloric testing produces nystagmus, a sign seen only in awake patients. The electroencephalogram (EEG) reveals a waking record.

The "locked-in" syndrome is an important condition to recognize. The patient appears to be in coma but has essentially all higher mental activity intact. The syndrome is most frequently related to basilar pontine destruction or infarction. There is an interruption of the descending corticobulbar and corticospinal tracts, resulting in quadriplegia and paralysis of lower cranial nerves. The patient is unable to talk, breathe, or move his extremities. Since the ascending reticular activating system is spared, however, arousability and wakefulness are present. There is also sparing of fibers controlling eye blinking and vertical eye movements. Thus, the patient's only means for communication may be using eye blinks (Morse code). The ramifications of not recognizing this disturbing clinical condition are obvious. Every patient, no matter how deep in coma he appears to be, should be asked to open and close his eyes, or to move them up and down.

The vegetative state appears clinically to be the opposite of the "locked-in" syndrome. The patient is actually in coma and unable to attain higher mental functions (wakeful unresponsiveness). Although the patient may visually track the examiner, there is essentially no other appropriate response. Sleep–wake cycles may have returned, but there is no return of higher mental activity. The syndrome occurs in the setting of severe cortical dysfunction with relative brainstem sparing (e.g., from anoxia).

It is not uncommon for patients with acute onset of global aphasia to be initially diagnosed as being in coma. The patient is indeed unable to comprehend, communicate, or carry out simple verbal commands. The diagnosis may be established by noting that he frequently appears to be awake and alert, with roving eye movements or deviation of the eyes to the left, and he most often has a right hemiplegia.

COMA

ANATOMY

In the evaluation of the comatose patient, it is necessary to consider the physiologic and anatomic abnormalities that result in decreased level of consciousness. Simply stated, coma results from bilateral, diffuse cerebral hemisphere dysfunction or involvement of the brainstem (midbrain and pons) ascending reticular activating system, or a combination of the two.

Coma is unusual with unilateral cerebral hemisphere disease unless there is a dysfunction of the other hemisphere or secondary pressure or destruction of brainstem structures. Most large cerebral hemisphere infarctions will result in a slightly decreased level of consciousness, but the patient can still be aroused to elicit some purposeful movements or higher mental activity. Exceptions may be patients with large, acute lesions affecting the dominant cerebral hemisphere. In contrast, profound coma may result from very small infarctions in the brainstem affecting the ascending reticular activating system.

A unilateral hemispheral mass lesion, such as a tumor, abscess, or expanding hemorrhage, will frequently present with unilateral focal neurologic symptoms and signs. Upon continued enlargement of the mass, there may be a compression of the contralateral cerebral hemisphere or a downward herniation of the ipsilateral temporal lobe, creating distortion and compression of the brainstem. At this point, coma will ensue. There is also the suggestion that horizontal displacement of the brain at the level of the pineal body may correlate more closely with levels of consciousness than downward displacement with brainstem compression.

Metabolic processes usually affect both brainstem and cerebral hemispheres to produce coma. This likely reflects a direct interference of the metabolic activity of the neurons. Initially, the patient is drowsy, but coma ensues as the metabolic process worsens.

ETIOLOGY

Coma is not an independent disease entity but a reflection of some underlying disease process. The causes of coma can be divided into two main categories: (1) those of primary central nervous system (CNS) disease and (2) those of metabolic or systemic depression (Table 5-1). The latter group contains the more common causes of a depressed level of consciousness.

Metabolic or systemic disorders generally cause depressed consciousness without focal neurologic findings. Primary CNS disorders may or may not produce focal abnormalities on examination. A previous neurologic injury, however, may render certain neurons more susceptible to a metabolic insult. A metabolic encephalopathy could thus produce focal neurologic findings. These signs may disappear after the metabolic disturbance has been corrected.

EVALUATION AND TREATMENT

Initial emergency treatment for a comatose patient is essentially the same as for all other medical emer-

TABLE 5-1. Causes of Coma

COMA SECONDARY TO PRIMARY BRAIN INJURY OR DISEASE

Infection

Meningitis	Nuchal rigidity; CSF shows pleocytosis, increased protein; glucose may be decreased
Encephalitis	May have focal findings; CSF shows mildly increased protein, increased lymphocytes, normal or slightly decreased glucose
Abscess	Focal findings; positive CT scan; history of ear or sinus infection; CSF shows mildly increased protein, increased cells, negative cultures

Tumor

Primary or metastatic	Focal findings; progressive course; papilledema

Infarction

	Usually no coma unless bilateral or acute, large, dominant hemisphere, or involving brain-stem reticular activating system

Hemorrhage

Subarachnoid	Sudden onset; headache; nuchal rigidity; vomiting; positive CT scan; bloody CSF
Intracerebral	Sudden onset; headache; nuchal rigidity; vomiting; focal findings; abnormal CT scan; history of hypertension

Trauma

Concussion, contusion	Positive history, evidence of injury on examination; uncomplicated concussion leaves no residual
Subdural hematoma	Depressed level of consciousness can occur before focal findings; may have trivial or no trauma history
Epidural hematoma	Lucid interval; skull fracture over middle meningeal artery

Seizures

	Convulsive or nonconvulsive status epilepticus; postictal progressive improvement in level of consciousness unless other factors are involved

COMA SECONDARY TO METABOLIC AND SYSTEMIC DISEASES

Exogenous Toxic Substances

Sedatives, hypnotics, antidepressants	Positive blood or urine screens; may cause pupillary abnormalities
Alcohol	Breath odor may not be apparent; seizures, delirium tremens on withdrawal
Acid poisons—methyl alcohol, paraldehyde	Metabolic acidosis; visual symptoms with methyl alcohol
Enzyme inhibitors—heavy metals, cyanide, arsenic, lead, salicylates	Lead encephalopathy common in children, not in adults

Endogenous Toxic Substances

Hepatic coma	Fetor hepaticus, jaundice, ascites, asterixis; triphasic waves on electroencephalogram
Uremic coma	Uriniferous breath; seizures; asterixis; increased BUN
CO_2 narcosis	Increased P_{CO_2}; positive physical chest findings, electrolytes
Endocrine—pituitary, thyroid, pancreas (diabetes), adrenals	Urine and serum osmolalities; thyroid studies

Hypoxia

Pulmonary disease, carbon monoxide intoxication, anemia	Abnormal blood gases; carboxyhemoglobin

(continued)

TABLE 5-1. (*continued*)

COMA SECONDARY TO METABOLIC AND SYSTEMIC DISEASES

Ischemia	
Decreased cardiac output	Congestive heart failure, myocardial infarction, arrhythmia, cardiopulmonary arrest
Hypertensive encephalopathy	Papilledema; proteinuria; headaches; seizures
Hypoglycemia	Reversed with D_{50} unless prolonged
Thiamine Deficiency	Wernicke's encephalopathy potentially reversible
Electrolyte Imbalance	Water, sodium, acidosis, alkalosis, calcium
Temperature Regulation	
Hypothermia	Exposure; myxedema; barbiturates; circulatory failure
Hyperthermia	Heat stroke; phenothiazines (neuroleptic malignant syndrome)

BUN = blood urea nitrogen; CSF = cerebrospinal fluid; CT = computed tomography.

gencies. An adequate airway should be established. Endotracheal intubation and artificial ventilation may be necessary. The cardiovascular status must be promptly evaluated, and shock and blood pressure should be controlled. The temperature should be noted, since hypo- or hyperthermia may play a prominent role in the identification of the underlying problem.

A history should be taken, but unfortunately this is often incomplete, nonexistent, or misleading. A search for "less likely" causes for the coma is necessary when the treatment procedures for the "obvious" cause from the history obtained do not change the patient's clinical status. Nevertheless, aggressive management of the unconscious patient includes an aggressive pursuit of the history. Friends or family of the patient often do not realize the value of the information that they can offer.

There should be a search for evidence of trauma. Battle's sign (purple and blue discoloration of the mastoid skin area), blood in the external auditory canal, or blood noted behind the tympanic membranes may signify a temporal bone or basal skull fracture. Raccoon eyes (purple discoloration of the eyelid and orbital regions) may signify orbital or basal skull fractures.

One should check carefully for nuchal rigidity, but several factors must be considered in doing so. If there is any suspicion of a cervical neck fracture, there should be no manipulation of the neck. In deep coma, nuchal rigidity may be lacking despite its presence in a lighter level of consciousness. Finally, some patients with a CNS infection or subarachnoid hemorrhage may not manifest nuchal rigidity initially in the course of their illness.

The odor of the patient's breath may indicate the cause for the coma. Alcohol gives its characteristic smell, hepatic coma is often associated with a musty odor, and a fruity or acetone smell is characteristic of ketoacidosis.

After a screening general physical examination, an orderly, systemic neurologic examination is undertaken. The goal of the neurologic examination is essentially to determine the presence, location, and nature of the underlying process creating the decreased level of consciousness and also to give some prognosis of the patient's condition.

Respiratory patterns yield information regarding the activity of different cerebral areas. When one develops bilateral cerebral hemisphere dysfunction (essentially, functioning at the diencephalic level), Cheyne–Stokes respiration may occur. This respiratory pattern is associated with periods of hyperpnea alternating with periods of apnea. There is a regularity to the respirations: first a gradual build-up of respirations to the level of hyperpnea, and then a gradual tapering off of respirations to apnea. The periods of apnea may last up to 30 seconds or more. It is believed that Cheyne–Stokes respiration relates to an abnormal response of carbon dioxide–sensitive respiratory brain centers. There is an increased ventilatory response to carbon dioxide stimulation, creating hyperpnea. After the concentration of carbon dioxide drops below the level at which the centers are stimulated, the apnea phase appears and continues until the carbon dioxide reaccumulates and the cycle repeats itself. Because sleep induces further cerebral depressing mechanisms, Cheyne–Stokes respiration may be seen in some patients during sleep, whereas they exhibit normal breathing patterns while awake.

Cheyne–Stokes respiration is, by itself, not a serious prognostic sign. Although it can be seen in focal primary CNS problems, it can also be seen early in many metabolic and systemic problems.

Central neurogenic hyperventilation appears when lower brain centers are involved; it is noted with dysfunction at the midbrain or the upper pons. There are continuous, regular, and rapid respirations up to 40 or 50 times per minute. Arterial blood gases reveal a respiratory alkalosis with decreased PCO_2 and increased pH. The PO_2 must be greater than 70 or 80 millimeters of mercury (mm Hg). If the PO_2 is not above that level, it raises the possibility of an extracerebral cause (hypoxemia) for the respiratory problem. Cardiac, pulmonary, and metabolic (e.g., diabetes, uremia, hepatic, salicylates) problems must be ruled out as possible causes of the hyperventilation.

Apneustic respiration, noted in lower pontine lesions, consists of a prolonged inspiratory phase with a pause at full inspiration. Cluster breathing, also signifying lower pontine damage, is characterized by a disorderly sequence of closely grouped respirations followed by apnea.

Ataxic respirations signify a lower pontine or medullary respiratory center problem. The breathing pattern is chaotic and haphazard with irregular pauses. It may, and usually does, lead to gasping and eventual cessation of breathing. Ataxic breathing is a forewarner of respiratory arrest, and prompt endotracheal intubation is necessary at the time of its discovery.

An examination of the pupillary responses, eye movements, and fundus must be undertaken. In a patient with a decreased level of consciousness, but who is not yet in coma, visual threat (forceful movements of the hand toward either side of the eyes) may be helpful. Blinking in response to a threat from one side, but not from the other side, suggests a hemianopsia. The abnormality would thus be in the cerebral hemisphere opposite to the side that did not blink. A funduscopic examination may reveal papilledema or retinal hemorrhages.

The pupillary response is recorded. The light reflex is mediated, in succession, through the optic nerve, the optic chiasm, the optic tract, the posterior diencephalon, and the Edinger–Westphal nuclei of the midbrain, and then to the sphincter pupillae by way of the parasympathetic nerve fibers in the oculomotor nerve (cranial nerve III). Thus, it is not surprising that the most significant abnormalities of the pupils are seen with dysfunction at the level of the midbrain or oculomotor nerve.

Diencephalic pupils, the result of bilateral hemispheral dysfunction, are small and reactive. The small size likely reflects sympathetic nerve dysfunction at the level of the takeoff of the sympathetic fibers from the hypothalamus.

Mid-position, unreactive (4 to 7 mm) pupils result from direct midbrain (tectal region) damage. The pupillary size likely reflects an involvement of both the descending sympathetic fibers and the parasympathetic fibers of the oculomotor complex.

A widely dilated, fixed pupil is usually seen as a result of direct oculomotor nerve involvement, with unopposed dilator sympathetic tone. In addition to the pupillary abnormalities, ptosis and extraocular muscle paralysis (especially adduction of the eye) are frequently present. Since the oculomotor nerve is strategically situated at the temporal incisura, temporal lobe herniation will result in a widely dilated, fixed pupil, and possibly total cranial nerve III paralysis.

Pinpoint pupils are seen with pontine damage but may be a transient finding for only the first 24 or 48 hours. The pupils are small and can be seen occasionally to react slightly to light if viewed through a magnifying glass. This is thought to relate to damage of the descending sympathetic tracts. Frequently, however, mid-position and fixed pupils are noted with pontine dysfunction.

Of great importance is the fact that metabolic processes do not alter pupillary response until late in their course, if at all. For example, a deeply comatose patient with no spontaneous or reflex movements and no respirations, but with reactive pupils, must be considered to be in metabolic coma until proved otherwise.

In addition, certain drugs can alter pupillary size and response. Opiates characteristically produce pinpoint pupils (reversed with naloxone). Atropine may result in widely dilated and fixed pupils. Various eyedrops may also alter pupillary size and reaction.

The position and movements of the eyes are observed, and certain procedures are undertaken to evaluate cerebral hemisphere and brainstem integrity. The neural pathways for the control of horizontal conjugate eye movements are outlined in Figure 5-1. Cortical control originates in the frontal gaze centers (Brodmann's area 8). Descending fibers controlling horizontal conjugate gaze cross the midline in the lower midbrain region and descend to the paramedian pontine reticular formation (PPRF) in the pons. The PPRF is thus the major area of confluence of pathways controlling horizontal eye movements. Neurons from the PPRF project to the nearby abducens nerve (cranial nerve VI) nucleus and thereby stimulate movement in the lateral rectus muscle of the eye ipsilateral to the PPRF and contralateral to the frontal

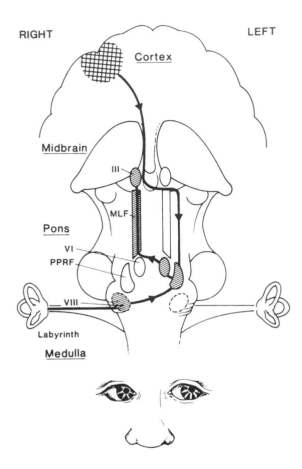

FIG. 5-1. Diagram of the conjugate vision pathways (nuclei and paths are shaded to include those important to left conjugate gaze). Fibers from the right frontal cortex descend and cross the midline, and they synapse in the left paramedian pontine reticular formation (PPRF). Fibers then travel to the nearby left cranial nerve VI nucleus (to move the left eye laterally) and then cross the midline to rise in the right medial longitudinal fasciculus (MLF) to the right cranial nerve III nucleus (to move the right eye medially). In addition to the cortical influence on the left PPRF, there is vestibular influence. With vestibular activation from the right, the left PPRF is stimulated, and the eyes conjugatively move to the left. Instillation of ice water into the right ear canal will test the integrity of this vestibular-PPRF-cranial nerve-VI-cranial nerve-III-circuit, and if the eyes move to vestibular stimulation, the brainstem from medulla to midbrain must be functioning.

gaze center. In addition, impulses from the abducens nerve nucleus cross the midline and ascend the median longitudinal fasciculus to the medial rectus nucleus of the oculomotor nerve (cranial nerve III) in the midbrain. This stimulates adduction of the eye ipsilateral to the frontal gaze center. Horizontal conjugate gaze is thus completed.

By following these pathways, it can be seen that stimulation of fibers from the frontal gaze center of one cerebral hemisphere results in horizontal, conjugate eye movements to the contralateral side. If one frontal gaze center or its descending fibers are damaged, the eyes will tend to "look" toward the involved cerebral hemisphere because of unopposed action of the remaining frontal gaze center. For example, a destructive lesion in the right cerebral hemisphere, involving descending motor fibers and frontal gaze fibers, will cause a left hemiplegia with head and eyes deviated to the right. In other words, the eyes "look" at a destructive hemispheral lesion and "look" away from the resulting hemiplegia.

By contrast, a destructive left pontine lesion, for example, will damage the left PPRF. The eyes, therefore, cannot go to the left and will tend to deviate to the right. Since descending pyramidal tract fibers cross the midline in the medulla, damage to the pyramidal tract fibers in the pons on the left results in a right hemiplegia. Thus, the eyes "look" away from a destructive pontine lesion but "look" toward the hemiplegia.

If the abducens nerve or nucleus is destroyed, there will be a loss of abduction of the ipsilateral eye (cranial nerve VI palsy). With destruction of the tract of the medial longitudinal fasciculus, disconjugate gaze results, with loss of adduction of the ipsilateral eye (same side as the tract of the medial longitudinal fasciculus). Abduction of the contralateral eye is preserved, but there is nystagmus. This type of disconjugate gaze abnormality is also termed *internuclear ophthalmoplegia* (see Chapter 23). The pathways for vertical eye movements are less well understood. Lower centers likely exist in the midbrain (pretectal and tectal) regions.

If a patient cannot follow verbal commands, two useful tests are employed to determine brainstem integrity. An oculocephalic (doll's head) maneuver is performed by turning the patient's head rapidly in the horizontal or vertical planes and by noting the movement or position of the eyes relative to the orbits. This maneuver should obviously not be performed if a cervical neck fracture is suspected. If the pontine (horizontal) or midbrain (vertical) gaze centers are intact, the eyes should move in the orbits in the direction opposite to the rotating head. An abnormal response (no eye movement with doll's head maneuver) implies pontine or midbrain dysfunction and is characterized by no movement of the eyes relative to the orbits, or by an asymmetry of movement.

Horizontal oculocephalic maneuvers are a relatively weak stimulus for horizontal eye movements. If a doll's head maneuver is present, it is not necessary to continue with oculovestibular testing. If, however, a doll's head response is lacking, ice water calorics should be performed, since it is a stronger stimulus than oculocephalic maneuvers.

Oculovestibular responses (ice water calorics) are reflex eye movements in response to irrigation of the external ear canals with cold water. The head is raised to 30° relative to the horizontal plane, and the external canals are inspected for the presence of cerumen or a perforated tympanic membrane. Fifty to 100 ml cold water is instilled into the canal (waiting 5 min between ears), and the resulting eye movements are noted. Ice water produces a downward current in the horizontal semicircular canal and decreases tonic vestibular input to the contralateral PPRF. Simplistically, one can think of this as an indirect means of stimulating the ipsilateral PPRF. Hence, after cold water instillation, there is a slow, tonic, conjugate deviation of the eyes toward the irrigated ear. In a waking patient, there is a correction of the eyes to the opposite side, resulting in a fast nystagmus away from the stimulated ear. In an unconscious patient, there is a loss of the fast-phase nystagmus, and only tonic deviation of the eyes is seen if appropriate pontine–midbrain areas are intact. Thus, if nystagmus is noted in a seemingly unconscious patient, the patient is either in a very light coma or in a hysterical coma.

A lack of oculovestibular responses thus suggests pontine–midbrain dysfunction. Ice water calorics can help to differentiate between the conjugate gaze weakness or paralysis caused by either cortical (cerebral hemisphere) or brainstem (pontine) damage. Oculovestibular responses should not be altered in patients with only hemispheral pathology.

Movement of the ipsilateral eye toward the irrigated ear, but no movement of the contralateral eye, suggests an abnormality of the contralateral medial longitudinal fasciculus (see Chapter 23).

Severe metabolic coma (e.g., after barbiturate overdose) may result in a lack of oculocephalic and oculovestibular responses. Reactive pupils may signify that the coma is of metabolic origin.

Ocular bobbing is characterized by a rapid downward eye movement with a slow return to the horizontal plane. This is seen most often in pontine destruction and is thought to relate to the loss of horizontal eye movements with preservation of midbrain-mediated vertical eye movement pathways.

Roving eye movements signify intact brainstem mechanisms for horizontal gaze. The movements should be distinguished from those seen in patients with seizures. In the latter, the eye movements are of a jerking quality and frequently tend to lateralize to one side. Referring to Figure 5-1, it can be seen that an irritative cortical focus in the area of the frontal gaze center will deviate the eyes away from the side of the lesion (and possibly toward a hemiplegia). Oculovestibular responses will usually be able to overcome the eye deviations because of the strong direct input into the pons, "bypassing" the cortical effects on eye movements.

Motor movements may be spontaneous, induced, reflex, or totally absent. It is important to note not only the type of response but also the symmetry of response. An asymmetrical induced motor movement may be the only indication of an underlying focal problem.

It may be necessary to observe the patient for several minutes to note the presence or lack of spontaneous or reflex motor movements. The position of the extremities (e.g., a persistent externally rotated leg secondary to weakness of that extremity) may indicate focal pathology.

The most favorable prognostic sign related to the motor system is symmetrical, spontaneous movements of all four extremities. Appropriate motor response to noxious stimuli (e.g., pain) signifies that sensory pathways are functional and there is at least partial integrity of corticospinal tracts. It is not necessary to use unusually noxious stimuli, but rather mild supraorbital pressure, pinching of the skin of the neck, or mild sternal pressure.

Reflex motor movements can frequently be elicited by light, painful stimuli; flexion of the neck; or during routine care of the patient, such as tracheal suctioning. Decorticate posturing consists of flexion of the arms, wrists, and fingers, and adduction of the upper extremities. In the legs, there is extension, internal rotation, and plantar flexion. Decerebrate (extensor) posturing consists of extension of the arms as well as adduction and hyperpronation of the arms. There may be opisthotonic posturing of the neck. The movement of the lower extremities is similar to that seen in decorticate posturing. Although not completely anatomically specific, bilateral decerebrate posturing is often seen in lesions of the midbrain and pons, while decorticate posturing often implies a higher corticospinal tract lesion. Decerebrate posturing, often seen secondary to structural processes involving or compressing the high brainstem, is generally a poorer prognostic sign than decorticate posturing. However, decerebrate posturing can also occasionally be seen in the setting of severe, although potentially reversible, metabolic encephalopathies.

A common mistake regarding the interpretation of motor responses is that of relating a withdrawal response in the legs as representing an appropriate cortical response. When the bottom of the foot is stroked, or a noxious stimuli is applied to the leg, there may be hip flexion, knee flexion, and dorsiflexion of the foot (triple flexor response). This signifies spinal cord reflex integrity and does not signify an intact cerebral response.

Asymmetrical extensor toe signs (i.e., flexion on one side, extensor response on the other) are of moderate value in localizing a focal cerebral lesion. Bilateral extensor toe signs can be seen in any form or at any level of coma and are, by themselves, neither prognostic nor localizing. For example, transient extensor toe signs are common in hypertensive encephalopathy.

LABORATORY EVALUATION AND TREATMENT

Following the establishment of an airway, assisting of respirations, and maintenance of circulation, certain laboratory tests and therapeutic measures are undertaken, often occurring simultaneously with obtaining a history and performing a neurologic examination.

Blood is drawn for a complete blood count (CBC), electrolyte, glucose, calcium, and blood urea nitrogen (BUN) determinations, liver function tests, arterial blood gas determinations, and a drug/toxin screen. Urinalysis and urine drug screening are performed. An electrocardiogram and chest roentgenograms are obtained. If hypoglycemia is suspected, or if the cause of the coma is uncertain, 25 to 50 ml of 50% dextrose in water is given intravenously (IV). Hypoglycemia is

an extremely important, potentially reversible cause of coma that, if not treated promptly, will lead to irreversible cerebral damage. For suspected opiate overdose, naloxone 0.4 mg IV is given and is repeated every 5 to 15 minutes as needed. Repeated infusions should be instituted if the response to glucose or naloxone is incomplete. Other medications can be given for specific drug overdoses when appropriate, such as intravenous flumazenil for benzodiazepine overdose. If chronic or acute ingestion of alcohol is suspected, thiamine should be given IV to treat or prevent the Wernicke–Korsakoff syndrome. Correction of any other underlying metabolic process (e.g., hyponatremia) must be undertaken. If there is significant evidence for increased intracranial pressure, intubation with hyperventilation, and the use of mannitol must be considered. Corticosteroids may be beneficial to reduce vasogenic edema related to neoplasms, but their effect is not immediate.

Seizure activity may be generalized or focal and necessitates prompt treatment and a search for a cause. Myoclonic jerks (symmetric or asymmetric rapid, brief movements of the extremities) are frequently seen in metabolic encephalopathies and are common following anoxia (e.g., after cardiac arrest). Unfortunately, myoclonic jerks in the setting of severe anoxic coma are often difficult to treat, and their appearance following anoxia is a poor prognostic sign.

It may be necessary to proceed with further neurologic studies if the cause of the coma remains unclear. Computed tomography (CT scan) will demonstrate intracerebral or extracerebral blood, mass lesions, infarctions, and abscesses, as well as skull fractures. Magnetic resonance imaging (MR scan) is less useful in the evaluation of the comatose patient. Patients will need to be left unattended for a longer scanning time. Unconscious patients are often on ventilators, which usually cannot be placed near the MR scanner. If a CNS infection or subarachnoid hemorrhage is suspected, a lumbar puncture is indicated, although a CT scan will identify most subarachnoid hemorrhages sufficient to cause coma. A CT scan should usually be obtained prior to the lumbar puncture to rule out a focal mass lesion or increased intracranial pressure.

The electroencephalogram (EEG) may be helpful in the diagnosis of an overdose from sedatives (excessive fast activity), hepatic or uremic encephalopathy (triphasic waves), hysteria (normal EEG), or in differentiating focal from diffuse disease. It can be used to rule out subclinical seizure activity as a cause for prolonged, unexplained coma. An EEG with no evidence of cerebral activity can be reversibly noted secondary to barbiturate intoxication (and occasionally other drugs) and also with hypothermia.

PROGNOSIS

Several studies that have dealt with postanoxic coma have revealed that the prognosis is generally better for the patient with spontaneous motor movements or appropriate movements in response to noxious stimuli, and those with pupillary reactions and oculocephalic or oculovestibular responses. Patients studied after cardiopulmonary arrest reveal that depth and duration of postarrest coma correlated significantly with poor neurologic outcome. Motor unresponsiveness, lack of pupillary responses, and lack of oculocephalic and oculovestibular responses were associated with a poor prognosis for neurologic functional recovery. In addition, the prediction of survival and outcome could be based on a loss of consciousness alone within 3 days after cardiopulmonary arrest. Those patients not awakening within 72 hours had the worst prognosis.

Prognosis for patients with metabolic encephalopathies or drug overdose cannot be based on the level of consciousness. For example, patients with barbiturate overdose in deep coma may have no spontaneous respiration, absent oculovestibular responses, and absent cerebral activity on the EEG, yet have a complete neurologic recovery.

QUESTIONS AND DISCUSSION

1. A 24-year-old man is brought to the emergency room with a decreased level of consciousness. Upon arrival, he suffers a respiratory arrest and is intubated. An examination reveals small, reactive pupils (2 mm), a lack of oculocephalic and oculovestibular responses, and no response to painful stimuli. Which of the following is correct?

A. The most likely diagnosis is a pontine hemorrhage.
B. A CT scan should be obtained immediately.
C. The pupils should be pharmacologically dilated to obtain a good funduscopic examination.
D. Neurosurgical consultation should be sought immediately to evacuate a subdural hematoma.
E. Drug screen and other blood tests should be obtained immediately, and glucose and naloxone should be given IV.

The answer is (E). Metabolic encephalopathies can result in a lack of oculocephalic and oculovestibular responses, with preserved pupillary responses.

2. Cheyne–Stokes respiration:

A. Is associated with irreversible brain disease
B. Is pathognomonic of midbrain dysfunction
C. Is characterized by sustained inspirations
D. May occur in noncomatose patients while they are asleep
E. Is associated with decerebrate posturing

The answer is (D). Cheyne–Stokes respirations are related to bilateral hemispheral dysfunction. During sleep, increased inhibitory influences may create this pattern of respiration.

3. A right hemispheral destructive lesion may produce:

A. Lack of caloric responses, eyes conjugately deviated to the left, and left hemiplegia
B. Right eye deviated to the right, left eye midline, and left hemiplegia
C. Eyes conjugately deviated to the right, left hemiplegia, and present caloric responses
D. Ocular bobbing and left hemiplegia
E. Present caloric responses, eyes conjugately deviated to the left, and left hemiplegia

The answer is (C). Eyes "look toward" a destructive hemispheral lesion. Caloric responses are preserved because the pathway for the oculovestibular responses does not involve hemispheral connections.

4. Lack of caloric (oculovestibular) responses bilaterally:

A. Signifies marked suppression of both cerebral hemispheres
B. Is pathognomonic of pontine hemorrhage
C. Is frequently associated with Cheyne–Stokes respiration
D. Can be seen in metabolic encephalopathy
E. Is always reversible

The answer is (D). Oculovestibular responses are mediated by brainstem (i.e., pontine) pathways. The responses are reversible if a metabolic encephalopathy is corrected in appropriate time.

5. Decerebrate posturing:

A. May be associated with central neurogenic hyperventilation

B. Is seen in patients with bilateral frontal lobe dysfunction
C. Consists of flexion of the arms and wrists
D. Signifies integrity of spinal cord and occipital lobe synapses
E. Is a good prognostic sign

The answer is (A). Decerebrate posturing, which partially consists of extension and hyperpronation of the upper extremities, is often associated with midbrain dysfunction (as is central neurogenic hyperventilation).

SUGGESTED READING

Bates D: Predicting recovery from medical coma. Br J Hosp Med 33:276, 1985

Buettner WW, Zee DS: Vestibular testing in comatose patients. Arch Neurol 46:561, 1989

Fisher CM: The neurological examination of the comatose patient. Acta Neurol Scand 45(suppl 36): 1, 1969

Hamel MB, Goldman L, Teno J, et al: Identification of comatose patients at high risk for death or severe disability. JAMA 273:1842, 1995

Hoffman RS, Goldfrank LR: The poisoned patient with altered consciousness: controversies in the use of a "coma cocktail." JAMA 274:562, 1995

Levy DE, Caronna JJ, Singer BH, et al: Predicting outcome from hypoxic-ischemic coma. JAMA 253:1420, 1985

Lewis SL, Topel JL: Coma. In: Weiner WJ and Shulman LM (eds): Emergent and Urgent Neurology, Second Edition. Philadelphia, Lippincott Williams & Wilkins, 1999.

Plum F, Posner JB: The Diagnosis of Stupor and Coma, 3rd ed. Philadelphia, FA Davis, 1980

Wijdicks EFM, Parisi JE, Sharbrough FW: Prognostic value of myoclonus status in comatose survivors of cardiac arrest. Ann Neurol 35:239, 1994

Young GB, Ropper AH, Bolton CF: Coma and Impaired Consciousness. New York, McGraw-Hill, 1997

Neurology for the Non-Neurologist, Fourth Edition, edited by William J. Weiner and Christopher G. Goetz. Lippincott Williams & Wilkins, Philadelphia © 1999.

C H A P T E R 6

Cerebrovascular Disease

Roger E. Kelley

Stroke is defined as an insult to the central nervous system on a primary vascular basis. This definition includes vascular insults of the cerebral hemispheres, the subcortical structures, the brainstem, the cerebellum, and the spinal cord. The terminology is increasingly important because of newer management strategies that are available. For instance, the term *brain attack* has been proposed to alert medical personnel that stroke is now recognized as a treatable illness that requires the same rigorous approach as heart attack. As for a heart attack, the sooner a patient is evaluated for symptoms of stroke, the more likely it is that more therapeutic options will be available.

Stroke is classified into two major categories: primary ischemic and primary hemorrhagic. Primary ischemic stroke accounts for approximately 80% of cases and includes cerebral embolism (approximately 30%), large artery thrombosis (approximately 30%), and small artery thrombosis, often referred to as lacunar-type stroke (approximately 20%). The second major category, primary hemorrhagic stroke, accounts for approximately 20% of cases and includes intracerebral hemorrhage (approximately 14%) and subarachnoid hemorrhage (approximately 6%). Spontaneous subarachnoid hemorrhage (SAH) is usually associated with either rupture of a berry aneurysm or bleeding from an arteriovenous malformation (AVM).

It is important to take a mechanistic approach toward acute stroke, as the mechanism of the insult directly impacts on management. This approach is outlined in Table 6-1. The terms *embolic* and *thrombotic* may well be an oversimplification of the true pathogenesis. For example, vascular dissection is a pathologic process in which there is a tear within the vessel intima that can result in acute thrombosis. The tear in the vessel is most commonly associated with trauma, although the degree of trauma can be quite trivial. The tear can occur with no apparent inciting factor, termed spontaneous cerebrovascular dissection. There can also be an underlying pathologic process associated with a predisposition toward vascular dissection, such as fibromuscular dysplasia. When vessel dissection is associated with thrombus formation, there can be vessel occlusion directly related to the clot, or there can be propagation of the thrombus with the potential for thromboembolism, with a piece of the clot migrating to the more distal intracranial circulation. This latter phenomenon can result in an infarction in the vascular distribution of the particular vessel involved—for example, a middle cerebral artery infarction. Thus, what initially appeared to be a simple process can actually be much more complicated from the standpoint of stroke pathogenesis. The same can be said for sinovenous thrombotic disease. This is a process usually associated with infection in children and with either pregnancy, hormonal manipulation, or a hypercoagulable state in adults. It was not listed as one of the more common explanations for stroke, but its timely recognition is certainly important from a management standpoint.

Transient ischemic attack (TIA) and minor stroke are now often used synonymously, and there are

TABLE 6-1. Major Mechanisms of Stroke

1. Large artery thrombosis
2. Small artery thrombosis (lacunar-type)
3. Embolic
   a. Artery-to-artery
   b. Cardiogenic
4. Vascular dissection
5. Hemodynamic
6. Mechanical obstruction
7. Sinovenous occlusion
8. Arteritis
9. Vascular anomaly
10. Hypertensive bleed
11. Bleeding diathesis
12. Amyloid angiopathy

practical reasons for this lack of delineation. It has been recognized for years that some patients do not completely recover within 24 hours from an ischemic insult (a TIA). On the other hand, patients with minor stroke often recover within several weeks, which has led to the term *reversible ischemic neurologic deficit* (RIND). Generally speaking, based on the results of recent clinical trials of thrombolytic and neuroprotective agents in acute ischemic stroke, the vast majority of patients with minor stroke demonstrate essentially complete recovery within 3 months with or without treatment. This is the reason that recombinant tissue plasminogen activator (rt-PA) is not recommended as acute stroke therapy unless the patient presents with a certain degree of neurologic deficit. This led to the use of the National Institutes of Health (NIH) stroke scale as an objective indicator of the degree of deficit at the time of presentation.

EPIDEMIOLOGY

Stroke afflicts approximately 500,000 people per year in the United States. It remains the third leading cause of death and the number one cause of chronic neurologic disability in adults. It is more common in men than in women, and in blacks than in whites. The incidence of stroke more than doubles for each decade beyond age 55. It is increasingly important to recognize stroke-prone individuals—patients who have a predisposition toward stroke based on genetic factors as well as on the presence of factors that promote atherosclerosis and other types of vessel wall

damage. It is important to recognize that patients with stroke often have coexistent coronary artery disease and that structural cardiac disease and certain cardiac arrhythmias can predispose to cardioembolic stroke. It is estimated, for example, that nonvalvular atrial fibrillation (NVAF) accounts for up to 75,000 strokes per year in the United States.

Factors that promote carotid atherosclerosis include hypertension, diabetes mellitus, and cigarette smoking. It has been generally assumed that elevated serum cholesterol played a smaller role in cerebral atherosclerosis than in coronary artery disease. However, recent studies have found that aggressive control of serum cholesterol level with "statin" drugs has a beneficial effect in reducing the risk of stroke. Hypertension is a major risk factor for stroke, with up to a fivefold enhanced risk of stroke, but only if the hypertension is not effectively treated. The risk can be brought down by at least 42% with effective long-term blood pressure control. Hypertension is a major contributor to both ischemic and primary hemorrhagic stroke. Hypertension is the most common cause of intracerebral hemorrhage (ICH). Chronic hypertension promotes not only large artery atherosclerosis but also small vessel (penetrating artery) wall damage, which is termed lipohyalinosis and which is believed to be one of the most common mechanisms for lacunar-type stroke.

Transient ischemic attack and minor stroke identify individuals who are at particular risk for a subsequent major cerebral infarction. It is estimated that one in three patients with TIA will have a major stroke within 5 years. The risk is particularly high for those patients who have been diagnosed with high-grade (i.e., 70% to 99%) carotid stenosis (Fig. 6-1). In addition, patients with recurrent stereotypic TIAs (i.e., a so-called crescendo pattern) appear to be at enhanced risk of completed infarction. Stroke itself is perhaps the greatest risk factor for further stroke. It is estimated that the recurrence rate for stroke is up to 12% per year. In one study, the 5-year recurrence rate for stroke was 42% for men and 24% for women.

The major and minor risk factors for stroke are outlined in Table 6-2. It is important to recognize that identification of stroke risk factors is an evolving process. For example, oral contraceptives have traditionally been cited as an important risk factor for ischemic stroke in women. The newer low-estrogen birth control pills are considerably safer, especially if the "pill" is avoided in women who are older, who smoke, or who have additional risk factors for vascular occlusive disease that amplify their risk.

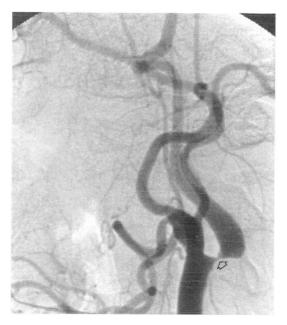

FIG. 6-1. High-grade internal carotid artery stenosis that occurs just at the origin of the vessel (*arrow*).

TABLE 6-2. Risk Factors for Stroke

Major risk factors
  Age
  Sex
  Race
  Genetic predisposition
  Diabetes mellitus
  Asymptomatic bruit
  Peripheral vascular disease
  Cigarette smoking
  Hypertension
  Polycythemia
  Sickle cell disease
  Transient ischemic attack and prior stroke
  Valvular heart disease
  Atrial fibrillation
  Cardiomyopathy
  Hypercoagulable state
Minor risk factors
  Hypercholesterolemia
  Oral contraceptives
  Migraine
  Obesity
  Physical inactivity
  Mitral valve prolapse
  Patent foramen ovale
  Bacterial endocarditis
  Marantic endocarditis
  Aortic arch atheromata

This concept of cumulative risk is very important when seeking to identify stroke-prone patients. NVAF, for example, is not a significant risk factor for ischemic stroke in patients who are less than 60 years old and have no coexistent risk factors. However, with advancing age, and in the presence of structural cardiac disease (e.g., significantly impaired left ventricular function), hypertension, or prior embolus, the risk of cardioembolic stroke in association with NVAF rises substantially. Overall, there is approximately a 3% to 5% annual risk of embolic stroke with NVAF, and the risk of recurrent stroke has been reported to be approximately 20% within 11 days of the initial event without treatment. The coexistence of valvular heart disease and atrial fibrillation is associated with a 17-fold increased risk of stroke with a recurrence rate, over time, of at least 50% without anticoagulant therapy. Similarly, acute myocardial infarct is associated with a 1% to 2% risk of embolic stroke. However, the risk is directly related to whether or not the myocardial damage represents a large anterior wall transmural infarction associated with wall motion abnormality, especially in the presence of associated thrombus formation and/or a ventricular aneurysm.

A number of uncommon causes of ischemic stroke tend not to show up in large epidemiologic surveys of stroke because of their relative infrequency. In studies of stroke in the young, however, there are instances of stroke related to mitral valve prolapse, paradoxical cerebral embolism secondary to patent foramen ovale, migrainous infarction, and stroke related to a hypercoagulable state [e.g., the presence of antiphospholipid antibodies (anticardiolipin antibodies and lupus anticoagulant), protein C deficiency, protein S deficiency, and antithrombin III deficiency]. Furthermore, there is a growing literature related to stroke secondary to atheroma of the aorta. Stroke should also be kept in mind in the presence of meningovascular syphilis in susceptible individuals, cerebrovascular dissection, endocarditis, atrial myxoma, and cerebral arteritis (which can occur in association with systemic lupus erythematosis and polyarteritis nodosa). Finally, stroke may be a complication of ingestion of illicit drugs such as sympathomimetic amines.

In addition, sympathomimetic amines can be responsible for ICH, as they can result in a sudden precipitous rise in blood pressure. ICH can also be seen in association with vascular malformations, berry aneurysms, bleeding diatheses, neoplastic disorders, anticoagulant therapy, amyloid angiopathy, and certain infectious processes such as septic embolism.

DIAGNOSTIC EVALUATION

The assessment of a patient who presents with symptoms of stroke is outlined in Table 6-3. It is important to distinguish routine assessment from more specialized testing, which is performed only if clinically warranted. The computed tomography (CT) brain scan allows ready distinction between primary hemorrhagic and primary ischemic stroke. This is extremely important from a management standpoint, and CT scanning remains superior to magnetic resonance imaging (MRI) in this respect. The use of rt-PA is predicated on the results of a noncontrast CT brain scan, on which there should be no evidence of blood. Furthermore, the use of this agent may do more harm than good, especially if there is an early infarction pattern, such as sulcal effacement or the presence of low density in the appropriate vascular territory, as this is associated with an increased risk of hemorrhagic transformation of the infarction (Fig. 6-2).

A contrast-enhanced CT brain scan is not indicated in acute stroke unless there might reasonably be an

TABLE 6-3. Diagnostic Evaluation of the Patient with Acute Stroke

Routine studies
  Noncontrast CT brain scan
  CBC, platelet count, PT, INR, PTT
  Serum chemistry profile
  Electrocardiogram
  Carotid/vertebral duplex scan
  Echocardiogram
  Heart monitor
Specialized studies
  Transcranial Doppler ultrasound
  Transesophageal echocardiography
  Contrast-enhanced brain scan (MRI, CT)
  Magnetic resonance angiography
  Cerebral arteriography
  Stress electrocardiogram
  Blood cultures
  Lumbar puncture
  Electroencephalogram
  Syphilis serology, ESR
  Sickle cell prep
  Platelet function studies
  Special clotting factor studies
  Antiphospholipid antibody titers
  Protein C and S levels
  Antithrombin III level

CT = computed tomography; CBC = complete blood count; PT = prothrombin time; INR = international normalization ratio; PTT = partial thromboplastin time; MRI = magnetic resonance imaging; ESR = erythrocyte sedimentation rate.

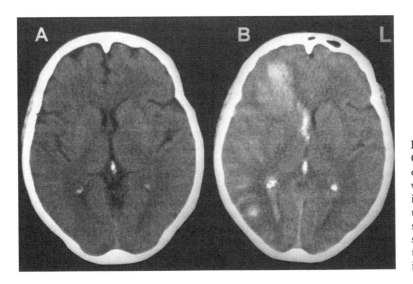

FIG. 6-2. A. Initial noncontrast CT brain scan in a patient who developed symptoms of stroke within hours of the scan. This initial scan is normal. **B.** Follow-up noncontrast CT brain scan, several days later, which demonstrates hemorrhagic transformation of the right hemispheric infarct.

alternative explanation for the clinical presentation, such as a neoplasm or an infectious process. Contrast enhancement can also be useful in the detection of vascular anomalies such as arteriovenous malformations (AVMs). If a contrast-enhanced study is necessary, it is advisable to have it performed with MRI, which uses agents that are potentially less toxic than the iodine-based contrast agents of CT. Potential complications of CT contrast agents include severe allergic reactions, including anaphylaxis, and nephrotoxicity.

Magnetic resonance imaging is more sensitive than CT brain scan for demonstrating the infarct, especially in the posterior fossa (Fig. 6-3). However, it is not necessary to demonstrate an infarct to diagnose an ischemic stroke; in most cases, it is not clinically justified, and it is certainly not cost effective. In addition, the specificity of MRI can be called into question. A number of patients have nonspecific areas of increased signal intensity on the T2-weighted and proton-density images. Those areas of abnormal signal intensity that do not have a clinical correlate (i.e., that are not associated with signs or symptoms of stroke) are of questionable clinical significance. They may be referred to as infarcts, ischemic demyelination, or white matter disease, and the clinician is often left wondering what this all means. On the other hand, a distinct area of hypodensity on the CT brain scan is generally much more specific for the presence of a stroke (Fig. 6-4), although it is quite possible to see "silent infarction" on the CT brain scan.

A complete blood count allows evaluation for polycythemia, which can be associated with increased blood viscosity, decreased cerebral blood flow, and a predisposition to ischemic stroke. On the other hand, a significant anemia raises concerns about the advis-

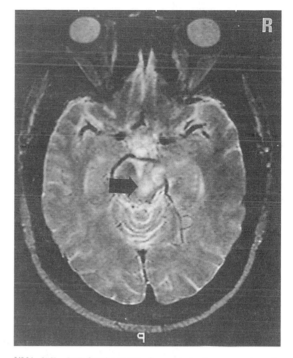

FIG. 6-3. MR brain scan demonstrates an extensive infarction of the right midbrain (*arrow*).

ability of any sort of therapy that can affect the coagulation parameters. An elevated white blood cell count raises suspicion about possible infective endocarditis or a lymphoproliferative disturbance, whereas a low white blood cell count may be indicative of

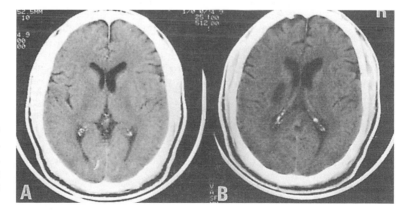

FIG. 6-4. A. Initially normal CT brain scan in a patient presenting with right hemiparesis. **B.** Follow-up CT brain scan, 3 days later, demonstrating a discrete left subcortical infarct.

immunodeficiency. It is important to have a baseline prothrombin time (PT), partial thromboplastin time (PTT), and platelet count to screen for a bleeding disturbance and to monitor the bleeding parameters in case anticoagulant therapy is initiated. The international normalization ratio (INR) is now the more reliable means of monitoring the level of anticoagulant therapy with warfarin. An elevated erythrocyte sedimentation rate (ESR) can be useful in screening for metastatic disease, atrial myxoma, endocarditis, or a connective tissue disorder. Syphilis serology may be indicated. The possibility of sickle cell disease necessitates a sickle cell preparation and possibly hemoglobin electrophoresis. A serum chemistry profile is also useful to determine whether there is a clinically significant alteration of blood glucose, serum sodium, serum calcium, renal function, or liver enzymes, which might impact on the clinical presentation or on management.

The routine performance of an electrocardiogram (EKG) in stroke patients underscores the importance of the heart in patients with symptoms of stroke. The heart is not only the most common source of cerebral embolus, but, in addition, patients with TIA are more likely to die of cardiac disease than stroke. If there is any evidence of cardiac disease by history, physical exam, or EKG, or if the patient is 45 years of age or younger, then further cardiac evaluation is in order *if* it might affect management. It is not justified to perform such a diagnostic assessment in a moribund stroke victim who has no chance of meaningful recovery.

Further cardiac evaluation should include two-dimensional echocardiography and, in selected cases, cardiac monitoring. Transesophageal echocardiography can be particularly useful for the assessment of a possible patent foramen with right-to-left shunt, when contrast is used. It can also be more sensitive for the detection of stasis of blood within the chambers of the heart, as well as for the evaluation of valvular heart disease, and to assess for the presence of atheromata of the aortic arch. Approximately one third of patients with ischemic stroke and TIA have significant coronary artery disease. This finding has led to the recommendation that such patients be routinely evaluated with a stress EKG.

Cerebral arteriography remains the gold standard for the accurate identification of extracranial or intracranial vascular stenosis, vascular dissection, cerebral arteritis, and sinovenous thrombosis, and for the determination of the nature and extent of vascular anomalies such as berry aneurysms and AVMs. Because cerebral arteriography is an invasive procedure with a significant risk of major complications, alternative vascular imaging techniques have been developed.

Ultrasound imaging of the cerebral circulation is now a standard procedure available at most medical centers. The most common imaging unit consists of B-mode (anatomic) imaging of the vessel wall characteristics, coupled with Doppler (physiologic) imaging of the flow characteristics of the moving column of blood. Such a combined unit is termed duplex imaging. Many units now have the ability to demonstrate the flow pattern in a color-coded fashion, termed color flow imaging. This represents superimposition of the color-coded Doppler flow velocity characteristics on the B-mode (gray-scale) image of the vessel wall. Although measurement of the peak systolic flow velocity remains the most reliable means of assessing vessel stenosis, the color flow images allow ready detection of hemodynamically significant flow-limiting stenotic lesions.

Noninvasive imaging provides an accurate assessment of the carotid bifurcation and the proximal vertebral arteries in most patients. In certain subjects, there are anatomic limitations that interfere with an adequate assessment. It is important to point out that the quality of noninvasive imaging can vary considerably between ultrasound laboratories.

Transcranial Doppler ultrasonography (TCD) allows noninvasive assessment of the intracranial circulation. There is an inverse relationship between the insonated vessel's diameter and the flow velocity. Detection of an elevated intracranial artery flow velocity can be of use in the evaluation of intracranial stenosis (e.g., middle cerebral artery stenosis), as well as in the detection of vasospasm, which can be seen as a complication of aneurysmal rupture. TCD can also be of use in determining which patients with sickle cell disease are at greatest risk for stroke, and it is of value in monitoring the resolution of cerebrovascular dissection in a noninvasive fashion.

Magnetic resonance angiography (MRA) is a noninvasive MR technique that can provide a fairly reliable assessment of the extracranial and intracranial circulation. This technique can be quite useful for screening purposes, but it has not evolved to the point where it can replace routine angiography. It tends to provide an overestimation of internal carotid artery stenosis at the origin of the internal carotid artery, and it remains susceptible to artifact. It allows detection of intracranial aneurysms greater than 3 to 4 mm in size, and it allows noninvasive monitoring of the response of AVMs to treatment as well as follow-up monitoring of cerebrovascular dissection. The latter can be enhanced when the MRA is performed in conjunction with TCD.

Lumbar puncture (LP) is not routinely indicated for stroke, but it can be of great value in certain conditions. The major contraindications to LP are the presence of mass effect by brain scan and the presence of any type of bleeding disorder that could promote an epidural hematoma. It is important to remember that an LP should not be performed in patients on anticoagulant therapy, especially if there is a therapeutic level of anticoagulation. There are several clear-cut indications for lumbar puncture, if it can be performed safely, including positive syphilis serology, an unexplained fever, evidence of meningeal irritation, or the presence of atypical features such as relatively young age with no obvious explanation of the stroke-like symptoms. A high-resolution CT brain scan generally allows adequate evaluation of a possible hemorrhagic lesion that would contraindicate anticoagulants or thrombolytic therapy. On the other hand, the sensitivity of CT scan in evaluating possible SAH is only 89% according to one study. Thus, the LP becomes mandatory if there is clinical suspicion of SAH despite a negative CT scan. Figure 6-5 demonstrates the only abnormality on a CT brain scan in a 54-year-old man who presented to the emergency room with the worst headache of his life. Cerebral arteriography demonstrated an anterior communicating artery aneurysm (Fig. 6-6).

Electroencephalography (EEG) is not routinely indicated in stroke. However, it can be useful to distinguish focal seizure activity from fluctuating symptoms of stroke or TIA. The absence of an abnormality on EEG in a patient with motor or sensory deficit secondary to stroke, and in the absence of

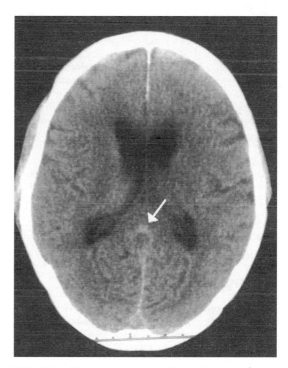

FIG. 6-5. This noncontrast CT brain scan demonstrates the subtle presence of blood within a subarachnoid cistern (*arrow*).

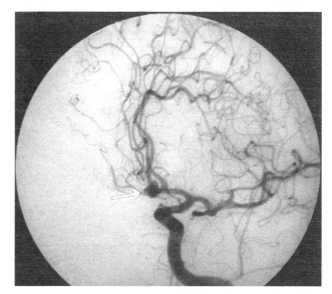

FIG. 6-6. A cerebral arteriogram performed in the patient whose CT scan was shown in Figure 6-5. This study reveals an anterior communicating artery aneurysm (*arrow*).

cortical impairment, supports a subcortical location for the stroke; this is most commonly seen in lacunar-type stroke.

Other studies that are useful, in selected instances, include fasting serum lipid profile, blood cultures if there is a fever or other reason to suspect bacterial endocarditis, platelet function studies, and a connective tissue screen if vasculitis is suspected. In addition, a lupus anticoagulant assay, anticardiolipin antibody titers, protein C level, protein S level, and antithrombin III level should be obtained if a prothrombotic state is being considered. In some instances, in addition to performing routine clotting studies, coagulation factor levels and bleeding time should be measured.

ISCHEMIC STROKE AND TRANSIENT ISCHEMIC ATTACK

PRESENTATION AND LOCALIZATION

Clinically, it does not usually take a great deal of acumen to diagnose a stroke. The differential diagnosis of stroke can include episodic TIA-like symptoms, which can be mimicked by focal seizures, radiculopathy, complicated migraine, and carpal tunnel syndrome. A mass lesion within the brain can produce TIA-like symptoms, including neoplasm, abscess, and subdural hematoma. Visual loss and headache in an elderly person should always raise suspicion for temporal arteritis. In certain patients with multiple sclerosis and motor neuron disease, the onset may be precipitous enough to raise the possibility of stroke.

Hemispheric cerebrovascular events can be associated with headache, alteration of consciousness, speech disturbance (including aphasia and dysarthria), homonymous hemifield visual deficits, cognitive impairment (which might include apraxia or agnosia), and contralateral motor and sensory dysfunction. Symptoms or signs referable to the brainstem or cerebellum include dysarthria, dysphagia, ataxia, diplopia, vertigo, nausea, various forms of nystagmus, and drop attacks, especially when seen in combination. Isolated symptoms such as vertigo or diplopia are usually not related to stroke, but a combination of manifestations is a more likely scenario for posterior circulation events. "Crossed" impairments in sensory and motor function, such as numbness on one side of the face and the other side of the body, are highly suspect for brainstem ischemia.

Certain clinical features are useful for cerebral localization. Infarcts involving the middle cerebral artery distribution typically result in aphasia, if the dominant hemisphere is affected, as well as contralateral motor weakness in which the lower two thirds of the face and arm are significantly weaker than the leg. Infarcts involving the anterior cerebral artery distribution typically cause significantly greater weakness in the contralateral leg than in the arm or face. An isolated homonymous hemianopia is usually localized to the contralateral posterior cerebral artery. Bilateral visual loss suggests ischemia involving the vertebrobasilar system, since the posterior cerebral arteries, which supply the occipital (visual) cortex, usually receive their primary blood supply from the basilar artery.

A paresis that affects equally the face, arm, and leg, with no evidence of sensory loss or cortical dysfunction, is characteristic of lacunar-type stroke. Traditionally, lacunar-type stroke implies *in situ* occlusive disease of a small penetrating artery, with special predilection for the arterial supply of the posterior limb of the internal capsule, resulting in "pure motor stroke" (Fig. 6-7). The most common lacunar syn-

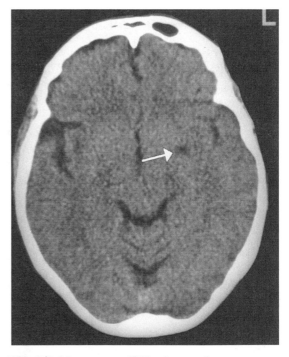

FIG. 6-7. Noncontrast CT brain scan demonstrates a left subcortical (lacunar-type) infarct (*arrow*).

TABLE 6-4. Most Common Lacunar-Type Stroke Syndromes and Associated Area of Involvement

LACUNAR SYNDROME	ANATOMIC LOCALIZATION
Pure motor	Posterior limb of the contralateral internal capsule or basis pontis
Pure sensory	Thalamus or parietal white matter
Sensorimotor	Posterior limb of the contralateral internal capsule
Clumsy hand—dysarthria	Basis pontis
Hemiparesis, hemiataxia	Midbrain or internal capsule

dromes and their most likely anatomic correlates are outlined in Table 6-4.

It is important to distinguish TIAs of carotid distribution from those of vertebrobasilar distribution. The manifestations of both are summarized in Table 6-5. The common carotid artery (CCA) bifurcates in the neck and gives rise to the external carotid artery (ECA) and the internal carotid artery (ICA). The ICA gives rise to the anterior and middle cerebral artery of the respective hemispheres. The ECA is a potential source of collateral blood supply when the ICA circulation is impaired. The two vertebral arteries give rise to the basilar artery at the mid-pons level.

The basilar artery proceeds rostrally to give rise to both posterior cerebral arteries, which join the circle of Willis via the posterior communicating arteries. The vertebrobasilar system supplies the brainstem, cerebellum, and occipital lobes, while the remainder of the cerebral hemispheres are supplied by the carotid circulation. The circle of Willis, which connects the anterior and posterior circulations, allows collateral reserve in instances where a particular system of vascular supply is impaired. Note that the circle of Willis is also the most common site of cerebral artery aneurysm formation.

PATHOGENESIS AND TREATMENT

In the initial evaluation of ischemic stroke or TIA, it is most important to assess the mechanism as quickly and accurately as possible. Major immediate questions include whether the patient is a candidate for thrombolytic therapy, whether there is symptomatic, high-grade (i.e., 70% or greater) ICA stenosis, whether there is a likely cardiogenic source of embolus, and whether the stroke is lacunar in nature. In addition, it is important to know whether cerebrovascular dissection, sinovenous thrombosis, or cerebral arteritis is the mechanism of the ischemia.

Recombinant tissue plasminogen activator is now available for acute ischemic stroke patients who can be evaluated clinically and by CT brain scan, and treated, within 3 hours of presentation. This 3-hour window is a very rigid rule, mandating that if the patient woke up with the deficit, it must be assumed that the stroke occurred when he last went to sleep. In addition, patients should not be treated if they present with severe neurologic deficits, an early large infarction

TABLE 6-5. Manifestations of Transient Ischemic Attack

CAROTID DISTRIBUTION	VERTEBROBASILAR DISTRIBUTION
Aphasia	Bilateral visual loss
Transient monocular blindness (amaurosis fugax)	Ataxia
	Quadriparesis
Hemiparesis	Perioral numbness
Hemisensory deficit	"Crossed" sensory or motor deficits
Homonymous hemianopsia in combination with motor or sensory deficit	Combination of two or more of the following:
	Vertigo
	Syncope
	Dysarthria
	Diplopia
	Nausea
	Dysphagia
	Drop attack, especially when seen in association with a motor or sensory deficit

pattern on CT brain scan, any evidence of a bleeding diathesis or severe metabolic disturbance, or marked blood pressure elevation, or if they have recently had major surgery, a prior stroke, or significant trauma. There is a 6.4% risk of ICH with rt-PA, and the consequences can be quite severe. On the other hand, there is clearly an improved functional outcome for treated patients at 3 months from the time of onset of the stroke. The benefits outweigh the risks when patients are carefully selected, and this selection process should prevent major intracranial bleeds in most instances. It is important that anticoagulant therapy and antiplatelet therapy not be given within the first 24 hours of the rt-PA intravenous infusion. The dose of rt-PA is 0.9 mg/kg, with 10% by intravenous bolus over 1 minute and the remainder infused over 1 hour. The maximum dose is 90 mg.

Anticoagulant therapy continues to be controversial in acute ischemic stroke. The major indication for immediate anticoagulation is a TIA or minor ischemic stroke in association with a presumptive cardiogenic source of embolus, assuming there is no contraindication by CT brain scan for its use. If the patient has clinical evidence of a moderate to severe infarction, by either clinical presentation or CT, it is advisable to wait 3 to 5 days and then repeat the CT brain scan to ensure that hemorrhagic conversion of the infarct has not taken place. Then, if it is decided to proceed with intravenous heparin therapy, a large initial bolus of medication should be avoided, and the PTT must be carefully monitored. If there is hemorrhagic transformation of the infarct, the physician should wait longer before deciding about anticoagulant therapy. In life-threatening circumstances, the benefits of starting heparin sooner rather than later must be weighed against the risks. One study that addressed this issue suggested that intravenous heparin could be given safely even when there is evidence of blood on the CT brain scan. However, this should be considered only in extremely carefully selected cases.

Intravenous heparin with subsequent warfarin maintenance also appears to be the optimal therapy in sinovenous thrombosis. This must also be done with extreme care because of the propensity for venous infarcts to demonstrate hemorrhagic transformation. There are also data that suggest that cerebrovascular dissection is best managed with acute anticoagulant therapy *if* the patient has not already suffered a major infarct. Once again, the concern with a major infarct is the potential for hemorrhagic transformation. Anticoagulant therapy is also the therapy of choice for cerebral ischemia in association with a prothrombotic state.

Recent data suggest that 160 to 300 mg of aspirin given acutely for ischemic stroke has a favorable effect on outcome. The benefit was rather small and at least one study raised concerns about an increased risk of brain hemorrhage. The International Stroke Trial (IST) assessed the subcutaneous administration of 5,000 to 12,500 units of heparin given twice a day. No overall reduction in risk of recurrent stroke or death was seen, but lower-dose heparin (or heparinoid) continues to be recommended in patients who have immobility after a stroke, in an effort to protect against deep vein thrombosis.

A number of general measures need to be taken for patients presenting with completed cerebral infarction (Table 6-6). In the acute setting, it is especially important to avoid relative hypotension. Agents that promote a precipitous drop in blood pressure should be avoided. Generally speaking, a systolic blood pressure of 160 ± 20 mm Hg or a diastolic blood pressure of 110 ± 10 mm Hg are reasonable values in the acute setting and do not require treatment. Aggressive blood pressure control has the potential to lower cerebral perfusion and this can promote extension of the infarct.

In lacunar-type infarctions, a good prognosis can be expected because of the small nature of the infarct. Extensive cardiac evaluation or carotid evaluation does not usually have to be considered. Instead, stroke-prevention efforts should be made. It is estimated that there is a 12% recurrence rate for lacunar-type stroke within the first year, and the outcome will be worse with each successive stroke. The major thrust should be toward reduction of risk factors that promoted the propensity for stroke in the first place: hypertension, smoking, diabetes mellitus, and hyperlipidemia. Over the long term, aggressive blood pressure control is clearly indicated, and this

TABLE 6-6. Guidelines for General Management of the Acute Stroke Patient

1. Stability of vital signs
2. Protection of airway with aspiration precautions
3. Assessment of swallowing capacity
4. Early mobilization as clinically indicated
5. Bowel program
6. Prevention of pressure sores
7. Anti-embolus measures
8. Rehabilitative therapy evaluation as indicated by deficit
9. Social service evaluation
10. Assessment for evidence of poststroke depression
11. Long-term management of risk factors for stroke

can have a very favorable impact on reduction of stroke risk.

If there is no ongoing cardiogenic source of embolus, antiplatelet agents appear to be the optimal choice of antithrombotic therapy. In one recent study, higher-dose warfarin therapy had an unacceptably high risk of bleeding complications when compared with aspirin. An ongoing study is comparing lower-dose warfarin to aspirin in the prevention of recurrent stroke. The optimal dose of aspirin remains controversial. Various studies have suggested that between 81 mg and 1,300 mg per day is effective. Overall, aspirin appears to reduce the risk of recurrent stroke by approximately 20% to 25%. The European Stroke Prevention Study reported that dipyridamole, at a dosage of 75 mg three times a day, augments the effectiveness of aspirin, and that 200 mg of long-acting dipyridamole twice a day confers some benefit even without aspirin. Ticlopidine is associated with approximately a 27% risk reduction of recurrent stroke. Ticlopidine has significant side effects, including a 1% risk of severe neutropenia. Its additional cost and the blood count monitoring necessary for its use makes it a second-line agent, primarily reserved for those patients who continue to have recurrent symptoms despite aspirin, or for those who are aspirin intolerant.

The first phase of the Stroke Prevention in Atrial Fibrillation (SPAF) study found that warfarin, at a dose that produced an INR of 2 to 3, reduced the risk of embolic events in NVAF by 67%. Surprisingly, one enteric coated 325-mg aspirin per day reduced the risk of vascular events by 42%. This led to the second phase of the study, in which aspirin and warfarin were directly compared without a placebo arm. The authors reported that the event rate per year was 1.3% for warfarin and 1.9% for aspirin in subjects 75 years of age or less. For subjects beyond 75 years of age, the event rate was 3.6% for warfarin and 4.8% for aspirin, but any benefit of warfarin was essentially negated by the heightened risk of bleeding complications. Although the results are subject to interpretation, warfarin remains the superior agent for patients who are at relatively high risk for embolus and who are at relatively low risk for bleeding complications. A follow-up study found that low-dose warfarin, even when given in combination with aspirin, was inferior to the dose of warfarin that resulted in the INR of 2 to 3. This superiority of adjusted-dose warfarin over aspirin in higher-risk patients was also observed in the European Atrial Fibrillation Trial. Unlike the primary prevention SPAF studies, this study looked at secondary prevention after a TIA or minor stroke. In

patients with mechanical heart valves, a higher dose of warfarin is warranted, with a recommended INR target of 3 to 4. This is also the case for the prevention of thrombosis in antiphospholipid antibody syndrome.

Carotid endarterectomy is the treatment of choice for symptomatic ICA stenosis of 70% to 99%. This is associated with a risk reduction of ipsilateral stroke of approximately 65%. The recommendation for this procedure is predicated on the medical stability of the patient, an arteriography suite with an acceptably low complication rate for the procedure, and the availability of a surgeon who achieves an acceptably low complication rate. In one recent study, there was no benefit from performing carotid endarterectomy for symptomatic stenosis in the moderate (i.e., 30% to 69%) range. The relatively high rate of complications associated with the surgical procedure, in this study, might have negated a potential benefit. The Asymptomatic Carotid Atherosclerosis Study reported a benefit of prophylactic carotid endarterectomy for stenosis of 60% to 99%. The absolute risk reduction was only 5.9% in this study, and the benefit was restricted to men. The results are subject to interpretation, but the best candidates for this approach appear to be relatively young patients who are excellent surgical candidates. It might be particularly useful for patients with bilateral higher-grade carotid stenosis, especially if there is evidence of progressive stenosis over time.

INTRACEREBRAL HEMORRHAGE

CLINICAL APPROACH

Among the possible causes for ICH (Table 6-7), the most common is hypertension. This is attributed to the formation of *Charcot-Bouchard microaneurysms*, observed as a sequela of long-standing, poorly controlled hypertension. The most common locations for hypertensive ICH are the basal ganglia, thalamus, pons, and cerebellum. It has been reported that only half of lobar hemorrhages are hypertensive in origin. An atypical location, atypical presentation, or lack of a clear-cut history of hypertension, should always point toward further diagnostic evaluation. Clinical or CT findings suggestive of a vascular anomaly or tumor should lead to angiographic investigation. This procedure is often best delayed until the hemorrhage has reabsorbed and the mass effect has resolved, unless the results will directly impact on patient management. Allowing time for the hematoma to reabsorb will allow better visualization of the

TABLE 6-7. Causes of Spontaneous Intracerebral Hemorrhage

1. Hypertension
2. Intracranial aneurysm
3. Arteriovenous malformation
4. Bleeding diathesis
5. Anticoagulant therapy
6. Illicit drugs (e.g., cocaine)
7. Mycotic aneurysm
8. Hemorrhagic metastasis
9. Bleed into a primary brain tumor
10. Bleed into a brain abscess
11. Arteritis secondary to connective tissue disease
12. Amyloid angiopathy
13. Hemorrhagic leukoencephalopathy
14. Idiopathic? cryptic arteriovenous malformation

vessels in the area of the bleed so that a possible vascular anomaly such as an AVM or aneurysm can be excluded.

Patients with ICH should be evaluated for evidence of head trauma, and bleeding parameters should also be obtained. There is increasing use of anticoagulant therapy for prophylaxis against cardiogenic emboli, and this translates into an enhanced risk of iatrogenic bleeds. In addition, a previous history of malignancy, especially lung cancer, breast cancer, thyroid carcinoma, melanoma, and renal cell carcinoma, should raise the suspicion of a hemorrhagic metastasis. Multiple lobar hemorrhages in an elderly patient, especially if there is a history of dementia, should raise the question of amyloid angiopathy. Illicit drugs such as cocaine can be associated with a precipitous rise in blood pressure, resulting in rupture of a previously undiagnosed vascular malformation. Such agents can also promote arteritis, which can lead to either ischemic or hemorrhagic stroke. Vasculitis with secondary bleeding is also a concern with systemic lupus erythematosis and polyarteritis nodosa.

An intracerebral bleed tends to be a precipitous event with no premonitory symptoms except, perhaps, headache. If hypertension is the mechanism, there is usually an impressively elevated blood pressure and often a history of poor compliance with antihypertensive medication. The bleeding tends to subside, in patients who survive, within 4 to 6 hours. This has been demonstrated by hyperacute serial CT scan in a number of recent series and the expansion of the hematoma is usually associated with deterioration of the neurologic status. The CT brain scan remains the definitive study for the documentation of ICH

(Fig. 6-8). The CT scan is also helpful from a prognostic standpoint. For example, the larger the hematoma, the worse the prognosis. The prognosis is also adversely affected by the presence of intraventricular extension of the bleed.

MANAGEMENT

The guidelines outlined for routine care of patients with ischemic stroke also apply to patients with hemorrhagic stroke. The major aspects of therapy for ICH concern treatment of the increased intracranial pressure, if present; protection of the airway, with institution of hyperventilation as the initial means to lower increased intracranial pressure; evacuation of the hematoma in selected cases; and aggressive control of elevated blood pressure. Recent studies have indicated that persistently elevated blood pressure in hypertensive ICH is deleterious. This appears to be related not only to a potential contribution to the extension of the hematoma, but also to the promotion of end-organ damage.

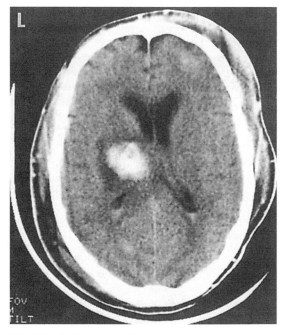

FIG. 6-8. Left thalamic hematoma, as demonstrated by CT brain scan, in a patient with long-standing hypertension.

Patients presenting in a stuporous or semicomatose state may still have a reasonably good prognosis if they are relatively young, and if they do not have progression of the neurologic deficit. For relatively small hematomas that are not in a critical location, such as the pons, the prognosis actually tends to be better than for infarction, as the affected tissue tends to be displaced rather than destroyed. Surgical evacuation of the hematoma, in selected cases, can result in dramatic improvement. This is most feasible for a lobar location, especially of the nondominant hemisphere, as well as for cerebellar hematomas *prior* to the development of long tract signs or respiratory compromise.

The management of significantly increased intracranial pressure is an emergent problem and requires aggressive management. The primary methods include the use of hyperventilation, as well as either mannitol or glycerol to combat cerebral edema. Dexamethasone was not found to be an effective agent in one controlled study. The presence of intraventricular extension is more likely to lead to complications such as ventriculitis and hydrocephalus. Progressive ventricular enlargement is often treated with ventricular shunting, but in most cases there is little or no benefit.

SUBARACHNOID HEMORRHAGE

INTRACRANIAL ANEURYSM

An intracranial aneurysm is an outpouching of the arterial wall, and its shape has led to the descriptive term *saccular* or *berry* aneurysm. These aneurysms are viewed as being acquired lesions, but they appear to originate from a congenital defect within the vessel wall. They tend to be located at vessel bifurcations or trifurcations, and the majority are found in the anterior circulation at the base of the brain, specifically at the circle of Willis. It is estimated that 20 to 30% of patients have multiple aneurysms. Genetic factors almost certainly play a role in the pathogenesis of cerebral aneurysms. This is supported by familial predisposition as well their association with inherited disorders of connective tissue such as polycystic kidney disease and Ehlers-Danlos syndrome.

Risk of aneurysmal rupture is associated with advancing age, cigarette smoking, hypertension, excessive alcohol consumption, and female sex. The mean age of aneurysmal rupture is approximately 50 years. The most common presentation is a particularly severe headache, which is not uncommonly associated with nausea and vomiting, and with evidence of meningismus. Syncope may actually be the most prominent feature at the time of onset, and this must be recognized. In addition, up to one half of patients have a premonitory severe or atypical headache within weeks of a major event, and this is felt to represent a "warning leak."

As mentioned previously, the CT brain scan is relatively sensitive for the detection of subarachnoid blood, but a small amount of blood may be quite subtle (see Fig. 6-5) or simply not seen. Larger aneurysms may be visualized by CT or MRI, especially when contrast is given. The ability to detect unruptured aneurysms with neuroimaging has led to a potential management dilemma. This is especially pertinent in view of the ability of MRA to noninvasively detect most aneurysms 5 mm or more in size. A study that evaluated the natural history of unruptured aneurysms reported that no patient with an aneurysm of less than 1 cm in diameter had a rupture during the follow-up period. On the other hand, 38% of patients with an aneurysm 1 cm or greater in diameter had eventual rupture. This study suggests that prophylactic clipping of aneurysms 1 cm or greater in diameter is clinically indicated.

Aneurysmal rupture carries a very worrisome prognosis. It is estimated that the overall mortality rate is up to 50%. This is impacted a great deal by the possible complications that can occur after the initial rupture (Table 6-8). Approximately 20% to 30% of patients with aneurysmal rupture will rebleed within the first 2 weeks, and the result will be fatal in 75% of instances. This has led to efforts to perform surgical clipping of the aneurysm early (i.e., within the first few days of presentation) if at all possible. This should effectively protect against rebleeding. If early surgery is not feasible, or if the patient's degree of neurologic deficit does not justify aggressive intervention, then surgery is delayed for 2 weeks or longer, depending on the patient's neurologic status. It is over this time period that the risk of

---

TABLE 6-8. Complications of Aneurysmal Rupture

1. Rebleeding
2. Vasospasm with secondary ischemia
3. Hydrocephalus
   a. Obstructive
   b. Communicating
4. Diffuse cerebral edema
5. Chemical meningitis
6. Subdural hematoma
7. Intracerebral hematoma

vasospasm, which can promote cerebral ischemia, is greatest. There is a relationship between the amount of subarachnoid blood visualized on CT brain scan and vasospasm. The calcium channel blocking agent nimodipine has been approved for use in preventing the cerebral ischemic complications of vasospasm, but there continues to be some controversy over the true efficacy of this agent. The recommended dosage is 60 mg every 4 hours for 21 consecutive days. Many medical centers have protocols in place to combat vasospasm. This involves serial TCD monitoring to detect early vasospasm. If there is evidence of vasospasm, interventional methods include relative hypertension, hypervolemia, and either intra-arterial papaverine infusion or endovascular balloon angioplasty.

ARTERIOVENOUS MALFORMATION

An AVM represents an anomaly of embryonal development in which there is a conglomeration of arteries and veins with no intervening capillaries. The prevalence of AVM in the general population is estimated at 0.14%, and most remain clinically silent throughout life. They are reported to be twice as common in men as in women. Although present at birth, they tend to become clinically evident most commonly between the ages of 10 and 40 years.

Approximately 50% of people who become symptomatic from an AVM have either ICH or SAH. It is the second most common cause of SAH after aneurysmal rupture. Approximately 30% of patients with AVM present with seizures, while the remaining 20% present with headache, focal neurologic deficit, or cognitive impairment. One quarter of patients with AVM who present with ICH will suffer serious morbidity or death, and the recurrence rate for hemorrhage is roughly 7% within the first year. Of patients with AVM who present with seizure, 1% will suffer ICH within 1 year. The headache that is associated with AVM can be very difficult to distinguish from migraine, and there is always the possibility that the two coexist.

Fortunately, the risk of rebleeding with an AVM is not analogous to that of aneurysmal rupture. This gives the clinician time to carefully plan optimal management. The most effective course is to surgically remove the AVM, if this is feasible. The feasibility of surgical extirpation is based on the size of the AVM, the nature of its feeding vessels, and the location. AVMs of the dominant hemisphere and those that are located within the deeper brain structures present a greater surgical challenge. In an effort to reduce the size of the AVM, and to diminish the number of feeding vessels, selective catheterization with injection of

silastic pellets has been used. This embolization procedure can be quite effective as an adjunct to surgery.

For inoperable AVMs, special irradiation techniques have been developed. These include Bragg-peak proton beam therapy, which requires a linear accelerator, and gamma irradiation, the so-called gamma knife. These therapies can reduce the risk of rebleeding and, in certain cases, there can be total obliteration of the AVM based on follow-up cerebral arteriography. The therapy is designed to reduce the lumen diameter of the feeding vessels and to promote thickening of the surrounding wall of the AVM. Routine radiation therapy is not effective for this endeavor.

QUESTIONS AND DISCUSSION

1. A 68-year-old right-handed woman presents with several episodes of transient aphasic deficit and right-sided weakness. Her noncontrast CT brain scan is normal and her routine blood work is unremarkable. Her EKG reveals newly documented atrial fibrillation. Important determinants of the advisability of long-term anticoagulant therapy include which of the following:

A. Effective suppression of the cardiac rhythm disturbance
B. Evidence of significantly impaired left ventricular function by echocardiography
C. Compliance of the patient
D. Presence of a bleeding diathesis
E. All of the above

The answer is (E). The determination of whether to proceed with long-term anticoagulation in nonvalvular atrial fibrillation is very dependent on benefits versus risks. The follow-up Stroke Prevention in Atrial Fibrillation (SPAF II) Study underscored the need for careful patient selection, as the benefit of warfarin therapy in older patients was, at least partially, offset by the risk of bleeding complications.

2. A patient presents to your emergency room with an acute right hemispheric ischemic stroke. The onset of symptoms was approximately 90 minutes prior to the time of presentation. Factors that would have an impact on whether the patient is a proper candidate for rt-PA would include all but the following (choose one):

A. Recent major surgery
B. Reasonably well controlled blood pressure at the time of presentation

C. Therapeutic anticoagulation with warfarin at the time of presentation

D. The severity of the stroke

E. A history of aspirin allergy

The answer is (E). Patients who are appropriate candidates for rt-PA must present and be treated within 3 hours of onset. The CT brain scan must reveal no contraindication to thrombolytic therapy. Patients who have had recent major surgery or trauma, who have an unacceptably high blood pressure, who have therapeutic anticoagulation at the time of presentation, or who have a major incapacitating deficit are not proper candidates for this therapy.

3. A 47-year-old woman presents to you with her third lacunar-type stroke within the past year. She has not been on therapy for cerebrovascular prophylaxis. She has long-standing hypertension and is a heavy smoker. The most effective means of prevention of recurrent stroke in this patient would include all but the following (choose one):

A. Effective blood pressure control

B. Antiplatelet therapy

C. Initiation of warfarin

D. Attention to diet

E. Cessation of smoking

The answer is (C). Warfarin is not established as an effective agent for the prevention of lacunar-type stroke. Its primary indication is for the prevention of cerebral emboli with a cardiogenic source. Antiplatelet therapy, usually with aspirin as the first choice, along with aggressive attention to risk factors for stroke, is the optimal approach at this time.

4. A 53-year-old woman presents to the emergency room with what she describes as one of her most severe headaches. She is afebrile, with an admission blood pressure of 156/96 mm Hg. Features that would raise the index of clinical suspicion for aneurysmal subarachnoid hemorrhage in this patient would include all but (choose one):

A. A well-documented history of migraine

B. A history of hypertension

C. A history of smoking

D. A history of polycystic kidney disease

E. Evidence of neck stiffness

The answer is (A). Risk factors associated with aneurysmal rupture include hypertension, smoking, female sex, and alcohol abuse. Patients with polycys-

tic kidney disease have a special predilection for cerebral aneurysm. Migraine is not directly associated with aneurysmal rupture, but, when the diagnosis of aneurysmal rupture is missed, the presenting headache is often attributed to migraine.

SUGGESTED READING

Broderick JP, Brott TG, Duldner JE et al: Volume of intracerebral hemorrhage. A powerful and easy-to-use predictor of 30-day mortality. Stroke 24:987, 1993

Dandapani BK, Suzuki S, Kelley RE et al: Relation between blood pressure and outcome in intracerebral hemorrhage. Stroke 26:21, 1995

Delanty N, Vaughan CJ: Vascular effects of statins in stroke. Stroke 28:2315, 1997

Diener HC, Cunha L, Forbes C et al: European Stroke Prevention Study 2. Dipyridamole and acetylsalicylic acid in the secondary prevention of stroke. J Neurol Sci 143:1, 1996

Executive Committee for the Asymptomatic Carotid Atherosclerosis Study: Endarterectomy for asymptomatic carotid artery stenosis. JAMA 273:1421, 1995

International Stroke Trial Collaborative Group. The International Stroke Trial (IST): A randomized trial of aspirin, subcutaneous heparin, both, or neither among 19435 patients with acute ischaemic stroke. Lancet 349:1569, 1997

Kelley RE: Understanding rt-PA therapy for acute ischemic stroke. Intern Med 18:20, 1997

The National Institute of Neurological Disorders and Stroke rt-PA Stroke Study Group: Tissue plasminogen activator for acute ischemic stroke. N Engl J Med 333:1581, 1995

Pessin MS, Estol CJ, Lafranchise F, et al: Safety of anticoagulation after hemorrhagic infarction. Neurology 43:1298, 1993

Schievink WI. Intracranial aneurysms. N Engl J Med 336:28, 1997

Stroke Prevention in Atrial Fibrillation Investigators. Warfarin versus aspirin for prevention of thromboembolism in atrial fibrillation. Lancet 343:687, 1994

The Stroke Prevention in Reversible Ischemia Trial (SPIRIT) Study Group: A randomized trial of anticoagulants versus aspirin after cerebral ischemia of presumed arterial origin. Ann Neurol 42:857, 1997

Neurology for the Non-Neurologist, Fourth Edition, edited by William J. Weiner and Christopher G. Goetz. Lippincott Williams & Wilkins, Philadelphia © 1999.

C H A P T E R	7

Headache Disorders

Joel R. Saper

Head, neck, and facial pain disorders (hereafter referred to as headache disorders) possess characteristic features that, in some ways, distinguish them from other painful disorders. Generally speaking, however, the headache disorders can be reconciled within the same model of assessment as that of other painful conditions.

GENERAL CONCEPTS OF HEADACHE DISORDERS

Seventy-six percent (76%) of women and 57% of men report at least one significant headache per month, and over 90% experience a noteworthy headache at least once in their lifetime. Over 90% of those who suffer from headache illnesses have never been seen by a specialist. The majority (67%) of headache patients in the United States use over-the-counter medications to find relief. Between 1980 and 1989, the prevalence of migraine (a primary headache disorder, see later) increased by 60%.

The *primary headache disorders* include such conditions as migraine, cluster headache, and tension-type headache. *Secondary headache disorders* are those associated with a variety of organic etiologies, and in which the pain is *secondary* to an identifiable, distinct pathologic processes of which head pain is a symptom. Over 300 organic disorders are capable of producing headache (secondary headaches). Nonetheless, over 90% of headaches reaching clinical significance are the result of one or more of the primary headache disorders.

Current classification of headache is based on the recently proposed classification of the International Headache Society (IHS). Thirteen categories of headache are subdivided into 129 subtypes.

Headache may present either in an intermittent fashion (periodic), in a recurring periodic fashion, or in a persistent, constant form. Although headaches such as migraine are generally intermittent and periodic, they may evolve or transform to a state of constancy. Similarly, headaches secondary to organic processes may begin intermittently and then evolve to a more constant form.

CONCEPTS OF HEADACHE PATHOGENESIS

Although muscular and vascular disturbances have been historically considered the fundamental physiologic alteration causing the primary headache disorders (e.g., migraine, tension-type), the most current concepts of headache pathogenesis provide compelling evidence that the primary headache disorders arise fundamentally from disturbances within the central nervous system. Supporting this "neurogenic" concept of migraine are the frequent presence of premonitory symptoms prior to the headache event, suggesting hypothalamic dysfunction; the presence of focal neurologic disturbance that cannot alone be explained by cerebral blood flow alterations; the numerous accompaniments to headache, which include autonomic and constitutional dysfunction; magnetoencephalographic alterations demonstrating cerebral neuronal disturbances during migraine; growing support and evidence for alterations of serotonin function in patients with migraine; and the demonstrable presence of inflammatory disturbances within the trigeminal vascular system, induced by alterations within the nervous system. Moreover, the primary headache disorders often respond therapeutically to drugs and other therapies that influence central serotonin function, independent of any direct vascular or muscular effects.

Recently, positron emission tomography (PET) scanning has shown the presence of an area in the brainstem that appears likely to represent the migraine "generator." Sumatriptan, while apparently able to reverse physiologic changes in other areas of the brain, was not able to turn off this "generator."

MIGRAINE

Migraine comprises an increasingly large number of headache presentations, ranging from typical, characteristic, periodic attacks, to a number of variant forms, including a daily persistent form. Growing support exists for the concept that migraine represents a broad clinical spectrum, or continuum, that on one end is an occasional intermittent migraine with aura (see later) and on the other end is a daily persistent pain similar to the traditional classification of chronic tension or tension-type headache. A basic central pathophysiologic disturbance appears to be fundamental to a broad range of clinical events and supports the concept that migraine is far greater in scope and in clinical manifestation than heretofore considered.

Migraine is a complex neurophysiologic disorder characterized by episodic and progressive forms of head pain with numerous neurologic and nonneurologic accompaniments and prodromal events. The attacks of pain are frequently accompanied by neurologic, autonomic, and psychophysiologic disturbances.

Formerly, migraine was classified into two major subgroups: *classic* and *common* migraine. *Classic migraine,* that form characterized by an aura of neurologically significant "pre-headache" phenomena, is now called (according to the IHS classification) *migraine with aura.*

Common migraine, attacks of migraine without clear-cut pre-headache neurologic symptomatology, is now referred to as *migraine without aura.*

Since the late 1970s, there has been increasing recognition of migraine's capacity to *transform* or *evolve* from intermittent attacks to daily or almost daily head pain. This "variant" form of migraine has been most recently termed *transformational migraine, progressive migraine,* or *pernicious migraine.* It represents the progressive form of an illness that, for reasons still uncertain, possesses the capacity to evolve from intermittency to persistency.

Migraine is an inherited disorder, currently thought to represent an autosomal dominant trait with incomplete penetrance. Sex distribution is approximately equal in childhood, but by adulthood migraine affects women over men in a ratio of approximately 2–3:1, a dominance thought to reflect the aggravating influence of estrogen on the central migraine mechanisms.

Subclassifications of migraine reflect specific migraine syndromes, including *ophthalmoplegic migraine, hemiplegic migraine, aphasic migraine, retinal migraine,* and others. Migraine itself may impart a stroke risk and lead to brain infarction. Major, as well as often prolonged disturbances of brainstem function, are well known, including dizziness (with or without vertigo and disequilibrium); nausea, vomiting, diarrhea, and anorexia; loss of consciousness; sudden mood change; and other often dramatic disturbances, including stupor, confusion, and frank ataxia.

The predisposition to migraine appears to be present throughout the life of the individual but manifests itself periodically or more frequently as a result of poorly understood internal and external factors. Among the events known to be capable of provoking an attack or series of attacks of migraine are hormonal alteration, emotional phenomena, sleeping disturbances, weather changes, certain types of drugs and food substances, and smoke and ambient air factors.

Unlike several other painful disorders, the most effective primary treatment for headache is based on a pharmacotherapeutic model. Nonpharmacotherapeutic interventions, such as biofeedback, stress management, discontinuing smoking, and day-to-day activity regulation, can be helpful but are not generally considered as effective as pharmacotherapy. They are often combined with pharmacotherapy for maximum therapeutic control.

There is another difference from the other painful disorders: Compelling evidence supports the idea that the excessive use of symptomatic medications, including analgesics and ergotamine tartrate, when used more than 2 days a week in patients with migraine, may provoke a progressive excitation of the headache disorder, leading to and inducing a transformation from intermittency to constancy. This phenomenon, called rebound, renders appropriate treatment ineffective until the offending drug has been entirely withdrawn and a period of physiologic stabilization occurs. Treatment of this phenomenon often requires hospitalization and parenteral therapeutic support.

Migraine may thus occur in an intractable, persistent form, accompanied by prolonged and severe pain, associated with anorexia, dehydration, and refractory nausea, vomiting, and diarrhea.

TENSION-TYPE HEADACHE

Although still controversial, many headache authorities believe that what has been traditionally called *tension headache,* or more recently *tension-type headache,* represents a variant form of migraine. Symptomatically, there is significant overlapping between the features of tension-type headache and migraine. A large number of patients with tension-type headache actually suffer superimposed periodic attacks of traditional migraine in addition to daily or almost daily pain.

Tension-type headache may have an intermittent or episodic form, as well as a chronic form. The chronic form, which occurs more than 15 days per month, may mimic or overlap with transformational migraine, described previously.

Tension-type headache, which many authorities believe represents a migraine form, may thus occur within at least the following three perspectives:

1. Many cases occur as a direct result of the transformation of migraine from intermittent, intense, periodic attacks to daily, or almost daily, constant headache. This evolutionary or transformational form may in some instances be induced by analgesic or ergotamine tartrate overuse (rebound) or may transform spontaneously without apparent external induction. A distinction between this and transformed migraine is not possible, and many believe they are the same disorder.

2. Tension-type headache may also manifest spontaneously without a preceding history of migraine. This has been referred to as *new onset, tension-type headache.*

3. Finally, tension-type headache may occur as a consequence of head injury, a phenomenon also seen with migraine.

MIGRAINE, TENSION-TYPE HEADACHE, AND COMORBIDITIES

It is now apparent that many migraine patients suffer from one (or more) of a wide spectrum of neuropsychophysiologic conditions in addition to headache. These disorders, currently referred to as "comorbid conditions associated with migraine," appear to coexist in migraine patients with a prevalence much greater than expected by chance alone. It is currently believed that these disorders share certain neurophysiologic commonalities with headache disorders, believed to reflect central (perhaps brainstem) or other brain neurotransmitter/receptor disturbances.

The most important of the comorbid conditions include depression, sleep disturbance, obsessive-compulsive disorders, bipolar disease, epilepsy, and panic and anxiety attacks. Others include personality disorders, chemical dependency vulnerability, irritable bowel syndromes, eating disorders, and mitral valve prolapse.

Difficult cases of migraine often require the diagnosis and treatment of these comorbid conditions, and in some instances this is a significant treatment and management challenge. Studies on the cost of headache suggest that these comorbid conditions may contribute significantly to the increased utilization costs in patients with headache. The comorbid conditions require coordinated treatment.

CLUSTER HEADACHE

Cluster headache, like migraine, is a devastating, painful affliction, primarily affecting men more than women, in which attacks lasting half an hour to an hour and a half occur daily for weeks, months, or years at a time. Up to eight or more attacks may occur per day.

The term *cluster headache* was originally used to describe the clustering or sequence of bouts of painful attacks in which the headache cycle occurs for a period of time (usually several months) and then spontaneously remits into a period of quiescence referred to as the *interim.* A chronic form of cluster headache in which an interim does not occur is now recognized.

The key clinical features of *cluster headache* include severe, periodic, painful attacks primarily localizing around the eye, temple, forehead, or cheek region. Focal tenderness in the ipsilateral occipitocervical junction is often noted.

Each attack is usually accompanied by ipsilateral lacrimation and nasal drainage, lid drooping, pupillary change, and conjunctival injection. Suicide has been noted to a higher-than-expected degree in men with cluster headache.

Treatment considerations are primarily those employing pharmacotherapeutic agents for both preventive therapy as well as symptomatic treatment.

FUNCTIONAL, CLINICAL, AND OPERATIONAL CLASSIFICATION OF HEADACHE

It is now possible to reconcile the primary headache disorders as well as the secondary forms into existing functional, clinical, and operational classifications of pain.

Functional Classification Based on Neuropsychiatric Model

1. The *primary headache disorders* are best classified as *neurogenic pain,* which by definition results from an excitation from within the central, peripheral, or autonomic nervous system, occurring in the absence of any specific identifiable noxious stimuli.
2. The *secondary headache disorders* are classified as nociceptive pain.

Clinical Classification Based on Pathogenicity

1. The *primary headache disorders* are classified as *primary pain* because they appear to result directly from physiologic disturbances, either nociceptive or neurogenic.
2. The *secondary headache disorders* are classified as *secondary pain.*

Operational Classification Based on a Bio-Psycho-Social Model

1. The *primary headache disorders* are classified as *acute, recurrent pain.* This pain may be peripheral or neurogenic, primary or secondary, and it may evolve to a persistent form, with or without periodic pain-free periods.
2. The *secondary headache disorders* are classified as *acute pain.*

HEADACHES AND CHRONIC PAIN

Chronic pain may be referred to as chronic, intractable pain or chronic, benign pain that exceeds simply "persistent pain" but that embodies a condition in which a malevolent and destructive influence occurs. Headache evolving into chronic pain is a self-sustaining process and is not, in and of itself, a reflection of an underlying acute somatic injury but rather a physiologic/pathologic disorder in its own right. It is chronic, long lived, and progressive. Pain perception is markedly enhanced, and pain behavior becomes maladaptive and counterproductive. Both the pain behavior and perception are grossly disproportionate to identifiable underlying noxious stimulation. In essence, it presents a bio-psycho-social phenomenon of maladaptive behavior with far-reaching medical, social, and economic consequences. It may arise from or be aggravated by inappropriate management of acute pain problems (such as inappropriate surgical intervention, and excessive administration and/or usage of addictive, dependency-producing medication) or result from a natural deterioration based on factors yet to be determined. Early detection and prompt effective intervention are essential to effective management.

FREQUENCY PATTERNS OF PRIMARY HEADACHES

Four patterns of headache occur, independent of specific diagnoses.

Minimal, slight, moderate, and marked headache may occur in intermittent, occasional, frequent, or constant forms.

Cycles or episodes of the first pattern may last moments, hours, days, weeks, months, or years, followed by periods of complete or almost complete remission.

Constant and persistent pain of varying intensities may last years, decades, or a lifetime.

Complex patterns of the first three patterns, in which varying intensities and frequencies of one form of headache occur with superimposed features of varying intensities and frequencies of another headache form (mixed forms).

CLINICAL FEATURES THAT DISTINGUISH HEADACHE ILLNESSES FROM MANY OF THE OTHER PAINFUL DISORDERS

Many headache illnesses are accompanied by dramatic, often stroke-like clinical phenomena that can be even more disruptive and disabling than the pain experience itself. Moreover, patients with headache syndromes are often compromised periodically or constantly by the effects of excessively used sedative medications administered appropriately and inappropriately for the treatment of headache.

Typical Accompaniments of Acute, Periodic Headache Events (i.e., Migraine)

1. Mental and cognitive impairment, including irritability, depression, forgetfulness
2. Visual disturbances (blurred vision, scotoma, hemianopsia, etc.)
3. Focal neurologic events, hemiparesis, hemisensory disturbance, aphasia, ataxia, dizziness with or without vertigo, diplopia, etc.
4. Nausea, vomiting, and diarrhea
5. Dehydration (from nausea, vomiting, diarrhea, anorexia, etc.)
6. Dramatic light and/or sound sensitivity
7. Sleep disturbance
8. Compulsive seeking of dark, quiet, cool environment with unavoidable tendency to sleep through the pain
9. Panic, hypomanic, and manic behavior manifested by moaning, crying, screaming, and anger outbursts (as seen in cluster headache)
10. Ptosis, eyelid drooping, pupillary disturbances (as in cluster headache)
11. Lacrimation and rhinorrhea (as in cluster headache)
12. Autonomic disturbances (hypertension, hypotension, bradycardia, tachycardia, pallor, orbital and facial swelling, pupillary disturbances, abdominal cramping, epistaxis, nasal stuffiness, etc.)
13. Alterations in the ability to carry on the events of daily living

Many of these symptoms persist beyond the period of pain itself and/or can occur hours, days, or longer in advance of an anticipated attack. Following an acute attack, a period of mental dullness, fatigue, and somnolence occurs, not dissimilar from that seen in the *postictal phase* of an epileptic seizure.

Diagnostic Considerations for Headache

Because the presence of a primary headache disorder, or at least any feature of the primary headache disorder, does not in and of itself exclude the presence of a separate, comorbid, distinct pathologic process, broad diagnostic considerations are required both initially and periodically. Moreover, when the patient is involved in an intense pharmacotherapeutic program, monitoring of blood levels, organ responses, and cardiac status is required for safety. Screening studies are necessary to determine the safety parameters for drug administration.

FACTORS TO BE CONSIDERED IN DETERMINING IMPAIRMENT/DISABILITY OF PATIENTS WITH HEADACHE

The following are the variables that are particularly important in determining and assessing the limitation imparted by the headache disorders:

1. Frequency of pain
2. Quality of pain (sharp, dull, piercing, boring, etc.)
3. Duration of pain
4. Intensity of pain
5. Function-limiting accompaniments

   Neurologic [hemiparesis, aphasia, visual (e.g., blurred vision, hemianopsia, diplopia)]

   Autonomic (nausea, vomiting, diarrhea, hypotension, anorexia, tachyarrhythmias, etc.)

   Mental, cognitive, and mood disturbances

   Others

6. Effects of medication
7. Relief requirements, such as seeking a dark, cool, quiet environment
8. Treatment requirements, such as the use of often compromising medications
9. Inability to carry on the activities of daily living

PRINCIPLES OF TREATMENT

Four principles are important in approaching the treatment of migraine.

First, one must determine the intensity of care that is required, based on the severity of the illness. The severity of illness implies not only the intensity of an individual attack but the frequency of the attacks and important accompaniments, including comorbid illness (e.g., psychiatric, neurologic) and the presence of confounding factors such as rebound phenomena.

Second, the clinician must determine whether the approach will be to use medication treatment exclusively, nonmedical therapy exclusively, or a combination of both.

Third, a decision must be made whether to treat the individual attacks (symptomatic, abortive) or whether the nature of the condition requires prophylactic treatment.

And fourth, what is the most appropriate setting for care to initially institute treatment (i.e., outpatient clinic or hospital)? This decision is based largely on the acuteness of the clinical presentation, the accompaniments, and the presence or absence of such clinical factors as drug toxicity, dehydration, rebound, and general intractability.

NONMEDICINAL THERAPY

There are relatively few means of symptomatically reversing a migraine attack without medication. Actions that can be taken include applying ice; taking refuge in a cool, quiet, dark environment; practicing biofeedback and relaxation techniques; and inducing sleep.

Nonmedicinal therapies that might, to a greater or lesser extent, have a prophylactic value include biofeedback and stress management training; discontinuance of smoking; maintaining the same schedule of activities from one day to the next; and avoiding foods and circumstances that may provoke headache. Treating other comorbid or confounding medical conditions (such as rebound) may be very helpful, if not critical.

PHARMACOTHERAPY OF MIGRAINE

Either a symptomatic or a preventive approach (or both) can be chosen. Applying both approaches simultaneously is necessary when attack frequency warrants preventive measures, but breakthrough headaches require symptomatic treatment. Even under the best preventive circumstances, acute attacks may occur.

Ideally, symptomatic therapy reverses or controls the headache and accompaniments once the attack has begun, whereas preventive therapy minimizes the frequency and intensity of anticipated attacks.

Symptomatic treatment alone should be chosen in the following circumstances:

1. When acute attacks occur no more than two times per week
2. When the use of symptomatic treatment is effective and not contraindicated by other health factors

Preventive therapy should be used in the following circumstances:

1. When attacks of migraine occur at a frequency greater than two per week

2. When, despite the infrequency of attacks, the devastating nature of the condition makes the use of daily (preventive) medication worthwhile
3. When symptomatic medications are contraindicated or ineffective

The following *general guidelines* should be employed in considering the treatment of migraine:

1. Provide sufficient, but not excessive, symptomatic treatment, perhaps allowing the patient to have alternatives for moderate and severe attacks, so that excursions to the emergency room are not necessary. Firm limits on frequency and usage are required.
2. Use nasal spray, rectal, or parenteral forms of symptomatic medication as alternatives for attacks that are not responsive to oral medication.
3. The use of nasal, rectal, or parenteral forms of medication are essential when attacks are accompanied by significant nausea or vomiting or when there is evidence, as is often the case, of delayed gastrointestinal absorption (gastroparesis), which can be present even in mild attacks.
4. If necessary, employ the use of adjunctive oral metoclopramide to reverse gastroparesis and improve absorption when oral symptomatic medications are administered.
5. Employ preventive treatment when criteria are met, and use symptomatic treatment for breakthrough attacks.
6. Develop a combination of symptomatic and preventive medication to establish ideal treatment outcomes.
7. Use preventive medication for several months, if effective, and then reconsider alternate treatment or the imposition of a "drug holiday."
8. Consider center-based care when treatment overuse or ineffective treatment occurs regularly, and prior to the development of complications or addiction/dependency syndromes.
9. Clinician availability is essential for advice for acute attacks not responsive to at-home treatment if patient compliance and an effective therapeutic relationship is to develop.

SPECIFIC TREATMENT APPROACHES

SYMPTOMATIC TREATMENT: THE AURA

The aura of migraine, when present, rarely requires treatment, and it is not certain that medications provide any meaningful benefit. There is anecdotal evidence that the use of sublingual nifedipine (10 mg) to reverse focal neurologic disturbances has been successful, but it is generally unnecessary, since the symptoms usually reverse within 10 to 20 minutes spontaneously. For severe, recurrent, neurologically dramatic aura, nifedipine may be advisable. Nifedipine may intensify the headache phase that is likely to follow. Anecdotally, aspirin has been used during the aura as a means of preventing stroke risk, although there are no data to suggest that this is effective or necessary.

SYMPTOMATIC TREATMENT: THE HEADACHE

For treatment of the headache, the following groups of medication can be used:

Moderate intermittent attacks

1. Simple analgesics, mixed analgesics, hydroxyzine
2. Nonsteroidal anti-inflammatory agents
3. Oral or nasal spray antimigraine medications (ergotamine tartrate, isometheptene [Midrin], oral or nasal spray sumatriptan,[1] dihydroergotamine [DHE] nasal spray, oral naratriptan,[1] oral zolmitriptan[1])

Moderate to severe intermittent attacks

1. Rectal NSAIDs (indomethacin)
2. Mixed analgesics (Fiorinal, Esgic, etc.)
3. Specific antimigraine medications (rectal ergotamine tartrate,[1] DHE nasal spray,[1] oral or nasal spray sumatriptan,[1] naratriptan,[1] zolmitriptan,[1] Midrin)
4. Mixed analgesics/opiate preparations (containing codeine, oxycodone, hydrocodone, etc.)

Severe intermittent attacks

1. Rectal ergotamine
2. Parenteral DHE/nasal spray DHE[1]

3. Parenteral sumatriptan/nasal spray sumatriptan
4. IM ketorolac[2]
5. Rectal barbiturate
6. Rectal opiates (morphine sulfate)
7. Rectal/parenteral neuroleptic (phenothiazine)
8. Nasal butorphanol[3]

Treatment of nausea, vomiting, and diarrhea

1. Oral, rectal/parenteral neuroleptics
2. Oral antidiarrheic agents

PREVENTIVE MEDICATIONS FOR MIGRAINE

The categories of drugs that have been found most useful in migraine prophylaxis are:

1. Beta adrenergic blockers
2. Calcium channel blockers
3. Antidepressants [tricyclic antidepressants, fluoxetine, monoamine oxidase inhibitors (MAOI)]
4. Ergot derivatives (methysergide, methylergonovine, ergonovine maleate)
5. Nonsteroidal anti-inflammatory drugs
6. Anticonvulsants (valproate, phenytoin, clonazepam)

Beta adrenergic blockers, the mainstay for many years for preventive treatment, include such important agents as propranolol and nadolol. This author prefers nadolol in a dose of 20–60 mg twice a day, provided blood pressure and cardiac rate are able to tolerate beta adrenergic blockade, and provided contraindications, such as asthma, congestive heart failure, Raynaud's phenomenon, and peripheral and cerebrovascular disease, are not present.

---

[1] Ergot derivatives, such as ergotamine tartrate and DHE, and the "triptans" should not be given to patients with coronary artery disease, severe hypertension, peripheral vascular disease, Prinzmetal's angina, or cerebral vascular disease. These drugs should be withheld until appropriate screening can occur to rule out occult disease in patients at significant risk, including those with significant hyperlipidemia, a family history of early heart disease, severe diabetes, or hypertension. These drugs should not be given to patients who are pregnant, and sumatriptan should not be given to patients taking MAOIs.

[2] Ketorolac should be restricted to no more than 3 days of usage in a row and should be given at the lowest possible dose of efficacy. Renal disease and gastrointestinal bleeding are risk factors. The drug should be withheld from anyone at high risk for renal disease, including patients who are dehydrated, have renovascular disease, have other major kidney ailments, or are particularly impaired physiologically. Dosages should be significantly reduced in the elderly population.

[3] Stadol Nasal Spray (nasal butorphanol) should not be used more than 2 days per week and should be avoided in patients with high risk for addictive disease or obsessive drug taking patterns, and in those with daily or frequent headaches. Overuse and physical dependency are potentially a problem. Withdrawal and absence symptoms can be severe.

Antidepressants, such as amitriptyline, nortriptyline, and others, have an important place in migraine prophylaxis. They can be used alone or in combination with beta adrenergic blockers or calcium channel blockers. Amitriptyline and nortriptyline are the most frequently used tricyclic antidepressants for headache phenomena. The value of serotonin specific receptor inhibitors (SSRIs) remains uncertain.

Calcium channel blockers have less efficacy than beta adrenergic blockers. However, verapamil, more than the other calcium channel blockers, may be effective in treating migraine (and cluster headache) and should be considered when beta adrenergic blockers have either failed or are contraindicated.

Recently, valproate in divided dosages totaling 1–2 grams per day has been found effective in the preventive treatment of migraine and daily chronic headache. This agent is recommended when first-line therapies such as beta adrenergic blockers, TCAs, and calcium channel blockers are not effective or contraindicated, and when the condition of the patient warrants this level of care.

Methysergide (Sansert) or methylergonovine (Methergine) are appropriate, as are MAOIs (specifically, phenelzine), when more aggressive treatment is required. Methysergide and methylergonovine are also useful in patients when hypotension is present, which would be aggravated by beta adrenergic blockade, calcium channel blockade, tricyclic antidepressants, or MAOIs. Ergot derivatives, when used preventively, should be discontinued after approximately 6 months for at least a 1-month drug holiday. It is also advisable to evaluate the patient for the presence of fibrotic lesions, including retroperitoneal fibrosis, pulmonary fibrosis, and cardiovalvular fibrosis. Recommended studies include chest x-ray, cardiac auscultation, and computed tomography scan of the abdomen with contrast enhancement, or MRI of abdomen with enhancement.

PRINCIPLES OF PREVENTIVE MEDICATION USE

The following principles should be employed:

1. Select the appropriate initial agent.
2. Increase dose at a reasonable pace, carefully monitoring for adverse effects, including changes in blood pressure, pulse rate, etc.
3. If ineffective after several weeks or months at therapeutic levels, add a complementary treatment or discontinue and begin another preventive treatment.
4. Combined preventive treatment is necessary in difficult-to-control cases.

COMBINATION PREVENTIVE TREATMENT

Combinations of medications are required for difficult-to-manage cases, when risk considerations allow combined usage. Careful monitoring and screening for cardiac, liver, and renal abnormalities and blood pressure and pulse abnormalities are mandatory. The clinician must be aware of additive effects, such as anticholinergic influence, vasoconstriction, and liver toxicity.

The following combinations may be used:

1. Beta adrenergic blocker and antidepressant
2. Calcium channel antagonist and antidepressant
3. Calcium channel antagonist and ergot derivative
4. Nonsteroidal anti-inflammatory agent with calcium channel antagonist or beta adrenergic blocker or antidepressant
5. An MAOI and appropriate tricyclic antidepressants, such as amitriptyline or nortriptyline. *(This combination must be used with special care, patient education, and monitoring, and when the clinician is well experienced in the use and administration of both MAOI and tricyclic antidepressants.)* When using amitriptyline or nortriptyline along with an MAOI (phenelzine), it is mandatory to either begin the tricyclic antidepressant and MAOI simultaneously, or to add the phenelzine to an existing regimen of amitriptyline or nortriptyline. Do not add amitriptyline or nortriptyline to an existing program of an MAOI.

The following combinations must be avoided because of serious adverse consequences when used together (Table 7-1):

1. Fluoxetine and MAOI (the serotonin syndrome with the risk of fatal outcome)
2. MAOI and meperidine (potentially fatal)
3. High-dose beta adrenergic blockade or calcium channel blockade and MAOI (severe hypotension)
4. Midrin (isometheptene) with MAOI (hypertension)
5. MAOI and Tegretol (hypertensive crisis)
6. Fluoxetine and lipophilic beta blockers (e.g., propranolol, metoprolol) (by inhibiting the P-450 enzyme system, may result in unexpected increases in blood levels, causing hypotension and heart block)

When switching from MAOI to fluoxetine, a wait of 3 to 5 weeks is mandatory after discontinuing the MAOI and before administering fluoxetine. When *(text continues on page 97)*

Table 7-1. Selected Drugs Used in the Pharmacotherapy of Head, Neck, and Face Pain[a]

DRUG NAME	MG/DOSE	STANDARD DAILY ADMIN.	NOTES
SYMPTOMATIC DRUGS			
Analgesics Excedrin[b]	—	varies	Avoid more than 2 days/wk of use
NSAIDs			
Naproxen sodium[b] (p.o.)	275–550	bid–tid	Avoid extended, daily use
Indocin SR	75	1 q day or bid	Avoid extended, daily use
Indomethacin (p.o.)	25–50	bid–tid	Avoid extended, daily use
Indomethacin supp.	50	bid–tid	Avoid extended, daily use
Meclofenamate (p.o.)	50–200	bid	Avoid extended, daily use
Ibuprofen[b] (p.o.)	600–800	bid–tid	Avoid extended, daily use
Ketorolac (p.o.)	10	qid	Avoid extended, daily use
Ketorolac (IM)	30	tid	Avoid extended, daily use. Appears particularly valuable when ergot derivatives and narcotics must be avoided and parenteral therapy is necessary. No more than occasional, short-term use is advisable because of renal toxicity, most likely in predisposed patients
Special Migraine Drugs			
Isometheptene[b] combinations (Midrin, etc.)	—	2 caps at onset, 1–2 q 30–60 min	Max 5–6 caps/day; 2 days/wk
Ergotamine tartrate[b] (ET)			
Oral (Cafergot, Wigraine, etc.)	1 mg ET, 100 mg caffeine	2 tabs at onset, 1–2 q 30–60 min	Max 4–6/day; 2 days/wk
Suppositories (Cafergot, Wigraine)	2 mg ET, 100 mg caffeine	⅓–1 at onset; may repeat in 60 min × 1	Max 2/day; 2 days/wk
Sublingual (Ergomar, Ergostat)	2 mg ET	1 at onset; may repeat after 15 min × 1	Max 2/day; 2 days/wk
Dihydroergotamine[b] (DHE)			
Intramuscular	0.25–1	0.25–1 mg SC, IM tid	Can be used 2–3 times/day in conjunction with antinauseant, analgesic, etc. IM more effective than SC
Intravenous	0.25–1		Can be used 2–3 times/day in conjunction with antinauseant, analgesic, etc. IM more effective than SC
DHE nasal spray[b]	1 mg	1 spray each nostril (½ mg/spray); may repeat in 15–30 min (4 sprays – 2 mg)	Use no more than 2–3 times/week, on separate days
Sumatriptan[b]			
(Parenteral)	6 mg SC	May repeat in 1 hr	Cannot be used within 24 hours of ergotamine-related meds or other triptans; should not be used in presence of cardiovascular, cerebrovascular, severe hypertension, Prinzmetal angina, or peripheral vascular disorders; no more than 2 doses in 24 hours; limit to 2 days/week usage

(continued)

TABLE 7-1. *(Continued)*

DRUG NAME	MG/DOSE	STANDARD DAILY ADMIN.	NOTES
(Oral)[b]	25–50 mg	1–2 at onset; may repeat at 2 hrs; max 100–200 mg/day	Cannot be used within 24 hours of ergotamine-related meds or other triptans; should not be used in presence of cardiovascular, cerebrovascular, severe hypertension, Prinzmetal angina, or peripheral vascular disorders; no more than 2 doses in 24 hours; limit to 2 days/week usage
(Nasal spray)[b]	5 or 20 mg	1 spray in 1 nostril; may repeat in 2 hrs; max 40 mg/24 hrs	Cannot be used within 24 hours of ergotamine-related meds or other triptans; should not be used in presence of cardiovascular, cerebrovascular, severe hypertension, Prinzmetal angina, or peripheral vascular disorders; no more than 2 doses in 24 hours; limit to 2 days/week usage
Zolmitriptan[b] (Oral)	2.5–5 mg	1 at onset; may repeat in 2 hrs	Cannot be used within 24 hours of ergotamine-related meds or other triptans; should not be used in presence of cardiovascular, cerebrovascular, severe hypertension, Prinzmetal angina, or peripheral vascular disorders. No more than 2 doses in 24 hours. Limit 2 days/week usage
Naratriptan[b] (Oral)	2.5 mg	1 at onset; may repeat in 2 hrs	Cannot be used within 24 hours of ergotamine-related meds or other triptans; should not be used in presence of cardiovascular, cerebrovascular, severe hypertension, Prinzmetal angina, or peripheral vascular disorders. No more than 2 doses in 24 hours. Limit 2 days/week usage
Rizatriptan[b] (Oral)	5–10 mg	1–2 at onset; may repeat in 2 hrs; max 40 mg/day	Cannot be used within 24 hours of ergotamine-related meds or other triptans; should not be used in presence of cardiovascular, cerebrovascular, severe hypertension, Prinzmetal angina, or peripheral vascular disorders. No more than 2 doses in 24 hours. Limit 2 days/week usage
Antinauseants/Neuroleptics Chlorpromazine Oral	25–100	bid–tid	Limit 3 days/wk, except for persistent nausea; avoid extended use; monitor for hypotension
Suppository	25–100	bid–tid	Limit 3 days/wk, except for persistent nausea; avoid extended use; monitor for hypotension

TABLE 7-1. *(Continued)*

DRUG NAME	MG/DOSE	STANDARD DAILY ADMIN.	NOTES
Intramuscular	25–100	bid–tid	Limit 3 days/wk, except for persistent nausea; avoid extended use; monitor for hypotension
Intravenous	—	—	—
Metoclopramide			
Oral—tablet, syrup	10–20	tid	Limit 3 days/wk, except for persistent nausea; avoid extended use; monitor for hypotension
Parenteral	10–15	tid	Limit 3 days/wk, except for persistent nausea; avoid extended use; monitor for hypotension
Promethazine			
Oral	25–75	tid	Limit 3 days/wk, except for persistent nausea; avoid extended use; monitor for hypotension
Intramuscular	25–75	tid	Limit 3 days/wk, except for persistent nausea; avoid extended use; monitor for hypotension
Perphenazine			
Oral	6–8	bid–tid	Limit 3 days/wk, except for persistent nausea; avoid extended use; monitor for hypotension
Intramuscular	5	bid	Limit 3 days/wk, except for persistent nausea; avoid extended use; monitor for hypotension
Droperidol			
Intramuscular	1.25–5	bid–tid	Limit 3 days/wk, except for persistent nausea; avoid extended use; monitor for hypotension
Intravenous	1.25–5	bid–tid	Limit 3 days/wk, except for persistent nausea; avoid extended use; monitor for hypotension
Antihistamines			
Hydroxyzine (p.o.)	50–100	bid–tid or at h.s.	Can be used as a symptomatic treatment
Cyproheptadine (p.o.)	2–4	tid–qid	Can be used as a symptomatic treatment
Steroids			
Prednisone	40–60	in 1 or divided doses	4–10 day program; avoid repeated use
PREVENTIVE DRUGS[c]			
Tricyclic antidepressants			
Amitriptyline	10–150	Divided doses or h.s.	Bedtime dose aids sleep disturbance
Nortriptyline	10–100	Divided doses or h.s.	Bedtime dose aids sleep disturbance
Doxepin	10–150	Divided doses or h.s.	Bedtime dose aids sleep disturbance

(continued)

TABLE 7-1. *(Continued)*

DRUG NAME	MG/DOSE	STANDARD DAILY ADMIN.	NOTES
Other antidepressants			
Fluoxetine	20	20–80 mg/day in divided doses	Actual efficacy for headache uncertain; Administer with care to patients using lipophilic beta blockers, such as propranolol, metoprolol, etc., or switch to hydrophilic beta blockers such as nadolol
Others (SSRIs, etc.)			Value for headache of numerous other antidepressants still under investigation
MAO inhibitors			
Phenelzine	15–30	15–60 mg/day in divided doses	Dietary and medicine restrictions mandatory
Beta adrenergic blockers			
Propranolol[b]	20–80	tid–qid (standard dose)	Monitor cardiac function, BP, pulse, lipids
Inderal LA[b]	80–160	bid	Monitor cardiac function, BP, pulse, lipids
Atenolol	50–100	bid	Monitor cardiac function, BP, pulse, lipids
Timolol[b]	10–20	bid	Monitor cardiac function, BP, pulse, lipids
Metoprolol	50–100	bid	Monitor cardiac function, BP, pulse, lipids
Nadolol	20–120	bid	Monitor cardiac function, BP, pulse, lipids. Metabolized by kidneys
Calcium channel blockers			
Verapamil	80–160	tid–qid	Monitor cardiac function, BP, pulse
Nimodipine	30–60	tid	Monitor cardiac function, BP, pulse
Diltiazem	30–90	tid	Monitor cardiac function, BP, pulse
Ergotamine derivatives			
Methysergide[b]	1–2	tid–5×/day	After 6-month treatment, review cardiac, pulmonary, and retroperitoneal regions for fibrotic changes; carefully observe contraindications
Methylergonovine	0.2–0.4	tid–qid	After 6-month treatment, review cardiac, pulmonary, and retroperitoneal regions for fibrotic changes; carefully observe contraindications
Anticonvulsants			
Valproate[b]	125–500	1–2 g/day in divided doses	Monitor hepatic and metabolic parameters carefully; consider dose reduction when used with antidepressants, lithium, verapamil, phenothiazines, other anticonvulsants; observe warnings carefully

TABLE 7-1. *(Continued)*

DRUG NAME	MG/DOSE	STANDARD DAILY ADMIN.	NOTES
Carbamazepine	100–200	300–1200 mg/day in divided doses	Monitor hepatic and metabolic parameters carefully; consider dose reduction when used with anticonvulsants, lithium, verapamil, phenothiazines, other anticonvulsants; observe warnings carefully; *reduces oral contraceptive efficacy*
Gabapentin	100–400	1600–2800 mg/day	Actual value for headache uncertain; may cause agitation and other CNS adverse effects
Others			
Baclofen (Lioresal)	10–20	tid–qid	Increase dose slowly and allow tolerance to develop
Lithium	150–300	bid–tid	Reduce dose in conjunction with verapamil and other calcium antagonists; monitor metabolic parameters
Oxygen inhalation	100% O_2 w/mask	7 liters/min for 10–15 min	Must be used at onset of attack of cluster headache; avoid around extreme heat or flame, such as cigarettes
Stadol nasal spray (butorphanol)	Limit use to no more than 2 dosage days/wk		Useful for acute migraine, but important side effects; dependency and addictive potential significant; avoid in patients with addictive or obsessive drug-taking patterns or history of drug overuse; avoid in patients with daily or almost daily headache; withdrawal symptoms can be severe

[a] Few of the medications listed in this table are either approved specifically for headache or have been shown by controlled studies to be effective for headache. Their inclusion reflects that they have been recommended from various sources as possibly useful for the treatment of some cases of headache.
[b] Approved by the FDA for the treatment of migraine, cluster headache, or tension-type headache.
[c] Avoid sustained use for more than 6 months without trial reduction.
Modified with permission from Saper JL, Silberstein SD, Gordon CD et al. Handbook of Headache Management. New York: Lippincott Williams & Wilkins, 1998.
bid = twice a day; tid = three times a day; h.s. = at bedtime; p.o. = orally; IM = intramuscularly; SC = subcutaneously; BP = blood pressure; CNS = central nervous system.

switching from fluoxetine to MAOI, a wait of 5 weeks is mandatory after discontinuing fluoxetine and before administering MAOI. Also, never switch from one MAOI to another without a 3- to 5-week interval.

REBOUND OR TOXIC HEADACHE SYNDROMES

The excessive and frequent use of symptomatic medications that include symptomatic ergot derivatives (ergotamine tartrate), analgesics, and perhaps high-dose nonsteroidal anti-inflammatory drugs results in a headache–medication cycle referred to as rebound headache or analgesic rebound headache. This is a self-sustaining clinical phenomenon, *rendering otherwise preventive medications ineffective until discontinuance and withdrawal of the offending agent occurs.* Withdrawal may require hospitalization and time to stabilize physiologic systems before preventive medications will be effective in reducing the frequency or intensity of attacks.

The key features of this syndrome include the following:

1. Insidious increase of headache frequency
2. Dependable and irresistible use of increasing amounts of offending agents at regular, predictable intervals
3. Failure of alternate medications or preventive medications to control headache attacks
4. Development of psychologic and/or physiologic dependency
5. Predictable onset of headache within hours to days following the last dose of symptomatic treatment
6. Awakening with a headache at the same time each day when this has not been a feature of past headache patterns

TREATMENT OF MENSTRUAL MIGRAINE

Menstrual migraine often requires aggressive and innovative treatments, combining preventive and symptomatic approaches. The following are recommended.

Symptomatic Medications:

1. NSAIDS/Midrin
2. Ergotamine tartrate (oral or rectal)
3. Parenteral DHE/nasal spray DHE
4. Parenteral, nasal spray, or oral sumatriptan, zolmitriptan, or naratriptan
5. Opiate or related analgesics (oral, rectal, or nasal spray)

Preventive Medications:

1. Standard preventive agents described previously
2. Short preventive course of DHE, ergotamine tartrate, or a triptan (4 to 5 days), just around the menstrual period
3. Hormonal manipulation (i.e., estrogen patch applied prior to headache onset)

Often a combination of preventive and symptomatic treatment is required. Preventive treatment should be started several days before predictable onset of headache vulnerability and continue 2 to 4 days after menses begins. An estrogen patch (Estraderm, 0.05 mg) should be administered several days prior to onset of menstrual headache, presumably to reduce the precipitous fall of premenstrual estradiol, thought to incite the headache.

TREATMENT OF INTRACTABLE, SEVERE MIGRAINE

Acute, intractable (persistent, progressive) migraine is defined as a sustained (persistent, non-self-limited), severe migraine and accompaniments, not effectively terminated by appropriate outpatient interventions. This condition requires continuing acute therapeutic treatment over a day or longer, sometimes as long as 8 to 10 days. Intractable, severe migraine is synonymous with that previously called *status migrainosis,* causing severe debilitation if the condition is protracted.

The clinical features of acute, intractable migraine can include:

1. Continuing, persistent, severe head, neck, or face pain
2. Progressive physical and emotional accompaniments, such as the following:

    Nausea, vomiting, anorexia, and diarrhea

    Dehydration

    Despair/depression

    Alteration of normal sleeping, eating, and activities of daily living

    Additional migraine accompaniments, including focal neurologic symptoms, malaise, and photosensitivity

3. Toxicity and/or withdrawal symptoms from excessive use of symptomatic medications

Treatment Principles

The treatment of intractable headache departs markedly from the treatment of more ordinary headache events. These patients often require parenteral pain therapy, rehydration, control of nausea and vomiting, removal of provoking factors, general psychologic and physiologic support, and monitoring, often in acute care settings. Rebound or analgesic toxicity is a common accompaniment. Dehydration may result from a combination of factors, including reduced fluid intake over days or weeks; increased fluid and electrolyte loss through emesis, anorexia, diarrhea, and polyuria; and diaphoresis.

Factors that contribute to acute, intractable migraine include drug-related causes, including rebound; endocrine disturbances, including estrogen replacement or the use of oral contraceptives; and the presence of comorbid, intracranial, cranial, cervical, or systemic disease, particularly if pathways of the trigeminal system or of the occipitocervical junction are involved. Head injury and severe, intense psychologic duress are other contributing factors.

Choosing the Proper Setting for Treatment

Emergency department treatment is appropriate in the following cases:

1. To treat moderate to severe intermittent headache, *unaccompanied by drug toxicity, dependency, or rebound*
2. To rapidly rule out severe neurologic or medical illness (e.g., subarachnoid hemorrhage)
3. When headaches are associated with acute suicidal potential

Emergency department services are inappropriate in the following cases:

1. For persistent, continuous intractable headache
2. For dehydration, electrolyte depletion, or hypotension that requires prolonged therapy or sustained monitoring
3. For toxic/rebound or dependency states that require days to weeks to resolve
4. For intractable nausea, vomiting, or diarrhea that may require many hours or days of treatment and that may recur
5. When concurrent medical illness influences or limits the effectiveness of treatment of headache
6. When there is a likelihood of delayed withdrawal, with potential for marked increase in pain, seizures, diarrhea, leg or abdominal cramps, etc.
7. When a pattern of multiple emergency department treatments is observed
8. When it is unlikely that emergency department therapy will be able to address the headache patient's needs promptly and effectively

Criteria for Hospitalization

The following criteria to justify hospital admission are based on the modified admission criteria established jointly by the Michigan Head–Pain & Neurological Institute in Ann Arbor, in conjunction with Blue Cross/Blue Shield of Michigan.

1. Moderate-to-severe, intractable headache, failing to respond to appropriate and aggressive outpatient or emergency department services, and requiring repetitive, sustained, parenteral treatment
2. The presence of continuing nausea, vomiting, and diarrhea

3. The need to detoxify and treat toxicity, dependency, or rebound phenomena, requiring monitoring services against withdrawal symptoms, including seizures
4. The presence of dehydration, electrolyte imbalance, and prostration, requiring monitoring and intravenous (IV) fluids for the presence of unstable vital signs
5. The presence of repeated, previous emergency department treatments
6. The presence of serious concurrent disease [e.g., subarachnoid hemorrhage, intracranial infection, cerebral ischemia, severe hypertension or hypotension]
7. The need to develop, simultaneously, an effective pharmacologic prophylaxis to sustain improvement achieved by parenteral therapy
8. The presence of confounding comorbid conditions
9. Concurrent medical and/or psychologic illness requiring careful monitoring in high-risk situations (e.g., severe hypotension, coronary artery disease)

Specific Treatment Protocols

In an Emergency Department Setting. In addition to supportive and monitoring measures, including the ruling out of comorbid disease, the following *parenteral* treatment protocols are appropriate:

1. Intramuscular or IV DHE (Table 7-2)
2. Ketorolac
3. Narcotics
4. IV phenothiazine (see later)
5. Antiemetics
6. Others (sumatriptan, zolmitriptan, or naratriptan)

Hospital Treatment. Parenteral protocols include the following:

1. IV DHE (see Table 7-2)
2. IV phenothiazines [chlorpromazine (7.5–15 mg in 25–50 cc saline, by drip or slow push for 2 min); given two or three times a day, with careful monitoring for orthostatic hypotension and other adverse effects for several hours after administration; IV diphenhydramine used if acute dystonic reactions occur]
3. Hydrocortisone (100 mg IV push, given every 6 hours for 24 hours, every 8 hours for 24 hours, and every 12 hours for 24 hours); regimen should be limited because of the potential for

adverse effects, including remote possibility of avascular necrosis of bone

Although pharmacologic therapy may interrupt the headache, many difficult- and chronic-headache patients require much more for sustained benefit. In addition to effective prophylaxis and symptomatic treatment of acute breakthrough headaches, behavioral therapies, treatment of obsessive drug-taking tendencies, frank psychotherapy, and family therapy are often required. Exercise programs, improvement in general health, dietary control, and stabilization of life activities are often required in difficult cases. Patients with personality disorders require ongoing limit-setting and "boundary" determination.

TABLE 7-2. Intravenous Protocol for Dihydroergotamine (DHE) Administration

Protocol

- Administer 0.25–0.5 mg IV "push" (test dose), over 2 minutes via heparin lock apparatus.
- If tolerated, administer DHE 0.5–1 mg IV "push" q 8 hours for 3–5 days.
- Administer 10 mg metoclopramide (IV[a] or IM) before DHE administration, if nausea occurs.
- Maintain for 3–5 days, if tolerated. May repeat program one time.

Guidelines for Use

1. Administer metoclopramide before or at DHE administration if necessary to control nausea. Discontinue if not necessary.
2. DHE is to be administered via 1–2 minute slow "push."
3. Most patients stabilize at end of day 3, but extension of program for 2–3 more days may be necessary.
4. Discontinue DHE via a 1–3 day gradual reduction program if patient is pain free for 2 days or fails to respond after 3 days.
5. Hospitalization is most appropriate for therapy, during which careful monitoring for blood pressure elevation, chest pain, severe nausea, etc. can be carried out, and necessary concurrent therapies can be administered, including establishment of an effective preventive program.
6. Discontinue or substantially reduce dose if severe nausea, chest pain, severe leg cramps, or other significant adverse reactions occur.

---

[a] 10 mg slow "IV push" or in 50 cc dextrose in water (D5W) over 20–30 minutes.

TREATMENT OF CLUSTER HEADACHE

The symptomatic treatment of cluster headache is limited because many of the therapies that are useful cannot be used daily. Oxygen inhalation can be effective, at 7 l/min, with 100% oxygen given via a mask at the onset of each attack. Indocin may be occasionally effective by rectal form but is generally not efficacious, except for variant attacks. Sumatriptan and ergotamine tartrate can reverse an attack but are not appropriate for daily usage. Intranasal capsaicin and intranasal lidocaine may have a role occasionally. Data are limited on their effectiveness. Parenteral treatments, such as DHE and ketorolac, may also reverse an individual attack, but chronic or sustained usage is a problem. Periactin (cyproheptadine), an antihistamine with serotonergic properties, may be used in some cases. Sedation and weight gain are common untoward effects.

Preventive treatment of cluster headache is the most appropriate intervention, since most attacks occur daily, and cycles last for weeks, months, or longer. A 7- or 10-day burst of prednisone at 60 mg a day with taper during the burst is recommended for difficult-to-break attacks. High-dose verapamil in dosages ranging from 120 mg three times a day to 160 mg four times a day (short-acting form) is highly effective in many individuals. Lithium at a dose of 150–300 mg three times a day can be used as primary prophylaxis or in conjunction with other agents, although an interaction with verapamil occurs and verapamil and lithium should be maintained at lower-than-usual dosages when they are used together. Valproic acid, methysergide, and methyleronovine are also effective in prophylaxis. Daily chlorpromazine may be useful in some individuals, and for refractory attacks, low-dose daily ergotamine has been used with severe limitations.

The effectiveness of these agents is individualized, and combination therapies are used in refractory cases. Some individuals with refractory headaches have used maintenance opioids for the duration of the cycle, but the ratio of risk to value is an important consideration.

Surgical intervention can be considered in patients with truly refractory attacks. Surgical considerations should be considered in chronic cluster headache patients, in those without remission for at least 1 year, and in those who are totally resistant to aggressive medical management for a "reasonable" period of time. Also, surgical intervention should be restricted to those patients who have strictly unilateral pain and who are physiologically stable, not prone to medication overuse, and otherwise medically and mentally healthy.

As previously described for migraine, hospitalization may be necessary for intractable cases.

COMPREHENSIVE CENTERS AND "HEADACHE SPECIALISTS"

Although comprehensive, multidisciplinary intervention is not available in most communities, this intensive treatment is appropriate for difficult and complex patients who have not responded to appropriate local and regional care facilities. Outcome studies from the Michigan Head–Pain & Neurological Institute in Ann Arbor have shown a sustained and noteworthy reduction in pain, depression, symptomatic drug use, and emergency room utilization, along with a return to work in a statistically significant and impressive number of patients who had previously been disabled prior to inpatient treatment. This study represented a 2-year prospective analysis of patients with daily, severe headache who were admitted to the hospital unit.

Criteria for referral to comprehensive centers include the following:

1. History of recurring, intractable acute-care needs or progressive, persistent headache
2. Multiple diagnostic and therapeutic interventions by qualified physicians without successful outcome
3. Evidence of excessive utilization of outpatient services, diagnostic procedures, or repeated hospitalizations for narcotic analgesics or other parenteral treatments
4. Uncertain or questionable diagnoses
5. The need for comprehensive, multidisciplinary services to address the multifactorial components of the patient's case, including confounding comorbid conditions

QUESTIONS AND DISCUSSION

1. Which of the following medications is not considered a treatment for cluster headaches?

A. Lithium
B. Methysergide
C. Prednisone
D. Verapamil
E. Inderal

The answer is (E). Beta blockers are not effective for the treatment of cluster headaches.

2. Which of the following medications is not appropriate for the prevention of migraine?

A. Valproic acid
B. Propranolol
C. Methysergide
D. Sumatriptan
E. Amitriptyline

The answer is (D). Sumatriptan is a symptomatic medication, the use of which should be restricted to 2 days per week. It is not generally considered a preventive drug.

3. The avoidance of rebound headaches in patients with recurring migraine requires limiting analgesic or ergotamine tartrate medications to no more than:

A. 1 day/week
B. 2 days/week
C. 4 days/week
D. 5 days/week
E. 3 days/month

The answer is (B). Use more than 2 days/week generally places patients at risk for rebound headache.

4. Which of the following conditions most closely mimics cluster headache?

A. Cyclical migraine
B. Transformational migraine
C. Hemicrania continua
D. Chronic paroxysmal hemicrania
E. Carotid dissection

The answer is (D). Chronic paroxysmal hemicrania is a possible cluster headache variant with attacks that are generally shorter in duration and responsive only to indomethacin.

5. Aside from natural progression, the most cited reason for the transformation from intermittent migraine to daily persistent pain is which of the following?

A. Stress
B. Hormonal changes
C. Overuse of analgesics or ergotamine tartrate
D. The presence of another medical condition
E. Weather changes

The answer is (C). Overuse of analgesics or ergotamine tartrate (more than 2 day/week) is cited in the literature as a key factor for the induction of transformation from intermittent migraine to daily or almost daily headache.

SUGGESTED READING

Dalessio D, Silberstein SD (eds): Wolff's Headache and Other Head Pain, 6th Edition. New York, Oxford University Press, 1993

Goadsby PJ, Silberstein SD: Headache (Blue Books of Practical Neurology). Boston, Butterworth-Heine-mann, 1997

Lance JW: Mechanisms and Management of Head-ache, 5th Edition. London, Butterworth-Heine-mann, 1993

Lipton RB, Stewart WF: Epidemiology and comor-bidity of migraine. In: Headache: The Blue Books of Practical Neurology. Boston, Butterworth-Heinemann, 1997, pp. 75–95.

Olesen J, Tfelt-Hansen P, Welch KMA: The Head-aches. New York, Raven Press, 1993

Raskin NH. Headache, 2nd Edition. New York, Churchill Livingstone, 1988

Rose FC (ed): Handbook of Clinical Neurology, Vol. 48. Amsterdam, Elsevier Science Publishers, 1986

Saper JR: Diagnosis and symptomatic treatment of migraine. Headache 37(Supp 1): S1, 1997

Saper JR, Silberstein DS, Gordon CD, Hamel RL: Handbook of Headache Management. Baltimore, Williams and Wilkins, 1992

Silberstein SD (ed): Intractable Headache: Inpatient and Outpatient Treatment Strategies. Neurology 42(Suppl 2), 1992

Weiller C, May A, Limmroth V, et al.: Brainstem acti-vation in spontaneous human migraine attacks. Nature Med 1:658, 1995

Welch KMA: Drug therapy of migraine. N Engl J Med 329:1476, 1993

Neurology for the Non-Neurologist, Fourth Edition, edited by William J. Weiner and Christopher G. Goetz. Lippincott Williams & Wilkins, Philadelphia © 1999.

| C | H | A | P | T | E | R | 8 |

Epilepsy

Donna C. Bergen

What is a seizure, and who can have one? A convulsive seizure is one of the most dramatic occurrences in medical practice and in everyday life. Although the physical characteristics and the electroencephalographic phenomena of convulsions are well known, the pathophysiology of seizures is still being investigated. No one really knows why an individual attack starts precisely when it does, or even why it finally comes to an end. Anyone can have a generalized (or tonic–clonic) convulsive seizure in appropriate circumstances (e.g., brain hemorrhage, severe hypocalcemia, certain drug intoxications). The vexing question considered here, however, is why and how some people have seizures that occur unpredictably and recurrently, without an acute cause. This disorder is called epilepsy.

Although not all aspects of seizures are understood, we know that seizures occur when groups of cerebral neurons behave abnormally. Different types of seizures probably have different neuronal mechanisms. The most closely studied seizure type is the *focal cortical seizure*. The production of focal epilepsy requires the occurrence of certain types of brain injury such as penetrating head trauma, cerebral infarction, or brain tumor. The cause of focal epilepsy is obscure in many cases.

Brain injury and subsequent gliosis (scarring) alter the electrical properties of certain neurons, changing both their electrical firing properties and their ability to recruit and synchronize other neuronal activity. The basic cellular abnormality underlying these changes is not clear but may involve increased membrane permeability to sodium and calcium, selective loss of vital inhibitory neuronal input, functionally disruptive distortions of neuronal and glial anatomy, and neuronal damage and synaptic reorganization caused by excitotoxic neurotransmitter activity.

The pathophysiology of nonfocal seizures is even more obscure than that of focal epilepsy. In these disorders the entire cerebral cortex appears to participate in the generation of tonic-clonic "grand mal" attacks as well as in the brief losses of consciousness called *absence seizures*. In the latter case, widespread, congenital abnormalities in neuronal connections or excitability are thought to underlie the disease.

A clear perception of the varied types of epilepsy is necessary not only to understand its pathophysiology but also to be able to diagnose and treat the disorder accurately and successfully.

Some definitions of a few rather loosely used terms may help at this point (Table 8-1). *Tonic–clonic seizures* are generalized, convulsive seizures. Such attacks may begin *de novo*, without focal onset, in patients with primary generalized epilepsy. They may also result from the spread of localized seizure discharges from a cortical focus. Except for the onset of the attack, such secondary convulsions may look like those of primary generalized epilepsy.

An *absence attack* refers to a brief episode of loss of awareness. The term is occasionally wrongly applied to the complex partial seizure, a focal seizure usually arising from the temporal lobe, described in the section on focal epilepsy.

TABLE 8-1. Treatment of Common Seizure Types

Partial (focal) seizures	Phenytoin
Simple partial	Carbamazepine
Complex partial	Valproate
	Gabapentin
	Lamotrigine
	Topiramate
	Tiagabine
Tonic-clonic seizures	Gabapentin
	Lamotrigine
	Topiramate
	Tiagabine
Absence seizures	Valproate
	Ethosuximide
	Lamotrigine
Myoclonic seizures	Valproate
	Lamotrigine

Although somewhat mysterious in etiologic terms, perhaps the easiest types of epilepsy to deal with clinically are *primary generalized epilepsies*. The typical patient often has a first-degree relative with one or more parts of the syndrome (including febrile seizures). The type of seizure seen in these syndromes varies and includes generalized tonic–clonic convulsions, absence attacks, and myoclonic seizures. Absence seizures are typically brief, lasting less than 15 seconds; they occur without warning or aura; and they consist mainly of an arrest of behavior and a loss of responsiveness and awareness. Automatisms are sparse, often limited to rhythmic blinking. The patient may not be aware of the attack, and the spells often occur in clusters or many times throughout the day.

Myoclonic seizures are also brief, although often more dramatic. They range in intensity from a few brief bilaterally synchronous jerks of the arms or head nods, to more violent muscular contractions that may cause the patient to fall. The patient is often unaware of an attack (myoclonic petit mal seizure) and is unable to describe it.

Generalized tonic–clonic seizures are the type of seizure best known by the layperson. In primary generalized epilepsy, an attack begins with a sudden loss of consciousness, sometimes with a loud cry and stiffening of the limbs and trunk: the tonic phase of the seizure. The patient is apneic and is usually cyanotic. After 15 to 30 seconds, this posture begins to be interrupted by short, rhythmic, bilaterally synchronous jerks of the arms and legs; breathing remains ineffec-

tual. After 30 to 45 seconds these clonic movements slow and then stop. The muscles are then flaccid, respirations are deep, rapid, and often stertorous, and consciousness slowly returns. After a single convulsion, most patients are awake after 10 to 15 minutes, but postictal confusion may persist much longer. Such an attack is without an aura or any focal neurologic sign such as strong adversive head and eye movements or postictal hemiparesis. Obvious physical stresses and physiologic abnormalities may accompany these attacks, including hypoxemia, acidosis, and autonomic disruptions such as cardiac arrhythmias and hypertension. Pulmonary edema can occur and may play a role in the syndrome of sudden death that occurs occasionally even in young, otherwise healthy patients with epilepsy.

Patients with primary generalized epilepsy have normal neurologic examinations, they are of normal intelligence, and they give no history suggesting prior brain injury. The electroencephalogram (EEG) shows normal background activity, often interrupted by bursts of generalized spike and wave discharges. The condition usually becomes symptomatic in mid childhood or adolescence, or occasionally earlier in the guise of febrile convulsions of infancy. Pharmacologic control is usually successful. The eventual remission rate in some syndromes, such as childhood absence, is high, probably approaching 80%. Primary generalized epilepsy is not a common form of seizure disorder in adults, accounting for about 10% of patients in large epilepsy clinics.

Although it may present in a similar fashion, the pathophysiology and clinical implications of focal (partial) epilepsy are profoundly different from those of the genetic disorders. First, the occurrence of focal seizures almost always implies the existence of focal brain disease. Second, an almost unlimited variety of focal seizure types may be seen, depending on the site of brain injury. As in the diagnosis of all forms of epilepsy, taking a meticulous history not only from the patient but also from witnesses to the seizures is essential, because it is the precise sequence of events making up the attacks that reveals the site of seizure onset in the brain, and the route and extent of seizure propagation through the brain.

For example, a patient with a meningioma growing over the right cerebral hemisphere may present with focal motor seizures of the left leg due to irritation of nearby cerebral motor cortex by the tumor. Such an attack may spread down along the precentral (motor) gyrus, involving the contralateral arm before stopping in 1 or 2 minutes. If intrinsic cerebral inhibitory mechanisms and appropriate pharmacology fail, such a seizure may spread suddenly into thalamic and other brain structures with strong, widespread axonal projections, and a generalized convulsion ensues. Unless the clinician obtains the history of focal onset of such an attack, a mistaken diagnosis of primary generalized epilepsy may be made, and a search for localized brain disease may be left undone.

A completely different symptom complex may be reported by the patient with temporal lobe injury, such as that following head trauma, anoxia, or complicated febrile convulsions. A temporal lobe (psychomotor, complex partial, limbic) seizure often begins with a subjective experience such as a sudden feeling of strangeness, or an abrupt sensation of nausea that appears to move upward from the epigastrium. If the seizure discharges remain confined to a small area of the temporal lobe, the attack may not proceed further and may end in 30 to 60 seconds. If it spreads throughout both sides of the limbic system, consciousness may be lost. The patient may stare vacantly or may appear to look about, is usually unresponsive, and often makes simple movements (automatisms) such as lip smacking, grimacing, or hand wringing. He or she may stand or sit still or may walk about aimlessly. Because of the intimate relationship between limbic cortical structures and the hypothalamus, autonomic signs are common in complex partial seizures: flushing, piloerection, borborygmus, and sweating are examples. Should the seizure stop at that point, the ictal phenomena also stop abruptly, but the patient may remain confused for several minutes or longer, and if the seizure has started in the speech-dominant hemisphere, language function may be temporarily impaired postictally. On the other hand, if the ictal activity spreads even further, or generalizes, a full-fledged tonic–clonic seizure occurs. Patients may be able to describe vividly the aura (onset) of such attacks, but many temporal lobe seizures give no recalled warning before a loss of consciousness occurs, and the physician must rely on witnesses for a full description of the episodes.

Focal epilepsy, with or without secondary generalization of the attacks, is by far the most common form of seizure disorder seen by the primary care physician and by most neurologists. Within that category, complex partial seizures are the most prevalent type. Many patients with partial seizures find complete relief from attacks with medication, but about 30% continue to have some seizures even with competent medical advice and optimal therapy.

The clinical picture becomes even more complex in the patient with multifocal or diffuse brain injury. Such a person may be subject to two, three, or sometimes even more seizure types. Generalized motor convulsions, focal seizures of any type, or absence attacks may all occur chronically. Additional patterns may also be present, often as fragments (tonic seizures) or distinctive types of episodes such as sudden losses of muscle tone with falling (akinetic seizures). Such patients often bear other stigmata of cerebral injury such as mental retardation or cerebral palsy. In these cases, seizures are usually difficult if not impossible to control with drugs and are almost always lifelong.

Epilepsy is thus a chronic if not permanent condition for most patients, demanding daily anticonvulsant therapy for years, and the toll taken on many aspects of patients' lives is high. Epilepsy carries a stain of fear and shame for many of their friends, colleagues, and even family members. Although this attitude is gradually softening, epilepsy is still a condition often hidden from those outside the family (and sometimes from those inside as well). When the condition is poorly controlled, it can dominate and define relationships between parents and children, spouses, and siblings. Children are often sheltered excessively by parents and teachers, and social maturation is delayed or prevented. Suicide rates are above average.

The employability of those with epilepsy is also reduced. Some employers are reluctant to have a person with seizures on the premises, fearing injury and liability. Others worry over potentially higher medical costs for the employee. Even obtaining medical insurance may be difficult.

Difficulty with driving makes appropriate employment even more elusive. State regulations vary, but usually the seizure patient who cannot demonstrate complete, long-term control of the attacks is prohibited from driving. Public transport and car pools are often inadequate resources, and this problem alone makes working a major challenge for many people who have epilepsy. A diagnosis of epilepsy thus has far-reaching implications for the life of the patient. It is, therefore, essential that the diagnosis be neither missed nor misapplied.

Epilepsy is diagnosed by the patient's history and not by head scanning, EEG, or neurologic examination. In cases where a seizure disorder is seriously suspected, the physician must spend adequate time with the patient and others, to acquire a clear impression of the nature of the attacks.

First, simply asking what the attacks are like often produces a vague description as the patient produces a composite picture of his experiences. Asking for an account of the last episode, or of the last one the patient recalls well, will more often evoke precise details and a coherent impression. Physicians should ask what the patient was doing when the attack began. They should inquire about the first thing that occurred when the attack started, and what happened next. They should also ask how the patient felt after the episode ended, and if any focal weakness or speech difficulty was present.

Second, physicians should also ask if all the attacks were similar, or if and how they varied. Seizures are highly stereotyped events, like broken records. Unless there is more than one seizure type, each type with its own stereotypy, significant variation in the pattern of attacks argues against epilepsy.

Third, physicians should ask if anything tended to bring on an episode. Aside from unusual cases of "reflex epilepsy," in which specific physical stimuli reliably provoke seizures, epileptic attacks characteristically occur without warning, one of their most frightening aspects. Attacks which always begin during an argument with a girlfriend, or exclusively at home and never at work, may represent emotional symptoms rather than epilepsy.

Fourth, the duration of each attack should be appropriate. Except for brief absence or myoclonic seizures, most seizures last 30 seconds to 3 minutes, with additional postictal periods depending on the type of seizure. Episodes that last many minutes to hours are usually not epileptic.

Fifth, what do witnesses see and how does the attack begin? Patients with clear auras at the start of a seizure ("Oh, I'm going to have a seizure") may sometimes have postictal amnesia for a focal onset that was obvious to onlookers. The physician should inquire if the patient was fully or partially responsive during an attack.

The unwitnessed attack of "simple" loss of consciousness may not be as simple when carefully scrutinized. A diagnosis of neurogenic syncope should not be missed, since the typical prodrome is almost always remembered vividly by the patient. Giddiness, weakness, sweating, nausea, and fading or graying-out of vision are highly suggestive of true syncope. Witnesses report the unsupported victim of syncope as crumpling or sliding to the ground, whereas the patient with convulsions usually falls stiffly. The diagnosis may be made more difficult by myoclonic jerks, later reported as seizure activity (so-called *convulsive syncope*). Urinary incontinence is not rare in syncope but tongue biting is, so that this sign usually implies a convulsion.

Stokes–Adams attacks must be differentiated from seizures. The usual attack of unconsciousness has no warning. Again, the patient is seen to fall suddenly and limply to the ground. A witness is vital, since the movements of a generalized convulsion are unknown to the patient but are easily described by onlookers.

Syncope from cardiac arrhythmias rarely causes incontinence or tongue biting. The attacks are usually short, and consciousness is regained quickly and completely.

Discriminating between absence and complex partial seizures may also be a diagnostic hurdle, but one that is easily cleared. The former is probably overdiagnosed and is much rarer than the latter. Even patients often name their seizures incorrectly: most patients presenting to an epilepsy clinic with self-proclaimed "petit mal" attacks in fact have complex partial seizures. Making the correct diagnosis is important, because only one of the two seizure types implies the presence of focal brain disease, and the therapies for the two types are different.

If a reliable witness can be found, the two seizure types can be accurately distinguished by the duration of the attack. Almost all absence seizures last less than 15 seconds, and many are briefer. On the other hand, most complex partial seizures continue over 30 seconds, with many lasting a minute or two.

The patient often reports an aura for complex partial seizures, although this is not always the case. There is never an aura in absence epilepsy, and often the attacks are so subtle that the family usually reports many more seizures than the patient notices.

The absence seizure has no aftereffects, whereas several minutes or more of confusion often follow a complex partial seizure. In the latter, postictal language difficulty or other focal neurologic signs may be reported.

If confusion still exists after these points have been checked, the EEG may help. Three per second spike and wave activity is seen in over 80% of untreated absence patients, especially if hyperventilation is performed. Focal temporal spikes may be seen in complex partial seizures, but there is a dismaying 50% false-negative rate in a single EEG in patients with the disorder.

PSEUDOSEIZURES

Sometimes the most difficult differential diagnosis is between a seizure disorder and pseudoseizures, or seizure-like episodes of psychogenic origin. Like organic seizures, pseudoseizures vary tremendously in presentation, from convulsive-like episodes to transient alterations in consciousness or sensation. Faced with this diversity, one must fall back on the general rules previously discussed. Attacks that do not follow the usual "rules of behavior" of epilepsy should not be labeled as a seizure.

Episodes tightly related to stress or personal events and circumstances should be particularly scrutinized. Patients with epilepsy also often relate a correlation between seizures and stress, but the relationship is a loose one. The immediate triggering of an attack by an argument, for example, is typical of pseudoseizures.

After applying these general guides, a meticulous comparison between the pseudoseizure and the specific type of epileptic attack mimicked can further solidify the diagnosis. For example, the person with pseudoepileptic "grand mal" seizures may report an awareness of his or her surroundings during the throes of the attacks, which is an impossibility for a person in a convulsion. Full consciousness and accurate orientation may be regained instantly after the "seizure," which does not occur in genuine grand mal epilepsy.

Ancillary signs may not be of much diagnostic help. Urinary incontinence and even bodily injury occur with surprising frequency in pseudoseizures. Tongue biting is unusual but not unheard of.

A witness can sometimes provide small but highly suggestive clues. The pseudo–grand mal attack, for example, may include such atypical motor features as head shaking from side to side, or alternating (not synchronous) extension and flexion of the arms. Weeping is typical of pseudoseizures.

Even ictal and psychotic or functional hallucinations can usually be distinguished from one another. Psychotic hallucinations are usually complex and highly meaningful, often including auditory commands to do specific things. Likewise, functional "hallucinatory" experiences are colorful and varied, whereas the ictal experience is stereotyped, is not usually emotionally charged or significant, and is relatively brief.

The most elusive diagnosis often involves the pseudo–complex partial seizure. Here, the physician must rely on the monotonously repetitive nature of the true complex partial seizure. The onset of the true complex partial seizure, for example, may include distortions of reality or psychic perceptions that are impossible for the patient to describe satisfactorily. Nevertheless, the patient will usually admit that the experience is always the same from episode to episode, and that once an attack starts, it proceeds in a predictable manner. On the contrary, the pseudoseizure is typically varied from attack to attack, one time including "déjà vu," another time including numbness of the hands, another time nausea and dizziness, and so on. In general, the more varied, elaborate, and colorful the events of the episodes, the less likely they are to be epileptic.

If an attack occurs in the hospital or office, drawing a serum prolactin level within 15 minutes, and another 2 hours later, may clinch the diagnosis. Virtually all patients having a grand mal seizure are found to have greatly elevated serum prolactin levels immediately after the episode. (The 2-hour specimen is used as a *post hoc* "baseline" value.) Many, but not all, complex partial seizures also cause such elevations, so that a positive prolactin test is a reliable sign of epileptic activity, but a negative test is not helpful.

Occasionally, the only accurate way to distinguish seizures from pseudoseizures is to record an attack on EEG. This is often done with simultaneous video recording, so that the electrophysiologic and clinical characteristics of an episode may be defined and preserved for review. It is important to note, however, that patients with pseudoseizures may also have real seizures.

TREATMENT OF EPILEPSY

Medical therapy is begun once a diagnosis of seizures has been firmly established. There are two major reasons to treat seizures: first, to prevent potential harm from the single attack, and second, to maximize the chances of eventual seizure control and remission of the disorder.

Patients sometimes question or even reject adequate medical treatment of "mild" seizures, for example, the occasional brief complex partial or focal sensory attack. Since the drugs themselves have certain undesirable side effects and risks, both the physician and the patient must be convinced that therapy is worthwhile. The answer to the dilemma must be found in the observation of the natural history of seizure disorders as a group. Many observations have shown the same thing: the natural history of most untreated seizure disorders is to get worse with time, and the remission rate for epilepsy is higher with early medical treatment. In addition, a commonly observed progression is the initial occurrence of short, relatively unobtrusive focal seizures that are followed later by convulsions. Every patient with focal seizures must be regarded as being at risk for convulsions.

The treatment of a single, apparently nonfocal grand mal convulsion is a debated therapeutic issue. Those who believe that no treatment is indicated unless a second seizure occurs point to repeated studies showing "only" a 30% to 35% recurrence rate after a single attack in some studies. Those who recommend treatment point to other studies with more rigorous patient selection criteria and longer follow-up, with recurrence rates up to 70%.

Once a decision for therapy has been made and the reason for the seizures elucidated and treated if necessary, the physician must choose the drug that he or she feels will give the highest chance of successful seizure control at the lowest risk. That drug is then started in an appropriate manner and is increased slowly to the point at which the seizures are satisfactorily controlled, or at which the patient suffers unacceptable dose-related side effects. If the latter occurs, the drug has failed and another drug should be chosen and started. The first drug should eventually be withdrawn after the second drug has reached therapeutic levels, the goal being monotherapy if possible and appropriate for seizure type.

The patient should be instructed to keep an accurate calendar of any attacks, including the time of day and circumstances in which they occur. Reports by memory are inaccurate and are subject to distortion by expectation as well as by the memory-blurring effect of anticonvulsants.

Anticonvulsant blood level monitoring has proved to be valuable in seizure management. It can aid decision making when a patient taking more than one drug becomes toxic. In addition, although the slavish pursuit of the usual "therapeutic level" may not always be sensible, such guides may be helpful in managing convulsive epilepsy, when the only alternative is dosage guess-work and waiting to see if an attack will occur. Drug levels are also beneficial in judging patient compliance. When drawn at the same time of day at the same laboratory, and without interference from other medications or illness, anticonvulsant blood levels are remarkably stable from sample to sample.

The initial choice of anticonvulsant must be guided by the seizure(s) under consideration. Primary generalized epilepsy may have several manifestations: absence, grand mal, or myoclonic seizures, or combinations of these seizure types. Absence attacks usually respond readily to valproate or ethosuximide. The grand mal seizures of primary generalized epilepsy are also usually well controlled by valproate, so that there is even a rationale for monotherapy in this condition. If ethosuximide is used for the absence attacks, however, a second antiepileptic drug such as diphenylhydantoin or carbamazepine must be added if grand mal seizures are present. Myoclonic seizures usually respond to valproate or lamotrigine.

Focal or grand mal attacks may be treated with carbamazepine, diphenylhydantoin, valproate, lamotrigine, gabapentin, topiramate, or tiagabine. Although the reasons are obscure, it has been repeatedly observed that failure of seizure control with one of these drugs does not ensure failure with the others, so that if unacceptable side effects, allergy, or ineffectiveness calls for the rejection of one drug, the others should be tried.

Treatment of the retarded or otherwise brain-injured patient with multiple seizure types or akinetic seizures is beyond the scope of this chapter and is usually challenging enough to require the assistance of a neurologist or epileptologist.

Although some general principles govern their use, the antiepileptic drugs vary enough in their metabolism, side effects, and interactions with other drugs that they require separate comment. First, primidone and phenobarbital are highly sedative, and only occasionally used now. Diphenylhydantoin avoids the sedative side effects of the barbiturates but brings problems of its own. Chronic but usually harmless laboratory abnormalities such as macrocytosis and elevated alkaline phosphatase are common. Allergic skin reactions from the common maculopapular eruption to the rare but devastating Stevens–Johnson syndrome may occur. Dose-related side effects are predictable and characteristic, consisting of nystagmus at low doses and ataxia at higher ones. Long-term side effects have been well cataloged and include gingival hyperplasia, hirsutism, osteoporosis, and, particularly in children, facial coarsening. Therapy is easily induced, and most people tolerate the immediate use of full doses. The half-life of about 24 hours allows single-dose daily use.

For most epileptologists, carbamazepine is the preferred drug for complex partial or grand mal seizures. It is generally well tolerated by patients but requires initial slow titration of dose to avoid complaints of light-headedness. Blood level measurements are essential with carbamazepine, because the same levels can be achieved by doses that vary threefold in different people. Dose-related side effects, consisting of blurred or double vision in most people, are easily monitored. Many patients show a transient, usually mild, leukopenia on induction, and severe leukopenia is a rare cause for stopping the drug. Serious side effects (most commonly toxic hepatitis) are no more frequent than with diphenylhydantoin or phenobarbital.

Valproic acid is generally tolerated well, but idiosyncratic side effects such as weight gain, reversible alopecia, and tremor can present a problem. The use of an enterically stable form (divalproex sodium) generally obviates the nausea and vomiting caused by the earlier version of the drug. Fatal toxic hepatitis has been reported, mainly in young children on polytherapy during the first 6 months of use. Blood levels of valproic acid tend to vary more than they do with other anticonvulsants, and they are less useful.

Recently several new antiepileptic drugs have become available for treatment of seizure disorders. Gabapentin is a derivative of gamma-amino-butyric acid (GABA), the main inhibitory neurotransmitter of the brain. Like the other new antiepileptic drugs, it is effective in partial and tonic–clonic seizures. Because gabapentin is not metabolized or protein-bound, it demonstrates no interactions with other drugs; it is therefore very useful in the elderly who are often taking a variety of other pharmaceuticals. It is a relatively safe drug; no safety monitoring is necessary. The most common dose-related side effect is drowsiness.

Lamotrigine is a powerful antiepileptic drug that must be introduced more slowly and at lower doses if valproate is also taken, due to pharmacokinetic interactions. Skin rashes, sometimes severe, have limited its use in children, but it is generally well tolerated in adults. Adding lamotrigine to carbamazepine usually requires lowering the dose of the latter to avoid diplopia and dizziness, and it is often best tolerated as monotherapy.

Topiramate has the advantage of multiple mechanisms of action. Like other GABA-ergic drugs, its most common dose-related side effects include alterations in thinking, confusion, and occasionally weight loss. Serious side effects, however, are extremely rare. The concomitant use of hepatic enzyme–inducing drugs such as phenytoin or carbamazepine significantly lowers the blood level of topiramate, a factor that must be considered when adding or subtracting these drugs.

The most recent major antiepileptic drug to be introduced in the United States is tiagabine, another GABA agonist. Like topiramate, its metabolism is briskly enhanced by enzyme-inducing drugs, and its dose must be managed accordingly. Three-times-a-day dosages are usual, although there is some evidence that its antiepileptic effect may outlast its rather short serum half-life. Confusion and difficulty thinking are common during dose escalation.

Although most of the new antiepileptic drugs have been approved for use as add-on therapies, there is no reason to think they are any less effective as monotherapy, and they are often used as such by most epileptologists. In addition, "therapeutic" blood levels may be underestimated by many laboratories, and doses of the newer antiepileptic drugs may generally be increased carefully as tolerated, without frequent monitoring of blood levels.

A novel treatment for chronic epilepsy is vagus nerve stimulation, recently approved for treatment of partial and tonic–clonic seizures. This pacemaker-like device is implanted subcutaneously, and it operates both by programmed, intermittent stimulation and by being switched on "by demand" when a seizure is felt or seen to begin. Clinical trials have shown a success rate similar to that of the new antiepileptic drugs in a population of intractable seizure patients.

Surprisingly, the effects of anticonvulsants on the maturing brain are almost entirely unknown, but animal experiments suggest that they may cause significant reduction in the development of normal neuronal complexity. Considering the well-demonstrated immediate and long-term harm of repeated seizures, however, their continued use in children with epilepsy is not questioned.

The point at which antiepileptic drugs may be safely stopped in a well-controlled patient is debatable. A time span of 2 to 5 years without any seizure or aura is cited by most experts as a reasonable time at which to consider a trial without drugs. The subject is complex, however, and the reader is referred to the Suggested Reading list for more information.

Although most patients with epilepsy are helped to achieve substantial control of seizures, many patients on optimal drug therapy continue to have seizures serious or frequent enough to cause major disruptions to life. Such patients should be referred to specialized treatment centers for investigation into possible surgical treatment. If seizures can be demonstrated to emanate from a surgically accessible focus that can be removed without the possibility of neurologic injury, significant relief or cure may be achieved.

QUESTIONS AND DISCUSSION

1. Patients with primary generalized epilepsy may have which of the following types of seizures?

A. Absence
B. Myoclonic
C. Grand mal
D. All of the above
E. None of the above

The answer is (D). Patients may have any combination of these seizures. Sometimes grand mal attacks are preceded or led into by clusters of absence or myoclonic spells.

2. The physiologic substrate of clinical seizure activity is:

A. Abnormal neuronal discharge
B. Hyperactive glial potentials
C. Repeated disturbances in cerebral blood flow
D. Autoimmune mechanisms

The answer is (A). In focal epilepsy, groups of hyperirritable neurons, perhaps released by loss of inhibitory input and affected by anatomic distortions, overact and are able to hypersynchronize the activity of other neuronal populations. This activity spreads and causes focal or even generalized seizures.

3. Some cause(s) of new epilepsy after adolescence is/are:

A. Brain tumor
B. Penetrating head injury
C. Cerebral infection
D. B and C
E. A, B, and C

The answer is (E). New onset of seizure disorder in adulthood demands a full investigation into the cause. Epilepsy is thus better regarded as a symptom rather than as a disease.

4. High blood levels of diphenylhydantoin are usually accompanied by:

A. Somnolence
B. Hair loss
C. Ataxia
D. Pulmonary edema
E. Weakness

The answer is (C). Ataxia is much commoner than somnolence. Sedation is caused by diphenylhydantoin only at extremely high levels, as would be caused by deliberate overdosing. Hair loss may occur with valproate, but not with diphenylhydantoin. Neither pulmonary edema nor muscle weakness is typical of diphenylhydantoin effect. Ataxia is seen in most patients with blood levels above 30 mg/dl.

SUGGESTED READING

Aird RB, Masland RL, Woodbury DM: The Epilepsies: A Critical Review. New York, Raven Press, 1984

Annegers JF, Shirts SB, Hauser WA et al: Risk of recurrence after an initial unprovoked seizure. Epilepsia 27:43, 1986

Bialer M, Johannessen SI, Kupferberg HJ et al: Progress report on new antiepileptic drugs. Epilepsy Res 25:299, 1996

Chadwick D: The discontinuation of antiepileptic therapy. In: Pedley TA, Meldrum BS (eds): Recent Advances in Epilepsy, Vol 2. Edinburgh, Churchill Livingstone, 1985

Dodrill C, Batzel LW: Interictal behavioral features of patients with epilepsy. Epilepsia 27(Suppl 2): 564, 1986

Fish DR, Smith SJ, Quesney LF, et al.: Surgical treatment of children with medically intractable frontal or temporal lobe epilepsy: Results and highlights of 40 years' experience. Epilepsia 34:244, 1993

King DW, Flanigin HF, Gallagher BB, et al.: Temporal lobectomy for partial complex seizures: Evaluation, results, and 1-year follow-up. Neurology 36:334, 1986

Laidlaw J, Richens A: A Textbook of Epilepsy, 2nd Edition. Edinburgh, Churchill Livingstone, 1982

Leppik IE, Goldensohn ES, Hauser WA, et al: Epilepsy through life: Recent advances in understanding and treating epilepsy during pregnancy, childhood, adulthood, and old age. Epilepsia 33(Suppl 4):S1, 1992

Morselli PL, Pippenger CE, Penry JK: Antiepileptic Drug Therapy in Pediatrics. New York, Raven Press, 1983

Prince DA: Mechanisms of epileptogenesis in brainslice model systems. In: Ward AA, Penry JK, Purpura D (eds): Epilepsy. New York, Raven Press, 1983

Resor SR Jr, Kutt H (eds): The Medical Treatment of Epilepsy. New York: Marcel Dekker, 1992

Reynolds EH: Mental effects of antiepileptic medication: A review. Epilepsia 24 (Suppl 2):S24, 1983

Schachter SC, Schomer DL (eds): The Comprehensive Evaluation and Treatment of Epilepsy. San Diego, Academic Press, 1997

Scheuer ML: Seizures and epilepsy in the elderly. In: Pedley TA, Meldrum BS (eds). Recent Advances in Epilepsy, No. 6. Edinburgh, Churchill Livingstone, 1995

Shinnar S, Amir N, Branski D: Childhood Seizures. Basel, Karger, 1995

Theodore WH, Porter RJ, Penry JK: Complex partial seizures: Clinical characteristics and differential diagnosis. Neurology 33:1115, 1983

Wyllie E: The Treatment of Epilepsy: Principles and Practice. Philadelphia, Lea & Febiger, 1993

Neurology for the Non-Neurologist, Fourth Edition, edited by William J. Weiner and Christopher G. Goetz. Lippincott Williams & Wilkins, Philadelphia © 1999.

C H A P T E R 9

Multiple Sclerosis

William A. Sheremata

Lawrence S. Honig

Brian Bowen

Multiple sclerosis (MS) is a disease characterized clinically by the appearance of relapsing–remitting or progressive neurologic deficits in multiple areas of the central nervous system (CNS) over time. While the cause is unknown, the dominant pathology is in the CNS white matter: major immune-mediated destruction of myelin sheathing is evident, with relative preservation of axons. MS is almost twice as common in women as in men, predominantly affecting them as young adults. In the United States, peak incidence is at about age 24 years. Multiple sclerosis is more common in northern regions of Europe and the United States, areas in which the prevalence is as high as 1 per 1,000 population. In these areas, it is the most frequent cause of chronic neurologic disability in the young and middle-aged population. Certain clinical presentations appear commonly, but there is a panorama of less common symptoms and signs.

Epidemiologic studies have long suggested that the risk of MS is in part related to geographic location in temperate zones during childhood years: Individuals born or migrating to warmer climates before the age of 15 appeared to have reduced risk. However, recent evidence makes it likely that much of the geographic distribution of the disease is more related to genetic predisposition of certain peoples than the latitude of their residence. Other evidence has delineated epidemics of MS in the Faroe Islands, Iceland, and Sardinia, raising the possibility that young adults might carry the risk of MS to disease-free populations. Such a process might suggest a viral etiology. Prior investigations of causative factors of MS have consisted of numerous "false starts," most notably with a variety of viral or nutritional hypotheses. Viruses that have been proposed to be involved in the etiology include influenza, measles, canine distemper, human T-cell lymphocytotropic virus-I (HTLV-I) and more recently human herpes simplex virus-6 (HHSV-6).

DIAGNOSTIC CRITERIA

When evaluating a particular clinical presentation, the minimal criteria for the diagnosis of MS should be borne in mind. MS remains a clinically diagnosed disorder, despite marked technical advances in laboratory and neuroimaging support.

Multiple sclerosis has been recognized as a disease entity since the middle of the last century when it was characterized by Charcot as a disease of white matter. While a variety of criteria were put forward in the 1950s, the Schumacher Panel in 1965 set forth criteria for two types of disease, defined as *relapsing–remitting,* and *chronic progressive.* According to the criteria, definite MS is diagnosed in patients (1) when two separate areas of the CNS are involved, with two or more attacks lasting 24 hours or more, at least 1 month apart, and when other diseases have been eliminated with reasonable certainty; or (2) when the patient has had a minimum of 3 months of progressive slow or stepwise progression. Subsequent revisions culminated in the 1983 Poser criteria, resulting from the Workshop on the Diagnosis of MS. These broadened the definition of MS by providing a role for supporting laboratory data, as shown in Table 9-1. Earlier definitions were supplemented by allowing "paraclinical" tests, such as evoked potentials, urodynamic and neuroimaging studies, and cerebrospinal fluid (CSF) examination, to support the clinical criteria elicited from history and neurologic examination. Presently, four standardized clinical courses of the disease are recognized: relapsing–remitting, secondary-progressive, primary progressive, and relapsing–progressive (Table 9-2).

CLINICAL PRESENTATION

Charcot originally described MS over a century ago, recognizing three types of disease: disseminated, brainstem, and spinal. The "spinal" form, now defined as primary progressive MS, was least common, occurring in about one of ten patients. Presently, it is recognized that the majority of the symptoms and signs of MS are attributable to spinal cord and brainstem involvement. In particular, motor and sensory signs in the limbs derive preponderantly from spinal cord lesions.

DISEASE ONSET

While early sensory symptoms are a hallmark of MS, the initial clinical presentation of MS is commonly that of a young person with the complaint that he cannot walk on a street without tripping over the curb or uneven sections of pavement. Alternatively, he may complain that one or both legs are heavy or numb. Objective signs of decreased motor strength vary greatly but occasionally may be severe. Also variable is the rate of progression of debility after the first awareness of difficulty. Interpretation of onset complaints, such as unexplained falling, depends in large part on the findings on neurologic examination. Some patients may not have complaints referable to the lower extremities, yet examination may reveal weakness and evidence of spasticity. On the other hand, patients who present primarily with sensory complaints and decreased well-being may initially lack objective findings.

Several studies have attempted categorical surveys of symptoms and signs occurring with the first attack of MS (Table 9-3). The findings of Kurtzke represent

TABLE 9-1. Criteria for the Diagnosis of Multiple Sclerosis (MS)

Clinically definite MS
  Two attacks and clinical evidence of two separate lesions.
  or
  Two attacks; clinical evidence of one lesion and paraclinical evidence[a] of another separate lesion. The two attacks must involve different parts of the central nervous system (CNS), must be separated by a period of at least 1 month, and must each last a minimum of 24 hours. However, certain historical information may be substituted for clinical evidence of one of the two lesions.

Laboratory-supported definite MS
  Two attacks; either clinical or paraclinical evidence[a] of one lesion, and cerebrospinal fluid (CSF) oligoclonal bands and/or increased CSF IgG.
  or
  One attack; clinical evidence of two separate lesions; and CSF oligoclonal bands and/or increased CSF IgG.
  or
  One attack; clinical evidence of one lesion and paraclinical evidence[a] of another, separate lesion, and CSF oligoclonal bands and/or increased CSF IgG.

Clinically probable MS
  Two attacks and clinical evidence of one lesion.
  or
  One attack and clinical evidence of two separate lesions.
  or
  One attack; clinical evidence of one lesion and paraclinical evidence[a] of another, separate lesion.

Laboratory-supported probable MS
  Two attacks and CSF oligoclonal bands and/or increased CSF IgG.

[a] Paraclinical evidence of a lesion - "The demonstration, by means of various tests and procedures, of the existence of a lesion of the central nervous system (CNS) that has not produced sign of neurologic dysfunction but that may or may not have caused symptoms in the past. Such tests and procedures include the hot bath test, evoked response studies, tissue imaging procedures (including CT and MRI of the brain and spinal cord), and reliable expert urological assessment, provided that these tests and procedures follow the guidelines and are interpreted according to the newly established criteria." Poser CM, Paty DW, Sheinberg L, et al: New diagnostic criteria for multiple sclerosis: Guidelines for research protocols. Ann Neurol 13:227, 1983.

a cross section of experience in the United States and Canada. Symptoms attributed to corticospinal tract lesions were found in 64% of patients, and sensory disturbances were present in 42%. Incoordination was recorded in 43% and an internuclear ophthalmople-

TABLE 9-2. Clinical Courses in Multiple Sclerosis

CLINICAL COURSE	DEFINITION
Relapsing–remitting	Episodes of acute worsening with recovery and a stable course between relapses
Primary progressive	Gradual, nearly continuous neurologic deterioration from the onset of symptoms
Secondary progressive	Gradual neurologic deterioration with or without super-imposed acute relapses in a patient who previously had relapsing–remitting multiple sclerosis
Progressive relapsing	Gradual neurologic deterioration from the onset of symptoms, but with subsequent superimposed relapses

Lublin FD, Reingold SC: Defining the clinical course of multiple sclerosis: Results of an international survey. *In* National Multiple Sclerosis Society (USA) Advisory Committee on Clinical Trials of New Agents in Multiple Sclerosis. Neurology 46:1907, 1996.

TABLE 9-3. Findings in the Original Attack of Multiple Sclerosis: Three Reports

Wilson (100 Cases)

SYMPTOM	CASES (%)
Motor	46
Sensory (paresthesias)	23
Cerebellar	10
Sphincter disturbances	9
Seizures	1

Wilson SAK: Neurology. London, Edward Arnold, 1940, p. 156.

McAlpine (Review of Published Reports)

SYMPTOM	CASES (%)
Motor	40
Optic neuritis	22
Sensory (paresthesias)	21
Diplopia	12
Vertigo	5
Bladder dysfunction	5

McAlpine D: Luindsden, Achesen. Edinburgh, Churchill Livingston, 1972, p. 135.

Kurtzke

SYMPTOM	CASES (%)
Motor (corticospinal)	64
Cerebellar (incoordination)	43
Sensory	42
Brain Stem	40
Visual	24
Internuclear ophthalmoplegia	13

Kurtzke JF, Beebe GW, Nagler B, et al.: Studies on natural history of multiple sclerosis IV: Clinical features of the onset bout. Acta Neurol Scand 44:467, 1968.

gia in 13%. Complaints related to other brainstem signs were present in 40%.

Only about a third of patients who present with a single symptom have neurologic findings limited solely to that symptom. For example, in patients with retrobulbar neuritis, almost half exhibit signs attributable to spinal cord or brain stem lesions. Similarly, "la belle indifference," emphasized by Charcot, is often noted in early MS. Rather than euphoria, this sign is evidence of an inappropriate emotional response to what should be a traumatic emotional experience. Blunted affect or inappropriate response to affliction can reflect denial of illness or depression but also can be important, although subtle, manifestations of other nervous system disease (e.g. frontal lobe dysfunction). These and other subtle observations may easily pass undetected but when noted can be helpful in reaching a correct diagnosis.

MOTOR AND SENSORY SYMPTOMS

Motor and sensory signs of central nervous system involvement in MS result primarily from spinal cord involvement, although lesions anywhere in the pyramidal tracts, including subcortical white matter, internal capsule, and brainstem, may cause weakness. Because the spinal cord is one of the most frequent sites responsible for motor symptoms, the lower extremities are more often affected than the upper extremi-

ties and may show early and symmetrical involvement. Predilection for the lower extremities may be understood as a consequence of greater disease in the longest fibers running from the upper motor neurons in the frontal motor cortex to the lower motor neurons in the spinal cord anterior horns: longer axons are likely to be more involved if lesions occur randomly throughout the neuraxis. With constant improvements in neuroimaging, it is now clear that patients frequently have asymptomatic brain lesions even though their symptoms may be entirely due to spinal cord lesions. Even so, early in the course of disease, it is not uncommon to find patients without evidence of cerebral disease.

Motor symptoms referable to the corticospinal tract are described by patients as heaviness, weakness, stiffness, gait abnormalities, failure of a body part to respond to command, or even as "numbness." Findings on examination include decreased strength, increased tone, hyperreflexia, clonus, and Babinski reflexes ("up-going toes"). Motor difficulties are often relatively mild and may be mistakenly considered peripheral in origin. Difficulty walking is a common symptom, although such problems may not only be motor, but also relate to sensory, visual, vestibular, and cerebellar dysfunction. It is important to examine all the muscle groups in both upper and lower extremities to detect changes in tone and strength. Amyotrophy is uncommon, although not uncommon in the late stages of disease, presumably the result of disuse. Focal amyotrophy may be a sign of root exit zone involvement by demyelinative lesions. It rarely poses a problem in the differential diagnosis of motor neuron disease. Radicular pain is probably a more common manifestation resulting from root entry zone lesions. Importantly, "silent" motor signs may frequently be elicited on examination, without having been noticed by the patient or being the subject of any complaints.

Sensory symptoms may be prominent without consistent objective findings on examination. Complaints of glove-and-stocking distributions of sensory deficits are common. Findings are much less prominent than are complaints. However, suspended sensory loss can be an important finding. Such relative decreases in pain and temperature sensation are found in the mid to lower thoracic dermatomes by careful examination in a substantial number of cases. Patients may report Lhermitte's phenomenon, consisting of an electric shock sensation, a vibration, or dysesthetic pain radiating down the back and often into the arms or legs, usually occurring on neck flexion. It is an important symptom, although nonspecific, since it is notable in many myelopathies including that of cervical spondylosis. Lhermitte's sign can often be elicited on examination and is thought to reflect the presence of posterior column plaques. Proprioceptive difficulty may be difficult to detect even when clinically significant, but careful examination can often document this difficulty.

OPTIC AND RETROBULBAR NEURITIS

Optic neuritis is associated with typical visual symptoms, including blurring or darkening of vision, scotomas, decreased color perception, and occasionally flashes. Pain often occurs and may be experienced or aggravated upon movement of the affected eye. The pain may be described as a dull ache, or as a sharp jab with eye movement. Pain may precede or accompany the appearance of visual loss, often calling attention to visual difficulty. Descriptions of visual losses vary among patients, with common descriptions including "a curtain coming down" as well as "blurring." A small proportion of patients will proceed to "black out" or "white out" of vision, with somewhat poorer prognosis for recovery of good vision. Objectively, large central scotomas may occur. As many as 50% to 80% of cases of retrobulbar neuritis may ultimately progress to clinically obvious MS, whereas only about one in ten cases of transverse myelitis is subsequently diagnosed as MS.

Swelling of the optic disc, or papillitis, may be evident on careful inspection of the nerve head during the acute presentation. When the patient is seen in consultation by a neurologist, without the benefit of a full ophthalmologic examination, this will be often designated as retrobulbar neuritis. A small scotoma is frequently detectable in the visual field even after recovery of good vision. Color desaturation is usually demonstrable, although Ishihara color plates may not be adequately sensitive. Paroxysmal retrobulbar neuritis may also occur, with repeated, yet only momentary, blurring or obscurations of vision. The recurrent visual difficulty may occur many times a day or only occasionally. However, the whole period of disturbed vision usually lasts 3 to 8 weeks, the approximate length of an exacerbation of MS.

When severe optic nerve involvement is combined with prominent deficits from a spinal cord lesion, the combination has been termed Devic's syndrome or neuromyelitis optica. This syndrome is gaining more attention with the recognition of genetic differences in Japanese patients with such presentations, as compared to patients with the European type of MS. The exact relationship of either isolated optic neuritis or transverse myelitis to MS or Devic's disease is not known, but it is suggested that the lesions of Devic's disease are typically necrotizing in type. The MRI lesions are typically more extensive in transverse myelitis and Devic's disease when compared to typical MS.

CEREBELLAR AND BRAINSTEM SYMPTOMS

Cerebellar lesions are common in MS, with signs occurring in approximately half of patients. Action (or intention) tremor is common, and although severe resting or postural tremor is infrequent, it may if present be totally disabling. The affected individual may be in a totally dependent state, constituting a major nursing problem (1% of our experience). In many patients, mild hand tremor is present and may compound other motor problems. Cerebellar gait disorders, often with titubation of the trunk or head, are common. Scanning dysarthric (syllabic) speech may result from bilateral cerebellar involvement.

Charcot's original triad of multiple sclerosis consisted of nystagmus, scanning speech, and upper extremity tremor, although few patients show this exact clinical complex. Brainstem or cranial nerve lesions occur with almost equal frequency as cerebellar signs, and include extraocular muscle abnormalities [diplopia, internuclear ophthalmoplegia (INO), cranial nerve or gaze palsies, or nystagmus], trigeminal neuralgia, facial palsies and myokymia, hearing and vestibular deficits (vertigo), and rarely glossopharyngeal neuralgia.

Diplopia occurs in 12% to 22% of patients and is secondary to demyelinative plaques involving the intramedullary portions of the sixth and third nerves or the medial longitudinal fasciculus (MLF; see later). An INO occurs in about 13% of patients as a result of lesions affecting the MLF in the brainstem. Bilateral INO is a pathognomonic sign of MS (although unilateral INO may be a sign of brainstem infarction). An incomplete bilateral INO is easily missed. The essential clinical finding is bilateral abducting nystagmus with adduction weakness. This may be asymptomatic, or it may be associated with transient diplopia or vertigo upon movement of the head or eyes. Fourth cranial nerve palsies are rare in MS.

Nystagmus is an important finding in MS. The majority of patients exhibit nystagmus, although it may not be obvious early in the clinical course. Eye movements may seem to be jerky, especially when visualized under a fluorescent light. As the examiner becomes presbyopic, care must be exercised not to miss this important sign, as the absence of nystagmus mitigates against the diagnosis of MS.

Trigeminal neuralgia (tic douloureux) occurs in about 1% of MS patients. Severe momentary lancinating jabs of pain in the distribution of the maxillary or mandibular divisions of cranial nerve V are the only symptom. The pain may prevent eating, since contact with trigger zones may predictably produce pain. The pain usually responds well to carbamazepine but subsequently may be refractory to this agent.

Facial myokymia involving the lower face is an important, although not common (1–5%), finding of MS. These adventitious movements are most often unilateral but may be difficult to see. Their presence may require some patience to detect but they argue strongly for a diagnosis of MS.

Hearing loss of some degree is more common among MS patients than in the general population. Severe hearing loss is rare, although it can occur at any time in the clinical course. Earlier literature suggested that losses were irreversible, but significant improvement often occurs on long-term follow-up of those with sudden severe onset of deafness.

Vertigo is a frequent symptom (10% to 15%) among patients and may be symptomatically associated with diplopia. Severe vertigo occurs in approximately 5% of patients, often noted early in the clinical course. For acute attacks, recovery after several weeks is usual.

Olfactory abnormalities have been reported in MS and are included in early drawings of olfactory lesions by Charcot. However, they have been less frequently reported in recent literature, and their explanation is not obvious. Some of the difficulty probably results from technical problems in assessing smell, and the widespread prevalence of decreased smell in the general population.

GENITOURINARY SYMPTOMS

Urinary retention, urgency, frequency, and stress or overflow incontinence are frequent in MS and may be acute presenting signs of the disorder. Bladder symptoms are more common in women. Retention is usually secondary to a hypotonic (hyporeflexic) bladder. While it may occur transiently early in the clinical course of MS, late in the illness it is usually permanent and requires catheterization as it is refractory to medical measures. Frequency and incontinence are more commonly associated with detrusor hyperreflexia and sphincter dyssynergia. Careful urodynamic studies may establish the type of bladder dysfunction, but these neurogenic bladders are often managed empirically, albeit frequently with only partial relief of symptoms. The end result of a hyperreflexic bladder often is a small contracted organ associated with incessant urinary frequency, repeated secondary infections, and often stone formation that results from excessive fluid restriction by the patient. In years past, urinary tract infection accounted for the majority of deaths in MS.

Sexual impotence is reported in as many as 30% of male MS patients. Etiologic factors include upper motor neuron and sensory spinal lesions, as well as secondary effects of bladder dysfunction, pharmacologic therapy, depression, and anxiety. When first recognized, it may be transitory, and it may exhibit apparent response to various proffered therapies; however, it often becomes refractory to medical treatment. Surgical management through implantation of a penile prosthesis frequently provides satisfactory results.

COGNITIVE DYSFUNCTION AND EMOTIONAL ASPECTS

Cognitive symptoms may arise in as many as 50% of MS patients. The cognitive changes may be categorized as those of subcortical dementia, with signs of slowed processing and memory retrieval, decreased motivation, and disturbed executive function, rather than frank amnesia, apraxia, or aphasia as seen in cortical dementias. Cognitive dysfunction becomes more prominent in patients with longer duration of disease, and it seems to correlate with increased degree of cerebral white matter disease, rather than with clinical disability. An electroencephalogram (EEG) may show mild background slowing. Long-latency evoked potentials, such as the auditory P300, show prolongation. Severe dementia is uncommon (5%). However, it is not infrequent that high-functioning executives or professionals with only relatively minor gait, sensory, or visual problems are unable to continue in their employment. Whether cognitive deficits or affective components are responsible for such problems is unclear.

Depression is documented in 60% or more of patients and indubitably contributes to disruption of personal and family life in addition to employment difficulties. Denial of illness, frustration, and anxiety may be compounded by fatigue. Many patients report major social difficulties following false reassurances that early symptoms are emotionally based. Apart from personal frustration and side effects from sedative drugs, family members and friends may reject patients' pleas for help. Thus, it is often more appropriate for the diagnostician to admit inability to provide or exclude a diagnosis on the basis of subjective complaints, and to recommend careful follow-up, than to provide diagnoses of "hysteria" or functional illness. Psychological counseling may also be better accepted in this context.

PAROXYSMAL SYMPTOMS

Symptoms that may last only seconds to hours occur in the course of MS. Such symptoms are not commonly recognized and may be ascribed to hysteria. They probably occur in considerably more than the 34% of patients documented to experience them. Paroxysmal symptoms include sensory symptoms, such as visual blurring, trigeminal pain, paresthesias, Lhermitte's phenomenon, and body pain; and motor symptoms such as dysarthria, dystonia ("tonic seizures or spasms"), choreoathetosis, ataxia, falling, and akinesia. Paroxysmal falling is unexplained by ataxia, motor phenomena, or epileptic seizures, and thus it is often not recognized for what it is. The majority of these paroxysmal conditions respond well to carbamazepine. In some cases, phenytoin, valproic acid, gabapentin, or acetazolamide have proven useful.

These transient symptoms of MS are often the source of diagnostic confusion because of their misinterpretation as transient ischemic attacks, epileptic seizures, cataplexy, convulsive syncope, or hysteria.

Epileptic seizures have been reported to occur in as many as 10% of MS patients with long-term follow-up, which approximates the frequency of seizures following other kinds of cerebral insults. However, the prevalence of epileptic seizures in the patient pool at any given time is actually much lower (12%), and it is likely that some reported "seizures" represent nonepileptic paroxysmal phenomena rather than epileptic convulsions. When epileptic seizures do appear early in the clinical course, it is a poor prognostic sign, especially so if status epilepticus occurs.

PAIN SYMPTOMS

Pain is not uncommon in MS. Usually it is of neurogenic origin rather than of a secondary musculoskeletal nature. Paroxysmal pains include those of paroxysmal dystonia and trigeminal neuralgia. The most common chronic pain is a dull tingling sensation, or painful paresthesia. Acute spinal exacerbations are often accompanied by a bandlike body-encircling pain, or by back pain, reflecting the level of the spinal cord lesion. High cervical plaques may acutely cause head pain. These spinal symptoms are likely due in part to root entry zone involvement, and they usually respond promptly to steroid treatment.

NATURAL HISTORY

Multiple sclerosis in most patients is characterized by the appearance of symptoms of CNS deficit over hours to days. New symptoms and most recurrent symptoms last from days to months. If symptoms persist a day or longer, they probably indicate the appearance of new loci of white matter disease. Evanescent symptoms are difficult to evaluate. They may indicate the presence of new pathologic lesions, but in many instances they are more likely to reflect adverse effects of physiologic changes on central conduction. Increased temperature is a well-known factor in increasing MS symptoms, but changes in blood ionic composition (pH, $[Ca^{++}]$, $[HCO_3^-]$) and other physiologic parameters can show pronounced effects on conduction in demyelinated fibers. The resulting paroxysmal phenomena may be due to ephaptic transmission (cross talk) or to ectopic generation of spontaneous potentials, as through mechanical deformation of damaged nerves.

The natural course of the relapsing–remitting form of the disease is part of a wide and unpredictable spectrum. Relapses may occur one or more times per year, or even monthly. On the other hand, some patients may have only one or a handful of attacks in a lifetime. Some people do not have recorded symptoms their entire life and then are found incidentally to have the pathology of MS at autopsy. In younger patients early in their disease, increased frequency and severity of attacks is often seen, sometimes with later "burning out." Recovery from an exacerbation usually occurs over days to weeks and occasionally continues over a period of months. Upon resolution of an exacerbation, neurologic signs may disappear completely, although meticulous examination usually will detect some residua. Subsequent exacerbations are sometimes more difficult to recognize, in part because the patient is less alarmed by them, and because new deficits can be more difficult to detect when superimposed on prior multifocal neurologic impairment. MS takes on a waxing-and-waning character, although deficits tend to accumulate, with many patients exhibiting progressively increasing disability.

Chronic progressive disease may be the presenting form of MS (primary progressive MS), or it may occur subsequent to varying durations of relapsing remitting disease (secondary progressive MS). When relapses occur after onset of slowly progressive illness, progressive–relapsing MS is diagnosed. Primary progressive and progressive–relapsing MS are more common among men, usually occurring after the age of 30. However, in about 10% to 20% of patients under the age of 30 at onset, relapsing–remitting illness evolves into a secondary progressive course. The occurrence of a rapidly progressive course carries a bad prognosis for life as well as function. Patients with this "malignant" or life-threatening form of illness (also called acute multiple sclerosis) may die from brainstem disease or status epilepticus, which reflects widely disseminated lesions. Improved management of these patients is resulting in a better prognosis. In addition, as patients with milder illness are recognized, the proportion of patients with a malignant presentation has statistically declined to about 5% of the total. Slowly progressive forms of illness may appear to plateau or "burn out" at times, although slow progression may be continuing, with the changes too gradual for easy recognition by the patient or clinical detection.

McAlpine found that after 10 years of disease, 80% of MS patients with relapsing–remitting disease had "unrestricted" neurologic function. Of these, 85% continued without severe disability for a further 10 years. More recent studies also show that lifespan expectancy is only slightly reduced in MS patients, representing at most a 7-year difference in younger patients compared to their non-MS cohort, and even less difference in older patients. Newer diagnostic techniques are allowing diagnosis of increasing numbers of patients with benign disease that might otherwise have gone undiagnosed, and they are allowing the assignment of different diagnoses for some patients with more severe diseases that might otherwise have been labeled MS. The net result of these forces is that inclusion and exclusion of these individuals, respectively, yields an overall "better" prognosis for the MS population.

CONTRIBUTORY FACTORS

Infections of the respiratory tract, particularly influenza, have been shown to increase the risk of exacerbation of MS. However, it has also been noted that MS patients have relatively fewer respiratory infections. Mechanisms that could account for this are unknown, but it might be related to immune activation. Urinary tract infections or other intercurrent illnesses also can cause temporary worsening of chronic symptoms and be associated with clear exacerbations.

Pregnancy itself appears to be associated with decreased MS disease activity, although the puerperium seems to be accompanied by increased risk of exacerbation, particularly in the months immediately following delivery. However, not all reports are consistent in this regard.

Trauma or surgery, even minor, seems to be associated with an increased risk of exacerbation of MS, as observed by many clinicians familiar with MS. However, a number of studies do not validate this association. An increased risk of exacerbation has been noted within the month following spinal anesthesia (but not after lumbar puncture alone).

Emotional stress may antedate MS exacerbations, as has long been recognized. The relationship of stress and immunemediated tissue responses has spawned a new field of investigation: psychoneuroimmunology. New findings have been published by a combined American and English effort demonstrating the role of major life stresses in aggravating MS. The findings support earlier findings by Canadian workers as well as our studies with a colleague now deceased (J. B. R. Cosgrove). Importantly, immune responses have been shown to reduce brainstem noradrenaline in experimental animals. It is possible that depression, known to be associated with altered control of CNS monoamines, may in MS be related to such changes.

VARIANTS OF MULTIPLE SCLEROSIS

Transverse myelitis may subsequently evolve into MS, but 90% of cases do not. Some cases will have disseminated involvement limited to the optic nerve (Devic's disease). Finding subclinical brainstem or optic nerve involvement makes a diagnosis of MS likely.

Neuromyelitis optica (Devic's disease) is a syndrome consisting of optic nerve and spinal cord demyelination. It may represent a related but separate entity from MS, since it occurs with similar or increased frequencies in Asia and South America, areas where MS is otherwise infrequently recognized. Moreover, disease onset occurs over a much wider age range.

Marburg's disease ("acute multiple sclerosis") is a rare form of demyelinating disease occurring in the very young. It has recently been shown to be due to the inability to synthesize adult isoforms of myelin basic protein, a structural protein of myelin. Fetal myelin appears to be unstable in postnatal life.

Malignant multiple sclerosis is more common when MS is associated with histocompatibility haplotypes HLA B7 and DR2. The prognosis of this grave type of presentation has been improved with aggressive immunosuppression. Early death previously occurred within weeks to months, but it may be avertable by aggressive measures.

Concentric sclerosis of Balo is a very rare disease (only about 40 cases have been described) that clinically follows a fulminant monophasic course compatible with acute multiple sclerosis, with death in weeks to months, but that is pathologically distinguished by concentric lamellar demyelinating lesions in the white matter.

Diffuse sclerosis of Schilder is an extremely rare chronic or subacute myelinoclastic disorder that can be separated from adrenoleukodystrophy (ALD) by careful pathologic studies as shown by Poser. Patients show one or two large demyelinative plaques characteristic of MS in the cerebral hemispheres.

Multiple sclerosis with demyelinative peripheral neuropathy is an uncommon clinical disorder. While morphometric and neurophysiologic abnormalities of peripheral nerve may occur in MS, they do not appear to have any clinical relevance. Severe demyelinative attacks on cranial nerve or spinal root entry or exit zones can result in apparent peripheral symptomatology. Cases of combined peripheral and CNS disease in MS must be clearly differentiated from adult-onset leukodystrophies (such as metachromatic leukodystrophy or adrenoleukodystrophy), where such combined involvement is characteristic. There may be common pathogenetic mechanisms in central and peripheral demyelination.

PATHOLOGY

Multiple sclerosis is an inflammatory disease affecting central nervous system white matter. Lymphocytes and monocytes penetrate the white matter surrounding small blood vessels, destroying myelin, and usually, but not always, sparing axons. Individual lesions are termed plaques and vary greatly in size. With time, perivenular lesions may coalesce, forming plaques several centimeters in size. Plaques are distributed throughout the neuraxis, as demonstrated radiologically and pathologically. They do tend to be conspicuous in the periventricular white matter, particularly adjacent to the frontal and/or occipital horns of the ventricular system. Spinal cord involvement is cardinal; the cervical region may have a particular predisposition. Optic nerves, chiasm, periaqueductal gray matter, and corpus callosum are also prominently affected.

Active plaques can be seen by microscopy to be less clearly circumscribed and very intensely cellular, particularly along the margin of active demyelination. While there is no agreement as to the subtypes of lymphocytes predominating in lesions, electron microscopic studies show that myelin is actively destroyed by the invading macrophages. These changes are associated with interstitial edema and swelling of astrocyte foot processes. Inactive (old) plaques are relatively acellular and are often intensely gliotic. The traversing axons are reduced in number and may disappear completely. These plaques are sharply demarcated from normal tissue. Areas of incomplete myelination referred to as *shadow plaques* are thin myelin sheaths and are now known to be areas of *remyelination*. They are more typically located in more superficial white matter at the graywhite junction.

PATHOPHYSIOLOGY

Experimental demyelination produces conduction delays, or blocks, and dispersion of impulses. This may impair normal physiologic responses. In acute lesions, the inflammatory reaction itself impairs axonal function. Function may resume when the inflammation subsides, but the axon, while regaining ability to conduct under optimal conditions, becomes hyperexcitable and prone to spontaneous discharge. Crosstalk (ephaptic transmission) and hyperexcitability may explain paroxysmal phenomena. The susceptibility of demyelinated axons to total conduction block with increased temperature or physiologic alterations satisfactorily explains the effects of heat, fever, and illness resulting in reappearance or aggravation of symptoms of MS.

IMMUNE RESPONSE

Altered immune responses have been detected in numerous studies. Lymphocytes are often present in modestly increased numbers in the CSF. In pathologic specimens of plaques, there are both helper (CD4$^+$) and suppressor/cytotoxic (CD8$^+$) T cells present in lesions, as well as macrophages that primarily have direct responsibility for the myelin damage. In addition to these cell types, which are not normally present in brain, MS plaques show a variety of cell surface molecules (histocompatibility antigens, T-cell receptors), adhesion factors (integrins), and soluble cytokines [β-interferon, γ-interferon, interleukins IL1 and IL2, tumor necrosis factor (TNF-α), and transforming growth factor-β (TGF-β)]. Immunoglobulin IgG is increased in the CSF of MS patients, and it frequently shows oligoclonal bands with reactivity to myelin proteins. The increased IgG apparently is mostly due to intrathecal synthesis, with occasional contribution from breakdown of the blood–brain barrier (BBB). Thus, findings have not implicated a particular arm of the immune response, nor do they necessarily implicate a single antigen in the nervous system as a specific target, although increasing attention is focused on myelin basic protein.

While considerable amounts of data suggest prominent involvement of an abnormal immune response in MS, the factors responsible for this are unknown. Viruses or other microorganisms have been fingered as responsible in part for provoking autoimmunity, without any conclusive evidence, and genetic background also seems important. Two hypothetical mechanisms that might explain the apparent autoimmunity of MS are that myelin might be damaged either as the consequence of "molecular mimicry," or as simply an "innocent bystander." Mimicry implies that myelin has structural similarity to some exogenous virus or substance, and thus it is attacked as an unfortunate side effect of the body's response to this outside insult. In the bystander model, an outside virus or factor causes CNS destruction and exposure, thus prompting an anti-self response.

GENETIC FACTORS

Histocompatibility antigens (HLA) have been extensively studied in MS. In Northern European popula-

tions, MS patients show significant overrepresentation of HLA haplotypes DR2, A3, and B7. In the Shetland and Orkney Islands, the entire population exhibits A3 and B7. The presence of both DR2 and B7 predict the likelihood of a malignant course for affected individuals. Other recent studies have confirmed that there is an increased risk for siblings of MS patients, apparently greatest for identical twins, lending credence to a role of genetic factors in the etiology of MS. Other genes are under active study including the TNF-alpha (TNF-α), TNF-β, and several identified mutations.

LABORATORY DATA

CEREBROSPINAL FLUID EXAMINATION

Examination of CSF obtained by lumbar puncture is important in the evaluation of patients. Cell counts reveal a modest increase in number of mononuclear cells (lymphocytes), generally between 5 and 100/μl. Total protein content is often normal but may be mildly elevated, although rarely greater than 100 mg/dl. IgG is very often elevated (>10.5% of total CSF protein). Increased intrathecal IgG synthesis, calculated from CSF and serum concentrations of albumin and IgG (expressed as IgG index or IgG synthesis rate) can be found in about 70% of patients. An increase in CSF IgG with normal CSF protein or albumin always indicates the presence of abnormal intrathecal IgG synthesis. Oligoclonal IgG bands, present in CSF but not serum, can be demonstrated by properly performed CSF agarose gel electrophoresis in 90% to 100% of MS patients at some point in their illness. However, bands are not specific for MS, as they may be found in various infectious or inflammatory disorders of the CNS. Myelin basic protein is increased in the CSF of most MS patients during acute exacerbations, although it may be technically difficult to detect because of specimen handling and assay problems, and it is nonspecific.

NEUROIMAGING STUDIES

X-ray computerized tomography is frequently quite unrevealing, although nonspecific-appearing white matter lucencies and ventriculomegaly may be seen. Active lesions, such as are present during acute exacerbation, often show contrast enhancement, particularly after administration of a double dose of intravenous contrast and with accentuation by delaying the contrast scan. However, magnetic resonance imaging (MRI) is so superior for visualizing plaques of MS that CT is not indicated except for the occasional acute attack in which other processes such as an intracranial bleed needs to be ruled out.

Magnetic resonance imaging is remarkably sensitive for visualizing cerebral lesions in MS. However, the findings (particularly without contrast) are not specific for MS: similar changes can be seen with microvascular disease and even normal aging. Thus, overreliance on brain images should be avoided during the diagnostic process. MRI images do bear a striking resemblance to gross sections of brain in their representation of normal anatomy and plaques.

Since the early 1980s, when the first clinical MR neuroimaging studies were performed, the high sensitivity of MRI compared to other imaging methods in detecting MS plaques in the brain and spinal cord has been evident. For years, the primary technique used to detect demyelination has been T2-weighted spin-echo MRI imaging (Figs. 9-1A and 9-2A). This technique, which is exquisitely sensitive to the presence of bulk water molecules, displays demyelinating lesions as hyperintense due to alteration in the local water distribution. These hyperintense lesions are well seen against a background of low signal from intact white matter. A drawback is that CSF in the ventricles and subarachnoid space is markedly hyperintense on T2-weighted images, and this tends to obscure periventricular lesions in the brain and peripheral white matter lesions in the spinal cord. Recently, another technique has become widely used. In this technique, called fluid-attenuated-inversion recovery (FLAIR), the signal from CSF (or other fluid-filled structures, such as a cyst or necrotic infarct) is suppressed without significantly altering the hyperintensity of brain parenchymal lesions (Figs. 9-1B and 9-1C). This has resulted in increased sensitivity in the detection of periventricular MS plaques.

In the late 1980s, an intravenous contrast agent, often referred to simply as gadolinium, was first used in clinical studies. In the brain or spine, this agent is deposited in areas of BBB breakdown, resulting in markedly increased signal intensity on T1-weighted spin-echo images (a technique analogous to T2-weighted spin-echo imaging) (Fig. 2B). Usually, the T1-weighted images are less sensitive in detecting plaques than the T2-weighted images, but when there is active breakdown of the BBB, as seen with acute demyelination, the lesions become more conspicuous as a result of gadolinium enhancement. The visibility of the enhancing lesions can be improved further by suppressing the signal from surrounding normal white matter. This is accomplished with another recent technique, called magnetization transfer (MT) imaging. On MT images without gadolinium, the suppression of normal white matter results in a mildly improved visibility of most plaques (Fig. 9-1D). On images obtained after gadolinium injection, the visibility of active enhancing plaques is markedly increased (Fig. 9-1E). Thus, MT improves detection of active lesions, particularly in the brain. As MRI imaging continues to evolve, newer techniques such as FLAIR and MT imaging are being incorporated into standard protocols and are providing increased sensitivity and specificity in the diagnosis and treatment of MS.

On T2-weighted images, demyelinating plaques appear as areas of increased signal (increased brightness in the recorded image) because of their increased water content. They are most commonly seen in the peri- and supraventricular white matter, but they can be present as single or multiple lesions of varying size anywhere in the white matter of the cerebral hemispheres, cerebellum, or brainstem, without abutting the ventricular system. Many patients scanned within the first few years after onset of MS do not show cerebral lesions by MRI, although a number of these patients can be shown to have MRI-demonstrable lesions in the spinal cord. Acute plaques, during disease exacerbation, whether in the brain or spinal cord, show marked contrast enhancement following injection of a gadolinium contrast agent. Serial scanning of MS patients at intervals of weeks to months has revealed that many cerebral white matter lesions of MS are stable, but that foci of abnormal signal may appear and disappear without accompanying clinical symptomatology.

It is important to be aware that brain and spinal cord MRI may appear normal in some cases. In primary progressive MS, which occurs in 10% of patients (30% of Irish and European Jewish populations) and where the brain may not be affected pathologically, brain and spinal cord MRI studies are normal except for mild atrophy of the superior cervical cord, which occurs later in the course of the illness.

EVOKED RESPONSES

Visual evoked responses are tested optimally by performance of a light and dark checkerboard pattern-reversal stimulus. Computer averaging of occipital scalp electrode potentials normally shows a major positive wave (P100) with a latency of about 100 msec, which varies somewhat with age and the stimulus parameters of each laboratory (e.g. frequency, check size, total subtended visual field, contrast ratio, and luminance). Prolonged latencies of the P100 wave

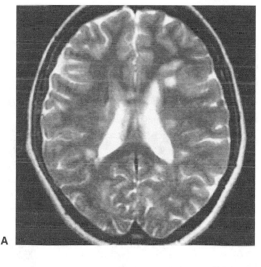

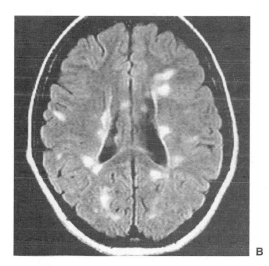

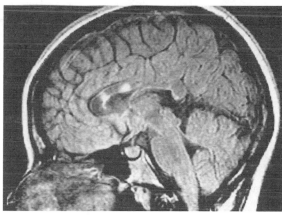

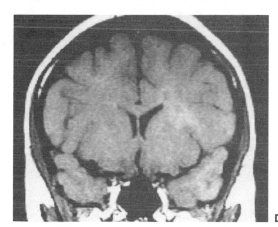

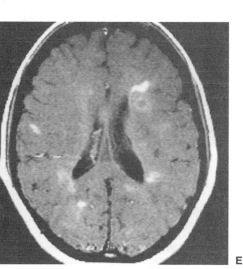

FIG. 9-1. MS involving the cerebral white matter. Axial T2-weighted spin-echo image **A.** and FLAIR image **B.** demonstrate bilateral periventricular white matter hyperintense lesions at the callosal–septal interface, characteristic of MS, are well shown on a midsagittal FLAIR image **C.** On a precontrast, coronal MT image **D.** from the same patient, left frontal periventricular white matter demyelination appears mildly hyperintense, compared to surrounding normal white matter. Acute demyelinating lesions appear even brighter because of contrast enhancement on the postcontrast axial MT image **E.**

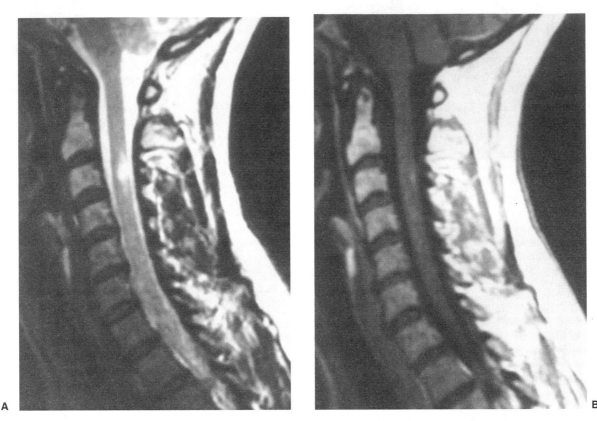

FIG. 9-2. MS involving the cervical spinal cord. Sagittal T2-weighted **A.** and postcontrast T1-weighted **B.** images of the cervical spine demonstrate an active demyelinating lesion involving the posterior columns of the spinal cord at C3.

are abnormal and, if monocular, specifically reflect prechiasmal disease. Abnormal findings are more prevalent with increased duration of MS, ultimately present in more than 75% of patients.

Brainstem auditory evoked responses (BAER) are obtained using auditory click stimuli. Seven waves can often be discerned, although only waves I through V are clinically useful. Normal results are specific to each laboratory because of dependence on parameters such as stimulus polarity, rate, intensity, and electrode placement. Increased latencies between waves I and V are seen in about 75% of patients with brainstem signs after many years of illness. Although increasing duration of illness makes abnormal BAERs more likely, these are the least sensitive evoked potentials for MS.

Somatosensory evoked responses are obtained by stimulating sensory or mixed nerves of an extremity (median, ulnar, posterior tibial, or peroneal). Short-latency (<50 msec) scalp potentials reflect conduction in the dorsal column (medial lemniscal) somatosensory system. Abnormalities in the response are sensitive for dysfunction of this system, although the studies and their interpretation can be technically difficult, especially in studies of the lower extremities; furthermore, positive findings are nonspecific as to disease process.

DIFFERENTIAL DIAGNOSIS

Dissemination of lesions in the nervous system over protracted periods of time is infrequently seen in other disorders. Rare cases of vascular disorders (principally systemic lupus erythematosus and vascular malformations) and neoplastic disease may occasionally resemble MS. Diagnosis is most difficult early in the clinical course. If only one CNS lesion is demonstrated clinically and radiologically, a diagnosis of MS cannot be established. Other paraclinical tests such as CSF analysis, and evoked potentials may be useful in confirming a laboratory-supported diagnosis of MS, and tests such as nerve conduction velocity may help lead to other diagnoses.

Disseminated encephalomyelitis and postinfectious encephalomyelitis are acute illnesses with disseminated central demyelination and MRI findings similar to that of MS. Most important, they are monophasic illnesses. If relapsing or progressive signs occur, the diagnosis of MS is likely.

Optic or retrobulbar neuritis may also occasionally result from inherited, nutritional, vasculitic, and ischemic syndromes. In young individuals, these latter include systemic lupus and syphilis. In such individuals, scotomas are often small and multiple in number. In addition, there is little subsequent change in these visual field abnormalities. Prognosis of isolated idiopathic optic neuritis is currently being prospectively studied in Europe. Preliminary results suggest that a large proportion of affected individuals eventually qualify for the diagnosis of MS. In addition, MRI reveals multiple brain lesions characteristic of MS in many otherwise asymptomatic patients with retrobulbar neuritis.

Brainstem signs such as bilateral INO are virtually pathognomonic of MS, but they may be mimicked by the ocular muscle weakness of myasthenia gravis, and by the ocular ataxia of fixed cerebellar lesions. Pontine gliomas may rarely be associated with an INO. Diabetes can produce isolated ocular palsies, but it rarely creates a problem in differential diagnosis. Trigeminal neuralgia, in combination with other brainstem signs, may be a manifestation of pontine gliomas and posterior fossa invasion by pharyngeal tumors. In these latter disorders, the corneal reflex is often diminished, an extremely rare finding in MS.

Familial spinocerebellar degenerations can occasionally be difficult to clinically distinguish from MS early in their presentation, especially when family history is unclear. These disorders have in common slow progressive (rather than episodic or acute) dysfunction, and autosomal dominance inheritance. They are much rarer than MS. Recently, however, two types of spinocerebellar degenerations (SCA-2 and SCA-6) have been shown to exhibit episodic increases in ataxia. Olivopontocerebellar degeneration is usually recognized by its dominant pattern of inheritance

and rather stereotypic presentation within a family. Friedreich's ataxia typically begins at an early age and has peripheral nerve involvement. The advent of neuroimaging has been helpful in differential diagnosis, since these disorders are not characterized by the presence of focal MRI lesions. In addition, CSF and visual evoked responses are usually normal in these disorders.

Compressive myelopathy has always been a major consideration in the differential diagnosis of patients with progressive myelopathies. The advent of MRI has eased the task of ruling out intervertebral disc herniations/protrusions (cervical spondylosis), syringomyelia, spinal canal tumors, and intraparenchymal neoplasms. However, spinal cord lesions having increased T2 signal, with or without contrast enhancement, must not be assumed to represent spinal cord tumors, as they may represent demyelinating lesions with edema. Retaking a complete history and performing other paraclinical tests in a search for evidence of disseminated disease is most helpful. Follow-up MRI examinations can reveal changes in spinal cord size and signal characteristics.

Transverse myelopathy is a term describing a spinal cord disorder appearing to involve a single level of spinal cord involvement. Transverse myelitis typically presents with subacute onset of weakness and numbness and progression to paraplegia within days to weeks. Subsequent partial or complete recovery suggests that the process is primarily demyelinative. Ischemic spinal cord disease can be associated with systemic lupus erythematosus, vasculitides, or disease of the radicular arteries. Acute spinal cord infarction usually has onset over minutes to hours, and it involves the lower thoracic dermatomes. It may be seen in those with diabetes, atheromatous vascular disease, or aortic aneurysms, and after aortic surgery. Because infarction usually involves only the anterior two thirds of the cord, these individuals have clear motor and sensory levels with sparing of proprioception. The occurrence of transverse myelopathy may herald the onset of Devic's disease or of multiple sclerosis. Devic's disease is diagnosed when one or both optic nerves and the spinal cord are affected but the brain is spared. The MRI changes in the spinal cord in transverse myelitis and Devic's disease are usually prominent but may require 2 or 3 weeks to evolve and affect several segments of the spinal cord in continuity. These changes differ from those seen in MS.

Tropical spastic paraparesis (TSP) was first described during the past century ("Jamaican neuropathy"). It has recently been shown to be caused by the human T-cell lymphocytotropic virus HTLV-I, and thus is now known as TSP/HAM (HTLV-I-associated myelopathy). This disorder shows a wide distribution with prevalence in the Caribbean region, tropical Central and South America, Japan, and Africa. It occurs, albeit uncommonly, in United States natives, and we have studied a number of patients who were recent immigrants. Clinically, it appears as an indolent progressive myelopathy with numbness and paraparesis. Onset in the third and fourth decade of life, and the chronic progressive nature of the illness are similar to MS. Although optic neuritis has been noted in some cases, prominent brainstem signs are infrequent. In addition, peripheral neuropathy may occur. Serum testing reveals antibody to HTLV-I. Only a small proportion (<1%) of seropositive individuals have neurologic disease. Infection is endemic among certain populations. Transmission modes are similar to those of HIV: through blood exposure (by transfusion or sharing contaminated intravenous needles), by sexual routes, or, less commonly, from mother to child.

Vitamin B₁₂ deficiency may cause subacute combined degeneration of the spinal cord. The symptoms of dorsal column sensory involvement and lateral column (corticospinal tract) upper motor neuron dysfunction can resemble MS. However B_{12} deficiency usually develops later in life; it is rare in the younger age groups in which MS commonly has onset. Furthermore, it is not usually difficult to clinically make the distinction between MS, which is often relapsing–remitting, and in which brainstem and optic nerve involvement occur, and B_{12} deficiency, which is usually chronic and progressive and features concomitant peripheral neuropathy, dementia (often with psychotic symptoms), and megaloblastic anemia. B_{12} deficiency can be ruled out by measurement of serum vitamin B_{12} levels. If these are borderline or low, studies of serum homocysteine and methylmalonate can confirm or refute functional B_{12} deficiency. Some MS patients may have borderline depressed B_{12} levels, but this is rarely functionally important. B_{12} deficiency may be the consequence of partial gastrectomy, tropical sprue, or autoimmune disease (pernicious anemia).

Vitamin E deficiency is a rare cause of myelopathy, frequently with spinocerebellar symptoms. It may occur in children or adults with malabsorption syndromes, but it may also be the result of genetic deficiency in the tocopherol receptor. Animal fat is our major source of this essential vitamin, and dietary elimination of animal fat has been found to produce experimental myelopathy in primates. Demyelination and motor neuron damage have been demon-strated. When suspected, serum tocopherol levels will exclude deficiency, unless there has been a very recent large intake of vitamin preparations.

Sjögren's syndrome has been reported to include some patients with progressive or relapsing CNS symptoms and brain MRI findings resembling MS. Sjögren's syndrome is a chronic inflammatory autoimmune disorder whose cardinal features are keratoconjunctivitis sicca (dry eyes) and xerostomia (dry mouth). Salivary gland biopsy is useful in revealing lymphocytic infiltration, and autoantibodies SSA and SSB (also known as anti-Ro and La) are usually present. Symptoms and signs of apparent peripheral neuropathy, actually a result of sensory neuronopathy (dorsal root ganglionitis), are common in Sjögren's syndrome. However, examination of the MS patient population shows that while up to one third may indeed have dry mouth and/or dry eyes, only a few have low titers of various autoantibodies, and only extremely few (<1% to 3%) meet diagnostic criteria for Sjögren's syndrome; in these few cases, it is likely a concomitant rather than etiologically significant diagnosis.

Lyme disease and neurosyphilis are infectious disorders that cause serial multifocal nervous system disease and thus can appear similar to MS. Lyme manifestations often include cranial neuritis, radiculoneuritis, peripheral neuropathy, and mild cognitive symptoms. Typically there is a pronounced chronic lymphocytic meningitis, with cell counts often higher than in MS. In rare cases, there is a chronic progressive clinical encephalomyelitis with sensory and motor abnormalities and brain MRI foci of increased T2 signal predominantly in white matter. Such cases have led to concern over diagnostic confusion of this treatable infectious disease with multiple sclerosis. However, even in Lyme seropositive patients, the two diseases may usually be distinguished by clinical course as well as by CSF antibody studies. Neurosyphilis may be of an active meningovascular type (with more active CSF than MS), or a chronic tabetic type with prominent dorsal column signs. Specific serum antibody tests can determine whether exposure has occurred to the pathogenetic spirochetal organisms *Borrelia burgdorferi* for Lyme and *Treponema pallidum* for syphilis. However, positive serum antibody tests do not indicate that a patient's symptom complex results from this exposure. CSF antibody tests can be useful for differential diagnosis in Lyme. Despite considerable interest in the overlap of Lyme disease symptoms with those of multiple sclerosis, it is now clear that the Lyme organism is only very rarely the cause of a truly MS-like clinical presentation. Antibody testing for Lyme requires the presence of a positive Western blot.

TREATMENT AND THERAPY

Treatment can be divided into disease-modifying and symptomatic categories. The former includes various therapies designed to modulate or suppress the immune response or its inflammatory end result. The latter includes a large armamentarium of neuropharmacologic agents that ameliorate dysfunction of different parts of the nervous system.

DISEASE-MODIFYING TREATMENT

Anti-inflammatory therapy with intravenous corticosteroids is presently the mainstay of treatment of significant acute exacerbations of MS. Acute symptoms may be alleviated, with significant shortening of the period of exacerbation. However, for a given attack, the extent of ultimate recovery is not altered. The most common treatment presently used is intravenous administration of methylprednisolone (Solumedrol) in doses of 500–1000 mg (or 10–15 mg/kg) daily for 5 days. Some patients may require hospital admission because of the severity of their neurologic symptoms. Intravenous steroids offer the advantage that they may be infused on an outpatient basis either in an ambulatory treatment unit or by a home-care agency. After intravenous steroid infusion, a tapered course of oral prednisone over 1 to 3 weeks usually is prescribed. In the past, some neurologists favored the less invasive alternative of a course of oral prednisone (0.5–1.0 mg/kg/day with taper over 2–4 weeks), rather than intravenous steroid administration. However, such oral-only regimens have been shown to have unfavorable outcome in the treatment of isolated optic neuritis and thus are now rarely used for demyelinating disease. Many experienced neurologists continue to favor the use of intravenous adrenocorticotropic hormone (ACTH; 80 U daily for 1–4 weeks). Administration of either steroids or ACTH may result in mood alterations, including euphoria and mania, and in psychotic symptoms. Euphoria may be more prominent among those patients with extensive brain involvement and can often be controlled by prescription of lithium carbonate. Most important, aseptic necrosis of the femoral head and other bones is a known complication of the use of steroids and is more common with intravenous use. This complication is unknown with ACTH.

Immunomodulating drugs have been used to modify the course of MS. For relapsing–remitting disease, three drugs, FDA labeled, have been shown to decrease exacerbation (relapse) rate, and there is some evidence that they may also affect disease progression. Two of these are closely related beta-interferons. Interferon β-1b (Betaseron) is injected subcutaneously every other day, while interferon β 1a (Avonex) is administered by intramuscular injection once per week. Both drugs are generally well tolerated, although side effects are more prominent with Betaseron (interferon β-1b) and notably include flulike symptoms; the former has also been the subject of reports of significant local skin reactions. A controversial topic is the development of neutralizing antibodies in response to interferon therapies (likely more so with β 1b than β-1a); these antibodies may correlate with some loss of responsiveness to therapy. From studies to date, it is also likely that interferon α will be effective in MS. Interferon γ is clearly *not* beneficial: It is the only known substance to *cause MS exacerbations.* Copolymer-1 (glatiramer acetate, Copaxone) is a synthetic amino acid copolymer that is injected subcutaneously daily; notable side effects include nearly universal injection-site reactions, and an acute anxiety-like reaction, with flushing and chest tightness.

Immunosuppressive agents in a variety of studies show modest efficacy in preventing disease exacerbations and deterring progression, and they are considered particularly helpful in cases of inexorably progressive disease. While not FDA-labeled for MS, studies have shown some efficacy for azathioprine (Imuran), methotrexate, and cyclophosphamide (Cytoxan), alone or in combination with steroids or ACTH. Other immunosuppressive therapies that have been investigated and found to be either without efficacy or with modest benefits outweighed by significant morbidity include plasma exchange in combination with cyclophosphamide, cyclosporine (Sandimmune), chlorambucil, linomide, total lymphoid irradiation (TLI), and oral myelin basic protein. Other immunomodulatory therapies still under investigation include mitoxantrone, cladribine, tacrolimus (FK506, Prograf), intravenous immunoglobulin (IVIg), and intravenous monoclonal antibodies directed against CD3, CD4, or CDw52 lymphocyte surface antigens. More specific experimental therapies also under investigation include other monoclonal antibodies including some against cell adhesion molecules (e.g., integrins), and vaccination against specific T-cell receptor V regions. Immunosuppressive therapies in MS patients are accompanied by some risk, particularly with regard to infection; these patients often already have compromised genitourinary and pulmonary systems. Patients with rapidly progressive disease should generally be referred to specialized centers.

SYMPTOMATIC TREATMENT

Physical and emotional rest have always been emphasized in the management of MS. Major life stress can aggravate MS but stress of any kind may transiently increase the symptoms of the illness and may be associated with exacerbations. Conversely, rest tends to ameliorate them. Apart from maintaining good health, patients should be encouraged to work within their physical limitations. Frustration may require psychologic counseling, although psychoanalytic therapy has not been productive in our patients. Since heat and overexertion can cause an increase in symptoms, and even cause acute exacerbations, use of air-conditioning and proper shelter is indicated. Fatigue can sometimes be improved with amantadine.

Spasticity is a major unremitting problem in many patients, and while physical therapy can be helpful, pharmacologic intervention is of much benefit. Baclofen (Lioresal) may be judiciously prescribed. Clonazepam (Klonopin) and other benzodiazepines, particularly when prescribed at night, can prevent spasms in the lower extremities. Similar small doses can also alleviate stiffness and spasms in the morning. Care should be exercised in prescribing baclofen or benzodiazepines since replacement of spasticity by weakness can result in greater handicap, and because of their sedating effects. Many patients find that carbamazepine (Tegretol) can alleviate paroxysmal leg spasms. Tizanidine (Zanaflex) is a new agent that can be very helpful with chronic spasticity. Its major advantage is that it does not induce muscle weakness in place of spasticity. Other drugs such as dantrolene (Dantrium), cyclobenzaprine (Flexeril) and other "muscle relaxants" are not especially helpful in the management of upper motor neuron spasticity.

Bladder dysfunction is very common. Acute urinary retention in the young patient often responds to sporadic catheterization. However, appropriate urologic care and follow-up is important. Hyperreflexic bladders are much more common. Oxybutinin (Ditropan) and propantheline (Pro-Banthine) are helpful in controlling nocturia but somewhat less so in the management of daytime urinary frequency. Dyssynergia occurs in the majority of patients and often is manifested as incomplete emptying. Failure to empty the bladder leads to increased risk of urinary infections and the risk of pyelonephritis. Timed voiding and fluid restriction are occasionally sufficient to achieve better emptying. Failing this, intermittent catheterization is always preferable to placement of an indwelling catheter because of the risks of infection. Urinary prophylaxis with antibiotic therapy is controversial. Many physicians avoid such suppressive therapy, even in cases of an indwelling catheter, because of the risk of selection of resistant bacteria, particularly *Pseudomonas* species, although nitrofurantoin (Macrodantin) or sulfamethoxazole/trimethoprim (Septa) is used by some patients with benefit. Acidification of the urine by ascorbic acid (24 g orally per day) with or without mandelic acid may be helpful without introducing risk of antibiotic-resistant bacteria.

Sexual dysfunction in men is often the product of spinal cord disease, but psychologic factors are equally important. Appropriate urologic and sleep studies may document the absence of morning erections, suggesting a neurourologic etiology. While penile prostheses may provide satisfactory results, a variety of injectable, and new oral pharmacologic approaches (sildenafil, Viagra) are now available to increase erectile function prior to attempted intercourse.

Physical therapy can improve gait and general level of functioning. Regular range-of-motion exercises can prevent contractures and maintain purposeful function in the upper extremities, especially during lengthy disability. Long-term maintenance therapy may be helpful in preventing patients from premature reliance on wheelchairs. Lightweight ankle/foot orthoses may be prescribed for drop-foot and can greatly assist in achievement of near-normal gait. Personal contact with the therapist may also be crucial in psychologic support of the patient.

QUESTIONS AND DISCUSSION

1. How is the diagnosis of multiple sclerosis made?

A. Clinical history and neurologic findings
B. Computerized tomographic examinations of the head
C. Cerebrospinal fluid examination
D. Magnetic resonance imaging of the brain
E. All of the above

The answer is (A). The diagnosis is always a clinical diagnosis. CSF and MRI are especially helpful procedures, but they do not replace history taking and neurologic examination.

2. Major disability in multiple sclerosis is usually due to:

A. Optic nerve involvement
B. Cerebral hemispheric lesions
C. Brainstem involvement
D. Spinal cord disease
E. All of the above

The answer is (D). Spinal cord lesions account for the majority of the disabling motor and sensory symptoms of MS. Brainstem and optic nerve deficits also figure importantly, with cerebral white matter involvement being less commonly symptomatic.

3. The three most useful laboratory tests to support the diagnosis of MS are:

A. Magnetic resonance imaging of the brain
B. Cerebrospinal fluid cell count
C. Cerebrospinal fluid immunoglobulin analysis
D. Visual evoked responses
E. Somatosensory evoked responses

The answer is (A), (C), and (D).

4. Trigeminal neuralgia:

A. Never occurs in young adults
B. Occurs in young adults only with pontine gliomas
C. Responds to most sedative drugs
D. Is treated only surgically
E. Usually responds well to carbamazepine

The answer is (E). While carbamazepine (Tegretol) is first-line treatment, phenytoin (Dilantin), and baclofen (Lioresal) are also useful in treatment. Surgery is a last resort.

5. Urinary frequency in multiple sclerosis:

A. Is rarely a significant problem
B. Is always a sign of infection
C. Predictably responds to propantheline (anticholinergics)
D. Requires careful evaluation and management
E. Should be disregarded

The answer is (D). Consultation and management by a urologist supplement the care by the attending physician. The major goal is to avoid damage to ureters and kidneys (hydronephrosis).

6. Treatment of multiple sclerosis:

A. Is a waste of time
B. Always requires the use of ACTH
C. Should take into consideration the patient's clinical status and disability

D. Should be limited to ACTH and physical therapy
E. Is limited to a low fat diet

The answer is (C). Management of the patient's psychologic reaction, clinical status, and disabilities must always be taken into consideration. Sometimes, the patient's most obvious disability is of least concern to him or her.

7. The risk of multiple sclerosis in the sister of a patient:

A. Is about 100 per 100,000
B. Is increased significantly
C. Is significantly decreased
D. Is increased only if HLA B7 is present
E. Is about the same as in any other community member

The answer is (B). Several studies have shown that the risk of multiple sclerosis is several times higher than by chance in a sibling.

8. Chronic progressive multiple sclerosis:

A. Has a good prognosis
B. May occur at any point in the illness but is more common after age 30
C. Is 10 times more common in women than in men
D. Most frequently arises between ages 20 and 30
E. All of the above

The answer is (B). Chronic progressive disease becomes more and more likely with age of onset after 30. It is also more common among men.

9. Which of the following statements concerning lumbar puncture are true?

A. It can cause exacerbations of multiple sclerosis.
B. When performed for spinal anesthesia, it may cause exacerbation.
C. It is helpful in establishing a diagnosis when oligoclonal bands are present.
D. It is helpful in establishing a diagnosis when IgG synthesis is increased.
E. It should not be performed because it is too risky.

The answer is (B), (C), and (D). Lumbar puncture, properly performed, is a safe diagnostic procedure. Risks of spinal anesthesia should be weighed carefully. CSF electrophoresis and immunoglobulin quantitation are helpful.

SUGGESTED READING

Adams CW: Color Atlas of Multiple Sclerosis and Other Myelin Disorders. Dobbs Ferry, NY, Sheridan Medical Books, 1989

Andersson PB, Goodkin DE: Current pharmacologic treatment of multiple sclerosis symptoms. West J Med 165:313, 1996.

Arnason BG, Toscas A, Dayal A et al: Role of interferons in demyelinating diseases. J Neural Transm 49 (Suppl):117, 1997

Bauer H, Hanefeld FA: Multiple Sclerosis: Its Impact from Childhood to Old Age. Philadelphia, Saunders, 1993

Compsten A, Ebers G, Lassman H et al: McAlpine's Multiple Sclerosis, 3rd edition. London, Churchill Livingstone, 1998

Dalgleish AG: Viruses and multiple sclerosis. Acta Neurol Scand 169 (Suppl):8, 1997

Dyment DA, Sadnovich AD, Ebers GC: Genetics of multiple sclerosis. Hum Mol Genet 6:1693, 1997

Halbreich U: Multiple Sclerosis: A Neuropsychiatric Disorder, 1st edition. Washington, DC, American Psychiatric Press, 1993

Hohlfeld R: Biotechnologic agents for the immunotherapy of multiple sclerosis: Principles, problems and perspectives. Brain 120:865, 1997

Kalb R, Scheinberg LC: Multiple Sclerosis and the Family. New York, Demos, 1992

Kurtzke JF, Beebe GW, Nagler B et al: Studies on natural history of multiple sclerosis IV: Clinical features of the onset bout. Acta Neurol Scand 44:467, 1968

Lauer K: On the diagnostic value of different CSF investigations in multiple sclerosis. J Neurol 231: 130, 1984

Noseworthy JH, Miller DH: Measurement of treatment efficacy and new trial results in multiple sclerosis. Curr Opin Neurol 10:201, 1997

Paty DW, Ebers GC: Multiple sclerosis. Philadelphia, FA Davis, 1998

Poser CM, Paty DW, Scheinberg L et al: New diagnostic criteria for multiple sclerosis: Guidelines for research protocols. Ann Neurol 13:227, 1983

Rao SM (ed.): Neurobehavioral Aspects of Multiple Sclerosis. New York: Oxford University Press, 1990

Rudick RA, Goodkin DE (eds.): Treatment of Multiple Sclerosis: Trial Design, Results, and Future Perspectives. London, Springer-Verlag, 1992

Schapiro RT: Symptom management in multiple sclerosis, 2nd edition. New York, Demos, 1994

Schumacher GA, Beebe G, Kibler RF et al: Problems of experimental trials of therapy in multiple sclerosis: Report by the panel on the evaluation of experimental trials of therapy in multiple sclerosis. Ann NY Acad Sci 122:552, 1965

Sibley W: Therapeutic Claims in Multiple Sclerosis: A Guide to Treatments, 4th edition. New York, Demos Vermande, 1996

Storch M, Lassmann H: Pathology and pathogenesis of demyelinating diseases. Curr Opin Neurol 10: 186, 1997

Thompson AJ, Noseworthy JH: New treatments for multiple sclerosis: A clinical perspective. Curr Opin Neurol 9:187, 1996

Neurology for the Non-Neurologist, Fourth Edition, edited by William J. Weiner and Christopher G. Goetz. Lippincott Williams & Wilkins, Philadelphia © 1999.

C H A P T E R 1 0

Parkinson's Disease

William J. Weiner

Lisa M. Shulman

Parkinson's disease is the most common akinetic rigid syndrome and the most frequently encountered extrapyramidal movement disorder. It is a neurodegenerative disease of unknown etiology that most often begins at 58 to 60 years of age. Approximately 10% to 15% of patients will have disease onset before age 50. As the population of the United States ages, the number of people at risk for the development of Parkinson's disease increases. Diagnostic and therapeutic knowledge is important not only because of the prevalence of the disorder but also because the pharmacology of Parkinson's disease has led to fundamental changes in the way investigators and physicians view central nervous system neurotransmitter function.

CLINICAL FEATURES

Parkinson's disease is characterized by a typical history of progressive neurologic disability and the following four major neurologic signs: resting tremor, cogwheel rigidity, bradykinesia, and impaired postural reflexes. It is often observed that by the time a patient presents to a physician for evaluation of this problem, the syndrome has been present for 1 to 2 years. Unilateral tremor involving a single limb is the most common presenting symptom and sign. However, careful history taking often reveals that dif-

ficulty buttoning shirts or blouses, fastening snaps, and cutting food with the proper utensils, and alterations in handwriting (Fig. 10-1), a feeling of stiffness, or a general feeling of overall slowness may have been noted up to 12 to 24 months earlier, and that these symptoms have gradually become worse. In addition, a patient may note that chewing food has become slow and laborious and that his voice fluctuates and seems to intermittently lose volume. Additional questions that help to illustrate the clinical problems in a patient with bradykinesia and impaired postural reflexes include inquiring whether or not the patient has difficulty rising from low, soft chairs or sofas, difficulty entering and leaving an automobile, difficulty turning from his back to his stomach or vice versa while lying in bed, or difficulty maintaining balance in a crowd. The patient may have noticed that occasionally he is unable to stop walking forward (propulsion) or backward (retropulsion). Family members may also report that the his face has changed and that he does not smile as much (masked faces; Fig. 10-2), that he seems to stare all the time (reptilian stare), that his posture has become stooped and flexed (simian posture; Fig. 10-3), and that he has become exasperatingly slow. It may take 30 to 90 minutes to dress in the morning and even longer to disrobe in the evening.

The elucidation of this history may make the diagnosis of parkinsonism evident. It is apparent that not all patients will present with all of these symptoms,

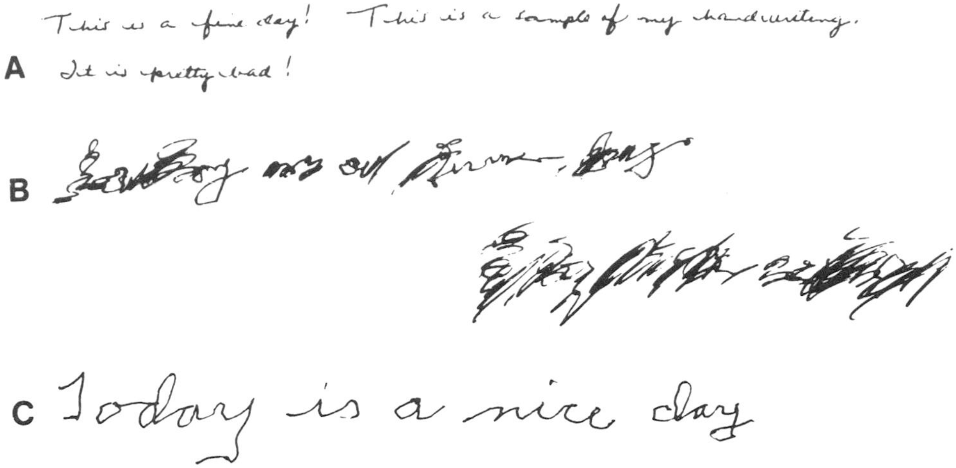

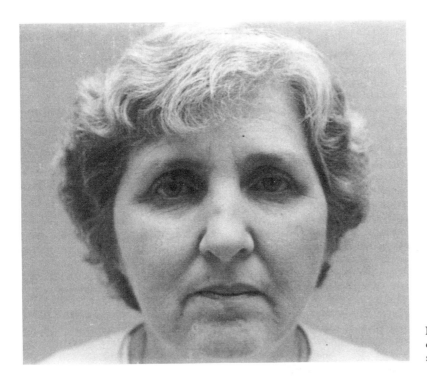

FIG. 10-1. **A.** This handwriting sample from a 55-year-old patient with untreated Parkinson's disease is a good example of the typical micrographic handwriting that is often characteristic of this condition. The handwriting samples shown in *B* and *C* are from a patient with essential tremor. **B.** Prior to treatment, the sample shows the typical large, sloppy script. **C.** This sample, taken from the same patient with essential tremor while being treated with propranolol (160 mg/day), shows obvious improvement. Changes in written script can provide excellent clues to the type of movement disorder that is present (see Chapter 11).

FIG. 10-2. Typical masked facies in a patient with Parkinson's disease.

and that a patient will occasionally present with only a single symptom and yet will have parkinsonism. Additional questions that may help determine the etiology of the syndrome are whether the onset of symptoms was abrupt or insidious; whether there has been a gradual progression of symptoms; whether there is a family history of neurologic syndromes; and whether there is concurrent drug use, past history of encephalitis, or exposure to various toxins including the use of street drugs.

Resting tremor is the most frequent presenting sign in these patients. The appearance of this tremor often precipitates the patient's visit to the doctor. The tremor is highly characteristic and consists of a low- to medium-amplitude, five-to-seven-cycles-per-second alternating movement. *Tremor* is defined as the involuntary rhythmic oscillatory sinusoidal movement that results from the alternating or synchronous contractions of reciprocally innervated antagonistic muscles. Resting tremor has been described as "pill rolling" because of the movement of the fingers and thumb. The tremor, however, may begin in the hands, legs, or face and most often appears unilaterally in a single limb. It will often progress to involve the second limb of the same side before becoming bilateral. With the exception of impaired postural reflexes, the major signs of parkinsonism appear most often as unilateral manifestations, often confusing the unfamiliar and raising inappropriate diagnostic categories. Careful observation of the tremor will reveal that it is a resting tremor that tends to be ameliorated when a purposeful movement is undertaken. A simple, quick way of assessing whether a tremor is primarily a resting or kinetic tremor is to have the patient perform a finger-to-finger and finger-to-nose maneuver and to observe the affected limb when it is posturally supported in a resting position. The patient with a resting tremor will perform these maneuvers and a marked amelioration of tremor will be observed during this time. The patient with kinetic tremor will be observed to have no tremor at rest but will develop typical dysmetric movements as the hand reaches the target object. When the limbs are observed in a totally supported and at-rest position, the patient with resting tremor will be seen to have the tremor, whereas those patients with kinetic tremor will not.

Cogwheel rigidity is a sign that can be present in a unilateral or bilateral distribution depending on the stage of illness. The patient does not complain of "cogwheeling." This sign is elicited by passive movement of the limb and neck through a full range of motion. When present, this sign is particularly elicitable when the neck is flexed and extended and when the elbow and wrist are fully flexed and extended. There is, in addition to increased tone, a characteristic rachet-like sensation felt with passive movement. This can often be observed but is more easily palpated by the examiner as the limb is flexed and extended. There are some patients in whom the initial symptomatology is cervical or low back discomfort, and the question of whether or not increased muscle tone is responsible for this symptom has been raised.

Bradykinesia, an additional characteristic sign, is certainly responsible for a great deal of the disability that is associated with parkinsonism. Slowness of voluntary movement is characteristic of this syndrome and accounts for the difficulty in such diverse activities as turning over in bed, rising from chairs, chewing food, dressing, walking, and numerous other activities of daily living. Some of these difficulties can be easily observed during an examination by watching the patient rise from a chair, walk to the examining room, and undress. Observe the general slowness with which the simplest maneuvers are undertaken. Again, this can initially be seen as a unilateral finding.

A final important sign in these patients is impaired *postural reflexes.* Postural reflexes refer to the ability of the patient to right himself and to keep from losing his balance when sustaining minor postural perturbances (e.g., being jostled in a crowd). In addition, these reflexes also encompass the ability of patients to turn around and change directions while walking without losing their balance and falling. These reflexes can be simply and effectively evaluated by observing the patient walk 10 to 15 steps and turn around. A patient with normal postural reflexes should be able to pivot and turn without taking extra steps. In parkinsonism, one will often observe that it takes the patient three to five steps to change direction. The second office test of postural reflexes includes a mild thrust to the chest wall with the admonition to the patient that he is not to step backward. The examiner must position himself, or have someone else positioned, behind the patient during this maneuver, because the response can vary from none, to taking one step backward, to taking seven to eight steps backward (retropulsion), to taking no steps but completely losing balance and falling (Fig. 10-4). Impaired postural reflexes with frequent falls are a source of severe disability in fully advanced parkinsonism because of associated morbidity (e.g., subdural hematomas, fractures of the hips or wrists). It should be noted that when postural reflex impairment is the predominant early manifestation of parkinsonism, the diagnosis more often than not is not true Parkinson's disease but one of the other neu-

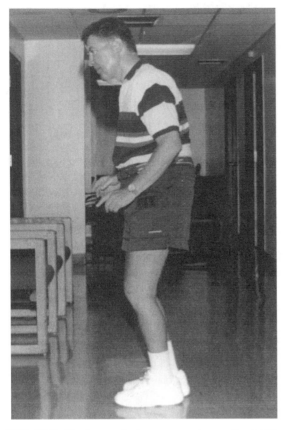

FIG. 10-3. Moderate simian posture in a patient with Parkinson's disease. Note the flexion of the upper extremities, of the upper trunk, and of the head. Facial masking is also apparent.

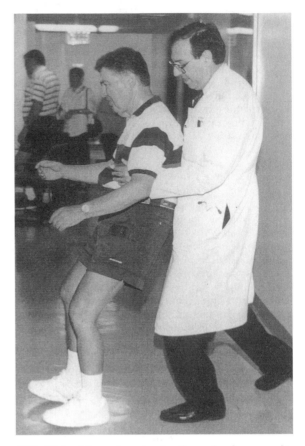

FIG. 10-4. A loss of postural reflexes is often seen in patients with Parkinson's disease. After instructing the patient to maintain his posture, the examiner has administered a backward thrust to the patient's chest. His postural response is quite poor: Rather than maintaining a fixed postural response to the thrust or taking one or two steps backward, the patient has lost his balance entirely and requires the assistance of the examiner to prevent him from falling to the ground.

rodegenerative disorders that produces parkinsonism, such as progressive supranuclear palsy (PSP).

This discussion of the symptoms and signs of parkinsonism should serve to remind the examining physician that there is no single pathognomonic sign of the disorder but that it is a constellation of symptoms and signs that results in this clinical diagnosis. There is no known biologic marker of Parkinson's disease and therefore there is no definitive laboratory or imaging study that confirms the diagnosis. The diagnosis is clinical and is dependent on the interpretation of the patient's history and neurologic examination. Furthermore, the diagnosis of parkinsonism does not necessarily mean that the patient has Parkinson's disease. Parkinson's disease is characterized by a specific

neuropathology. The substantia nigra (a pigmented midbrain nucleus) bears the brunt of the pathologic changes, with depigmentation, neuronal loss, and the presence of intracytoplasmic inclusion bodies (Lewy bodies). Patients who present with tremor, rigidity, bradykinesia, and impaired postural reflexes but who do not have this specific neuropathology are diagnosed as having an akinetic rigid syndrome or parkinsonism but not Parkinson's disease.

PHARMACOLOGY

Early studies demonstrated that there were regional concentration differences in dopamine in different areas of the brain. The corpus striatum (a basal ganglia nuclear group) was determined to have a high concentration of dopamine. Neurochemical investigation of the brains of patients who died with Parkinson's disease were conducted and the corpus striatum concentration of dopamine was low compared with the dopamine concentration in nonparkinsonian corpus striatum. This finding was the first definitive biochemical lesion in an adult-onset degenerative disorder of the extrapyramidal system. Parkinson's disease could now be defined by loss of dopamine in the corpus striatum and degeneration of the substantia nigra. Further study revealed that the high concentration of dopamine in the corpus striatum was not located in the neurons of the striatum but was anatomically situated in the presynaptic terminals of neurons whose origin was the substantia nigra. In other words, there exists an anatomic pathway between the substantia nigra and the corpus striatum. The nigrostriatal pathway utilizes dopamine as its neurotransmitter, and it became clear that the progressive loss of substantia nigra neurons was accompanied by a progressive loss of dopamine in the striatum. Since the projection pathway was degenerating and the dopamine is anatomically located within the projection pathway, it is not surprising that dopamine was progressively lost in this disorder.

The series of discoveries that led to the knowledge that Parkinson's disease was associated with the loss of a specific regionally located neurotransmitter (dopamine) was a remarkable advance in our understanding of adult-onset neurodegenerative disorders. In 1967, enormous quantities of levodopa (4 to 8 g/day) was administered to Parkinson's disease patients and the remarkable therapeutic response was observed. For levodopa to have a therapeutic effect, it must cross the blood–brain barrier and be decarboxylated to dopamine. The enzyme that decarboxylates dopa to dopamine is ubiquitous and also decarboxylates several other aromatic amino acids. This enzyme, termed *aromatic amino acid decarboxylase* or *dopa decarboxylase,* is found in several extracerebral locations, including the gastrointestinal tract, liver, and kidney. When orally administered, levodopa is absorbed, acted on by the extracerebral decarboxylase, and converted to dopamine, which cannot cross the blood–brain barrier. If levodopa is administered alone, enormous quantities are required to overcome the peripheral decarboxylase systems and achieve a

therapeutic benefit. The use of a peripheral decarboxylase inhibitor (carbidopa) with levodopa results in a much lower dose of levodopa needing to be administered to achieve a central effect.

Another important enzyme that plays a role in determining how much levodopa circulating in the blood can reach the brain is catechol-*O*-methyltransferase (COMT). COMT methylates levodopa and reduces the effective concentration of levodopa available for transport into the brain. COMT inhibition has just been introduced as a therapeutic maneuver to enhance levodopa availability for transport into the brain and thus increase central dopamine activity.

Since the replenishment of the neurotransmitter dopamine in the striatum results in remarkable clinical improvement in patients with Parkinson's disease, there is an implication that the neural substrate that dopamine acts on (the striatal dopamine receptors) is essentially intact in this disorder. The dopamine receptor sites are divided into five different subtypes, but there are two main families: the D_1 and D_5 group and the D_2, D_3, and D_4 group. Dopamine receptor agonists must have D_2 activity for them to be effective in the treatment of Parkinson's disease. The dopamine receptor agonists that are available to treat Parkinson's disease include the ergot derived (bromocriptine and pergolide) and the non-ergot derived (pramipexole and ropinirole). Pramipexole and ropinirole were both introduced for the treatment of Parkinson's disease in 1997. Although all of the dopamine receptor agonists have D_2 activity, they have somewhat different profiles of activation for the various dopamine receptors. Therefore, there are variations among individual patients in regard to which agonist is the most efficacious. Although the number of antiparkinsonian medications grows steadily, levodopa remains the gold standard of therapy, the most potent drug for Parkinson's symptoms.

TREATMENT

All medications currently used to treat Parkinson's disease provide symptomatic relief only, and do not alter the underlying pathogenesis of the disorder; in other words, the natural progression of Parkinson's disease continues despite current treatment. The treatment of each patient with Parkinson's disease should be highly individualized to provide acceptable symptomatic relief. If a patient's symptoms are very mild and causing no impairment in the activities of daily living, delay of treatment may be the appropriate choice. If a patient's symptoms are mildly troublesome, with tremor as the predominant feature, low-dose anticholinergics (e.g., trihexyphenidyl, bentropine) may be all that is required. The anticholinergics are useful because the striatum contains high levels of both dopamine and acetylcholine, and the dopamine deficiency state in the striatum of patients with Parkinson's disease produces a relative cholinergic hyperactivity. Anticholinergics exert their beneficial effect by partially correcting this apparent cholinergic excess. Anticholinergics must be used with caution in older patients, since they can induce memory dysfunction and confusion. In older men, anticholinergics can lead to urinary hesitancy and retention.

Amantadine is also useful in the treatment of early Parkinson's disease and can be helpful for early bradykinesia. Amantadine has anticholinergic activity, mild dopaminergic activity, and antiglutaminergic activity. Amantadine may also be useful in treating drug-induced dyskinesia in more advanced Parkinson's disease. Combined treatment with anticholinergics and amantadine may provide symptomatic relief for a short period of time. Alternative therapies for patients with early troublesome symptoms include monotherapy with the dopamine receptor agonists (pramipexole or ropinirole) or low-dose carbidopa–levodopa with a COMT inhibitor (tolcapone or entacapone). The progression of the disease process will eventually result in the need for more powerful dopaminergic stimulation.

The use of levodopa as a precursor loading strategy to increase central dopamine and to ameliorate Parkinson's disease has been one of the remarkable therapeutic advances in neurology. However, high-dose levodopa administration without the addition of a peripheral dopa decarboxylase inhibitor, such as carbidopa, produces anorexia, nausea, and vomiting. These symptoms occur because of the high levels of circulating peripheral dopamine that are present as a result of extensive extracerebral decarboxylation, and which result in the stimulation of the area postrema, the emesis center. The development of peripheral dopa decarboxylase inhibitors in large part ameliorated these problems and led to the development of combination therapy with levodopa and carbidopa. This drug is available in fixed ratios of 10:100, 25:250, and 25:100 with the numerator indicating the milligram dose of carbidopa and the denominator, the milligram dose of levodopa. The most important advantage of this drug is the ability to administer less levodopa to obtain the same central effect. This results in a reduction of nausea and vomiting. In fact, the ease of administration of carbidopa–levodopa (Sinemet) therapy both for the patient and the treating physician

has resulted in its being used almost exclusively in the treatment of patients with Parkinson's disease who require levodopa. Carbidopa–levodopa in a controlled-release formulation (Sinemet CR 25/100, Sinemet CR 50/200) provides a slower and longer-lasting effect of levodopa. Sinemet CR preparations are particularly useful to treat motor fluctuations, night-time bradykinesia resulting in sleep disruption, early morning painful dystonic cramps, and early morning severe bradykinesia.

There are now four dopamine receptor agonists available to treat Parkinson's disease (Table 10-1). All four are direct-acting dopamine receptor agonists that have been demonstrated to be effective in the treatment of Parkinson's disease. Since dopamine receptor agonists exert their effect on the striatal dopamine receptors (which presumably are not involved in the substantia nigra degenerative process), it was felt that they would perhaps be effective when carbidopa–levodopa fails and that they might not produce the same toxic effects as carbidopa–levodopa. Clinical experience with all four has shown that they are effective not only in the treatment of Parkinson's disease but also in ameliorating motor fluctuations in patients treated with carbidopa–levodopa. Bromocriptine and pergolide are most often used in practice as adjustments to therapy with carbidopa–levodopa in more advanced patients with Parkinson's disease. Pramipexole and ropinirole have been approved for use in both early and late Parkinson's disease. Preliminary evidence suggests that pramipexole and ropinirole are both effective and well tolerated in early Parkinson's disease, and these agents may become more widely used as first-line therapy in early Parkinson's disease. There is great interest in determining whether or not early treatment with pramipexole or ropinirole is better than early treatment with carbidopa–levodopa in terms of preventing long-term complications of therapy such as dyskinesias, motor fluctuations, and psychosis. Clinical trials are currently in progress testing this hypothesis.

TABLE 10-1. Dopamine Receptor Agonists for the Treatment of Parkinson's Disease

GENERIC	TRADE NAME
Bromocriptine	Parlodel[a]
Pergolide	Permax[a]
Pramipexole	Mirapex[b]
Ropinirole	Requip[b]

[a] Ergot derived.
[b] Nonergot.

Selegline (Eldepryl), a monoamine oxidase type B inhibitor, inhibits the catabolism of dopamine and promotes dopaminergic activity. Selegline has also been used in early Parkinson's disease and has been shown to delay the need for carbidopa–levodopa. There has been considerable discussion as to whether or not this effect in early Parkinson's disease is "neuroprotective" or simply symptomatic. The evidence strongly suggests that the effect of selegline in this situation is symptomatic.

Tolcapone (Tasmar) and entacapone (Comten) are the first COMT inhibitors to be approved for the treatment of Parkinson's disease. COMT inhibitors must be administered in combination with levodopa, resulting in increased bioavailability of levodopa to the brain. COMT inhibitors may enhance dopaminergic side effects, therefore downward titration of carbidopa–levodopa may be required, particularly in patients who already have dyskinesia. Tolcapone and entacapone have been shown to be effective in patients experiencing motor fluctuations. Both drugs are easy to administer and their therapeutic efficacy can be quickly ascertained. The Food and Drug Administration (FDA) has determined that hepatotoxicity associated with tolcapone requires stringent liver function monitoring and informed consent if this drug is prescribed. Entacapone, as of now, is not reported to be associated with liver toxicity. It should be noted that all of the various classes of anti-Parkinson's medications may be used in combination, particularly in the advanced patient with complex symptoms.

COMPLICATIONS

Although there is no question that carbidopa–levodopa is the mainstay of therapy in this disorder, numerous problems are associated with its use (Table 10-2). However, it should be recognized that several long-term follow-up studies of patients with

TABLE 10-2. Toxicity Associated with Chronic Levodopa Therapy

Central toxicity	Dyskinesias
	Motor fluctuations
	"On–off" phenomenon
	Sleep disturbances
	Psychiatric disturbances
Peripheral toxicity	Nausea and vomiting
Mixed central and	
peripheral toxicity	Orthostatic hypotension

Parkinson's disease who were treated with these agents showed that at the end of 5 and 6 years of treatment, most were either no worse than prior to treatment or better than before they were treated. This finding is extraordinary because prior to levodopa treatment in Parkinson's disease, the prognostic outlook was dismal.

In recent years, a controversy concerning the use of carbidopa–levodopa has arisen. Some argue that, despite its clear therapeutic effect, levodopa is toxic to dopaminergic neurons. Others dispute this concept for lack of evidence.

Several major side effects are associated with the use of levodopa and carbidopa–levodopa, including drug-induced dyskinesias, drug-induced psychiatric problems, and motor fluctuations. Levodopa-induced dyskinesias are striking long-term complications of this therapy. The dyskinesias are most often choreic. Chorea consists of irregular, unpredictable, brief jerky movements that flit from one body part to another in a continuous random sequence. Occasionally, levodopa-induced *dyskinesias* are dystonic in quality. Dystonia describes movements that are dominated by sustained muscle contraction, frequently resulting in twisting repetitive movements and abnormal postures. The dyskinesia may involve the lingual, facial, and buccal regions, the limbs, and the axial musculature. It is dramatic to see patients with this drug-related disorder, because they were previously always characterized by their slowness and poverty of movement. The chorea seen in this setting is quite similar to the chorea seen in Huntington's disease or tardive dyskinesia.

Levodopa-induced dyskinesias are quite frequent and are seen in more than half the patients at the end of 5 years of carbidopa–levodopa treatment. The severity of the chorea may increase with continued treatment, and the dose of levodopa required to elicit chorea may decrease with time. A reduction in dosage will invariably ameliorate this drug-induced movement disorder. Although the chorea may be severe, the parkinsonian patient rarely complains, and the family or the physician is usually the first to notice the chorea and become concerned about it. This common response to the movement disorder is probably best explained by the fact that often while a patient is choreatic they are still able to voluntarily move around with relative ease, and given their choice all parkinsonian patients would rather be choreatic and mobile than bradykinetic. Levodopa-induced dyskinesia can in some patients be as disabling as bradykinesia.

The *psychiatric side effects* of long-term dopaminergic therapy include altered sleep patterns, vivid nightmares, auditory and visual hallucinations, paranoia, and psychosis. While there may be a continuum in the expression of these side effects, with the increasing severity of each complication being dose- and treatment-duration-related, there are also reports that such a continuum does not represent an individual patient response. Whether or not single patients display the entire psychiatric spectrum of complications or the spectrum represents a wide range of responses to chronic dopaminergic treatment, it is certain that the following complications are drug-related and are frequently seen. These drug-related complications (alterations in sleep patterns beginning with increasing insomnia, day-night reversal, and vivid nightmares; visual hallucinations; increasing paranoia; and paranoid psychosis) can be ameliorated by dosage reduction.

The simplest approach to drug-induced psychosis in the setting of Parkinson's disease is to reduce the dosage of antiparkinsonian medications, and particularly to generally reduce the administration of other medications that depress the nervous system, including sedatives, hypnotics, anxiolytics, anticholinergics, and muscle relaxants. When this is not sufficient to relieve hallucinations and delusions, the use of antipsychotic medications is indicated in order to continue the Parkinson's medications at a level to maintain the patient's motor function. There are several atypical neuroleptic drugs now available that can reduce or abolish psychosis with less potential for extrapyramidal side effects. Clozapine (Clozaril) is the only neuroleptic that does not produce any adverse motor effects, while olanzapine (Zyprexa) and quentiapine (Seroquel) have reduced extrapyramidal side effects as compared to the traditional neuroleptics, which should be avoided in parkinsonians.

Fluctuation in motor performance is an additional complication of chronic carbidopa–levodopa therapy. After a variable period of treatment, patients note that the beneficial effects of the drug begin to wear off before they are due to take their next dose ("wearing off" or end-of-dose akinesia) and that they may be very akinetic in the morning before the first dose of medication (morning akinesia). One or more doses often do not seem to work. Later, particularly in patients on multiple overlapping doses of carbidopa–levodopa, the fluctuations from a mobile state or "on" to "off" with obvious parkinsonism may appear random with no obvious relation to dosage timing. The transition between relatively normal function to complete reemergence of the parkinsonian state can occur in several minutes and it can persist for up to 3 to 4 hours. Sudden, rapid, unpredictable fluctuations between these two extremes have been termed

the *on/off phenomenon*. Clinically, these fluctuations can be striking, and the dramatic nature of these transitions can occasionally be observed during an office evaluation. A patient may be seen in a severely parkinsonian state ("off") with marked cogwheel rigidity, resting tremor, severe akinesia to the degree that the patient is unable to rise from a chair, and impaired postural reflexes to the point of falling or being unable to stand. During 5 to 6 minutes, the same patient may turn "on" and be observed to be able to stand and sit without any difficulty, to be without cogwheeling, to have no tremor, and to be able to walk relatively normally and not look at all parkinsonian. The observer who is unfamiliar with these rapid transitions is astounded by these fluctuations, and the uninformed observer may believe that the severe parkinsonian state, or "off," may reflect a nonorganic problem of an emotional nature.

This perplexing problem seems to be related to alterations in central dopamine receptor-site responsiveness and to fluctuating levels of available neurotransmitter. There are many therapeutic maneuvers to employ in a patient with motor fluctuations, including increasing the antiparkinsonian medication dose or dosing frequency, adding the controlled-release formulation of carbidopa–levodopa, adding a dopamine receptor agonist, adding a COMT inhibitor, or implementing a restricted protein diet. New medications should be added one at a time. Both levodopa and the dopamine receptor agonists (bromocriptine, pergolide, pramipexole, ropinirole) must be initiated at a low dose and then gradually titrated upward to the therapeutic range while the COMT inhibitor, tolcapone or entacapone, is initiated at an effective dose. The restricted protein diet is particularly effective in those patients who report a relatively dramatic effect of diet on their response to carbidopa–levodopa. Levodopa shares the same gastrointestinal transport system as other amino acids, and high protein meals result in greater competition for the uptake system and lower the amount of levodopa available to the central nervous system. In patients who note loss of efficiency of carbidopa/levodopa when it is administered with a protein meal, the restricted protein diet may provide smoother motor response throughout the day.

The symptoms of Parkinson's disease remain responsive to the effects of levodopa throughout the duration of the illness; however, as the disease advances, the degree of symptom relief is less satisfying and the complications of motor fluctuations, dyskinesia, and hallucinosis emerge. The proper timing of the initiation of levodopa therapy concerns many clinicians. Common sense should rule this decision with the administration of levodopa when the patient's ability to carry out daily functions is significantly impaired. There is no benefit to withholding treatment until full disability ensues.

These problems associated with chronic dopaminergic agonist therapy in Parkinson's disease have led to the therapeutic recommendations already discussed. However, there are many patients who require long-term carbidopa–levodopa treatment and who also have these severe side effects. At present, the therapeutic decisions involve balancing drug-related side effects against drug-induced improvement. However, this approach eventually leads to the double-bind situation in which the patient requires increased levodopa to improve his/her parkinsonism, but decreased levodopa to decrease his/her dopaminergic toxicity syndrome. The introduction of dopamine receptor agonists can often be useful in this situation. Dopamine receptor agonist administration provides dopaminergic stimulation of the postsynaptic striatal dopamine receptors and also allows a reduction in carbidopa–levodopa dose. In some patients, this titration of doses up and down respectively will provide relief from drug-induced side effects and will provide continued motor improvement.

SURGERY

Although ablative surgery has been used in Parkinson's disease for over 50 years, there has recently been a resurgence of interest in surgical approaches, primarily because of increased understanding of the basal ganglia physiologic circuits involved in the production of the signs and symptoms of Parkinson's disease. Pallidotomy utilizing updated stereotaxic techniques has been widely reintroduced to treat advanced Parkinson's disease. In this procedure, a small lesion is made by the neurosurgeon in the globus pallidus in an attempt to disrupt the physiologic outflow of the basal ganglia and relieve the symptoms of Parkinson's disease. Some centers have reported a 20% to 25% improvement in the motor symptoms of Parkinson's disease, and resolution of dyskinesia in selected patients. Neurosurgical complications include intraparenchymal hemorrhage, cerebral vascular accident, and altered mental status. Some neurologists believe that the degree of motor improvement after pallidotomy does not justify the procedure, although most agree that severe uncontrollable dyskinesia is relieved by pallidotomy.

Another surgical procedure that has recently received approval for use in Parkinson's disease patients is deep brain stimulation (DBS). DBS is a neurosurgical stereotactic procedure in which a stimulating electrode is placed in a selected brain region (target) and wires are subcutaneously passed from the target to an electronic stimulator that is subcutaneously implanted in the chest wall (analogous to a cardiac pacemaker). The stimulator can be turned off and on by the patient with the use of a magnetic "wand." DBS is currently approved for electrode implantation and stimulation of the Vim nucleus of the thalamus. It may be useful for tremor suppression in patients with uncontrolled tremor. However, the other symptoms of Parkinson's disease (bradykinesia, rigidity, loss of balance) are not relieved by this procedure. There is considerable interest in the investigation of different target sites, such as the globus pallidus or subthalamic nucleus, for DBS. Preliminary results suggest that DBS in these sites may be beneficial for a wider range of Parkinson's symptoms. Further studies are in progress.

There has been considerable interest in the role of fetal tissue (mesencephalon) implants in the treatment of Parkinson's disease. This concept involves the transplantation of the dopamine-producing mesencephalon cells from an aborted fetal brain into the brain of the patient with Parkinson's disease. Although there have been reports that some Parkinson's disease patients who have received fetal tissue implants have improved, there is insufficient data available to form conclusions regarding the safety and efficacy of this procedure. Further research is required to answer a myriad of questions, including what anatomic area within the brain of the Parkinson's disease patient should receive the implant, how many fetal brains are needed for each transplantation procedure, which Parkinson's disease patients will benefit from the implants, and whether the disease process will affect the transplanted dopaminergic cells. There are currently two double-blind studies in progress to respond to the question of whether or not human fetal transplantation has a role in the treatment of Parkinson's disease. There is also interest in porcine fetal transplants to avoid some of the problems associated with human fetal cell transplantation.

DRUG-INDUCED PARKINSONISM

Drug-induced parkinsonism can be precipitated by any drug that decreases central dopaminergic transmission. Drugs that block the dopamine receptor (e.g., neuroleptics, metoclopramide) or deplete central dopamine (e.g., reserpine) often result in parkinsonian symptomatology. Parkinsonism induced by drugs can mimic all of the features seen in idiopathic Parkinson's disease. Akinesia is usually the most common sign, and resting tremor is seen less often. Other features that may help distinguish drug-induced parkinsonism from Parkinson's disease include a clear history of ingestion of a compound known to interfere with central dopamine activity, a relatively short time between the previous degree of parkinsonian symptoms and significant disability (about 1 to 2 months as opposed to 6 to 12 months), bilateral presentation instead of unilateral presentation of symptoms and signs, and the presence of other drug-related motor abnormalities (e.g., tardive dyskinesia, see Chapter 11).

The diagnosis of drug-induced parkinsonism requires a high index of suspicion. Once the diagnosis is made, treatment should be directed to stopping the offending drug. In almost all patients with this syndrome, the parkinsonism will resolve. If active treatment is required, anticholinergics, amantadine, and levodopa–carbidopa have been successfully used. In patients in whom drug-induced parkinsonism does not resolve, idiopathic Parkinson's disease may have been unmasked.

FURTHER CONSIDERATIONS

Although the etiology of Parkinson's disease remains unknown, there have been recent attempts to alter the progression of this disorder. This approach to treatment, sometimes referred to as "neuroprotective," have been based on interfering with both exogenous and endogenous oxidative processes in the parkinsonian brain with the antioxidants vitamin E, vitamin C, and deprenyl. These oxidative processes may contribute to dopaminergic cell death, and these drugs, through different mechanisms, may slow the process. A very large, well-controlled study indicated that vitamin E (2,000 units/day) did not slow progression of Parkinson's disease. This same study demonstrated that selegline had mild symptomatic effects in Parkinson's disease, and this confounded the issue of whether the effect of selegline in early Parkinson's disease was neuroprotective or symptomatic. Additional follow-up of these patients has demonstrated that selegline is not neuroprotective. Vitamin C in doses of 1,500–3,000 mg per day has been proposed as an additional antioxidant treatment, but vitamin C has never been properly tested. At present, there is no proof that a "neuroprotective" therapy exists for Parkinson's disease. Research in this area continues, and it is hoped that it will be successful.

The levodopa treatment era in Parkinson's disease has also led to broadening the scope of what is considered to be the central nervous system dysfunction seen in this disorder. Although James Parkinson did not originally describe mental deterioration as part of the illness, it has become increasingly apparent that dementia is often associated with Parkinson's disease. There is evidence from the pre-levodopa era to suggest that 25% to 30% of patients with Parkinson's disease were eventually institutionalized because of dementia and not because of incapacitating motor performance. However, the increased longevity and maintenance of communicative abilities in patients with Parkinson's disease have led to the observation that dementia is often seen as Parkinson's disease progresses. Recent studies confirm earlier observations that as many as 25% of patients with Parkinson's disease may develop dementia. Dementia must be differentiated from drug-induced altered mental states, since the former is not amenable to treatment but the latter is.

There is considerable interest in other nonmotor symptoms of Parkinson's disease including depression, apathy, fatigue, anxiety, and sleep disruption. Present studies indicate that all of these nonmotor symptoms of the disease are much more frequent than previously understood. Pramipexole (Mirapex) has antidepressant effects and may be helpful in patients with prominent nonmotor symptoms.

Any drug or degenerative process that interferes with central dopaminergic activity can lead to parkinsonism. The dysfunction of the dopamine system may involve the nigral (presynaptic) neuron or the striatal dopamine receptor (postsynaptic). Drugs or degenerative processes that affect not the presynaptic nigrostriatal dopaminergic pathway but the striatal dopamine receptors may result in the same clinical signs. The latter situation is sometimes referred to as *postsynaptic parkinsonism*. Examples of postsynaptic parkinsonism include drug-induced states and metabolic disturbances that result in calcification of the basal ganglia (often not seen on skull films but visible by computerized tomography or magnetic resonance imaging) and familial striatonigral degeneration. Since the pathology in these syndromes is located primarily within the striatum and involves the dopamine receptors, it should not be surprising that carbidopa–levodopa therapy has less effect in these disorders. Several additional syndromes that may have elements of both pre- and postsynaptic dopaminergic dysfunction include olivopontocerebellar (OPC degeneration, PSP, and the Shy-Drager syndrome. Clinical clues to the diagnosis of these syndromes, in addition to the variable response of the parkinsonian features to levodopa, include the presence of a marked intention tremor (OPC), the failure of voluntary conjugate gaze (PSP), and the presence of severe orthostatic hypotension (Shy-Drager).

QUESTIONS AND DISCUSSION

1. A 62-year-old right-handed man went to his physician with the following problems. He has noticed for the last 6 months that his handwriting had been changing and that it appears small and cramped. In addition, he has the feeling that his right hand is not as strong as it used to be, and he notices occasionally that he has to struggle to button his shirt. The week prior to his visit, his wife noticed that his right hand appeared to be shaking when he was resting quietly in an easy chair.

The most likely diagnosis in this patient based on history alone is:

A. Parkinson's disease
B. Wilson's disease
C. Huntington's disease
D. Dystonia

Neurologic findings present on examination might include which of the following?

A. Bilateral limb chorea, linguofaciobuccal dyskinesias
B. Resting tremor of the right hand, cogwheel rigidity of the right upper extremity
C. Fixed dystonic posturing of the right hand
D. Kinetic tremor of the right hand
E. Three-step retropulsion, two to three extra steps in turning maneuvers

The answer to the first part of the question is (A) and the answer to the second part is (B) and (E). This is a typical history of Parkinson's disease characterized by slow progression of the disability and a predominantly unilateral presentation of the symptoms and signs. In addition, the handwriting is described as cramped and small (micrographic). The feeling of weakness in an involved extremity is a common complaint, although there is not often any objective sign of weakness. The presence of unilateral signs of tremor and cogwheel rigidity is typical. The additional finding on examination that the postural reflexes are also impaired (retropulsion is present and there are increased steps on turning maneuvers) is an indication that a thorough examination of this patient will reveal additional signs of neurologic dysfunction.

2. A 59-year-old right-handed woman has a 5-year history of left upper extremity resting tremor. She has been treated with carbidopa–levodopa for the last 4 years. Although she states that originally her tremor was much improved, she has been having difficulty with increasing involuntary wild "dancelike" gyrating, nonpurposeful movements of the left upper and lower extremities. In addition, her husband relates that occasionally the patient remarks that there are visitors in the house when that is not so. Closer questioning of the patient about this reveals that she often sees people who are not really there. She speaks lucidly about this and recognizes that they are not real. The correct diagnosis in this patient would be:

A. Dystonic posturing of the left upper extremities
B. Tardive dyskinesia
C. Parkinson's disease and dopaminergic toxicity
D. Wilson's disease and dopaminergic toxicity

The answer is (C). The patient's initial presenting complaint is the spontaneous appearance of a unilateral resting tremor that is relieved by dopaminergic agents. This is a characteristic early presentation of unilateral Parkinson's disease, and the additional information that dopaminergic therapy ameliorated the symptoms suggests the diagnosis of Parkinson's disease. The patient's present complaints can be diagnosed as part of the chronic dopaminergic toxicity syndrome and in particular as dopaminergic-induced chorea and hallucinations. Choreiform movements that are induced by dopaminergic therapy in patients with Parkinson's disease are not phenomenologically distinguishable from the chorea seen in many other choreatic states. The hallucinations reported by this patient are also typical, since the most common hallucinosis seen in this setting are nonthreatening visual hallucinations.

Answer (A) is incorrect because dystonic postures and movements are not wildly gyrating. (B) is incorrect because there is no drug history of neuroleptic medication, and tardive dyskinesia is by definition secondary to chronic neuroleptic ingestion. (D) is incorrect because Wilson's disease does not produce initial onset of neurologic symptoms so late in life. The average age of onset of Wilson's disease presenting with neurologic symptomatology is 19 years.

The most appropriate therapy in this patients would be:

A. Raising the dose of carbidopa–levodopa
B. Addition of an anticholinergic

C. Reduction of the dose of carbidopa–levodopa
D. Administration of an atypical neuroleptic if levodopa reduction is not possible

The correct answer is (C) and (D). The patient's current problem of dyskinesias and hallucinations are secondary to chronic dopaminergic agonism, and the most appropriate therapy would be to reduce the dose of this drug. In all instances, these two drug-induced effects will be ameliorated when the dose is reduced. When the dose of the dopaminergic agents is reduced or the agents are discontinued, the patient's parkinsonian features will reemerge. In this case, if the patient's only symptom is resting unilateral tremor or mild parkinsonism, it would be wise to alter pharmacologic therapy.

If reduction in levodopa dosage results in excessive motor dysfunction with functional impairment, the addition of an atypical neuroleptic may be necessary. First, confirm that the patient is not taking other types of medications that may significantly contribute to confusion and psychotic ideation, such as sedatives, tranquilizers, and anticholinergics. If the drug regimen is simplified but the psychotic symptoms persist, choose either clozapine, olanzapine, or quetiapine for their antipsychotic effects. Use the lowest effective dosage to avoid extrapyramidal adverse effects. If drug-induced dyskinesia remains severe in spite of maximal reduction of antiparkinsonian medications, pallidotomy may be considered.

Answer (A) is incorrect because this is a drug-induced syndrome, and raising the dose of the drug will not ameliorate the problem but will exacerbate it. (B) is incorrect because anticholinergics will not improve chorea and are likely to increase the psychotic symptoms.

3. A 65-year-old right-handed man presents with difficulty seeing the food on his plate. His family says that his problem has been getting worse for the last 12 months and that the patient also has difficulty walking up stairs. In addition, he describes that he is having difficulty buttoning his shirt, rising from a chair, and turning over in bed. The family also reports that his facial expression has changed (he does not smile as much) and that a tremor of his left hand is occasionally noted. Examination reveals that there is a resting tremor of the left hand, cogwheel rigidity in the left upper extremity is present, and postural reflexes are mildly impaired. Additional findings include increased extensor tone in the neck and marked impairment of voluntary conjugate gaze. The patient is unable to look down voluntarily, and there is also moderate impairment of upward gaze. In addition, right and left lateral gaze are not normal. The correct diagnosis in this patient would be:

A. Wilson's disease
B. Huntington's disease
C. Parkinson's disease
D. Progressive supranuclear palsy (PSP)
E. Shy-Drager syndrome

The answer is (D). PSP is an idiopathic midbrain and brainstem degenerative disorder that is characterized by parkinsonian features and progressively impaired voluntary conjugate gaze. This patient is described as having parkinsonian features (resting tremor, cogwheel rigidity, impaired postural reflexes, and mild bradykinesia) and is also having markedly impaired conjugate gaze. A useful office maneuver to determine whether the gaze dysfunction is supranuclear or nuclear is the doll's head procedure. In this maneuver, the head is passively flexed and extended, and in a separate maneuver it is rotated to the right and to the left while the passive motion of the eyes is observed. In a patient with a supranuclear gaze dysfunction, the eyes will move reflexly and conjugately in an appropriate direction. This maneuver and its physiology are discussed in greater detail in Chapter 5 on the examination of the comatose patient.

Answer (A) is incorrect because of the late onset of neurologic symptoms and the type of eye movements observed. (B) is incorrect because of the late onset of neurologic symptoms and because the movement disorder is not that seen in adult-onset Huntington's disease. Although definite parkinsonian features are present, (C) is incorrect because of the additional findings of disturbed volitional gaze. (E) is incorrect because the syndrome, although often having parkinsonian features, is characterized by the presence of severe orthostatic hypotension.

4. The degenerative cellular pathology seen in Parkinson's disease is localized primarily in the:

A. Cerebral cortex
B. Thalamus
C. Cerebellum
D. Substantia nigra
E. Corpus striatum

The loss of cell bodies and their projection systems in the correct answer to the first part of this question results in what biochemical lesions?

A. Loss of acetylcholine in the striatum
B. Loss of dopamine in the striatum
C. Loss of dopamine in the cerebral cortex
D. Loss of acetylcholine in the cerebellum

The answer to the first part of the question is (D) and the answer to the second part of the question is (B). Parkinson's disease is pathologically characterized by depigmentation, Lewy bodies, and cell loss in the substantia nigra. The destruction of the nigral striatal projection system results in the loss of dopamine in the striatum. Dopamine is the neurotransmitter used by this system, and the dopamine within the striatum is primarily contained within the axonal terminations of the nigral neurons. These are not seen well histologically, and hence the striatum does not show major pathologic changes in parkinsonism.

SUGGESTED READING

Cotzias GC, Van Woert MH, Schiffer LM: Aromatic amino acids and modification of parkinsonism. N Engl J Med 276:374, 1967

Fahn S, Green PE, Ford B, Bressman SB: Handbook of Movement Disorders. Philadelphia, Current Medicine, 1998

Hohen MM, Yahr MD: Parkinsonism: Onset, progression, and mortality. Neurology 17:427, 1967

Jankovic J, Marsden CD: Therapeutic strategies in Parkinson's disease. In: Jankovic J, Tolosa E (eds): Parkinson's Disease and Movement Disorders, 3rd Edition, p 191. Baltimore, Williams & Wilkins, 1998

Lang AE, Weiner WJ (eds): Drug-Induced Movement Disorders. Mt. Kisco, NY, Futura, 1992

The Parkinson Study Group: Effect of deprenyl on the progression of disability in early Parkinson's disease. N Engl J Med 321:1364, 1989

Weiner WJ, Lang AE: Parkinson's disease. In: Movement Disorders: A Comprehensive Survey. Mt. Kisco, NY, Futura, 1989

Neurology for the Non-Neurologist, Fourth Edition, edited by William J. Weiner and Christopher G. Goetz. Lippincott Williams & Wilkins, Philadelphia © 1999.

CHAPTER 11

Hyperkinetic Movement Disorders

Stewart A. Factor

William J. Weiner

Strange, abnormal involuntary movements are the hallmarks of a number of neurologic diseases; they are collectively termed hyperkinetic movement disorders (also referred to as dyskinesias). In such conditions, the movements are easily visible, and intelligent observation allows the clinician, in most instances, to suggest the proper diagnosis or class of disorders. The characteristic tremor of Parkinson's disease, which is present at rest but lacking during volitional movements, is such an example (see Chapter 10). In this chapter, six other neurologic diseases will be described. All are dramatic visually because bizarre and abnormal involuntary movements are their major descriptive neurologic feature. The non-neurologist will certainly encounter these patients in an office practice and will identify them in public (e.g., in parks, trains, shopping centers). The disorders discussed are dystonia, essential tremor, Huntington's disease, Wilson's disease, Gilles de la Tourette's syndrome, and tardive dyskinesia.

DEFINITIONS

Dystonia: Involuntary sustained muscle contractions producing twisting or squeezing movements and abnormal postures. Dystonia can have stereotyped, repetitive movements that vary in speed from rapid to slow, and that may result in fixed postures from the sustained muscle contractions.

Tremor: Involuntary rhythmic oscillating movement that results from the alternating or synchronous contraction of reciprocally innervated antagonist muscles. Tremor may be classified according to its prominence during activity or at rest.

Chorea: A state of excessive, spontaneous movements, irregularly timed, nonrepetitive, randomly distributed, and often with a flowing "dancelike" quality that involves multiple body parts.

Tics: Repetitive, brief, rapid, involuntary, purposeless, stereotyped movements that involve single or multiple muscle groups. The tic can be a patterned sequence of coordinated movements that may be complex or simple.

Myoclonus: Rapid, shocklike, arrhythmic (usually), and often repetitive involuntary movements. Myoclonus can be classified by location: focal, multifocal, or generalized and by etiology.

DYSTONIA

Dystonia has a number of unusual but characteristic features. At onset, the movements may occur in association with a specific voluntary action by the involved muscle groups (such as in writer's cramp) or with any type of movement with these muscles, so-called action-induced dystonia. It may occur in one body part with movement of another (overflow dystonia). In addition, dystonia may be present at rest. Dystonic movements typically worsen with anxiety, heightened emotions, and fatigue, whereas they decrease with relaxation and disappear during sleep. There may be diurnal fluctuations in the dystonia, which manifest as little or no involuntary movements in the morning followed by severe disabling dystonia in the afternoon and evening. One particular form of dystonia with onset in childhood is characterized by this feature and by its response to small doses of levodopa (dopa-responsive or Segawa's dystonia). Other features of dopa-responsive dystonia (DRD) include a general association with onset at age 6, foot dystonia in childhood, and parkinsonism in adults. It has been linked to two chromosomes: (1) chromosome 14—the gene codes for an enzyme in the biosynthetic pathway of biopterin (GTP cyclohydrolase) and is dominantly inherited—and (2) chromosome 11—the gene codes for tyrosine hydroxylase, the rate-limiting step in catecholamine metabolism, and is recessively inherited. The resulting deficiency of biopterin, a cofactor in catecholamine synthesis, leads to decreased levels of dopamine, which explains the long-term responsiveness of patients to levodopa.

Dystonia may occur in nearly any muscle group. The following terms are utilized to describe dystonia in varied distributions. When the upper face and eyelids are involved and the eyes are involuntarily kept closed the patient is said to have *blepharospasm*. When the lower face, lips, and jaw are involved and the patient presents with involuntary opening or closing of the jaw, retraction or puckering of the lips, and repetitive contractions of the platysma, he is experiencing *oromandibular dystonia*. *Pharyngeal dystonia* is associated with dysphagia, dysphonia, or dysarthria and is typically action induced. *Lingual dystonia* may occur at rest, presenting as sustained or repetitive protrusion of the tongue or upward deflection of the tongue against the hard palate, or it may be action induced via speaking or eating. *Laryngeal dystonia* (involving the vocal cords) causes *spasmodic dysphonia* in which the speech is tight, constricted, and forced, or more whispery, depending on whether the adductor or abductor muscle groups are involved. The smooth flow of speech is lost and certain sounds are held longer and overemphasized. Spasmodic dysphonia is typically action induced by speech, and it most commonly involves the adductor muscles of the larynx. Abductor dysphonia resulting in a soft whispery voice is less common.

Dystonic contractions of the neck muscles, referred to as *spasmodic torticollis* or *cervical dystonia*, result in torticollis, retrocollis, anterocollis, or laterocollis. In spasmodic torticollis, rapid jerking and twisting neck movements may accompany sustained posturing of the neck. Some patients may appear to have a fixed abnormal neck posture without the spasmodic movements. The shoulder on the side of the head-tilt is typically elevated. Dystonic movements of the arms (*brachial dystonia*) most commonly present as pronation of the arm, often behind the back. The movements are often action induced as in writing (*writer's cramp*), manipulating a musical instrument (*musician's cramp*), and other occupational maneuvers. *Truncal* or *axial dystonia* manifests as lordosis, scoliosis, kyphosis, tortipelvis, or opisthotonus. Dystonic movements of the legs (*crural dystonia*) may occur with action or at rest, and they present most commonly with equinovarus posturing of the foot while walking, twisting of the foot, or increased elevation of the leg when walking. The knee usually maintains a hyperextended position with crural dystonia. It is interesting that some patients are able to walk backwards or run without incident, but when they attempt to walk normally, the dystonia recurs. Certain combinations are fairly common and make up specific syndromes that will be discussed later in this section.

Patients with dystonic disorders often discover ways to suppress or hide the movements using an interesting array of tricks. These usually consist of postural alterations or counterpressure maneuvers that are primarily sensory in nature. Examples include touching an eyebrow in blepharospasm, which leads to eye opening, or the classical *geste antagonistique,* where a finger placed lightly on the chin will neutralize neck-turning in spasmodic torticollis. There are also motor tasks that may deactivate dystonia, including singing by patients with blepharospasm or oromandibular dystonia, and dancing by patients with cervical or truncal dystonia. Typically, these tricks lose their effectiveness as the disease progresses.

The pathophysiology of dystonic movements and behind the usefulness of tricks remain a mystery. However, in recent times some clues have emerged, although it is beyond the scope of this chapter to describe them in detail. Briefly, it is believed that dystonia is the result of a basal ganglia lesion. This is primarily based on work involving cases of secondary dystonia. There appears to be a decreased output from the primary output nucleus of the basal ganglia, medial globus pallidus. There are two pathways from putamen to medial globus pallidus that dictate what this output would be—the direct and indirect pathways—and they have opposite effects. An overactivity of the direct pathway, or underactivity of the indirect pathway, could lead to dystonia. The decreased output somehow leads to a loss of reciprocal inhibition mechanisms for muscle contraction controlled at the brainstem or spinal levels. This allows antagonist muscle groups to contract at the same time, resulting in dystonia. There also appears to be sensory and motor cortical involvement. Sensory involvement is suggested by the usefulness of sensory tricks and studies demonstrating abnormalities in sensory fields in thalamus and cerebral cortex in patients with dystonia. Physiologic studies have also demonstrated that motor cortex is hyperexcitable and that there is decreased activation of these regions. It is possible that certain patterned or learned tasks (tricks), both sensory and motor, interrupt the production of dystonia through alterations in cortical activity, which in turn changes input of direct or indirect pathways to medial globus pallidus. How all these findings fit together to explain dystonic movements remains to be elucidated.

Dystonia is often misdiagnosed as hysterical or psychiatric in origin. The basis for this arises from its typical features, including the varied, often bizarre, movements and postures, the fact that they are often action induced, the worsening of dystonia with stress and improvement with relaxation, the diurnal fluctuations, and the effectiveness of various sensory tricks. Knowledge of the unusual characteristics of dystonic disorders will be helpful in avoiding a misdiagnosis.

CLASSIFICATION

Classification of dystonia has generally been based on (1) age of onset, (2) distribution of movements, and (3) etiology. Use of the first two items in the patient's initial assessment can lead to consideration of etiology. The age of onset classification separates patients into three subgroups: childhood (0 to 12 years), juvenile (12 to 20 years), and adult (older than 20). Childhood onset typically carries a worse prognosis than the older groups because of the more likely possibility of generalization of the movement disorder.

The distribution of dystonia is categorized as either focal, multifocal, hemi-, or generalized. Focal dystonia refers to dystonia in a single body part. Multifocal dystonia includes dystonic movements in more than one body part yet not fulfilling the criteria for generalized dystonia; segmental dystonia is a form of multifocal dystonia in which contiguous body parts are affected. In hemidystonia, an arm and a leg on the same side are involved. Finally, generalized dystonia refers to the presence of dystonia in at least one leg, the trunk, and an additional body part (cranial, cervical, or brachial), or both legs and the trunk. This classification is important in formulating a proper

diagnosis. For example, hemidystonia is almost always the result of an infarction or space-occupying lesion, whereas generalized dystonia is more than likely idiopathic. Generalized dystonia clearly has a worse prognosis than focal dystonia or hemidystonia.

Classification by etiology has undergone substantial change in the last few years, primarily because of the linkage (or nonlinkage) of many types of dystonia to a variety of genes. Table 11-1 demonstrates the latest scheme, first introduced at the Third International Dystonia Symposium in 1996. The primary dystonias [also known as idiopathic torsion dystonias (ITD)] are defined as syndromes in which the sole manifestation is dystonia, with the exception that tremor may be present as well. It is considered to be neurochemical in origin rather than degenerative. It has been discovered that primary dystonia is genetically and clinically heterogeneous and thus the various categories. Dystonia genes are depicted by

TABLE 11-1. Classification of Dystonia

Primary dystonia
   Early-onset dystonia (Oppenheim's dystonia):
      chromosome 9q—DYT1
   Adult-onset familial torticollis
   Adult-onset familial cervico-cranial dystonia:
      chromosome 18p—DYT7
   Mixed adult and childhood-onset dystonia:
      chromosome 8—DYT6
   Adult-onset sporadic focal dystonia
Dystonia—plus syndromes
   Dopa-responsive (Segawa's) dystonia: chromosome
      14q & 11p—DYT5
   Myoclonic dystonia
Secondary dystonia (see Table 11-2)
Hereditary and degenerative diseases
   Degenerative disorders
      Parkinson's disease
      Huntington's disease
      Progressive supranuclear palsy
      Hallervorden–Spatz disease
      Olivopontocerebellar atrophies
      Lubag (Filipino X-linked dystonia parkinsonism):
        chromosome X—DYT3
   Hereditary metabolic disorders
      Wilson's disease
      Leigh's disease
      GM 1 and 2 gangliosidoses
      Hexosaminidase deficiency
      Leber's optic neuropathy with dystonia

Unmapped genes include DYT2 (autosomal recessive dystonia) and DYT4 (whispering dysphonia family).

the symbol DYT (followed by a number) by the Human Genome Organization/Genome Database. DYT designations have been assigned to a variety of dystonic syndromes either clinically defined and unmapped, linked primary dystonias, or others not classified as primary (see Table 11-1). Seven genes causing dystonia have been mapped to human chromosomes, and three are for primary dystonias, and these will be discussed in more detail.

The second category comprises the dystonia-plus syndromes. These are also considered to be neurochemical in origin, but they have features other than dystonia (e.g., DRD patients have parkinsonian features). The third category is secondary dystonia, which develops as the result of an environmental insult (Table 11-2) and will be discussed in more detail in a later section. The fourth category includes hereditary–degenerative syndromes that have dystonia as part of the clinical spectrum. Of these, Parkinson's disease, Wilson's disease, and Huntington's disease are discussed in separate sections or chapters.

TABLE 11-2. **Secondary Forms of Dystonia**

Drugs
    Dopamine antagonists (i.e., haloperidol, thoridizine, compazine)
    Dopamine agonists (i.e., levodopa, bromocriptine)
    Antidepressants (tricyclics, SSRIs, lithium)
    Antihistamines
    Calcium channel blockers
    Stimulants (cocaine)
    Buspirone
Vascular disease
    Basal ganglia infarction
    Basal ganglia hemorrhage
    Arteriovenous malformation
Neoplasms
    Astrocytoma or glioma of the basal ganglia
    Metastatic neoplasm
    Cervical spinal cord tumor
Others
    Head trauma
    Thalamotomy
    Anoxia (in adulthood or perinatal)
    Meningitis (fungal or tuberculosis)
    Syringomyelia
    Colloid cyst of the third ventricle
    Münchhausen syndrome
    AIDS (toxoplasmosis abscess of basal ganglia, PML)

SSRI = selective serotonin reuptake inhibitors; PML = progressive mutlifocal leukoencephalopathy.

PRIMARY INHERITED DYSTONIAS

Dystonia is typically the only neurologic abnormality in patients with primary dystonia (although many may also have tremor) and any distribution of abnormal involuntary movements may be observed. The primary dystonias characteristically have an insidious onset and are progressive in nature. Initially, the movements may be action induced, later occurring at rest and producing fixed and sustained postures. The disorder ultimately plateaus and may remain at this level of severity for life. Five criteria for the diagnosis of primary dystonia were established by Herz in 1944 and are still applicable today. These include (1) the development of dystonic movements or postures, (2) a normal perinatal and developmental history, (3) no precipitating illnesses or exposure to drugs known to cause dystonia, (4) no evidence of intellectual, pyramidal, cerebellar, or sensory deficits, (5) negative results of investigation for secondary causes of dystonia (particularly Wilson's disease). Two factors are indicators of a poor prognosis: onset in childhood and onset in a crural distribution. Poor prognosis in dystonia refers to an increased disability, since life span is not shortened in this disorder. A majority of crural dystonia patients have onset of disease in childhood or early adulthood (referred to collectively as early-onset disease). Different phenotypes occur among different ethnic groups, suggesting that certain clinical presentations may represent distinct genetic entities.

The classical early-onset primary dystonia is DYT1 dystonia. It is the most severe and the most common form of hereditary dystonia. This disorder was called dystonia musculorum deformans by Oppenheim, who first described the syndrome in 1911. It has recently been suggested that this disorder be renamed *Oppenheim's dystonia*. DYT1 dystonia is inherited in an autosomal dominant pattern, with a 30% to 40% penetrance. The gene, located at chromosome 9q34, was recently identified. The gene abnormality is a unique three–base pair deletion in the coding portion of the transcript. The resulting protein, *torsinA*, is characterized by the loss of one of a pair of glutamic acid residues in a conserved region of a novel ATP-binding protein. The function of this protein and its role in altering basal ganglia function to cause dystonia remain to be elucidated. There is a high prevalence of early-onset dystonia in Ashkenazi Jewish families, with over 90% due to a single founder mutation in the DYT1 gene. This mutation has been traced back over 350 years to Lithuania, and the current gene frequency is approximately 1 in 2,000. In most, but not all, non-Jewish families with early-onset dystonia, the disease is also due to the same DYT1 mutation that has arisen independently in varied populations. Thus, apparently, only one variation in the encoded protein can give rise to the DYT1 phenotype.

The clinical spectrum of early-onset DYT1 dystonia is similar in all ethnic populations and fairly consistent. Onset of symptoms occurs at an average age of 12 years, but most patients have onset before age 28. The initial presentation is with limb onset, usually leg (crural dystonia). The presence of leg or foot dystonia is the best predictor of a DYT1 mutation. The foot is often twisted and plantar flexed while ambulating, and the patient usually toe-walks. All patients ultimately have leg involvement. The disorder may start in the arm (possibly as writer's cramp), although less frequently. In these cases, the age of onset is a little older than crural onset and the patients are less likely to end up with generalized dystonia. Generally, early-onset dystonia progresses by spreading across or down, and this occurs over approximately 5 years, with 50% of patients becoming either bedridden or wheelchair bound. Spasmodic dysphonia occurs in about 5%, cervical involvement is rare, and cranial involvement is not seen. Onset in the neck or vocal cords in early-onset patients, even if they are of Ashkenazi Jewish descent, is rarely caused by the DYT1 gene. These patients rarely generalize. Late-onset (>28 years old) craniocervical dystonia generally indicates that the patient does not have DYT1 dystonia. In adult life, the patient often stabilizes and may even improve to some degree, but the disorder does not spontaneously remit. There may be remissions early in the disorder and these may last hours to years. Most, if not all, recur, usually in the same distribution.

Linkage studies involving several large families with adult- or mixed-onset dystonia of a variety of distributions have excluded the DYT1 locus. However, dystonia families have been linked to two other possible genes. DYT6 has been linked to chromosome 8 in two Mennonite families from the midwestern United States with an autosomal dominant form of dystonia. The phenotype of these families includes a broader age of onset (5 to 38 years; mean, 19) and an onset distribution that includes limbs and cervical or cranial areas. There is frequent spread to cranial muscles, and there are apparently few patients whose dystonia becomes generalized. In some, the dystonia even remains focal. Thus, while some of the patients appear identical to those with DYT1 dystonia, there are obvious differences when examining the complete family. In addition, there are differences from typical adult-onset craniocervical dystonia, because DYT6 dystonia that starts in these regions commonly spreads to the limbs, but the former syndrome does not.

The DYT7 gene has been linked to chromosome 18p in a family from northwest Germany. This family has an autosomal dominant form of adult-onset craniocervical dystonia. The average age of onset was 41, and most patients had focal cervical dystonia (spasmodic torticollis). Some had cranial involvement as well. In the same town, apparently sporadic cases of spasmodic torticollis were also studied and they shared allelic characteristics with the family, suggesting that they also had an autosomal dominant form with reduced penetrance.

ADULT-ONSET SPORADIC DYSTONIA

Adult-onset ITD is the most common of all types of dystonia. It presents more commonly with brachial, truncal, and craniocervical dystonia and only rarely with crural dystonia. Only 18% of these patients progress to generalized dystonia, with even a smaller percentage becoming wheelchair bound or bedridden. The dystonia usually remains in the body part where it presented as a focal dystonia, but it may spread to a contiguous body part on rare occasions, becoming segmental in distribution. The course is typically benign, and remissions occur in approximately 20% of patients.

CRANIOFACIAL DYSTONIA

Blepharospasm–oromandibular dystonia syndrome was first described by Henry Meige in 1910 and is often referred to as Meige's syndrome. Blepharospasm and oromandibular dystonia may occur independently in this syndrome, but the combination is more frequent. They may also be accompanied by pharyngeal, laryngeal, or cervical dystonia. Blepharospasm in isolation (referred to as essential blepharospasm) is more common than oromandibular dystonia. Blepharospasm is often preceded by eye irritation, photophobia, and increased blinking frequency. It may start in one eye and spread to the other or start in both. Approximately 12% of these patients are functionally blind because of their inability to voluntarily open their eyes. Features that aggravate blepharospasm include looking upward, stress, fatigue, watching television, walking, driving, talking, and even yawning. Sensory tricks utilized by patients to open their eyes include forced raising of the eyelids, pressure on the superior orbital ridges, and rubbing the eyelids. In addition, some find that forced jaw opening, neck movements, whistling, and wearing dark glasses are helpful. Some patients use eyeglasses with eyelid crutches to hold the lids open.

Oromandibular dystonia is frequently accompanied by tongue protrusion, soft palate dystonia, and nasal flaring. It may be aggravated by talking, chewing, or swallowing. Sensory tricks utilized include pressing on the lips or teeth with fingers, pressing on the hard palate with the tongue, or putting a finger in the mouth. Meige's syndrome typically affects women more commonly than men, and presents in the sixth decade of life. The onset of the disorder often begins with blepharospasm, which is later followed by oromandibular dystonia and pharyngeal dystonia. Other dystonic movements in other body parts may occur in some patients, and hand tremor similar to essential tremor may also be an associated problem. The severity of the dystonia fluctuates from day to day and disappears with sleep. Spontaneous remissions have been observed but are rare.

SPASMODIC TORTICOLLIS

Spasmodic torticollis is the most common of adult-onset focal dystonias, making up about 40% (Fig. 11-1). The age of onset is in the fourth or fifth decade (mean, 41) and women are more frequently affected than men by about 3 to 1. The disorder is characterized by abnormal involuntary neck movements, abnormal postures of the neck and shoulders that are often painful, and hypertrophy of involved neck muscles. Pain is present in about 80% of patients, and hypertrophy is seen in all. Initially, some patients do not perceive their dystonia, and it is brought to their attention by others. This suggests that a problem with perception of head position exists. The movements may be only intermittent at first and associated with specific actions. Most patients deteriorate during the initial 5 years and then symptoms stabilize. The condition may ultimately be characterized by fixed dystonic postures that are present at rest, worsen with action, and improve in sleep. Spontaneous remissions occur in 10% to 30%, most commonly in the first year. All patients relapse but few have a second remission. Rotation of the neck (torticollis) is the most common posture seen (with neither side being particularly more common), with lateral flexion (laterocollis), flexion (anterocollis), and extension (retrocollis) also occurring in various combinations. Spasmodic (dynamic) movements are not present in all patients despite the commonly used term *spasmodic torticollis*. In fact, they occur in only 10% to 15%. Factors that may exacerbate torticollis include emotional stress, fatigue, walking, working with the hands, and attempting to look in the opposite direction of the dystonic contractions. When the patient tries to overcome the movements and look in the opposite direction, he may experience a high-amplitude, jerky tremor referred to as dystonic tremor. Some patients

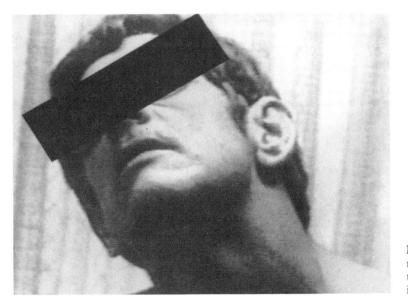

FIG. 11-1. Spasmodic torticollis resulting in a fixed cervical posture with extension, lateral flexion, and rotation to the right.

present with bi-directional torticollis, because at varying times the head may turn in different directions and muscles of both sides of the neck may be involved. Many of these patients present with head tremor. The tremor varies in amplitude, and if there is little directional change in the neck along with tremor, the patients are frequently misdiagnosed as having essential tremor. The distinction is important because dystonia does not respond to antitremor medications but does respond to botulinum toxin and other dystonia therapies. This tremor can be distinguished from essential head tremor by the presence of subtle changes in posture, a jerky nonrhythmic quality, and muscle hypertrophy along with improvement with sensory tricks. Head tremor is present in approximately 40% of torticollis patients. Sensory tricks usually involve the use of a light touch or pressure to the chin or cheek with fingers (*geste antagonistique*) or other objects such as a pen or eye glasses, and holding the back of the head with the hand or leaning the head against a wall or a headrest. This lessens the head tilt and tremor and relaxes the muscles for variable durations of time. After a while, the tricks lose their effectiveness. Spasmodic torticollis may be associated with Meige's syndrome, writer's cramp, and essential tremor, and it has also been observed in patients with generalized dystonia. Complications of prolonged torticollis occur in one third to one half of patients and include degenerative osteoarthritis of the cervical spine along with the expected sequelae of radiculopathy or myelo-

pathy. These may represent emergent situations for torticollis patients and lead to permanent neurologic deficits.

WRITER'S CRAMP

Writer's cramp (Fig. 11-2) is a dystonic spasm that is induced by a specific task (action-induced or task specific dystonia). When these cramps occur with a single type of action (such as writing), they are referred to as simple writer's cramp, but when the spasms occur with a variety of activities, they are referred to as dystonic cramps. Writer's cramp occurs in both men and women and the age of onset ranges from 20 to 70 years. These patients present with a change in handwriting that becomes sloppy and illegible. Some patients squeeze the pen tightly and press down hard on the writing surface, which results in a jerky writing motion and tearing of the paper. In others, the fingers splay and pull away from the pen involuntarily. The act of writing is painful in most patients. Initially, the dystonic contraction occurs with persistence of task, but, as the disorder progresses, it occurs with initiation of the task. Initially, other tasks performed with the same hand are normal, but later these too may become involved, and then the patient is said to have dystonic cramps. The disorder is usually asymmetric at first, but in those patients who learn to write with the opposite hand, the disorder may become bilateral (about 25% of patients) years after the change in hands. When some patients write with the unaffected hand,

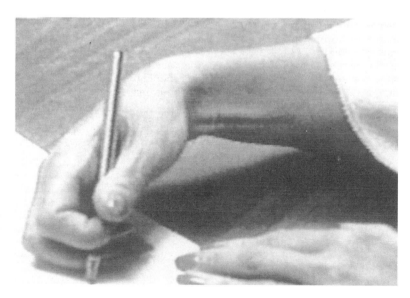

FIG. 11-2. Writer's cramp is an action-induced dystonic spasm, resulting, in this patient, in wrist flexion, metacarpophalangeal joint extension, extension of the thumb, and flexion of the distal interphalangeal joints, leaving the patient with an inability to continue writing.

the affected hand exhibits involuntary spasms—so-called mirror dystonia. Writer's cramp may be associated with essential tremor and may be related to the syndrome of primary writing tremor, which is thought by some to be a variant of essential tremor. Some other occupational cramps that have been reported include pianist and violinist palsy, golfer's palsy, and dart-thrower's palsy. The common factor in all of these disorders is the occurrence during the performance of a well-learned motor (manual) task and perhaps the overuse of the hand with that particular task. In writer's cramp, there appears to be co-contraction of agonist and antagonist muscles, perhaps related to loss of reciprocal inhibition. Patients generally have an otherwise normal neurologic exam, and this disorder is usually resistant to therapy.

SECONDARY DYSTONIA

To make a diagnosis of ITD, one must rule out known causes of dystonia [i.e., secondary or symptomatic dystonias (see Table 11-2) and hereditary degenerative diseases (see Table 11-1)]. Clues to the diagnosis of a secondary dystonia can be uncovered with a thorough history and physical exam, and radiologic and laboratory testing. Usually, there are examination findings suggestive of dysfunction of other parts of the central nervous system (CNS), including the cranial nerves, pyramidal system, cerebellar system, and higher cortical function tasks, in addition to the dystonia. There is usually an obvious onset to the dystonia, and dystonia is present at rest from the start in secondary cases. The presence of hemidystonia almost always suggests a focal lesion such as a tumor, infarction, abscess, or arteriovenous malformation (AVM) in the basal ganglia. In those patients with a single nonprogressive event such as an infarction or trauma, the dystonia will usually stabilize and not be progressive. The examiner should be cautious, however, because secondary dystonia may mimic idiopathic dystonia quite closely. For instance, stroke in the basal ganglia may cause a case of typical-looking torticollis. This is particularly true with respect to neuroleptic-induced (tardive) dystonia. In adult-onset patients, tardive dystonia may take on features identical to those of adult-onset ITD. Torticollis is the most frequent type. Clues that one may be dealing with tardive dystonia include more retrocollis, a more phasic or dynamic form of torticollis, and the co-occurrence of typical tardive dyskinesia. These patients also less frequently give a history of the effectiveness of tricks and do not seem to get head tremor. Finally, a lack of muscle hypertrophy may suggest a drug-induced dystonia.

An important feature of secondary dystonia, which examiners must be aware of, is that dystonia may have a delayed onset after a cerebral insult. In adults, the most frequent cause of delayed-onset dystonia is cerebral infarction. The duration of the delay can vary from weeks to years and is often associated with an improvement of the original neurologic deficit. In children, the most frequent cause of delayed-onset dystonia is perinatal trauma or hypoxia. The reason for the delay is unclear but it has been postulated that the dystonia in these circumstances is a result of neuronal sprouting stimulated by the original injury. A history of perinatal difficulties must be ruled out if a diagnosis of ITD is to be made.

As will be discussed later, the most important disorder to rule out in a new-onset dystonia patient, particularly a young-onset one, is Wilson's disease. Therefore, a screen for Wilson's disease and an imaging study of the brain should be performed on all dystonia patients, and then the rest of the work-up should be tailored to the individual patient's needs. It has been suggested that secondary dystonia occurs mainly in genetically susceptible individuals. This was thought to be particularly true in tardive dystonia because it appears to be very similar clinically to primary dystonia. A recent study has demonstrated that these patients are not carriers of the DYT1 gene, suggesting that genetic susceptibility is not a necessary component of tardive dystonia. Similar work needs to be done for other, particularly adult-onset, dystonia genes.

PATHOLOGY AND NEUROCHEMISTRY

Dystonia is considered to be the result of basal ganglia dysfunction. Since there have been only a few cases of ITD reported with autopsy results (and most of them were without abnormality), the pathologic–anatomic basis of this movement disorder has been related almost exclusively to cases of symptomatic dystonia. Anatomic locations in published cases have most commonly included the putamen, and to a lesser extent the caudate nucleus and the thalamus. These findings have been supported by radiologic studies. In those rare cases of ITD with pathologic abnormalities, the microscopic changes were observed in the brainstem. In one case of generalized dystonia, neurofibrillary tangles were found in the locus ceruleus and other brainstem nuclei. In one case of Meige's syndrome, neuronal loss was observed in multiple brainstem nuclei. Whether these abnormalities relate directly to the clinical syndrome remains to be proven. In Lubag, the X-linked dystonia–parkinsonism syndrome (DYT3) seen most commonly in the Philippines, the characteristic pathology is gliosis in a mosaic pattern seen primarily in the putamen and caudate nucleus. These patients have severe craniocervical dystonia and many of them generalize. This finding supports the concept of dystonia being a basal ganglia disorder.

The neurochemical basis of dystonia is unclear. It has been suggested that the abnormality in this disorder is in the dopamine or acetylcholine systems. Clinical evidence to suggest these hypotheses includes the onset of dystonia after treatment with dopamine receptor antagonists, and the response of dystonia to anticholinergic medications. In addition, the discovery that DRD is acutely responsive to small doses of levodopa and that it is caused by two genes involved in the biosynthesis of dopamine support a dopaminergic hypothesis. Recently, a noradrenergic imbalance in the lower portion of the brainstem involving the lateral tegmentum of the medulla oblongata and locus ceruleus has been hypothesized. In some areas, norepinephrine is elevated, while in others the levels are diminished. Norepinephrine is a neurotransmitter that, among other actions, inhibits cholinergic neurons. A deficiency in norepinephrine might explain the response of dystonia to anticholinergic medications. This finding is particularly interesting because the location of the DYT6 gene is in a region of chromosome 8 that contains the genes for alpha-1 and beta-3 adrenergic receptors. Other theories have included alterations in gamma-aminobutyric acid (GABA) or cerebral somatostatin. GABA alterations in the motor cortex have been implicated in the abnormalities of activation and inhibition in this region demonstrated by physiologic testing and positron emission tomography (PET).

Recently, it has been suggested that dystonia may be the result of a deficiency in activity of mitochondrial complex I, the first protein of the respiratory chain. This was considered a possibility because a mitochondrial complex I deficiency was seen in the hereditary disorder Leber's optic neuropathy with dystonia. The cause of the deficiency was a mitochondrial DNA mutation. Since then, three different studies have been reported on platelet mitochondrial function in the primary dystonias, with varied results. One study indicated that the deficiency was in all types of dystonia, and severity of dystonia correlated with severity of the deficiency. Another reported that the complex I deficiency was present only in the focal dystonia. The third indicated that no deficiency was present in this or any dystonia group. Further studies are required to clarify the role of mitochondrial dysfunction in dystonia.

TREATMENT

In the absence of a clear understanding of the etiology and neurochemistry of dystonia, medical treatment has been less than satisfactory. As a result, a number of therapeutic modalities have been tested, and varied responses have been observed. Approximately half of patients respond to medical therapy. The most widely accepted group of medications utilized in the treatment of dystonia is the anticholinergic group. Fahn, in an open label trial, found high doses of either trihexiphenidyl or ethopropazine (no longer available in the United States but available in Canada as Parsitan) to be beneficial in ITD. Twenty-three children and 52 adults were treated. The doses were gradually increased until a favorable response was observed or side effects occurred. Significant improvement was seen in 61% of children and 38% of adults. The average daily dose of trihexiphenidyl in children and adults was 41 mg and 24 mg, respectively. Adults were less tolerant of the anticholinergic side effects than the children. Side effects include blurred vision, dry mouth, urinary difficulties, constipation, sleep pattern alteration, forgetfulness, weight loss, personality changes, and psychosis. The longest duration of efficacy in children and adults was 13 years and 7 years, respectively. Severity of disease is not a good predictor of response to the anticholinergics, but patients with hemidystonia (due to a focal lesion) did not respond well. This result was later confirmed by a double-blind study with trihexiphenidyl. Tetrabenazine, a dopamine-depleting agent, has been found to be effective in a double-blind trial in patients with Meige's syndrome and a variety of other movement disorders including other types of dystonia. This drug is not available in the United States, but reserpine, another dopamine-deleting drug, is available and effective in approximately 30% of patients. The side effects of most concern with dopamine-depleting agents are depression, which can be severe, come on suddenly, and have a protracted course, parkinsonism, orthostatic hypotension, and gastrointestinal problems. The effectiveness of dopamine antagonists such as haloperidol have been inconsistent and studies utilizing these drugs have been inconclusive. Because of the threat of tardive dyskinesia, these drugs should be avoided. Mixed results with baclofen, carbamazepine, and the benzodiazepines have been observed, but these are frequently utilized nevertheless, especially in patients unresponsive to anticholinergics.

Numerous surgical techniques have been utilized with less than adequate results. Stereotaxic thalamotomy with the ventral tier of the thalamus as the target is the most common technique. The ventralis oralis posterior (VOP) and the ventralis intermedius (VIM) are the main targets. Modern techniques include the use of stimulation and electrophysiologic cellular recording and mapping to improve localization. These techniques have improved morbidity and mortality, which is one reason these surgical techniques enjoy a resurgence. The results continue to be varied. It appears that secondary, unilateral cases respond best, while primary cases show a response that is more modest. Bilateral procedures of this type can still result in pseudobulbar palsy, dysphagia, and gait disorder. More recently, a new target has been studied in dystonia patients. It has been shown that stereotactic posteroventral pallidotomy can eliminate dyskinesia and dystonia in patients with advanced Parkinson's disease. This prompted the evaluation of this technique in patients with generalized dystonia. This surgery is safer than thalamotomy, and results in a small number of patients have been significant. In one particular case, the improvement was delayed and reached a maximum in 3 months. It is likely that this procedure will receive a more in-depth evaluation in the coming years.

In blepharospasm and Meige's syndrome, myectomy of the periocular muscles has been utilized, also providing mixed results. The surgery consists of the extirpation of the lid protractors and strengthening of the lid retractors. Recurrence of blepharospasm weeks to months after this procedure is not unusual. In torticollis, selective peripheral denervation is a technique under investigation at numerous institutions. Results have indicated that the primary posture of the neck improves, but there is a decrease in range of motion and muscle atrophy occurs. Some patients experience a recurrence of the torticollis with involvement of different cervical muscles.

One other technique being utilized to treat generalized dystonia is intrathecal baclofen, which is delivered to the intrathecal space through an inserted catheter with a continuous pump. This has been highly effective in treating spasticity of spinal and cortical origin. In the small number of dystonia patients treated, results have been modest at best, although there has been the occasional case of severe dystonic crisis that improved dramatically. Possible side effects include respiratory depression from baclofen overdose, catheter malfunction, and pump infection.

Intramuscular injection of botulinum toxin remains the treatment of choice for focal dystonias, particularly in the craniocervical distribution. Botulinum toxin is one of the most lethal toxins known to man. Of eight subtypes produced by the anaerobic organism *Clostridium botulinum,* three have been linked to human botulism: types A, B, and E. Botulinum toxin A (Botox) has been utilized therapeutically since 1980. At that time, its usefulness in strabismus was demonstrated. In 1990, Botox was approved by the U.S. Food and Drug Administration (FDA) for treatment in blepharospasm, strabismus, and hemifacial spasm secondary to cranial nerve VII compression. Its use is now more widespread than that as it is routinely utilized to treat all types of focal dystonia: blepharospasm, oromandibular dystonia, spasmodic torticollis, spasmodic dysphonia, and other facial dystonias. Botox acts presynaptically at the cholinergic neuromuscular junction. It is endocytosed into the nerve terminal and then blocks the release of acetylcholine from vesicles. Its blockade of the neuromuscular junction results in weakness and atrophy of the muscle and a decrease in muscle spasms. Botox is administered by direct intramuscular injection. All side effects are local, secondary to its primary effect of weakening muscles. In blepharospasm, Botox is injected into the orbicularis oculi with two injections in the upper lid, and one injection in the canthus and lower lid. In addition, one or two injections are given in the frontalis muscle in the forehead, if necessary. The total dose is 15 to 40 units per eye. After 3 to 7 days, improvement is seen with moderate to marked functional improvement in 70% to 90% of patients. The response lasts 2 to 4 months, so that treatment is needed three or four times per year. Side effects include ptosis, diplopia, and increased tearing, all of which are transient. Spasmodic torticollis is probably the most common disorder treated with Botox at this time. Multiple studies have shown significant improvement in 60% to 90% of patients treated. Treatment requires an average of about 275 units per treatment and, as with blepharospasm, response occurs in 3 to 7 days and lasts 3 to 4 months. Patients require two to four treatments per year. Neck muscles injected are chosen based on the presence of hypertrophy, spasm, and pain, and in relation to the posture itself. Some investigators have suggested using electromyographic (EMG) techniques as an additional guide to injection, but not all treating neurologists find it necessary. This author uses EMG in complicated cases and in patients who do not experience an adequate initial response. Side effects are transient and include neck weakness, dysphagia, dry mouth, and a "flulike" syndrome. Spasmodic dysphonia of the adductor type, previously poorly responsive to any therapy, responds dramatically to Botox. Both unilateral and bilateral techniques have been utilized. The bilateral method is preferable because lower doses (0.65 to 5 units per side) can be utilized. The thyroartenoid muscles are approached though the neck with EMG guidance. The only adverse effects are a breathy, whispery voice and dysphagia, which improve over days to weeks. Injection is required two to four times per year. Treatment of oromandibular dystonia is also frequently successful. Injections can be made into the pterygoid muscles (medial or lateral) with EMG guidance, the masseters, temporalis, and digastric muscles in varied combinations depending on whether the patient has jaw opening, closing, or lateral deviation as the main manifestation. Seventy percent to 90% of patients improve. Side effects are dysphagia and weakness of the soft palate, which allows fluid to be regurgitated through the nose. Limb dystonias (e.g., writer's cramp) respond with less consistency because the resulting weakness of the hand muscles may be more troublesome than the cramps themselves. Nevertheless, some patients find them useful. Most neurologists feel that Botox is the treatment of choice for most focal dystonias because of greater efficacy than standard medical therapies and fewer side effects. Resistance to Botox has been a concern for years, especially in cervical dystonia patients who receive higher doses. It is believed that the patients develop antibodies that neutralize the toxin and make it ineffective. Not all resistant patients have measurable levels of antibodies, but this may be a reflection of the lack of reliability of currently available tests. The best way to assess resistance is to evaluate the patients clinically after treatment. Sometimes just the sternocleidomastoid is injected, with 75 to 100 units, and it is examined 2 weeks later for atrophy. If no atrophy occurs, the patient is resistant. A similar test involves the injection of a frontalis muscle (one side). After an injection of 15 to 20 units, if the folds on the forehead remain the same (and symmetrical) and the patient can raise his eyebrow and wrinkle his forehead, then he is resistant.

The occurrence of resistance has led to the testing of other types of botulinum toxin. It seems that the various types are antigenically distinct, so that resistance to one does not mean resistance to all. Thus far, two other types have been tested. Type F is useful but its effect only lasts about 3 weeks. Type B is completing its phase three trials in spasmodic torticollis at the time of this writing and will probably be available in 1999. At doses of 5,000 to 15,000, patients have a significant response with a duration similar to that seen with type A. The degree of response is similar whether the patients are or are not resistant to type A. Physicians administering Botox should be very familiar with the disorders treated, mechanism of action, and effective doses of Botox for each disorder, and with the anatomy of the area injected. As expected, the disorders treated with Botox have expanded beyond dystonia. Spasticity, achalasia, and anal and urethral sphincter disorders respond well to these injections. Botox has also been used cosmetically for facial wrinkles.

ESSENTIAL TREMOR

Tremor may be characterized by its prominence only in certain activities or postures, and it may be the sole manifestation of a disorder or a part of a syndrome. It is generally classified by its anatomic location, frequency, etiology, or, most frequently, in relation to rest, posture, and action. Resting tremor refers to tremor while the body part is at rest. The classical rest tremor is that seen in Parkinson's disease. Postural tremor refers to tremor occurring while the body part is maintaining posture against gravity, the most common being that seen in essential tremor. Finally, kinetic tremor refers to tremor during goal-directed movements, as in cerebellar disease. Recognizing these differences can be helpful in making a diagnosis. A listing of tremors classified by position is provided in Table 11-3. Since essential tremor (ET)

TABLE 11-3. Differential Diagnosis of Tremor

Rest tremors
  Parkinson's disease
  Secondary parkinsonism
  Hereditary chin quivering
  Severe essential tremor
  Drug-induced (neuroleptics)
Postural tremors
  Physiologic tremor
  Essential tremor
  Neuropathic tremor (Roussy–Lévy syndrome)
  Cerebellar head tremor (titubation)
  Dystonic tremor
  Drug-induced tremor (lithium, valproate, neuroleptics, caffeine, theophylline, tricyclic antidepressants, amphetamines)
Action tremors
  Classical cerebellar tremor (multiple sclerosis, infarction)
  Primary writing tremor
Mixed tremors
  Wilson's disease
  Rubral tremor
  Psychogenic tremors

is the most common cause of tremor and is a disorder primarily of tremor, it will be the major subject of this discussion.

CLINICAL FEATURES

Essential tremor is a monosymptomatic disorder of the nervous system that occurs in a sporadic or familial form with autosomal dominant inheritance. A senile form with onset after age 65 has also been described, but these patients generally are classified as sporadic. ET is considered to be the most common movement disorder, and it occurs equally in men and women. It is characterized by a postural tremor, with or without a kinetic component, that is most evident in the upper extremities. The kinetic component is seen in finger-to-nose testing, although it is often not as dramatic as in cerebellar disorders, and tremor at rest occurs rarely (in 5% to 10% of patients) in the most severe cases where the patient has a long duration of disease. The frequency of tremor ranges from 4 to 12 Hz. A maneuver to potentiate tremor during physical exam is to have patients hold the finger tips of their two open hands close together without touching, while holding their elbows out like wings. This maneuver can also bring out a more proximal distribution. One could also perform a cup test: the patient holds a full cup of water and pours it into another cup. The onset of ET can be at any age from birth to 90, with a mean of about 45 years. Those patients with a family history appear to have an earlier age of onset (age 40) when compared to sporadic cases (age 51). ET usually affects the fingers and hands first, and then it moves proximally. Tremor may occur bilaterally in the hands simultaneously, or in one hand at a time. When bilateral, it may be symmetric or asymmetric. Though hemitremor has been observed, it occurs only on rare occasions. When tremor is asymmetric, it usually is worse in the dominant hand. Handedness in ET is distributed according to population norms. Tremor may spread to the head and neck. Approximately 50% to 60% of patients with ET have head involvement and in some instances head tremor is the sole manifestation. Head tremor may present as a vertical nod (yes-yes) or as a horizontal nod (no-no). Voice tremor occurs in approximately 25% to 30% of patients with essential tremor. The voice is characterized by rhythmic alteration in intensity at the same frequency as the hand tremor. Head and voice tremor tend to be more frequent and severe in women than in men. Tremor in the head or voice should strongly suggest a diagnosis of ET and not Parkinson's disease. Less frequently, tremor occurs in the jaw, face (lips, tongue), trunk (if present while standing only, this is referred to as orthostatic tremor), and legs (15%). There are also task-specific tremors (i.e., primary writing tremor), which many believe to be variants of ET. One other nontremor feature in ET patients has been the deterioration of tandem walking. This feature worsens with advancing age.

Essential tremor is a slowly progressive disorder that remains stable in some patients for prolonged periods of time before progression is noticed, or it progresses continuously. It is not unusual for patients to seek medical advice after having the tremor for one or two decades. Initiation of a specific posture may aggravate the tremor early in the course. Later it is aggravated by many different movements or postures. It disappears during sleep and worsens with anxiety, fatigue, temperature changes, local pain, aminophylline, and possibly hunger. Alcohol characteristically improves the tremor (in 74% of those who drink any alcohol). A substantial proportion of cases are functionally disabled, with 20% having impaired job performance and requiring early retirement. This is why the term *benign* has been eliminated from the name. Other patients are very embarrassed by the tremor and impose social isolation upon themselves.

Essential tremor is a clinically heterogeneous disorder that may go unnoticed by the patient, may simply represent an embarrassment, or may actually be disabling, leading to difficulties with writing, drinking, using kitchen utensils. Currently, at least 5 million people in the United States have had this disorder diagnosed. As many as 13% of individuals over 65 probably have ET. There are many people with this problem who have not bothered to seek medical care and therefore have gone undiagnosed.

GENETICS

Essential tremor is an autosomal dominant disorder with 100% penetrance. At least 60% of cases have a clear genetic component. This may be an underestimate, as some sporadic cases may represent nonrecognition. Recently, genetic mapping has resulting in the linking of ET to genes on two different chromosomes. In one study, 16 families with 75 affected individuals from Iceland were examined using a genome-wide scan with 350 markers. The result was linkage to chromosome 3q13. The mutation in this gene (referred to in the paper as FET1) apparently accounts for the disease in 80% of Icelandic families stricken with ET.

The second study evaluated one large American family that originally hailed from the Czech republic. This family had 18 affected members with pure ET.

Utilizing similar methods, these authors discovered linkage to a locus on chromosome 2p22-p25. Genetic anticipation was suggested in the family because onset in each successive generation was progressively younger. Anticipation is usually associated with a CAG trinucleotide repeat and, in fact, repeat expansion detection analysis in this family revealed the presence of just such a mutation, but it remains unclear if there is a direct linkage between this CAG repeat and the ET gene. These findings indicate that a single highly penetrant gene is sufficient to cause ET. It also demonstrates that ET may be a genetically heterogeneous disorder.

PATHOLOGY AND PATHOPHYSIOLOGY

Since ET is neither life threatening nor life shortening, the opportunity for a postmortem examination of the CNS is not frequent. In those patients who have been examined pathologically, there is no distinctive CNS pathology. Recent PET studies have demonstrated an increase in regional cerebral blood flow in the cerebellum (bilateral) and red nucleus, indicating that the neuronal circuitry involving these regions may be the location of the abnormality. One study also demonstrated increased glucose metabolism in the inferior olivary nucleus of the medulla. This structure may be the source of the rhythmic discharge causing the tremors. This notion is supported by the fact that lesions in the cerebellum and thalamus may stop tremor.

Another interesting pathophysiologic postulate is that ET represents an exaggeration of physiologic tremor. Physiologic tremor is a normal phenomenon that can be recorded in all people by the use of an accelerometer and can be observed clinically in some normal individuals (at 8 to 12 Hz). Physiologic tremor can be seen in almost everyone when the hands are held out and a sheet of paper is placed over the fingers. The tremor starts at a frequency of 6 Hz and increases to a frequency of 8 to 12 Hz in childhood. It then decreases again with age. Possible physiologic mechanisms include inherent properties of motor neuron firing, oscillations in the stretch reflex causing synchronization of motor neuron discharges, or a supraspinal rhythmic input to the motor neurons. This tremor is known to be exacerbated by anxiety, emotional stress, thyrotoxicosis, caffeine, and other stimulants. Some believe that physiologic tremor may be a *forme fruste* of ET, and that both originate from the same neuronal oscillators. Thus, ET begins as enhanced physiologic tremor and then progresses in severity over time. However, evidence has been presented that physiologic tremor and essential tremor are different. This controversy remains unresolved.

DIFFERENTIAL DIAGNOSIS

The diagnosis of ET is a clinical one (see Table 11-3). The most common misdiagnosis in ET patients is Parkinson's disease. The two disorders can usually be differentiated by careful history and physical exam. The tremor of Parkinson's disease occurs at rest, whereas the tremor of ET is a postural and kinetic tremor. Patients with parkinsonism have rigidity, bradykinesia, micrographia, and postural and gait difficulties, and ET is associated with none of these. Other than the tremor, neurologic examination is normal. The handwriting of a patient with ET is usually large and tremulous. Sometimes a handwriting sample alone can lead to the correct diagnosis. Some studies have demonstrated an increased prevalence of Parkinson's disease in families of ET patients, an increased prevalence of ET in parkinsonian patients, and an increased prevalence of Parkinson's disease in ET patients, suggesting that an association of some kind exists. The nature of this association remains a mystery.

Postural tremor is frequently present in patients with ITD. This tremor can be indistinguishable from ET. A family history of ET is not uncommon in these disorders. Some investigators have indicated that this frequent association between postural tremor and dystonia is indicative of some sort of link between ET and idiopathic dystonia, but linkage of ET to the DYT1 gene has been ruled out. Tremor is particularly frequent in patients with spasmodic torticollis and Meige's syndrome. In spasmodic torticollis, head tremor is present in approximately 40% of patients, and misdiagnosis is frequent. In addition, approximately 20% of torticollis patients have a hand tremor similar to that seen with ET. It is important to differentiate between these disorders because treatments differ.

Postural and kinetic tremor secondary to cerebellar lesions can be differentiated from ET because of the presence of other signs of cerebellar dysfunction and the difference in severity (cerebellar tremor is generally much more disabling). There are three types of cerebellar tremor: (1) the classical cerebellar kinetic intention tremor, (2) cerebellar outflow rubral tremor, and (3) head titubation. The classical tremor appears with goal-related movements most evident at the beginning and end of the movement. It is much slower than ET, 2 to 5 Hz, and of wider amplitude. The lesion usually includes the dentate nucleus (most common in stroke patients). Outflow tremor is present at rest, when maintaining posture, and with action. Amplitude and frequency are similar to the classical tremor, and the lesion includes the outflow pathway from dentate nucleus to the thalamus, with the most common location of the lesion in the midbrain including the red nucleus. This type of tremor is seen most commonly in young patients as a manifestation of multiple sclerosis and in the elderly as the result of a stroke. Finally, titubation is a head tremor similar to the head tremor of ET. It is generally the result of bilateral cerebellar lesions.

EVALUATION

As noted, the diagnosis of ET is based on findings in the history and physical. If the patient presents with the typical picture as described, then no laboratory or imaging studies are necessary, with the exception of thyroid function studies since hyperthyroidism can worsen the already-existing tremor or cause an enhanced physiologic tremor that may appear similar to ET. Any patient with a sudden-onset tremor, unilateral tremor, or other complex features that do not appear to fit with ET or Parkinson's disease should be studied further with imaging studies and a screening for Wilson's disease. The diagnosis of Wilson's is extremely important because it will be fatal if undiagnosed. Finally, any person presenting with tremors must have his medications examined carefully, as many can induce tremors of varying types.

TREATMENT

The treatment of choice for ET is the beta-blocker propranolol (standard and long-acting formulations). It is particularly useful in controlling postural and kinetic tremor in the upper extremities and may make a significant difference to the patient in terms of being able to feed himself or write legibly. This may be true even though propranolol usually does not abolish the tremor but may only decrease its amplitude with little or no effect on frequency. There are often markedly inconsistent therapeutic results with 40% to 70% of patients showing a decrease in amplitude by 50% to 60%. There does not appear to be a correlation between plasma concentration of propranolol or its metabolites and a reduction in tremor. There are no apparent features that separate responders and nonresponders, but some investigators have found that tremors with lower amplitude and higher frequency respond less well. The dosage of propranolol may range from 80 to 320 mg per day;

it begins to exert its effect 2 to 6 hours after a single dose and the effects may last as long as 8 hours. Withdrawal from propranolol may result in a rebound increase in amplitude of the tremor, which may last longer than a week. The site of action of propranolol, whether central or peripheral, has not been fully established. There are certain groups of patients with ET in whom the use of propranolol is contraindicated. They include patients with chronic obstructive lung disease, asthma, and congestive heart failure, in whom propranolol can cause dyspnea and wheezing. In these instances, the substitution of a different beta antagonist, metoprolol, may result in amelioration of the tremor and no bronchospastic symptoms. Metoprolol is a beta-receptor antagonist that is relatively selective in its action; however, patients who do not respond to propranolol also do not respond to metoprolol. It has been suggested that the selectivity of this agent is lost when higher doses are used, and at higher doses bronchospastic symptoms may re-emerge. Acute side effects of beta-blockers include bradycardia and syncope, while chronic problems include fatigue, impotence, and depression.

Primidone, an anticonvulsant, may be as effective as propranolol in the treatment of ET. The major problem is acute adverse effects, which are frequent (30%) and include vertigo, a general ill feeling, unsteadiness, nausea, ataxia, and confusion. These side effects clear spontaneously after 1 to 4 days, so patients should be encouraged to stick with the drug during this time. It has be observed that lower doses (50 to 250 mg/day) are as effective as the higher doses and are better tolerated. As with propranolol, the response has varied from patient to patient and the reason for this is unknown. Plasma levels of primidone and its metabolites do not correlate with responsiveness. It is likely that a combination of primidone and propranolol will be more effective than each drug used alone.

A majority of those patients who respond to medical therapy will respond to either propranolol or primidone, and these patients can be managed long term. However, those patients who do not respond or are unable to tolerate these agents are extremely difficult to manage and should be referred to a neurologist well versed in the management of tremor patients. The neurologist will in all likelihood attempt to treat the tremors with other less frequently utilized medications or surgical therapy.

One of the features of the clinical history that an adult with ET often reports is the salutory effect of alcohol on the tremor. In fact, alcohol may be the most effective agent, as 75% of patients respond quickly and dramatically. The occasional use of alcohol in patients with ET is a reasonable recommendation. Benzodiazepines, particularly alprazolam and clonazepam, have also been demonstrated to be successful in treating essential tremor. A major side effect of this class of medications is sedation. Other agents useful in some patients with ET include methazolamide and acetazolamide, gabapentin, phenobarbitol, and clozapine. The last-named drug seems to have a general tremorolytic action, improving tremors in ET, Parkinson's disease, and multiple sclerosis. At low doses (<50 mg per day), there was reduction in amplitude and frequency. The one disadvantage of using this drug is the need to monitor white blood counts, since 1% of patients develop agranulocytosis. There are a number of other new treatments under investigation for essential tremor. Of greatest interest is Botox injection directly into contracting muscles. Pilot studies have been completed in patients with head, hand, and voice tremors, with moderate to marked functional improvement and tremor reduction in approximately 70% of patients.

As noted, 30% to 60% of patients do not respond to medications. Many have severe tremor and it is these patients in whom surgery needs to be considered. Stereotaxic thalamotomy of the ventral intermediate (VIM) nucleus has been utilized for 30 years with varying levels of success. Some patients experience a dramatic resolution of tremor, but in about 20% of patients, recurrence is observed. Persistent side effects from unilateral thalamotomy are uncommon but include dysarthria, dysphagia, and limb paresis. Complications from bilateral surgery occur in over 25% of cases and include speech impairment, mental status change, involuntary movements, and gait disorder. This bilateral procedure is not recommended.

During thalamotomy, stimulation is utilized to optimize placement of the lesion. It was found that this stimulation reduced tremor. This finding led to the consideration of using chronic stimulation of the VIM in treating tremors, otherwise known as deep brain stimulation (DBS). Chronic stimulating electrodes are implanted through a burr hole in the skull; they are placed utilizing stereotactic techniques for magnetic resonance imaging (MRI) or computed tomography (CT) imaging, and connected to a pulse generator. During the surgery, the patient is awake and the stimulator is tested. If it reduces tremor, it is kept in place permanently and the pulse generator is implanted subcutaneously in the subclavicular area. In a minority of patients, placing the electrode alone will reduce tremor as the result of a microthalamotomy. The stimulator can be controlled with an external magnet that can turn it on and off. It is recommended that patients keep it off at night to avoid the development of tolerance and to preserve the battery. Significant improvement has been observed in blinded evaluations and maintained for 1 year. In one study, efficacy was seen up to 8 years. Over 30% of ET patients experience complete resolution, and 90% demonstrate moderate to marked improvement in writing, pouring, drinking, and other activities. DBS improves all types of tremor (resting, postural, and kinetic) and it improves disability correlated most closely with improvement of postural type. Surgical complications have included intracerebral hemorrhage, subdural hematoma, and postoperative seizure. Stimulation-related complications include transient paresthesias, which occur in all patients at the time the stimulator is turned on, headache, gait disequilibrium, limb paresis, dystonia, and dysarthria. These problems disappear with time. Bilateral implants are not associated with the high morbidity of thalamotomy. The stimulation parameters (voltage, frequency, and pulse width) do not require significant adjustments over time. The advantages of DBS over thalamotomy include reversibility (minimal destructive lesions), adaptability (can change stimulus parameters to improve efficacy and decrease side effects), and the ability to perform bilateral procedures with much less risk. Drawbacks include the cost of the stimulators, implantation of foreign matter, need to replace battery, possibility of breakage, malfunction, and infection. This procedure has already begun to replace thalamotomy.

HUNTINGTON'S DISEASE

Huntington's disease (HD) is a chronic degenerative disorder of the CNS characterized by involuntary movements (most notably chorea), psychiatric symptoms, and progressive cognitive deterioration. Prevalence in the United States is approximately 12 per 100,000 population. There are two places in the world where it is much more frequent: Maracaibo, Venezuela (where most of the genetic research was conducted) and Moray, Scotland. It is inherited in an autosomal dominant pattern and commonly presents in adult life. The word *chorea* is derived from the Greek word for dance (*choreia*) and was originally used to describe the dancelike gait and continual limb movements of infectious forms of chorea (Sydenham's chorea or St. Vitus dance). The term *chorea* now is applied to a class of abnormal involuntary movements as defined at the beginning of this chapter. Choreiform movements disappear during sleep and are often exacerbated by nervousness and emotional distress.

CLINICAL FEATURES

A patient with HD may manifest his or her disease initially with chorea, psychiatric features, or dementia, although eventually all of these abnormalities are seen. HD may begin any time from the first to seventh decade but most commonly presents between ages of 35 and 42. The onset of chorea is almost always insidious with a few irregular movements of the face and limbs. Patients find themselves to be fidgety and clumsy. The typical history includes slight clumsiness or restlessness that progresses to "piano playing" movements of the fingers and facial grimacing. Family members will notice a peculiar gait associated with irregular involuntary hand movements. The patient may try to mask the involuntary facial movements by chewing gum, and limb movements by sitting on their hands. The muscles remain strong and the ability to initiate movements remains preserved, but the carrying out of a continuous movement is frequently impeded by the superimposition of the chorea. The reflexes are frequently brisk but patients rarely have the Babinski sign until the final stages of the disease. The voice is often affected by this condition and abnormalities of respiratory and articulatory muscles may lead to severe dysarthria and erratic, sometimes explosive, speech. As the disorder progresses, the chorea may diminish and rigidity and dystonia may ensue. On some occasions, other movement disorders, including dystonia, parkinsonism, and myoclonus, may predominate instead of chorea. Approximately 5% of patients have onset in childhood. Sixty percent of these patients have parkinsonian features, not chorea. This has been referred to as the Westphal variant. There is an increased incidence of seizures in children with HD (30% to 60%). These patients progress more rapidly than adult cases and die in an average of 9 years. Childhood-onset cases more frequently inherit the disease from their fathers, and this relates to the type of genetic abnormality found in the HD gene (further discussion to follow).

Progressive intellectual deterioration can be manifested as a personality change, depression, or dementia. Some patients show more emotional than intellectual decline, becoming irritable, excitable, and even apathetic over time. Inattention, poor concentration and judgment, and eventual memory loss progress until the patient is overtly demented.

Voluntary movement difficulties include abnormal ocular motor function, gait difficulties, and loss of finger and hand dexterity. The ocular motor difficulties include impairment of fixation, increased ocular reaction time with an obvious latency before the movement is initiated, loss of smooth pursuit movements, and an inability to look toward an object without accompanying head movements and blinking. Optokinetic nystagmus is generally abnormal. These findings are frequently observed early in the course of the disease. The gait abnormality is not solely the result of choreiform movements. The gait, which has characteristics of both basal ganglia and cerebellar dysfunction, has a stuttering and dancing character to it. The patient also exhibits a wide-based stance, swaying motions, decreased arm swing, spontaneous knee flexion, and a variable cadence. One other interesting feature of HD is the inability to maintain tongue protrusion.

In general, Huntington's patients live from 10 to 30 years (average, 17) with the disease and usually die from pulmonary causes (aspiration pneumonia), cardiac disease (ischemic heart disease), trauma-related injuries (subdural hematoma) from multiple falls, or nutritional deficiencies. Slower progression of disease is associated with an older age of onset of HD and heavier weight at onset. Patients inheriting the disease from their mothers also tend to have a slower progression. Since the discovery of the gene, it has been shown that HD is more clinically heterogeneous than originally thought. For instance, patients with late-onset chorea and no dementia have been shown to have the HD gene. The final stages of the disease include a loss of ambulatory function, severe dysarthria, dysphagia with the threat of aspiration, and dementia. The loss of functional capacity and rate of progression can be correlated in some patients with the degree of caudate nucleus atrophy seen on CT or MRI scan and caudate nucleus hypometabolism as measured on PET.

Clearly, the clinical picture of HD is variable and some patients have more chorea than mental changes, but the reverse is also possible. This can lead to difficulties with diagnosis. Since HD is an inherited, progressive, debilitating disorder with no cure, accurate diagnosis is of the utmost importance. In the patient with adult-onset chorea, dementia, and a positive family history, the diagnosis can be made easily. However, in patients with chorea and even dementia who have no family history, the diagnosis of HD requires acquisition of a gene test. If a patient has chorea but a definite lack of family history, the chorea may be due to some other etiology. However, studies of patients with a sporadic form of chorea resembling HD have shown that a majority of these patients do indeed have the HD gene. A recent follow-up study of 49 patients suspected to have HD on clinical grounds but without family history revealed that 75% do indeed have the disease. This finding is less common in patients with atypical features. Dementia and emotional symptoms are not essential for the diagnosis and are not considered sufficient evidence of HD in a family, but a history of family members hospitalized for these reasons in middle age or because of neurologic problems helps to raise the index of suspicion in patients with typical choreiform movements. There are a number of disorders that present with chorea and make up the differential diagnosis for HD (Table 11-4).

Since the discovery of the gene, presymptomatic patients have been studied in an attempt to find out when the earliest features begin. It is interesting to note that these patients can be perfectly normal even with psychometric testing. Subtle changes in motor skills, including movement time, movement time with decision, and auditory reaction time, have been described in patients considered to be at risk, asymptomatic gene carriers. Cognitive changes (measured via psychometric testing) have also been described in some reports as very early features in patients otherwise considered to be asymptomatic. The CAG trinucleotide repeat length significantly correlated with these test performances.

GENETICS

Huntington's disease is inherited as an autosomal dominant disorder with 100% penetrance. Children of an affected parent have a 50% risk of developing the disease. The emotional impact of the disease on children is profound. Children must watch as a parent deteriorates slowly, inexorably, while facing the prospect of inheriting the same disorder. Enormous advances have been made in the last decade regarding the genetics of HD. In 1983, the discovery of a DNA marker (polymorphism) linked to the HD gene on the short arm of chromosome number 4 raised the possibility of presymptomatic and prenatal testing. The test was quite complicated, comparing the genetic markers (DNA polymorphisms) in affected and unaffected family members, and requiring blood samples from many relatives with and without the disease.

In 1993, the actual gene was isolated (see following for details), and this simplified the process dramatically. Now, all that is required is blood from the patient only. The availability of such a test has raised a number of ethical questions, most fundamental of which is why should predictive testing be performed for an illness without a cure or an effective means of therapy. The impact of revealing to a young healthy person the rather bleak future of HD may be devastating. The results could be marital difficulties leading to disruption of the family and divorce, loss of employment, and psychiatric problems including suicide. Reasons for genetic testing are numerous. In symptomatic patients, it is now the gold standard from a diagnostic point of view. Its use will avoid a very costly work-up for other causes of chorea. In asymptomatic people, it will allow for personal and family planning and relieve uncertainty, and in both groups it will prepare patient and physician for treatment possibilities (e.g., clinical trials or new treatments, which may not be too far down the road). Many people now have realistic hopes that research in genetics and pathogenesis will lead to useful therapies and possibly a cure soon. There are also legal and social issues related to predictive testing that need to be addressed. Early studies showed that approximately 75% of at-risk patients would be interested in participating in predictive testing, but with the advent of such testing this was found to be a gross overestimation.

For many of the reasons noted, HD genetic testing is not to be taken lightly. One can image the devastating effect of a positive result on a young asymptomatic person and his or her family, but, surprisingly, a negative result can also cause havoc. Some people live their lives and make decisions based on the probability that they will incur HD. When they find they are negative, they experience regrets, and this can have a significant impact on family relationships. In addition, there is guilt for being gene negative while other family members suffer with the disease. This may cause the subject to either spend inordinate

---

TABLE 11-4. Differential Diagnosis of Huntington's Disease

1. Benign hereditary chorea
2. Senile chorea
3. Familial Alzheimer's disease with myoclonus
4. Creutzfeld–Jacob disease
5. Wilson's disease
6. Neuroacanthocytosis
7. Tardive dyskinesia in a psychiatric patient
8. Basal ganglia or subthalamic infarction
9. Parkinson patients treated with levodopa
10. Dentato-rubro-pallidal-luysian atrophy (DRPLA) (chromosome 11)
11. Choreoathetotic cerebral palsy
12. Chorea gravidarum
13. Recurrence of Sydenham's chorea in adulthood
14. Other drug-induced choreas (oral contraceptives, anticonvulsants, stimulants, antidepressants, anticholinergics, calcium channel blockers, buspirone)
15. Hyperthyroid chorea

amounts of time helping the affected sibling, or to distance himself. The testing process needs to be performed at a testing center equipped with the appropriate team of personnel in the specialties of genetics, neurology, psychiatry, psychology, social work, speech therapy, and nutrition, for both testing and treatment. The goals of such a program are to ensure that an informed decision is made, to prepare the subject for the result, and to ensure that an adequate support system is in place. The program must have maximal control over whether the patient and his family receive this irrevocable information (because of its profound impact), it must provide the opportunity for the subject to withdraw, and it must be able to ensure confidentiality. In most centers, the process of genetic testing for asymptomatic patients begins with an initial visit with a genetics counselor followed by evaluations from neurology, psychiatry, speech therapy, and sometime psychology. This takes place over a 4- to 8-week period. Occasionally, a second genetic visit is required. Once all evaluations are complete, the team meets and decides if testing can be safely performed or if it needs to be delayed. The subject then comes in for blood to be drawn and returns for results. Results are never given by phone or mail. In early symptomatic patients, the process is fairly uniform, but in advanced cases, and where a diagnosis is not clear, many of the steps are skipped depending on decisions made by the testing team. Testing should be avoided under the following circumstances: when not requested by the patient but requested by an employer, insurance company, prison, court, or the military; if the subject is less than 18 years of age (debatable); if prenatal testing is requested; if there is no informed consent; and if the subject has a poor support system.

The HD gene is called IT15 (IT = interesting transcription) and the gene product has been referred to as huntingtin. The abnormality within the gene is a polymorphic trinucleotide repeat sequence [(CAG)n] that is expanded and unstable. The instability leads to variations (expansion) in length between generations, especially if the father carries the gene. In normal individuals, this sequence repeats up to 29 times. Repeat lengths of 30 to 34 could lead to paternal transmission if expansion occurs, and lengths of 35 to 39 represent an intermediate- or reduced-penetrance situation. In HD, there are 40 or more copies. Longer segments appear in juvenile cases, suggesting that there is an inverse correlation between repeat length and age of onset of symptoms. It also appears to expand with each additional generation. This could lead to the phenomenon of anticipation, when the disease occurs at younger ages with each generation. There is also a correlation of repeat length and severity of disease and severity of pathology. There are no differences in repeat length in those patients presenting with neurologic or psychiatric symptoms.

The CAG trinucleotide repeat expansion in the gene results in a polyglutamine stretch within the protein. The normal function of huntingtin and the effect of the mutation on that function is unknown. The protein is widely expressed outside the brain in muscle, liver, heart, lung, and testes. Within the brain, both normal and mutant proteins are expressed in both affected and unaffected regions to various degrees, so expression does not predict vulnerability. On a cellular level, huntingtin is a cytoplasmic protein associated with vesicle membranes and microtubules. Localization of huntingtin within cells is changed in HD patients. There is decreased staining for the protein in nerve endings and increased perinuclear staining, which indicates that one function may relate to retrograde transport and protein degradation of cellular components. It also binds (via the polyglutamine stretch) to an important glycolysis enzyme (glyceraldehyde-phosphate dehydrogenase), which may lead to decreased mitochondrial function, decreased ATP formation, and, in turn, increased glycolysis and increased lactate. These changes relate to proposed pathophysiologic mechanism of cell death. In general, it is believed that huntingtin causes the disease process through a gain of function toxicity, not a loss of function. It does so possibly by binding to a "huntingtin-associated protein" (HAP-1). The discovery of the function of the huntingtin protein will lead to a better understanding of the neurobiology and pathogenesis of HD. The ultimate result would be a rational therapeutic intervention. These are the challenges of the next decade.

PATHOLOGY, NEUROCHEMISTRY, PATHOGENESIS

Postmortem examination of brain tissue from patients with HD reveals characteristic pathologic abnormalities. Grossly, the caudate nucleus and cerebral cortex are atrophied. On microscopic examination, there is severe neuronal loss (especially medium spiny neurons) and gliosis in the striatum, with the caudate nucleus being more affected than the putamen. Neuronal loss and gliosis may be seen in a wider distribution, and in advanced cases brain weight may decrease as much as 30%. Occasionally, patients come to postmortem examination with well-documented chorea and no pathologic changes.

Postmortem studies have also revealed that levels of many neurotransmitters, biosynthetic enzymes, and receptor binding sites are abnormal. Those that appear to have the most significance, as far as pathophysiology is concerned, will be discussed. Gamma-aminobutyric acid (GABA) levels have been found to be diminished in the striatum and globus pallidus. The levels of glutamic acid decarboxylase (GAD), the synthetic enzyme of GABA, have also been found reduced in the same areas. Both are found in the medium spiny neurons of the striatum. Levels of both are normal in other parts of the brain. GABA is an inhibitory transmitter that is released by the striatonigral pathways to modulate the outflow of dopamine from the nigrostriatal pathway. The result of the diminished GABA levels is a relative increase in dopamine activity. GABA is also the transmitter in neurons projecting from striatum to the globus pallidus. There are actually two projections: one to the external segment (the so-called indirect pathway) and the other to the internal segment (the direct pathway). Recent studies have shown that the projection to the external segment (also containing enkephalins) are first to degenerate. The result is decreased activity of the major output nucleus of the basal ganglia, the internal segment of the globus pallidus.

Somatostatin is a neuropeptide that has been studied in HD. It is known to be widely distributed throughout the brain including the basal ganglia and cerebral cortex. A three- to fivefold relative increase in somatostatin levels has been discovered in the caudate, putamen and globus pallidus in HD patients as compared to controls. Investigations suggest that somatostatin enhances release and action of dopamine and may therefore contribute to the functional dopamine excess and symptomatology in HD. It appears that somatostatin-producing neurons in the basal ganglia are selectively spared, suggesting that cell death is selective both in terms of regions and cell type. Striatal cholinergic interneurons also appear to be spared. Numerous other neurochemical abnormalities have been discovered in HD patients. These include diminished levels of substance P, cholecystokinin, met-enkephalin, and angiotensin-converting enzyme, plus an increase in neuropeptide Y. All these abnormalities are seen in the basal ganglia. The significance of these neurochemical changes is unclear at this time.

The pathogenesis of the selective neuronal degeneration in the striatum remains unknown. However, in the last few years, there is an increasing body of evidence pointing to a defect in mitochondrial energy metabolism. The evidence includes (1) glucose hypometabolism in the brain; (2) increased lactate concentrations in the basal ganglia and cortex; (3) altered activity of mitochondrial complex II-III and IV in caudate and putamen, with sparing of this activity in spared brain regions; (4) increased lactate-to-pyruvate ratios in cerebrospinal fluid of HD patients; and (5) abnormal energy metabolism in muscle of HD patients. It has been suggested that the mutant huntingtin protein may alter oxidative metabolism through its binding to the glycolytic enzyme described previously.

This energy defect may mediate cell death through excitotoxicity and possibly free radical formation. Progressive mitochondrial impairment brings about an increased vulnerability of neurons to normal endogenous levels of glutamate. Presumably, the decreased ATP formation leads to failure of the sodium–potassium pump (ATPase), membrane depolarization and easy activation of the n-methyl-d-aspartate (NMDA) type of glutamate receptors. This results in an influx of calcium ions, triggering the formation of free radicals, which the mitochondria can no longer take up, and oxidative cellular damage. In animal models, the cell damage caused by mitochondrial toxins is blocked by NMDA antagonists, which supports this scenario. An increase in markers for oxidative damage in HD supports the notion that free radicals play some role.

TREATMENT

DOPAMINERGIC ANTAGONISTS

Since one aspect of the basic pathophysiology in this disorder is related to relative striatal dopaminergic overactivity, the mainstay of symptomatic therapy for chorea remains dopamine receptor antagonists. Phenothiazines (e.g., chlorpromazine) and the butyrophenones (e.g., haloperidol) share the property of dopaminergic receptor blockade and are the accepted mode of therapy in HD for those patients requiring symptomatic relief of chorea. The amelioration of chorea is felt to relate to blockade of striatal dopamine receptors, whereas amelioration of the often-severe psychotic behavior may relate to dopamine receptor antagonism in the limbic system. Treatment with these agents should be limited to patients with disabling chorea and/or psychosis, and even in these cases it should be used as sparingly as possible. Therapy with these agents commonly results in sedation, lethargy, and depression. Of further concern is the risk of tardive dyskinesia. Also, it has been observed that a decrease in chorea secondary to neuroleptics does not significantly improve the patient's total functional capacity. Some patients actually have reported an overall improvement with discontinuation of these medications. Other agents that decrease striatal dopaminergic activity include reserpine and alpha-methylparatyrosine. Historically, reserpine was the first agent reported to be of use in the treatment of chorea. A rauwolfia alkaloid, reserpine acts to block intravesicular neurotransmitter reuptake and thereby it depletes the brain of dopamine. Because it also acts to deplete central norepinephrine and serotonin stores, reserpine's activity is not specific, but it is still used in the treatment of Huntington's disease because it has a less severe side-effect profile than dopamine antagonists. Tetrabenazine is another dopamine depletor that may be useful in HD. Alpha-methylparatyrosine inhibits tyrosine hydroxylase and thereby prevents the synthesis of dopamine and norepinephrine. After intravenous administration of this agent, amelioration of choreic movements in patients with HD has been noted. More recently, there has been an interest in using the atypical neuroleptic clozapine to treat HD. This drug is less likely to cause parkinsonism and tardive dyskinesia (see tardive dyskinesia section for details) and may be a better choice for that reason alone. The drug has been used to treat psychosis and chorea with mixed results. It has not been successful in improving functional capacity. Side effects of sedation and confusion limited the dose in some patients, and agranulocytosis may occur in 1% of treated patients. This drug has been utilized in only a small number of patients and further study is needed.

GABA AGONISTS

Replacement therapy with GABA and GABA analogs has been attempted. Sodium valproate, which inhibits GABA transaminase and raises central GABA concentration, has been tried alone and with GABA agonist supplementation, but no amelioration of chorea was noted. Isoniazid, when given with pyridoxine, also acts as a GABA transaminase inhibitor and in preliminary studies has been reported to lessen involuntary movements in a few patients with HD. This has not been confirmed in other studies. Although GABA levels are decreased in the basal ganglia of patients with HD, therapeutic maneuvers to address this transmitter change have not been successful.

GLUTAMATE ANTAGONISTS AND MITOCHONDRIAL ENHANCERS

Based on what is currently believed to be the pathophysiologic mechanism of cell degeneration in HD, a number of glutamate antagonists are being tested. The first study using this strategy was a large, long-term, controlled trial utilizing baclofen. Baclofen inhibits release of glutamate and aspartate and exerts a protective effect against potent excitotoxins in animal models. It was hypothesized that baclofen might slow the progression of HD, but results did not bear this out. A small trial with remacemide, a glutamate NMDA receptor antagonist, demonstrated safety in HD patients and possibly some indication for a symptomatic effect. It is currently being tested in a large multicenter trial for HD. Other drugs in early phases of study include ketamine and riluzole. Finally, coenzyme Q 10 (ubiquinone) is also being studied as a treatment for HD. This compound occurs naturally in mitochondria and shuttles electrons between complexes I, II, III, and it functions as an antioxidant and a respiratory chain activator. Studies in HD patients showed a 35% decrease in lactate levels in the cerebral cortex, and they returned to baseline 15 months after stopping the drug. The relevance of these findings to symptomatic improvement and slowing disease progression remains to be proven. It is safe, and it is being tested in HD as another treatment arm in the remacemide trial. Idebenone, another respiratory chain enhancer and antioxidant that protects against glutamate toxicity in animal models, failed to affect progression or cognition in 100 patients after 1 year of treatment.

PSYCHIATRIC THERAPY

Although the foundation of therapy in HD remains pharmacologic, psychiatric research has yielded a number of therapeutically pertinent observations. Psychiatric care is important to the management of behavioral problems implicit to the disease, whether they are related to psychotic or demented behavior. The management of these problems, from a behavioral viewpoint, is not specific to HD, and the same environmental restrictions and general supportive care administered for other psychotic and demented patients are required.

Aspects of HD that present unique psychological dilemmas appear to stem from the situations that result from genetic testing. Asymptomatic carriers must live the rest of their lives anticipating the onset of an as yet incurable disease. This frequently requires long-term psychological counseling and sometimes treatment with antidepressants. Gene-negative patients may also require psychiatric therapy. If they expected to get the disease and find that they will not, they may regret many life decisions, sometimes threatening the family unit, and they may feel guilt related to those siblings who are affected. This, too, may require long-term psychiatric follow-up and antidepressants. It appears that serotonin reuptake inhibitors are very helpful in these situations, and in treating the depression and aggressive behavior that are manifestations of HD.

WILSON'S DISEASE

Wilson's disease (WD) or hepatolenticular degeneration is a rare neurologic disorder of copper metabolism with a prevalence of approximately 5 to 20 per million population, and higher in countries with increased consanguinity. It is autosomal recessive with the gene locus located on chromosome 13q14. In 1993, the WD gene (designated ATP-7B) was cloned, and it was discovered that the gene coded for a copper-transporting protein. The abnormal protein has decreased function, leading to failure of the liver to excrete copper into the bile. More than 25 gene mutations have been identified to this point. Some mutations leave some residual transporter function, while others leave none at all. It is believed that those with the residual function have a later onset of disease while patients with no transporter function have an earlier onset. However, the exact relationship between phenotype and each mutation remains to be elucidated.

Accumulation of copper ultimately causes signs and symptoms that are neurologic, psychiatric, hepatic, or ocular in nature, but they may occur in variable combinations, making WD a difficult disorder to recognize. The importance of recognizing WD cannot be overstated because it is a treatable and often reversible disorder that, if not diagnosed, inevitably results in death. There is no question that the only way to make the diagnosis is to always keep it in mind. Approximately 75% of deaths due to WD today result from a lack of proper diagnosis.

CLINICAL MANIFESTATIONS

Approximately 40% of WD patients present with neurologic signs and symptoms. The most common is a speech disorder or extrapyramidal disorder beginning at 18 to 20 years of age. WD has a slowly progressive course, often with a single symptom predominating for months or even years before other manifestations appear. However, there may be a sudden dramatic worsening of what appears to be a stable neurologic deficit. Incoordination involving fine finger movements such as handwriting and typing is frequently an early manifestation. It may be subtle at first but worsens as the disorder progresses. Tremor is also a common early manifestation. It may occur at rest, so that when associated with rigidity, bradykinesia, and/or gait difficulty, WD may mimic Parkinson's disease. The tremor may also be postural or kinetic in nature. When severe, it takes on a flapping quality at the wrist with high-amplitude oscillations and a "wing beating" appearance at the shoulder, often resulting in significant disability. Focal or generalized dystonia is also a common and predominant symptom of WD. Some patients present with just bradykinesia and rigidity without tremor. Chorea is rare but may result in movements and a gait disorder that resemble Huntington's disease. Spasticity and ataxia are rarely seen. Dysarthria is a consistent feature of WD. It is sometimes associated with dysphagia, and frequently patients show frustration because of their difficulty communicating. Often patients develop a characteristic facial expression with retraction of the upper lip, the mouth constantly agape, and upper teeth protruding. This gives the patient the appearance of grinning, or a "vacuous smile." Approximately 6% of patients have had generalized seizures. Seizures are not an early feature: Most patients have them after the initiation of therapy with penicillamine. It is hypothesized that these seizures occur in relation to copper mobilization. Seizures also could be a prelude to death if they go untreated with standard anticonvulsant therapy. A majority of the symptoms are exacerbated by emotional stress and ameliorated by calm and sleep. There is also an acute dystonic form of WD. These patients appear ill, and they have a high fever, significant muscle rigidity, rapid emaciation, and confusion, a picture that can be confused with a neuroleptic malignant syndrome. This acute presentation could be a preterminal event so proper diagnosis is of utmost importance. Because of the protean nature of WD, it is very important to consider this diagnosis in all patients under the age of 40 presenting with movement disorders.

Approximately 25% of WD patients are seen first by psychiatrists for a wide range of emotional difficulties. At least 50% of patients overall have psychiatric manifestations early. There are no psychiatric manifestations that are specific for WD and diagnoses may range from adolescent adjustment reactions to depression and schizophrenia. The most common features include abnormal behavior, such as irritability, incongruous behavior, aggression, and personality change. Depression and cognitive impairment are also common, but schizophreniform psychosis is rare. Psychiatric problems may be seen in a pure form without neurologic deficits, making differentiation from the primary psychiatric disorders quite difficult. However, there frequently are neurologic findings in association with the psychiatric symptoms, and this clinical situation should raise the index of suspicion that WD may be the cause of the patients problem. In fact, psychiatric symptoms are more closely related to the presence of neurologic features than hepatic. Some patients with psychiatric manifestations treated with neuroleptics, who later develop movement disorders, are misdiagnosed as having a primary psychiatric disorder and tardive dyskinesia. Again, a raised index of suspicion will allow for making a correct diagnosis. In one study, personality change and irritability appeared to be more frequent in patients with bulbar and dystonic features. With neuropsychological testing, asymptomatic patients appear to be normal, whereas neurologically impaired patients have clear changes. To diagnose this treatable illness, some have advocated that all patients admitted to psychiatric wards under the age of 30 should be screened for WD.

Hepatic disease may be superimposed on neurologic manifestations or, as in 30% to 50% of patients, may be the presenting problem. Hepatic disease usually presents at an earlier age than the neurologic symptomatology of WD (approximately age 10). There are four different presentations for hepatic WD. First, there may be a transient acute hepatitis that resolves spontaneously. This is often misdiagnosed as infectious mononucleosis, or viral hepatitis because patients present with the typical hepatic symptoms and signs such as jaundice, malaise, and anorexia. The second presentation is that of a fulminant hepatitis, which is seen in adolescents and which presents with sudden onset of jaundice and ascites progressing relentlessly to hepatic failure and death. A history of fulminant hepatitis in a sibling of a patient suspected as having WD is significant. Third, and most common, is a chronic active hepatitis that presents with weakness, anorexia, jaundice, malaise, and abnormal liver function tests. Finally, patients may present with cirrhosis. A family history of cirrhosis may be an important diagnostic point. Hepatic WD patients may be psychologically and neurologically normal.

Nearly all patients with WD and neurologic symptoms exhibit a Kayser–Fleischer (KF) ring in the cornea. This is a golden or greenish-brown ring that represents copper deposition in Descemet's membrane. The ring is seen easily around the limbus in patients with light-colored or blue eyes but may be quite difficult to see in those with brown eyes. A slit lamp examination should be performed by an experienced oph-

thalmologist in order to accurately diagnose a KF ring in all those suspected of WD. Although a KF ring is not pathognomonic for WD, its presence is important in the diagnosis. It fades with adequate chelation therapy.

Another unusual ocular manifestation of WD is the sunflower cataract. This is a disc-shaped opacity with frondlike radiations, that is often described as a "cataract like the rays of the sun."

Other possible manifestations of WD include Coomb's-negative hemolytic anemia; skeletal changes, including pathologic fractures from metabolic bone disease and hypertrophic osteoarthropathy; renal disease, including gross hematuria, stones, tubular and glomerular disease, and the Fanconi syndrome; and cardiac symptoms including arrhythmia and cardiomyopathy.

NEUROPATHOLOGY

The lenticular nuclei are involved bilaterally and symmetrically. The lesions vary from softening and discoloration to frank cavitation. Other areas less significantly involved include the subcortical white matter, cerebellum (most commonly the dentate nucleus), and other nuclei that make up the basal ganglia. Excess copper is distributed throughout the CNS. Neuronal loss is observed in the basal ganglia and, to a lesser extent, in the cerebral cortex.

PATHOGENESIS

Excessive accumulation of copper leads to organ system dysfunction and clinical stigmata of WD. Ceruloplasmin, a copper-containing polypeptide, is deficient in 95% of patients with WD. The relationship between deficient ceruloplasmin, the pathogenesis of WD, and the WD gene mutation is unknown. Ceruloplasmin has a number of specific activities at a cellular level; however, the loss of these actions does not appear to be related to the pathogenesis of the disorder. Treatment with ceruloplasmin is not effective, and during chelation therapy the ceruloplasmin level may rise, fall, or remain the same and is, therefore, of no value in following treatment adequacy. Biliary excretion of copper in WD is impaired and copper accumulates in the liver, binding to thiol and carboxyl groups on copper-storage proteins. The copper binding alters both structure and function of storage proteins, disrupting normal cellular activity in a variety of ways. When storage reaches capacity, excess copper begins to move into extrahepatic storage sites. This explains why KF rings may not be seen in hepatic WD.

DIAGNOSIS

It can never be said enough that a high index of suspicion is very important in making the diagnosis of WD. This is especially true when evaluating patients 40 years or younger who present with extrapyramidal disorders, psychiatric disorders (especially when associated with neurologic signs and symptoms), and hepatic disease. In addition, a family history of WD (particularly a sibling) or hepatic disease at a young age should alert the physician to a possible diagnosis of WD. Once suspected, the diagnosis of WD can be confirmed using four tests: (1) a slit lamp examination for KF rings—the specificity of KF rings for patients with neuropsychiatric WD is nearly 100%; (2) a serum ceruloplasmin level (usually low in WD); (3) 24-hour urinary copper excretion (usually elevated in WD); and (4) a liver biopsy with quantitation of copper concentration—the most definitive of all tests (copper levels above 250 µg/g of dry tissue considered diagnostic). Clinical evaluation and the first three tests are usually sufficient to make the diagnosis of WD in symptomatic patients, and liver biopsy is generally not required. A normal serum ceruloplasmin (often utilized to screen for WD) by itself should not convince the treating physician that WD is ruled out, since 5% to 20% of WD patients have normal levels. In a patient with a neuropsychological presentation, absence of a KF ring indicates that he probably does not have WD. If ceruloplasmin level is low, examination for KF ring must be performed. If ceruloplasmin is normal and KF ring is present, a liver biopsy should be performed to make the diagnosis. Hepatic WD is the most difficult presentation to diagnose because ceruloplasmin may be falsely elevated or normal in WD hepatitis and a KF ring may be absent. If confusion remains after serum ceruloplasmin levels, slit lamp examination, and 24-hour urinary copper concentration, then liver biopsy is required.

Wilson's disease is inherited as an autosomal recessive disorder, so each sibling of a WD patient has a 25% chance of having the disease. All siblings of WD patients should be screened. If they have WD, treatment will prevent the onset of clinical stigmata. The at-risk siblings should have slit lamp examination, 24-hour urinary copper, and ceruloplasmin determination, along with physical and neurologic exams at regular intervals. If a KF ring is present, ceruloplasmin level is low, and urinary excretion of copper is elevated, the diagnosis of WD is clear and liver biopsy is not required. However, if the serum ceruloplasmin level is low but KF ring is absent, the patient may be a heterozygote for WD and a liver biopsy will be necessary to make a definitive diagnosis. Ten percent to 20% of heterozygotes have low serum ceruloplasmin levels, but these patients do not require treatment. With the recent discovery of multiple polymorphic DNA markers close to the gene on chromosome 13, multilocus linkage analysis makes possible accurate and informative testing of potential carriers in families with WD. With these techniques, one could discriminate between carriers and presymptomatic patients. Advantages of this technique include its noninvasive nature and early (possibly prenatal) diagnosis. Neuroimaging techniques are not diagnostic in WD, but typical lesions can be observed. On CT scanning, cortical and brainstem atrophy are seen in nearly all patients. Hypodensity of the head of the caudate and putamen are seen early, and cavitation of the putamen is seen late in some patients. Sometimes, hypodensities are seen in other areas including cerebellum, brainstem, thalamus, and cerebral cortex. These lesions do not enhance with contrast. On MRI scanning, hypointense lesions are observed in the lenticular nucleus, thalamus, caudate nucleus, cerebellum, brainstem, and subcortical white matter on T1-weighted images, and hyperintensity on T2 (Fig. 11-3). On the other hand, the accumulation of copper leads to areas of hypointensity adjacent to the hyperintense regions (see Fig. 3B). These changes are seen in all patients with neurologic symptoms and represent edema, gliosis, or cystic lesions.

TREATMENT

Once the diagnosis of WD is confirmed, treatment should be instituted without delay. There is now a choice of agents to try, in particular, chelating agents such as D-penicillamine or zinc sulfate. D-penicillamine, a chelating agent with thiol groups to bind copper and remove it from organ systems via urinary excretion, has been the treatment of choice, but this is now being challenged. Certainly, the largest and longest experience in treating WD is with this drug. It has a rapid action in mobilizing and clearing the copper. One to 2 g should be given in four divided doses on an empty stomach to ensure maximal absorption. Pyridoxine, 25 mg/day, should be added because of an antipyridoxine effect of penicillamine. Improvement occurs from 2 weeks to 1 year after the institution of therapy. The variation in response results from the size of the abnormal body pool of copper, the size of the initial penicillamine dose, patient compliance, and the variation in strength of copper binding from patient to patient. There is no set pattern as to which symptoms clear first, but dystonia tends to be more resistant than tremor, while dysarthria and the characteristic smile typically

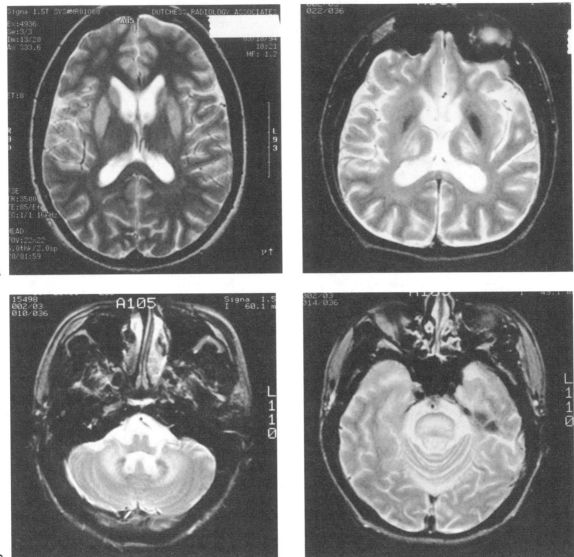

FIG. 11-3. A. T2-weighted MRI scan of a patient with early symptomatic Wilson's disease, demonstrating hyperintensity in the caudate nucleus and putamen. **B.** T2-weighted MRI scan of a more advanced patient with hypointensity in the striatum. The same scan as seen in **B**, showing hyperintensity in the dentate nucleus of the cerebellum **C.** and the pons **D**.

remain. Improvement of psychiatric manifestations is unpredictable. Sequelae resulting from irreversible structural damage to the liver or brain will remain unchanged and generally they are known by 2 years after the initiation of therapy. Seventy-five percent to

80% of WD patients will respond successfully to penicillamine. In the first 2 months of therapy, complete blood count, urinalysis, and liver enzyme levels should be examined frequently. Some WD patients initially worsen with penicillamine therapy during the first

2 weeks to 2 months. The actual frequency of this occurrence is unknown. In addition, a small percentage of WD patients continue to progress and die despite treatment. The reason for this is unknown. In one case, an asymptomatic WD patient had onset of neurologic symptoms after initiation of penicillamine.

Adverse effects of penicillamine are many and occur early and late. Early adverse effects include hypersensitivity reactions, fever, rash, adenopathy, leukopenia, thrombocytopenia, collagen vascular disorders, and bone marrow suppression. If any of these reactions are severe, therapy should be interrupted until symptoms subside. Then prednisone should be given, followed by the reinstitution of penicillamine. Late adverse effects occurring after a year of therapy include nephrotic syndrome, agranulocytosis, thrombocytopenia, Goodpasture's syndrome, pemphigus, myasthenia gravis, elastosis perforans serpiginosa, and dermopathy. Serious intolerance to penicillamine occurs in only 3% to 5% of patients, and these patients require alternative therapy. Trientine, like penicillamine a copper-chelating agent, is the alternative chelation therapy of choice. The dosage is 1 to 1.5 g/day. Adverse effects include collagen vascular disorders and iron deficiency anemia. British anti-Lewisite (BAL) is another chelating agent utilized in WD; however, its use is limited by severe toxic effects and the fact that it is only available for intramuscular injection.

Two newer therapies have been reported in the literature. Zinc sulfate, approved by the FDA in the United States in 1997, induces excretion of copper via the gastrointestinal tract by increasing the concentration of metallothionein in the bowel mucosa by 25-fold. As the tissue content of this protein increases, the proportion of copper in the cells increases. Then, as the mucosal cells are sloughed and lost in the stool, copper is lost also. Metallothionein levels also rise in the liver; this increases liver copper levels, but the copper is stored in a nontoxic form. Initially, it has a slower effect on copper metabolism than the chelating agents. The dose is generally started at 100 to 200 mg three times a day in adults, 50 mg twice a day in children, and the ultimate daily dose ranges from 300 to 1,200 mg/day. Patients are generally monitored by following free plasma copper levels (total plasma copper minus 0.3% of ceruloplasmin levels) and urinary copper levels. The first tests should be performed within the first 2 weeks, and if no change is seen then the dose is increased. The final dose is individualized. Zinc is less toxic than penicillamine and does not cause a paradoxical initial worsening of symptoms as penicillamine can. The side effects have been gastrointestinal irritation, elevation of serum amylase, and decrease high-density lipoprotein. Rarely, copper deficiency can occur, leading to leukopenia and anemia. It has been used successfully as both initial treatment and maintenance, with some patients followed over 30 years. The treatment of choice recently has been a matter of debate. Some feel that we should stick with the old reliable remedy of chelation therapy, based on decades of experience (since the 1950s). Others argue that zinc sulfate is the appropriate choice because it is equally effective, is much better tolerated, and does not cause a paradoxical worsening. There have been no formal controlled trials to examine this issue. It seems zinc has become the treatment of choice in presymptomatic patients and pregnant ones.

The other new treatment is tetrathyromolybdate. This compound has been utilized in animals to prevent copper accumulation in the liver. It prevents absorption of copper in the gastrointestinal tract and removes serum copper from the toxic pools by forming complexes with copper and albumin. It has a rapid action in relation to copper metabolism and does not cause a worsening of symptoms. The daily maintenance dose is 40 mg twice a day. Side effects include bone marrow suppression. Few patients have been treated to this point, and there is no evidence that it is any better than zinc. It is still considered experimental. Copper-rich foods should be avoided, including shellfish, chocolate, nuts, mushrooms, and liver.

Frequently, patients who are stable or, more commonly, asymptomatic will be tempted to stop their chronic medication. It may become difficult for asymptomatic patients to connect their good health to their chronic medication. Discontinuing chelation therapy invariably results in disaster for these patients, many of whom die of fulminant hepatitis within 3 years. It is the physician's job to reenforce the need for medication and to inform these patients of the disastrous results that lie ahead should the medication be stopped. Response to medication should be monitored utilizing urinary copper levels and serum free-copper levels. Chelating agents will cause an increase in urinary copper output before a decrease is seen.

Liver transplant is sometimes the only treatment alternative in patients with fulminant hepatitis and cirrhosis with liver failure. The 1-year survival rate is about 80% and the 5-year, 40% to 70%. These numbers are quite respectable, especially in this situation, where all the patients will otherwise die.

GILLES DE LA TOURETTE'S SYNDROME

Gilles de la Tourette's syndrome (GTS) is a disorder dominated by tics and behavioral abnormalities. Tics are classified according to whether they are motor or vocal, simple or complex. Simple motor tics are abrupt, brief, purposeless, isolated movements involving individual muscle groups and out of a background of normal activity. Examples of simple motor tics are eye blinks, head jerks, and shoulder shrugs. Complex motor tics are more coordinated, sequential, and complicated movements that may appear purposeful (resembling normal acts) but are inappropriately intense and timed. Examples of complex motor tics include eye deviation, facial grimacing, hand shaking, touching, jumping, hitting, kicking, squatting, copropraxia (obscene gestures), and echopraxia (mimicking the movements of others). Sometimes, a cluster of simple tics will appear to be complex. Simple vocal tics are a variety of inarticulate noises and sounds. Examples include sniffing, snorting, barking, throat clearing, and grunting. Complex vocal tics are actually linguistically meaningful utterances. They can include the utilization of words ("no-no"), phrases ("oh boy"), or even sentences. Classical forms of complex vocal tics include palilalia (involuntary repetition of words or sentences), echolalia (involuntary repetition of words or sentences just spoken by another person), and coprolalia (involuntary utterances of curse words). This latter phenomenon is perhaps the best known feature in GTS, but it occurs in less than 10% of cases. Vocal tics in general tend to occur at phrase junctions in speech and can cause blockage or hesitation of speech patterns.

Other forms of tics have recently been defined. Generally, motor tics are clonic or rapid in nature. When they are slow, twisting, and result in brief sustained postures (resembling dystonia), they are referred to as dystonic tics. Sensory tics are patterns of somatic sensations that have been variously described as a pressure, a tickle, a temperature change, or an uncomfortable feeling, localized to specific body regions and resulting in dysphoric feelings. These uncomfortable sensations may provoke a motor or a vocal tic. This indicates that the tic itself may actually be a voluntary movement (sometimes referred to as "unvoluntary"). The uncomfortable sensation is usually relieved by this movement, but relief is only temporary. As such, these movements are often repeated. An example of a sensory tic is a burning sensation or pain behind the eye leading to an eye blink or an eye deviation.

Tics have a number of characteristic features that help to differentiate them from other movement disorders. They are usually suppressible to some extent. Often, when patients with GTS come into the physician's office, their history of tics is a better indication than just observation, because patients can suppress tics well in the office. In addition, tics tend to wax and wane, so they can vary in intensity over time. They also tend to change location over time. More frequently, tics begin in the eyes with eye blinking and then move so that there are neck movements or shoulder shrugs or other types of movements. This suggests a tendency to migrate in a rostral-to-caudal fashion. Patients will often describe an inner tension or urge that is relieved by the tic itself. When patients suppress the tics, the inner tension grows and there will often be a flurry of tics once the suppression is released. Patients will often give a history of having few tics during work but having a flurry of them once they return home at the end of the day. Tics, in general, increase with stress, anger, and excitement, and decrease with relaxation and sleep.

CLINICAL SPECTRUM OF TIC DISORDERS

Tic disorders represent a continuum from a mild transient form to a potentially devastating neurobehavioral disorder. Studies of large families have indicated that various types of tic disorders occur in individual families and that they all appear to represent varied severity of a single disease. Transient tic disorder is probably the most common and mildest form of the disorder. It is defined by a duration of less than 12 months. As such, the diagnosis is often retrospective. In these patients, tics are usually the simple motor type. Chronic multiple tic disorder is a more severe form than transient tic disorder. In this case, patients have multiple motor or vocal tics but not both. Multiple motor tics are much more common. The duration of this disease is greater than 1 year. Gilles de la Tourette's syndrome represents the full expression of the disorder. Diagnostic criteria for GTS include the presence of multiple motor tics, at least one vocal tic, onset before the age of 21, and duration of disease greater than 1 year. Chronic multiple tic disorder and transient tic disorder most likely just represent mild forms of GTS and thus represent partial expression of the disorder. In its most severe form, GTS is a chronic, complex, fluctuating disorder. Although coprolalia, echolalia, intellectual dysfunction, and psychopathology are common manifestations of the disorder, they are not required for diagnosis. Coprolalia is distinguished from emotion-driven swearing by its cadence, volume, and context. When it occurs, it can be mild and transient as well.

Gilles de la Tourette's syndrome is more common in males than females (3:1 ratio) and has an age of onset between 3 and 21 years (with an average of about 6). It is often sudden in onset. Estimates of the prevalence of this disorder are probably significantly lower than actual prevalence, because, in the milder cases, a large percentage are unaware that they have a tic disorder, and in many the tics are not bothersome so they do not seek medical assistance. Spontaneous remissions occur rarely, and GTS is generally thought of as a life-long disorder. The natural history of the disease is that it reaches its maximal level of disability in adolescence and then in adulthood it tends to diminish in severity. Adults seem to manage tics better than adolescents and so are less bothered. Despite the continued presence of tics, adult tics are often mild and inconsequential. The severity of tics in childhood has no bearing on the severity in adulthood, as even the most severe cases can improve or even disappear. Moderate to severe tics in late adolescence, however, can be an indication that patients will have more severe tics in adulthood. In general, despite difficulties in school at young ages, most people with tics are employed or go on for further education as young adults and become very well adjusted. The need for treatment also diminishes in adulthood.

ASSOCIATED BEHAVIORAL DISTURBANCES

Obsessive compulsive disorder (OCD) is present in as many as 70% of cases. This behavioral disorder appears to be linked genetically to GTS and may, in fact, represent an alternate expression of this disorder. Symptoms can result in significant stress and disability. Examples of compulsive symptoms include ordered arranging habits; rituals of decontamination, including repeated hand washing; checking rituals (locks on doors or cars and stove switches); and ritualistic counting. Obsessive thoughts can often intrude on conscious thoughts and interrupt daily routines. Examples include fears and images of injuries to loved ones, fear of contamination with germs or dirt, feelings of responsibility for misfortune of others, and feelings of doubt that one has performed tasks that are already completed. One could see how obsessive thoughts and compulsive symptoms can go together. Compulsive behavior and tics, particularly complex ones, can overlap and one can see how difficult it might be to differentiate them. OCD symptoms, like tics, can wax and wane and increase with stress.

Another common behavioral disturbance is attention deficit hyperactivity disorder (ADHD). In these patients, the disorder can result in a short attention span, restlessness, poor concentration, diminished impulse control, and hyperactivity. It may be present in up to 60% of children and it is not uncommon for

ADHD to precede the onset of tics. ADHD seems to be more common in those patients with severe tic disorder. Stimulant medications that are generally utilized for primary ADHD may actually provoke or exacerbate tics in up to 50% of those treated. In these cases, it is difficult to know whether the tic is primarily due to the drug or the patient has GTS.

Other behavioral abnormalities include learning disabilities, aggressiveness, anxiety, panic disorder, depression, mania, conduct disorders, phobias, dyslexia, and stuttering. These disorders have been found to be 5 to 20 times more common in GTS than in the general population. It is difficult to know whether these disorders are secondary to the primary aspects of the disease (tics, OCD, ADHD) or whether they can stand on their own. Finally, sleep disorders are present in about half the patients. Problems include somnambulism, night terrors, nightmares, sleep initiation, and maintenance.

DIAGNOSIS

The diagnosis of GTS is generally based on clinical symptoms: there are no diagnostic laboratory tests. Because the features can be so varied, there is often a delay in diagnosis, perhaps as long as 12 years. Many patients diagnose themselves. In the last few years, a number of television shows have discussed the disorder or have characterized a person with it. When patients see these shows, they recognize their own symptoms and make an appointment with the physician. There are a few other diseases that cause actual tics. They have been seen in patients with stroke, tumor, head trauma, peripheral trauma (neck or face), encephalitis (and postencephalitic syndrome of encephalitis lethargica), and carbon monoxide poisoning. Locations of lesions from these disorders include frontal lobe, temporal lobe, and basal ganglia. The most common cause of secondary tics is the chronic use of neuroleptic medications (tardive tics). These patients usually have onset in adulthood and a clear history of neuroleptic exposure prior to the onset of the disorder. Other drugs that cause tics include anticonvulsants (phenytoin, carbamazepine), stimulants (including cocaine), and antihistamines. Finally, tics can be a manifestation of chronic neurodegenerative disorders; examples include Huntington's disease and neuroacanthocytosis.

GENETICS AND PATHOPHYSIOLOGY

Segregation analysis of multiple large families has suggested that GTS is an autosomal dominant disorder.

It has variable expressivity, including transient tic disorder, chronic multiple tic disorder, GTS, and OCD. It also is sex influenced as males are affected more than females. These studies have been supported by twin studies. Gene search utilizing the linkage analysis methodology has thus far been unsuccessful. These methods have been useful in finding the gene for rare autosomal dominant diseases such as Huntington's disease. However, GTS appears to be very common. This might suggest that GTS is genetically heterogeneous or that nongenetic etiologies exist or both. These possibilities would sabotage any chance that a GTS gene could be found. In addition, certain findings have challenged the notion that GTS is autosomal dominant. First, bilineal transmission is apparently common in this disorder, possibly because of a phenomenon referred to as assortative mating, in which people with the same clinical features are attracted to one another, perhaps because they do not find their clinical symptoms unappealing. Second, it has been suggested that genomic imprinting, in which gene expression is altered by whether the gene is inherited from the father or mother, may play a role in GTS. This phenomenon remains to be proven.

Despite clear genetic influences, there appear to be nongenetic factors that influence the form and severity of the disorder. Such factors have included maternal life stresses during pregnancy, gender of the child, severe nausea and/or vomiting in the first trimester, and birth weight.

The neuroanatomic location of the abnormality resulting in GTS is unknown. It is suspected from cases of secondary tic disorders, PET, and single photon emission computed tomography (SPECT) studies that the basal ganglia (particularly striatum), midbrain, frontal and medial temporal lobes, and limbic structures may be involved. One particular study suggested that basal ganglia–limbic circuitry is most important. In particular, there was decreased metabolism in left caudate and both thalami associated with covariate decreases in the lenticular nuclei, temporal cortex, and midbrain that correlated with disease severity. Postmortem studies have not resulted in any specific pathological findings. More recent studies using sophisticated morphometric MRI methods have found reduced lenticular volume and a loss of the left-sided predominance of the lenticular nucleus in adults and children with GTS. Other studies reported a loss of right caudate volume and a loss of the normal caudate asymmetry. There also has been an increase in measured cross-sectional area of the corpus callosum in GTS compared to controls, suggesting an abnormal development of corpus callosum in GTS.

This supports an abnormality of lateralization in GTS. The actual role of these findings in the development of GTS remains to be elucidated.

The biochemical basis of GTS is also not clearly understood. However, there is evidence to suggest that increase in activity of the dopamine systems is directly involved. This evidence includes (1) response to dopamine antagonist medications, (2) response to dopamine-depleting medications (reserpine, tetrabenazine), (3) exacerbation of tics with levodopa and stimulants (pemoline, amphetamine, methylphenidate), (4) the occurrence of tardive tics, and (5) the presence of alterations in dopamine metabolites in the cerebrospinal fluid of patients with GTS. Two hypotheses related to this increase in dopamine stimulation have been suggested. The more prominent one is that there is dopamine receptor supersensitivity in the basal ganglia, similar to that described in tardive dyskinesia; some forms of evidence support this. There is also the possibility that there is an increase in dopamine input into the striatum; some lines of evidence that support this as well. Further studies are required. Other neurotransmitter systems have been evaluated as well. Of most interest in the recent literature is the study of alterations in the opiate system. Dynorphin levels have been found to be reduced in the lateral globus pallidus of a patient with GTS on neurochemical evaluation. Further studies are ongoing to decipher the potential impact of these alterations.

TREATMENT

Effective pharmacologic treatment is available for GTS and its many behavioral manifestations. Patients should be evaluated by a team of specialists who can approach the disorder from many sides. This team should include a neurologist, a psychiatrist, and a social worker. It may be found that many patients with this disorder do not need treatment at all as their symptoms are mild and well controlled. If the symptoms are not disruptive or disabling, then patients should be treated supportively only. Some patients may do well with some behavioral therapy such as relaxation training and self-monitoring. Pharmacologic treatment should be utilized only in those patients who are disabled by their symptomatology. The team approach to evaluating patients can dictate which group of symptoms requires treatment (i.e., tics or behavioral disorder). Treatment should be directed toward the specific symptoms that are most disabling. With regard to tics, dopamine antagonist medications (neuroleptics) are the most effective drugs available. Doses of haloperidol ranging from 0.25 to 2.5 mg/day at bedtime can be effective in up to 80% of patients. Side effects, however, can limit its usefulness; these include sedation, dysphoria, weight gain, tardive dyskinesia, acute movement disorders (akathisia, acute dystonia, parkinsonism), depression, poor school performance, and school phobias. Other neuroleptic medications with fewer side effects are now available. Pimozide can be utilized at a dose of 1.5 to 10 mg/day. This drug can cause prolongation of the QT interval, which ultimately can lead to cardiac dysrhythmias. Electrocardiogram is required at baseline and then should be followed. Fluphenazine, stelazine, and thioridazine are other neuroleptics that can be utilized. In some patients, rotating two or three of these medications can be extremely helpful to prevent tolerance or breakthrough of tics during treatment. In recent years, atypical neuroleptics have been available. Clozapine, the first of this group, has been utilized in a limited number of GTS patients. The results have been mixed, but this and other atypicals should be considered because they are generally associated with few extrapyramidal side effects. Clonidine is another medication that has been utilized in GTS. This drug is an alpha-2 adrenergic agonist that inhibits presynaptic norepinephrine release. Studies have found that it can be useful in tics but more so for behavioral aspects of the disorder. Its efficacy in tics is controversial. Daily doses range from 0.15 to 0.5 mg. Side effects of this medication include sedation and low blood pressure. Clonidine is a good first-line drug because of its better side-effect profile. Other agents utilized with some success, which have not been studied in controlled trials, include clonazepam, reserpine, tetrabenazine, calcium channel blockers, and opiate antagonists. For facial and cervical tics, especially dystonic tics, carefully placed intramuscular Botox injections may be useful. In some patients, the injections decrease the number of tics and their severity, eliminate the associated urge to perform the tic, and decrease the pain that results from the tics.

When treating OCD, behavioral modification techniques can be useful, but pharmacologic intervention is often necessary. Recently, it has been found that fluoxetine, a bicyclic antidepressant that blocks serotonin uptake, can be extremely useful at doses of 20 to 60 mg/day. Clomipramine, sertraline, paroxetine, and fluvoxamine are other selective serotonin reuptake inhibitors that have been utilized in primary OCD with favorable results and may be useful in GTS. As mentioned, ADHD can be disabling in GTS. The standard therapies for primary ADHD, stimulant medications (such as methylphenidate, dextroamphetamine, and pemoline), can intensify tics and are relatively contraindicated in these patients. It is recommended that behavioral therapy and educational approaches be utilized first. If pharmacologic therapy is needed, the first drug to be utilized should be clonidine. Another drug that has recently been recommended for this problem is desipramine, a tricyclic antidepressant. If these medications are ineffective in controlling these symptoms and if the ADHD is much more disabling than the tics, then stimulant medications can be utilized. The patients should be informed that the tics may intensify with this treatment. Escalations in doses of stimulants should be performed gingerly.

TARDIVE DYSKINESIA

Tardive dyskinesia (TD) is an iatrogenic movement disorder related to treatment with dopamine receptor antagonist drugs (neuroleptics and antiemetics). The term *tardive* was coined to describe two features of the illness: (1) that it occurs after chronic therapy with these drugs (the cut-off has been arbitrarily set at 3 months), and (2) that the disorder is persistent. In recent years, the chronic exposure requirement has come into question as some cases have occurred shortly after initiation of therapy. Persistence of the dyskinesia remains a characteristic feature. Over the last decade, it has become increasingly clear that a number of variants of tardive dyskinesia exist. The most common is the classical TD syndrome, characterized by stereotypic or choreiform movements, which makes up at least half of all tardive syndromes. Others have been classified by the movement disorder that dominates the clinical picture—tardive dystonia, tardive akathisia, tardive tics, and tardive myoclonus. Although all these variants occur under the same conditions and they are frequently present at the same time, there are clear differences beyond clinical phenomenology (including natural history and pharmacology), and separation of these syndromes is important from a practical standpoint as well as for research protocols. For the remainder of this section, it is the classical TD syndrome that is referred to specifically, since most of our knowledge of TD is related to this particular disorder.

CLINICAL FEATURES

Tardive dyskinesia occurs in approximately 20% of patients treated with neuroleptic medications. The incidence of new cases increases with increasing duration of therapy: 5% at 1 year, 10% at 2 years, 15% at 3 years, 20% at 4 years. Approximately 10% of patients end up severely disabled. Classical TD is characterized by patterned, stereotypic orobuccolingual (OBL) chewing-type movements or dyskinesias. The tongue often has a writhing-type movement that will result in pushing out of the cheeks (bon-bon sign) but may also have stereotypic repetitive protrusions (referred to as fly catcher's tongue). They vary in severity from extremely mild (where the patient may be totally unaware of the movements and they simply look like an exaggeration of normal movements such as lip wetting), to severe enough to cause dysarthria and dysphagia requiring a feeding tube. On examination, the tongue movements tend to decrease with protrusion. In addition, patients can have jaw movements (opening, closing, deviations), facial grimacing, blepharospasm, cheek retraction and puffing, pouting, puckering, and lip smacking. Choreiform movements may also be present in limbs (piano playing movements of the fingers) and in the axial regions (with dancelike movements). Involvement of intercostal and diaphragm musculature results in respiratory dyskinesia. These patients have grunting, sighing, air gasping, and belching sounds as part of their picture, and they may become short of breath because of irregular breathing patterns. If severe, mechanical ventilation may be necessary. Respiratory dyskinesia usually occurs in conjunction with OBL and affects about 15% of TD patients. Another interesting type of choreic movement involves pelvic thrusting and twisting movements (so-called copulatory dyskinesia). It has been suggested that this particular pattern is more frequently associated with metoclopramide therapy, but this remains to be confirmed. TD movements may be increased or brought out by activating tasks such as testing dexterity maneuvers (finger or toe tapping, rapid alternating movements) and walking. Anxiety and fatigue also increase the movements.

The natural history of TD is that it reaches its maximal levels fairly quickly. In 50%, the movement disorder is persistent. In those patients where the inciting agent is removed, TD may gradually disappear but this may take years (as long as 5 years). The course may be one of persistence or fluctuations in severity. In some patients with choreiform movements, the continued administration of neuroleptics will result in a progressive movement disorder. In these patients, OBL dyskinesias may spread to involve the axial, limb, or diaphragmatic musculature. Another example of progression might be an increase in the severity and amplitude of the individual choreiform movements. For these reasons, as well as some theoretical reasons that are discussed when prevention and treatment of TD is presented, the use of a neuroleptic to treat TD is unwarranted. The fact that a large percentage of patients who develop this syndrome have an irreversible problem is an indication of the serious nature of this disorder.

Early descriptions and discussions about patients who might be predisposed to the development of TD define those patients as being female, chronically institutionalized, brain damaged, and psychotic. Many of these supposed preconditions have been abandoned, the most important being the concept that there had to be major preexistent psychiatric disease for a patient to develop TD. Unfortunately, it has been repeatedly demonstrated that after exposure to chronic administration of neuroleptics, patients with previously normal psychiatric and neurologic histories can and do develop TD. Nevertheless, there are factors that seem to increase a patient's risk for the development of this disorder. Age is the most consistent of risk factors for TD. After the age of 40, there is a dramatic rise in relative risk. There appears to be a direct relationship between age and severity and an inverse correlation between age and remission rate. Other possible patient-related risk factors include female gender, diagnosis of affective disorders, and history of drug-induced parkinsonism. There are also a number of treatment-related risk factors, including the use of depot formulations of neuroleptics and duration of exposure to these drugs.

PATHOPHYSIOLOGY

Based on anatomic models of basal ganglia function, it has been shown that hyperkinetic movement disorders (e.g., chorea) are the result of a decrease in the activity of the internal segment of the globus pallidus with a resulting loss of inhibition of the thalamus and increased stimulation of the motor cortex. This could come about through changes in the nigrostriatal dopamine system where this transmitter can have an inhibitory or stimulatory effect. Investigations have focused on alterations in dopaminergic function as a possible mechanism for TD. It has been proposed that the chronic administration of neuroleptics results in a chronic blockade of striatal dopamine receptor sites, and that this chronic blockade ultimately induces alterations in the sensitivity and number of dopamine receptors. Clinical data that support this notion include the exacerbation of TD with dopaminergic medications, suppression of TD with dopamine antagonists, and enhancement of the movements with anticholinergics. In the most simple conceptual terms, it has been proposed to be a chemical denervation supersensitivity. Although choreiform movements may begin when the neuroleptic is chronically administered without a change in dosage, the most common clinical setting in which the movement disorder begins is after the dosage is lowered or discontinued entirely. This latter setting is in keeping with the postulate of lowering the pharmacologic blockade of the dopamine receptor and allowing normal dopaminergic mechanisms to resume their interaction with the already sensitized receptor. Although there is much evidence in animal models to support this notion, there have been inconsistencies. For this reason, evaluation of other neurotransmitter abnormalities and mechanisms in the presence of TD have been evaluated, such as a decrease in GABA activity in the basal ganglia. Both animal studies and human studies have indicated that this is a possibility. An increased release of GABA from the external globus pallidus neurons innervating the subthalamic nucleus could ultimately result in decreased output from the internal segment of the globus pallidus. Some studies have indicated that an overactivity of norepinephrine is present and that decreased activity of serotonin (both of which modulate dopamine transmission) may also occur. Finally, there has been some suggestion that a decrease in acetylcholine activity in the striatum might play a role.

Another possible pathophysiologic mechanism for TD is related to direct neurotoxicity by neuroleptic medications. It has been theorized that the blockade of dopamine receptors results in an increase in dopamine turnover. This, in turn, results in the formation of increased free oxyradicals that ultimately damage striatal neurons. Neuroleptics may also be toxic to mitochondrial complex I. Finally, a comparison of the pharmacology of typical neuroleptic medications with atypical neuroleptics that do not cause TD (e.g., clozapine) has led to other theories, in particular one that involves the uncoupling of D1 and D2 receptors.

PREVENTION

As in all iatrogenic disorders, prevention is better than treatment. This is especially true in the case of TD, in which the syndrome itself may be irreversible. There are a series of simple steps that may help to limit the development of TD in the general population. First of all, the number of subjects at risk should be limited. This implies that these agents (the neuroleptics) should be employed only in the major psychiatric illness in which they are indicated, including

schizophrenia and Gilles de la Tourette's syndrome. These agents should not be employed for minor episodes of anxiety, restlessness, insomnia, or other minor psychiatric disturbances. The development of TD does not depend on any preexistent brain damage or psychiatric history, and patients who are normal psychiatrically can develop TD if exposed to neuroleptic agents. A second and a third means of decreasing the incidence of TD would be to limit the dose of neuroleptic employed and to limit the duration of treatment with the neuroleptics. All of these recommendations are common-sense approaches and seem realistic, although there is little clinical information in the literature to confirm these concepts. After all, if TD develops as a result of chronic neuroleptic blockade of the dopamine receptor, limiting the dose of neuroleptics employed, and therefore limiting the amount of blockade, may well be a contributing factor to the prevention of TD. In the same manner, limiting the duration of blockade by limiting the duration of treatment with neuroleptics may also decrease the incidence of tardive dyskinesia. It is always wise clinically to limit the dose of a pharmacologic agent to the symptoms being treated or controlled. Neuroleptic administration is no exception, and the dose of neuroleptic administered should be tailored to each patient. When neuroleptics are totally withdrawn from patients with relapsing psychosis, the relapse rate is significant. However, an initial episode of psychotic behavior does not necessitate the chronic life-long administration of neuroleptics. Another point in attempting to decrease the incidence of TD in the population is to avoid the concomitant use of anticholinergic and neuroleptic administration on a chronic long-term basis. The problem of chronic administration of neuroleptics and anticholinergics concomitantly is that there is some retrospective clinical evidence that patients who are on both neuroleptics and anticholinergics have a slightly greater risk for the development of TD than those on neuroleptics alone. The only reason for the concomitant use of anticholinergics and neuroleptics is to treat drug-induced parkinsonism. Drug-induced parkinsonism is a transient phenomenon that usually resolves within 3 months. If the patient develops it and is treated with anticholinergics, at the end of 3 months the anticholinergic should be slowly withdrawn to assess whether or not continued antiparkinsonian therapy is required. In addition, if the drug-induced parkinsonism has abated there is no point in administering a pharmacologic agent that is no longer indicated. Since the use of anticholinergics in the first place is directed towards the treatment of drug-induced parkinsonism, and since drug-induced parkinsonism in most cases is transient and reversible, it seems unwise to chronically administer an anticholinergic with a neuroleptic, even if the concomitant use of these drugs represents only a small increase in the risk factor for the development of TD.

An additional approach that may help to limit the development of TD is the early recognition of the syndrome and discontinuation of all neuroleptics, if that is psychiatrically possible, when the first abnormal movements are detected. In many instances, the continued administration of neuroleptics in the face of developing TD may result in progression of the syndrome. The best chance of both stopping the progression and reversing the TD thus resides in early detection of abnormal movements. A final approach to the prevention of TD relates to the use of antipsychotic agents that do not cause this syndrome, so-called atypical neuroleptics. Clozapine, the first of this class of drugs, appears to have less effect on the nigrostriatal pathways and, in addition, has more preference to D1 than D2 receptors, among other pharmacologic characteristics. Typical neuroleptics have a preference for blockade of D2 receptors, and it is alterations in these receptors that are thought to be important in the formation of TD. Clozapine does not cause D2 dopamine receptor supersensitivity and causes significantly fewer chewing-type movements than standard neuroleptics in animal models, indicating that there is less risk for TD. Clinical trials have indeed demonstrated that this drug is much less likely to cause the syndrome. There has not been a case of new-onset TD in a patient treated with clozapine who never received treatment with a standard neuroleptic. Clozapine has been approved for use in patients who have psychosis that does not respond to typical neuroleptics and in cases where typical neuroleptics are contraindicated. The presence of TD represents such a contraindication. If these movements are found early and the neuroleptics stopped, the TD could reverse and disappear. If clozapine is then utilized, TD can be further prevented. There are some drawbacks to this medication. The most important is related to its ability to cause an agranulocytosis. For this reason, a weekly white blood count is required for patients on the drug. Recently, two other atypical neuroleptics have been approved in the United States for treatment of psychosis, olanzapine and quetiapine fumarate. It is too early to tell if these medications will carry the same low risk for TD that clozapine does. As more of these agents become available, the incidence of TD could diminish significantly.

TREATMENT

The management of a patient who has already developed TD is a difficult clinical task. Medical therapies are frequently inadequate. The first approach to all of these patients should be careful review of whether the neuroleptics that have been and are being administered are psychiatrically indicated. In many instances, there is no major psychiatric indication for the use of these agents. If this is true, these neuroleptic agents should be gradually tapered off. In many patients, the movement disorder initially becomes worse when the neuroleptics are discontinued. This should not be surprising because, if TD is related to increased dopamine receptor site sensitivity secondary to chronic neuroleptic blockade, and if the patient is having involuntary movements (indicating dopamine receptor site sensitivity alteration is already present) while on the neuroleptics, and the drug is discontinued with abolition of the blockade, the abnormally sensitive dopamine receptor would be exposed to normal dopaminergic physiology. The result, intuitively, is an increase in the involuntary movements. This time period is often difficult to manage because the patients often do become worse. This should not be confused with worsening of the disease process itself, and generally speaking, this rebound of TD on withdrawal of the neuroleptic may persist for only 2 to 6 weeks. However, at the end of this time, one is able to assess the extent of the baseline disorder. The chronic syndrome has been reported to be irreversible in 30% to 50% of cases, depending on the age of the patient. Pharmacologic intervention in this choreiform movement disorder is based on what has already been discussed with regard to pathophysiologic mechanisms. The general pharmacology of chorea is such that agents that decrease dopaminergic activity within the brain will decrease chorea. Consequently, agents such as reserpine or tetrabenazine, which deplete the brain of dopamine, will ameliorate the chorea seen in tardive dyskinesia. Doses of reserpine from 1 to 9 mg/day are reached with a gradually increasing dosage schedule. Side effects of these agents are of concern and include orthostatic hypotension, parkinsonism, depression, and gastrointestinal problems. This is frequently the first line of treatment in TD. Other major drugs that interfere with dopaminergic activity include neuroleptics. However, despite the fact that if the neuroleptic dosage is raised the chorea in TD can be ameliorated, this is an incorrect approach because it will place the treating physician in a position of using the causative agent to treat the disorder. This situation should definitely be avoided. The only time that neuroleptics should be used to treat TD is if the TD is life threatening, and this is rare. Use of atypical antipsychotic medications (e.g., clozapine) has actually been associated with improvement of TD symptoms. Results of several studies have indicated that clozapine has an active therapeutic effect on TD, with some patients having complete resolution of symptoms. However, carefully controlled trials have not been done to confirm these findings. Thus, if the patients require continued antipsychotic medication, the use of clozapine will not only remove the risk of worsening the TD but may also lead to an improvement. Therefore, the use of clozapine is strongly recommended as treatment of choice in this situation, with discontinuation of all standard neuroleptics. The recommended dosage ranges from 100 to 900 mg/day, and the side effects more commonly seen include sialorrhea, orthostatic hypotension, weight gain, and seizures.

Dopamine agonist medications, such as levodopa or bromocriptine, have also been utilized based on the dopaminergic hypersensitivity hypothesis. It is felt that use of these agents would downregulate and decrease the sensitivity of dopamine receptors, and theoretically this would eventually lead to improvement of these symptoms. It is expected that treatment with these drugs will initially worsen TD before improvement occurs. Studies have shown variable results with these agents and, in general, they should be utilized with caution. Other pharmacologic approaches to the treatment of TD are based on manipulation of other neurotransmitter systems that may be abnormal in TD. As previously discussed with regard to the dopaminergic–cholinergic balance in both parkinsonism and chorea, increasing cholinergic activity will decrease chorea, and interfering with cholinergic activity (anticholinergics) may increase chorea. On one hand, anticholinergic medications have no role in the treatment of TD. On the other, there has been interest in the use of cholinergic agents in the treatment of chorea. Several attempts at a precursor loading strategy have been made using drugs such as choline and lecithin. These agents have not provided effective therapies. The use of a variety of GABA agonist medications, including valproate, diazepam, clonazepam, and baclofen, has also been disappointing: some patients do respond, but which will do so cannot be predicted. Noradrenergic antagonists, such as propranolol and clonidine, have been somewhat successful in some patients but this needs to be confirmed in larger control studies. Propranolol decreases neuroleptic blood levels and clonidine decreases the release of norepinephrine. These drugs are safe and are reasonable choices in the treatment of TD. Recent studies have indicated that vitamin E, an antioxidant, can improve TD symptoms. This may occur through the blockade of free radical damage to cells that may result from long-term neuroleptic use. Because of its safety, vitamin E is an excellent choice for first-line treatment. Finally, for facial and cervical distribution (especially if the tardive movements are dystonic), intramuscular Botox injections can be very useful, especially in those with refractory symptoms. This disorder can remain refractory to all treatments in many instances, and, as stated previously, it is far better to prevent the development of TD than to have to manage and treat it.

QUESTIONS AND DISCUSSION

1. Match the neurologic term with the appropriate description:

A.	Tremor.	**1.**	Excessive, spontaneous movements irregularly timed, nonrepetitive, randomly distributed and "dancelike"
B.	Chorea.	**2.**	An abnormal sustained posture
C.	Dystonia.	**3.**	Involuntary, rhythmic, oscillating movement resulting from alternating or synchronous contraction of reciprocally innervated antagonist muscles
D.	Tic.	**4.**	Patterned sequence of coordinated movements that may be simple or complex

The correct matches are (A) and (3), (B) and (1), (C) and (2), (D) and (4).

2. A patient presents with sustained involuntary eye closure and forced involuntary mouth opening. Which diagnoses are to be considered?

A. Meige's syndrome
B. Idiopathic torsion dystonia
C. Adverse effect of neuroleptic medication
D. Wilson's disease

All answers are correct. The description is that of Meige's syndrome. Meige's syndrome may be a manifestation of adult-onset idiopathic torsion dystonia or an adverse effect of neuroleptics. The latter may mimic the former quite closely. Dystonia may be a manifestation of Wilson's disease, a diagnosis that should be considered if the patient is under 30 years old when the syndrome occurs.

3. A 19-year-old patient complains of the recent onset of shaking, which occurs when he lifts a cup to drink or tries to retrieve food with a fork. When his index fingers are approximated, the tremor worsens. A sister has a history of liver disease. This description suggests:

A. Essential tremor
B. Huntington's disease
C. Wilson's disease
D. Parkinson's disease

The answers are (A) and (C). The description is that of a postural and kinetic tremor. This may be seen in essential tremor, which may be familial or sporadic and frequently occurs in adolescence or early adult life. Wilson's disease must also be considered in all patients under the age of 30 with any movement disorder, especially if there is a family history of liver disease.

4. Agents that might be effective in abating essential tremor would include:

A. Alcohol
B. Clozapine
C. Amphetamine
D. Propranolol
E. Primidone

The answers are (A), (B), (D), and (E). The last two agents are frequently used treatments for essential tremor. Amphetamines may induce a tremor similar to essential tremor or worsen an already present tremor.

5. A patient presents with a generalized choreiform disorder that began at the age of 45. He denies any neurologic or psychiatric problems prior to the onset of his current problem and never received neuroleptic medications. He denies a family history of any similar movement disorder, but his mother was institutionalized at the age of 55 for psychiatric reasons. What is this patients possible diagnosis?

A. Huntington's disease
B. Parkinson's disease
C. Essential tremor
D. Idiopathic torsion dystonia

The answer is (A). Huntington's disease is an autosomal dominant disorder with onset typically in middle age. Although psychiatric symptoms are insufficient for making a diagnosis of Huntington's, a family history of a parent with psychiatric disease in a patient with a choreiform disorder may be very suggestive. The diagnosis can be made through genetic testing.

6. Which of the following is not inherited in an autosomal dominant fashion?

A. Idiopathic torsion dystonia
B. Huntington's disease
C. Essential tremor
D. Wilson's disease
E. Gilles de la Tourette syndrome

The answer is (D). Wilson's disease is inherited as an autosomal recessive disorder.

7. Botulinum toxin is utilized in therapy for which of the following?

A. Spasmodic torticollis
B. Strabismus
C. Tics
D. Blepharospasm
E. Tremor

The answer is, All. Botulinum toxin therapy is accepted as safe and effective in strabismus, focal dystonias, and dystonic tics. Recent studies suggest that it is also useful in tremor.

SUGGESTED READING

Bressman SB, de Leon D, Kramer PL et al: Dystonia in Ashkenazi Jews: Clinical characterization of a founder mutation. Ann Neurol 36:771, 1994

Factor SA, Friedman JH: The emerging role of clozapine in movement disorders. Mov Disord 12:483, 1997

Fahn S: The varied clinical expressions of dystonia. Neurol Clin 2:541, 1984

Huntington's Disease Collaborative Research Group: A novel gene containing a trinucleotide repeat that is expanded and unstable on Huntington's disease chromosomes. Cell 72:971, 1993

Hoogenraad T: Wilson's Disease. London, WB Saunders, 1996

Jahanshahi M, Marion M, Marsden CD: Natural history of adult onset idiopathic torticollis. Arch Neurol 40:548, 1990

Jankovic J, Brin MF: Therapeutic uses of botulinum toxin. N Engl J Med 324:1186, 1991

Koller WC, Busenbark K, Miner K: The Essential Tremor Study Group: The relationship of essential tremor and other movement disorders: Report on 678 patients. Ann Neurol 35:717, 1994

Koller W, Pahwa R, Busenbark K, et al: High-frequency unilateral thalamic stimulation in the treatment of essential and parkinsonian tremor. Ann Neurol 42:292, 1997

Lang AE, Weiner WJ: Drug-Induced Movement Disorders. Mount Kisco, NY, Futura, 1992

Marsden CD, Obeso JA, Zarranz JJ, et al: The anatomical basis for symptomatic dystonia. Brain 108:463, 1985

Singer HS, Walkup JT: Tourette syndrome and other tic disorders: Diagnosis, pathophysiology, and treatment. Medicine 70:15, 1991

Weiner WJ, Lang AE: Movement Disorders: A Comprehensive Survey. Mount Kisco, NY, Futura, 1989

Neurology for the Non-Neurologist, Fourth Edition, edited by William J. Weiner and Christopher G. Goetz. Lippincott Williams & Wilkins, Philadelphia © 1999.

C H A P T E R   1 2

Neurologic Complications of Alcoholism

William C. Koller

Although alcohol is able to alter almost every organ system, its effects on the nervous system are of particular importance because multidimensional and severe neurologic complications are common in alcoholics. The neurologic complications of alcoholism have been classified by Victor under the five headings contained in the following list. In this review we will follow this classification.

Alcohol intoxication
   Drunkenness
   Coma
   Pathologic intoxication
Withdrawal syndrome
   Tremulousness
   Hallucinosis
   Seizures
   Delirium tremens
Nutritional disease secondary to alcoholism
   Wernicke-Korsakoff syndrome
   Polyneuropathy
   Optic neuropathy
   Pellagra
Disease of uncertain pathogenesis associated with alcoholism
   Cerebellar degeneration
   Marchiafava-Bignami disease
   Central pontine myelinolysis
   Cerebral atrophy
   Myopathy
Neurologic disorders associated with cirrhosis
   Hepatic stupor and coma
   Chronic hepatocerebral degeneration

ALCOHOL INTOXICATION

The manifestations of acute alcoholic intoxication are well known. Although alcohol is a central nervous system depressant, initially intoxication is associated with varying degrees of excitation and uninhibited behavior. Speech is increased and often slurred. The gait becomes ataxic. With further drunkenness, drowsiness, stupor, and coma may occur. It should be stressed that alcohol intoxication can indeed cause coma and even death.

In a certain population of patients, alcohol has an even more excitatory effect. This reaction has been variously labeled a pathologic intoxication or an acute alcoholic paranoid state. Although this state is not well studied, it is said to consist of irrational and destructive behavior that follows the ingestion of only small amounts of alcohol. The patient usually has no recollection of the episode. The mechanism underlying this paradoxical reaction is not known.

Most symptoms of alcohol intoxication are related to its depressive action on neural function. The early stimulatory effect of alcohol is thought to be caused by depression of subcortical structures that inhibit cerebral activity, thus resulting in stimulation. The usual manifestations of intoxication require no specific therapy. Mild stimulants (coffee, analeptics) may be of some help. Coma caused by alcohol intoxication requires the maintenance of respiration and blood pressure, if necessary. This supportive care is no different from that required in the treatment of coma from other causes. Pathologic intoxication requires the use of restraints and the parenteral administration of sedatives (e.g., phenobarbital or amobarbital).

ALCOHOL WITHDRAWAL SYNDROME

A variety of neurologic symptoms may occur in the chronic drinker after a period of relative or absolute abstinence from alcohol, termed the abstinence or withdrawal syndrome.

The most common manifestation of the withdrawal syndrome is tremulousness or "the shakes." This occurs after several days of drinking and frequently appears in the morning after the short abstinence that occurs during sleep. Associated symptoms consist of general irritability, mild autonomic hyperactivity, anorexia, nausea, and vomiting. The patients are clear mentally, although they tend to be inattentive with poor recollection of past events. Tremor is generalized and of a fast frequency. The severity of the tremor tends to increase with activity and emotional stress, and to decrease in a quiet environment. The tremor, overalertness, and autonomic instability may last for several days.

The second major symptom of the withdrawal syndrome is disordered perception and hallucinosis. This may occur in 10% to 25% of tremulous patients. Initially, there may be nightmares and disturbances of sleep. Illusions occur as sensory and visual information are distorted and misinterpreted. True hallucinations may be purely visual or auditory in type, mixed visual and auditory, and occasionally tactile or olfactory. Visual hallucinations often take the form of human, animal, or insect life. The feeling that bugs are crawling on oneself (formications) is an example of such hallucinations. Auditory hallucinations may be either acute or chronic. They are usually vocal in nature, with God or friends often speaking directly to the person. The voices are most often maligning and reproachful and may disturb and threaten the individual. Suicide may even be attempted in an effort to escape the verbal abuse. Hallucinations usually begin during the first day after the cessation of drinking and may last as long as a week. Initially, most patients do not recognize that they are hallucinating and it is only when the hallucinations cease that they acknowledge their previous hallucinations.

Chronic auditory hallucinosis presents a unique feature of this condition. In a small number of patients, the auditory hallucinations continue, and a schizophreniform personality evolves, with paranoid ideations and disordered thoughts. It has been suggested that repeated attacks of acute auditory hallucinosis may lead to the chronic form.

The third main symptom of the abstinence syndrome is withdrawal seizures. The majority of seizures, or 'rum fits,' occur within 8 to 48 hours of the cessation of drinking, with a peak incidence between 12 and 24 hours. Most often, withdrawal seizures are single, but several in a row may also occur. The seizures are usually generalized motor seizures with loss of consciousness. Rarely, status epilepticus may occur. A focal seizure in an alcoholic patient should lead to a search for focal disease (e.g., subdural hematoma). It should also be mentioned that people with a seizure tendency may have their seizures potentiated by a short abstinence period (e.g., overnight) after drinking. During the period of high-risk seizure activity, the electroencephalogram (EEG) may be transiently abnormal. The patient may be unusually sensitive to stroboscopic stimulation and may respond with either generalized myoclonus (photomyoclonus) or a generalized seizure (photoconvulsion). Other patients show diffuse abnormalities compatible with a mild encephalopathy.

Treatment of withdrawal seizures does not in most cases require anticonvulsants. The seizures are usually brief and do not recur. The long-term administration of anticonvulsants in patients with generalized withdrawal seizures is not reasonable because of poor patient compliance and because starting a drinking spree usually also means the abandonment of all medications. Since sudden withdrawal from drugs can be associated with withdrawal seizures, cessation of drugs as well as alcohol may in fact increase the risk of seizures.

The fourth manifestation of the withdrawal syndrome is delirium tremens. This term should be reserved for the rare, serious state of profound confusion, with vivid hallucinations, tremors, sleeplessness, and signs of increased autonomic nervous system activity, including fever, tachycardia, dilated pupils, and profuse sweating. Of 266 consecutive admissions of alcoholic patients to the Boston City Hospital, only 5% had delirium tremens. Although this can be a serious condition with a mortality rate of 5% to 10%, delirium tremens in most cases is benign and short-lived, lasting several days. The patient usually has no recollection of the events of the delirious period. Hyperthermia and peripheral vascular collapse are the usual causes of death. Intercurrent infection or injury tend to worsen the prognosis.

The mechanism of the withdrawal syndrome is unknown. Nutritional deficiency does not appear to play a primary pathogenic role. A depression of serum magnesium is often found during the withdrawal period and may increase the susceptibility to seizures, although it is probably not responsible for the entire syndrome.

The management of alcohol withdrawal begins with a careful search for infection or associated injury, such as subdural hematoma or meningitis. Lumbar puncture, a brain scan, and often an EEG are indicated. The major medical complications include water and electrolyte imbalance, vascular collapse, pneumonia, cirrhosis, gastritis, and hyperthermia. Specific treatment includes the following:

Maintenance of fluid intake and electrolyte balance. High volumes of fluids can be lost because of hyperthermia and sweating. Careful and continuous monitoring of intravenous fluid needs must be continued for several days.

Thiamine and multivitamin administration. Thiamine in a dose of 50 to 200 mg intramuscularly may be given, and thiamine may be added to the intravenous bottles. When the patient is on a diet, 100 mg thiamine twice a day orally is recommended.

Hypoglycemia. Blood glucose must be checked frequently because hypoglycemia is a complication of alcoholic binges, especially in the patient with inadequate hepatic function.

Control of agitation. The hallucinating, agitating patient can be dangerous to himself as well as to hospital personnel. A well-lighted room and the presence of a responsible family member helps to maintain the patient's contact with reality. Sedatives may be needed to control agitation: chlordiazepoxide is often recommended in doses of 25 to 100 mg intramuscularly every 3 to 4 hours as needed. It is important to check to see if the patient is awake before administering sedatives, and sedative orders should not be written on a continual basis. Accumulative dose effect can be seen with delayed metabolism of such drugs. These drugs are administered to calm the patient without putting him to sleep, so no sedative should be given to the sleeping patient.

NUTRITIONAL DISEASES

Several of the neurologic complications of alcohol on the nervous system are thought to be caused by the nutritional deficiency that occurs secondary to chronic alcoholism. These diseases include Wernicke's encephalopathy, Korsakoff's psychosis, polyneuropathy, alcohol amblyopia, and pellagra. In the alcoholic patient, caloric intake is supplied by alcohol, and there is an increased demand for B vitamins, which are necessary to metabolize the carbohydrate load imposed by alcohol. These nutritional diseases can also be seen in the nonalcoholic person in a variety of settings and hence are not exclusively seen in this patient population.

WERNICKE–KORSAKOFF DISEASE

Wernicke's disease is a neurologic syndrome characterized clinically by the triad of eye movement disorders, ataxic gait, and mental status changes. The ocular disturbances usually consist of nystagmus, paralysis of the lateral recti, or paralysis of conjugate gaze. Nystagmus, which may be either vertical or horizontal, is the most frequent abnormality. When cranial nerve VI paralysis occurs, it is usually bilateral, although not symmetric. The ataxia involves both stance and gait, and it may be so severe in the acute stages that the patient cannot stand up. The walk is broad based and ataxic; heel-to-shin testing is severely compromised. Three main types of mental symptoms may be observed. First, the most common change is that of a quiet, confusional state. The patient is apathetic, inattentive, and indifferent to his surroundings. Spontaneous speech is minimal, and communication is difficult. Second, the symptoms of delirium tremens or its variants may be present (i.e., disorders of perception). Third, there may be a selective abnormality of memory, termed Korsakoff's psychosis (see later).

The principal pathologic changes consist of paraventricular lesions in the thalamus and hypothalamus, in the mammillary bodies, in the floor of the fourth ventricle, and in the periaqueductal region of the midbrain. These lesions tend to be symmetric. Microscopic examination reveals capillary proliferation, often with necrosis of parenchymal structures and at times discrete hemorrhages, particularly in the mammillary bodies.

Korsakoff's psychosis is characterized by a selective memory deficit. The disordered memory is manifested by an impaired ability to recall events and other information that had been well established before the onset of the illness and a dramatically impaired ability to acquire new information. Remote memory tends to be better preserved than recent memory. Cognitive impairment (e.g., of mathematical skills and abstract thinking) may also be present. The patient may show little spontaneity and initiative. Confabulation, although frequently referred to as a main symptom of Korsakoff's psychosis, is not essential for the diagnosis.

The biochemical basis of Wernicke–Korsakoff disease appears to be a thiamine deficiency. The ophthalmoplegia, nystagmus, and ataxia can be reversed by the administration of thiamine alone. The ocular signs are the most sensitive to thiamine. Although the confusional state appears to clear with thiamine treatment, the memory deficit and confabulation are much less responsive. These symptoms recover slowly if at all. Korsakoff's psychosis has a poor prognosis, with only 20% of patients having significant recovery. An index of thiamine deficiency can be estimated by the blood transketolase activity. Transketolase is one of the enzymes in the hexose monophosphate shunt and requires thiamine-dependent cocarboxylase as a cofactor. Treatment with thiamine should be started immediately with 50 mg intravenously and 50 mg intramuscularly.

It should also be mentioned that Wernicke's syndrome can be precipitated by giving alcoholic patients intravenous solutions containing sugar without any vitamin supplements. The carbohydrate load may diminish marginal thiamine stores and induce the syndrome. As a rule, alcoholic patients seen in an emergency room or office should be given thiamine in an attempt to prevent the Wernicke-Korsakoff syndrome.

POLYNEUROPATHY

A common effect of chronic alcoholism is peripheral neuropathy. The extent and severity of the polyneuropathy in alcoholism is extremely variable. Some patients are asymptomatic, although sensory and motor loss and hyporeflexia may be found on examination. Many patients complain of weakness, paresthesia, and pain. Other patients may be so severely affected that they cannot walk. Symptoms usually evolve insidiously, with initial distal symptoms that progress proximally. The legs are affected exclusively, or more severely and earlier than the arms. Both motor and sensory symptoms often occur concomitantly. Paresthesias may be described as burning or as dull and constant. Examination discloses various degrees of motor, sensory, and reflex loss. Signs are, for the most part, symmetric, more severe in the distal portions of the limbs, and often confined to the legs. The main pathologic change in alcoholic neuropathy is degeneration of the peripheral nerves. Both myelin and axons are destroyed. There are no specific histologic changes that distinguish this type of neuropathy from that of other causes.

The pathogenesis of polyneuropathy in alcoholics may be the result of a nutritional deficiency, since neuropathy does not occur in chronic alcoholism if the diet is supplemented by B vitamins. The precise nutritional factor responsible has not been fully identified. Alcoholic patients with neuropathy should be treated with daily B vitamins. Physical therapy may be helpful. Even with these therapies, recovery from alcoholic neuropathy is often slow and incomplete.

ALCOHOL AMBLYOPIA

Alcohol amblyopia is characterized by the complaint of blurred vision and the finding on examination of a reduction of visual acuity and the presence of central scotomas indicative of an optic neuropathy. These changes develop gradually over several weeks and are always bilateral and generally symmetric. If untreated, irreversible optic neuropathy may occur. This type of amblyopia may also be seen during nutritional deficiency from other causes (e.g., in prisoners of war). Deficiency of several B vitamins (riboflavin, thiamine, vitamin B_{12}) has been implicated. Although pathologic changes have not been well documented, reported changes include degeneration of the optic nerves and at times degeneration of the chiasm and optic tract. Treatment should consist of a good diet and the administration of B vitamins. Improvement usually occurs with this regimen, although in long-standing cases the response may be minimal, and the patient remains with severe visual compromise.

PELLAGRA

The neurologic complication of pellagra is an encephalopathy. Fatigue, insomnia, and irritability commonly occur, and occasionally a confusional psychosis is present. Alcoholic pellagra, like pellagra of other causes, is known to be caused by a deficiency of nicotinic acid. Since the enrichment of bread with niacin began, this condition has become rare.

Pathologic changes consist of degeneration of the large cells of the motor cortex. Other central nervous system areas, such as the spinal cord, may also show changes. Treatment consists of a nutritious diet and the administration of niacin.

ALCOHOLIC DISEASES OF UNKNOWN PATHOGENESIS

There is a diverse group of neurologic and muscle disorders of unknown etiology associated with chronic alcoholism. These disorders do not specifically appear to be caused by nutritional deficiency.

ALCOHOLIC CEREBELLAR DEGENERATION

Alcoholic cerebellar degeneration is a common and highly characteristic syndrome. This disorder occurs most frequently in men. Clinically, patients demonstrate a wide-based gait, varying degrees of trunkal instability, and ataxia of the legs with relatively preserved upper extremity coordination. Infrequently, other neurologic symptoms such as nystagmus and dysarthria occur. Most often the syndrome evolves subacutely over a period of several weeks and then stabilizes. In general, these cerebellar symptoms cannot be distinguished from the ataxia associated with Wernicke's disease, although they are usually more chronic and severe and are not associated with the behavioral signs of the latter condition.

The pathologic changes are as distinctive as the stereotyped clinical syndrome. Marked and restricted degeneration of all neurocellular elements, particularly the Purkinje cells, occurs in the anterior cerebellar lobe and superior aspects of the vermis. In more advanced cases, there are additional paravermal changes in the anterior lobe. Although cerebellar degeneration is thought by some to be caused by a nutritional deficiency, vitamin therapy is usually of no benefit.

MARCHIAFAVA–BIGNAMI DISEASE

Marchiafava–Bignami disease is a rare complication of chronic alcoholism. Although it was first described in Italian men addicted to red wine, it may occur in a variety of settings, including in the nonalcoholic person. The clinical features are varied. For the most part, symptoms resemble those of frontal lobe disease with dementia, confusion, seizures, and apathy. Bilateral frontal lobe signs, such as a grasp-and-suck reflex, may occur, and rigidity and tremor may also be present. The clinical picture is therefore one of a gradual and progressive dementia. The diagnosis is usually made at autopsy because of the particular degeneration of the central portions of the corpus callosum. Other fiber tracts may also be affected. This is a rare condition, and many more common causes of altered mental states in alcoholic patients exist (hepatic encephalopathy, cerebral cortical atrophy, Wernicke–Korsakoff disease, subdural hematoma, and so forth).

CENTRAL PONTINE MYELINOLYSIS

Central pontine myelinolysis is a distinctive syndrome that occurs as a rare complication of chronic alco-

holism, as well as in other conditions such as carcinoma. Clinically, spastic bulbar paralysis and quadriplegia occur. This syndrome tends to occur in undernourished alcoholic patients who usually have weight loss, nausea and vomiting, and electrolyte disturbances, particularly hyponatremia.

The pathologic picture consists of a large symmetric lesion of necrosis at the center of the basis pontis. Nearly all myelin sheaths are destroyed, with the axis cylinders being preserved. Thus, like Marchiafava–Bignami disease, the lesion consists mainly of demyelination. In the past, the diagnosis of central pontine myelinolysis was made at postmortem examination.

CEREBRAL CORTICAL ATROPHY

Postmortem neuropathologic examination in alcoholic patients frequently discloses diffuse cortical atrophy and ventricular enlargement. These changes can often be visualized with computed tomography. The clinical correlate of these structural changes is imprecise. Although many of such patients are demented, some show very little cognitive or neurologic impairment.

ALCOHOLIC MYOPATHY

Alcohol is able to cause dysfunction of both cardiac and skeletal muscle. Several different types of myopathic syndromes affecting skeletal muscle exist and can be divided in acute and chronic myopathies. In the acute group, the first involves painless proximal weakness that develops during or shortly after heavy drinking and is associated with hypokalemia. Treatment with potassium supplements will reverse the disorder. The more dramatic myopathy involves sudden, severe pain, tenderness, and diffuse edema of the muscles. Renal damage and hyperkalemia usually exist. Myonecrosis is reflected in high serum muscle enzymes (creatine phosphokinase, aldolase) and myoglobin in the urine. Recovery usually occurs, but renal damage may be permanent. Another myopathic syndrome is characterized by muscle cramps without marked weakness and may be rather asymmetric. Muscle enzyme levels are elevated. The chronic form of myopathy associated with alcohol is rather uniform. It presents as a slowly progressive and painless weakness with atrophy of the proximal muscles as the hallmark. If the patient stops drinking alcohol and eats a normal diet, this condition often improves.

DISORDERS SECONDARY TO CIRRHOSIS OF PORTAL SYSTEMIC SHUNTS

Two neurologic disorders (hepatic coma and acquired hepatocerebral degeneration) often occur in the presence of severe alcohol-induced liver disease.

HEPATIC ENCEPHALOPATHY AND COMA

Hepatic coma, or acute hepatic encephalopathy, is an episodic disorder of consciousness associated with severe liver disease (i.e., cirrhosis). Initial mental confusion precedes progressive drowsiness and coma. The confusional state is frequently associated with characteristic liver flap or asterixis. The sign may be observed in a variety of metabolic encephalopathies, and although common in hepatic encephalopathy, is not diagnostic.

The EEG, which is frequently abnormal in the early stages of the disease, may show characteristic paroxysms of bilaterally synchronous slow waves. Triphasic waves, an indication of a metabolic disturbance, may be present.

The pathogenesis of hepatic encephalopathy is poorly understood. A disturbance of nitrogen metabolism with an increase in ammonium is frequently present because protein metabolism is altered by liver disease. However, the severity of the hyperammonemia often correlates poorly with the extent of the mental status changes. Neuropathologic changes in hepatic coma reveal a diffuse increase in the number and size of the protoplasmic astrocytes in the cerebral cortex, lenticular nuclei, thalamus, substantia nigra, and dentate and pontine nuclei. Nerve cells are basically unaffected.

The treatment of hepatic encephalopathy aims to reduce the intestinal production of ammonia. If gastrointestinal bleeding is present, it must be arrested as quickly as possible. Gastric aspiration is indicated if the bleeding is from the upper gastrointestinal tract, and cleansing enemas may be of additional value. Administration of any narcotics, sedatives, or tranquilizers containing ammonia or amino compounds should be stopped. The diet must be altered to a low protein content with an adequate calorie supply. Multivitamins should be given as well. Oral administration of poorly absorbed antibiotics decreases the intestinal bacteria and hence diminishes ammonia production and absorption. Neomycin, 4 to 6 g/day in divided doses, may be given orally for this purpose. The poorly absorbed ketohexose lactulose has been reported to be effective in decreasing encephalopathic symptoms. The drug is thought to act by producing a more acidic colonic pH, thus enhancing the movement of ammonia from blood into stool. Importantly, infections, especially those of the central nervous system, should be searched for vigorously, since patients with hepatic encephalopathy may have additional secondary causes of central nervous system compromise. Electrolyte imbalance, especially hypokalemia and alkalosis, must be avoided, so careful monitoring of fluid and electrolyte balance is essential. Levodopa has been reported to result in transient clearing of consciousness in patients with hepatic encephalopathy. It has been proposed that levodopa crosses the blood–brain barrier and alters central neurotransmitter concentrations, producing a more normal transmitter profile.

ACQUIRED HEPATOCEREBRAL DEGENERATION

This condition refers to the symptoms that may develop after a patient has experienced several episodes of hepatic coma. Clinical features include tremor, asterixis, choreic movement, myoclonus, dysarthria, ataxia of gait, and impairment of intellectual function. The condition may evolve over months or years with increasing neurologic deficit. The EEG usually reveals a diffuse slow wave abnormality. Hepatic function in these patients is grossly abnormal, with jaundice, ascites, esophageal varices, and elevated serum ammonium levels being present. Portacaval shunts are always present. Although the symptoms may resemble those of Wilson's disease, the lack of family history, Kayser-Fleischer rings, or disordered copper metabolism facilitates differentiation. Although the pathogenesis of this condition is unknown, there appears to be a close relationship between the acute form of hepatic coma and the chronic irreversible hepatocerebral lesions. Many attacks of hepatic coma usually precede the development of the hepatic cerebral syndrome. Astrocytic hyperplasia occurs in both conditions. Hyperammonemia is common to both disorders.

Pathologic findings are localized mainly to the cortex and consist of necrosis and gliosis. Microscopically, there is hyperplasia of protoplasmic astrocytes seen in many areas of the brain. Nerve cells may appear swollen with chromatolysis (Oplaski cells). Similar cells are seen in Wilson's disease.

QUESTIONS AND DISCUSSION

1. A 30-year-old man, a known alcoholic, comes to the emergency room complaining of abdominal pain, and a diagnosis of pancreatitis is made. An intravenous solution of dextrose 5% in water is started, and the patient is admitted to the hospital. Hours later, the patient is noted to be confused, and nystagmus and ataxia are now noted on physical examination. What is a possible explanation for the symptomatology the patient has developed while in the hospital?

Answer: It is probable that the patient developed Wernicke's syndrome from intravenous glucose administration, which further decreased his marginal stores of thiamine. Thiamine deficiency is responsible for Wernicke's syndrome. It is important that alcoholic patients be given thiamine, and multivitamins should be added to all intravenous solutions for alcoholic patients.

2. A routine neurologic examination of an alcoholic patient admitted 10 days previously for detoxification now reveals the following findings: no ankle jerk, loss of vibratory sensation in the lower extremities, mild distal weakness in the legs, inability to perform tandem gait, and dysmetria on heel-to-shin examination. What is your diagnosis and what should you do diagnostically or therapeutically?

Answer: Examination revealed evidence for a sensorimotor neuropathy (hyporeflexia, motor and sensory abnormalities) and a midline cerebellar syndrome (poor tandem gait). These abnormalities are not uncommon in chronic alcoholic patients and are so characteristic that other causes are much less likely. The patient should be given multivitamins, although full functional recovery would not be expected.

3. A chronic alcoholic patient has a focal seizure consisting of shaking of the left side of the face and the left arm, lasting several minutes. These spells began 1 week after admission. The patient was admitted for tremulousness and hallucinosis. Those symptoms were gone by the sixth day of hospitalization. Do these seizures represent "withdrawal seizures"?

Answer: Withdrawal seizures or "rum fits" characteristically occur between 8 and 48 hours after the ces-

sation of drinking. The majority occur 12 to 24 hours after the reduction of drinking. These seizures are of the generalized motor type without a focal character. Focal seizures should always raise the possibility of focal pathology (e.g., subdural hematoma, tumor, and so forth), and the patient should undergo radiographic evaluation (i.e., computed tomography of the head).

SUGGESTED READING

Adams RD, Foley JM: The neurological disorder associated with liver disease. Res Publ Assoc Res Nerv Ment Dis 32:198, 1953

Adams RD, Victor M, Mancall EL: Central pontine myelinolysis. Arch Neurol Psychiatry 81:154, 1959

Dreyfus PM, Victor M: Effects of thiamine deficiency on the central nervous system. Am J Clin Nutr 9:414, 1961

Morris J, Victor M: Alcohol withdrawal seizures. Emory Med Clin North Am 5:827, 1987

Ragan JJ: Alcohol and the cardiovascular system. JAMA 264:377, 1990

Spillane JD: Nutritional Disorders of the Nervous System. Baltimore, Williams & Wilkins, 1947

Victor M: The alcohol withdrawal syndrome. In: Seixas F, Eggleston S (eds): Alcoholism and the central nervous system. Ann NY Acad Med 215:210, 1973

Victor M: The pathophysiology of alcoholic epilepsy. Res Publ Assoc Res Nerv Ment Dis 46:431, 1968

Victor M, Adams RD: The effect of alcohol upon the nervous system. Res Publ Assoc Res Nerv Ment Dis 32:526, 1953

Victor M, Adams RD, Collins GH: The Wernicke-Korsakoff Syndrome. Philadelphia, FA Davis, 1971

Victor M, Adams RD, Mancall E: A restricted form of cerebellar degeneration occurring in alcoholic patients. Arch Neurol 1:577, 1959

Neurology for the Non-Neurologist, Fourth Edition,
edited by William J. Weiner and
Christopher G. Goetz. Lippincott
Williams & Wilkins, Philadelphia © 1999.

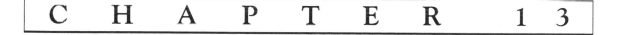

Peripheral Neuropathy

Morris A. Fisher

CLINICAL FEATURES AND SCIENTIFIC BACKGROUND

The peripheral nervous system (PNS) encompasses those parts of the nervous system that lie outside the confines of the brain, brainstem, and spinal cord. As such, it consists of those portions of the primary sensory neurons, lower motor neurons, and autonomic neurons that are outside the central nervous system (CNS). By definition, therefore, the PNS includes the cranial nerves, the spinal nerves with their roots and rami, the peripheral nerves, and those aspects of the autonomic nervous system that are outside the CNS.

The concept of the PNS is artificial, because all of its parts are connected with CNS structures and are therefore subject to pathologic processes that affect the CNS. Nevertheless, there are disease processes that seem to involve preferentially or primarily the PNS, and it is therefore useful to consider this system as a nosologic entity.

All parts of the PNS are associated with Schwann cells or the comparable ganglionic cells, the satellite cells. This anatomic commonality may account for some of the pathologic aspects of the PNS. More significantly, the normal functions of all parts of the PNS are dependent on the normal functioning of the nerve cell bodies from which the motor and sensory axons originate. Since the foot is supplied by nerve fibers whose cell bodies lie at the level of the upper lumbar vertebrae, the physiologic mechanisms involved in maintaining normal nerve function are considerable. There is a constant transport system

from the nerve cell bodies to their most distal axonal projections, and this system is necessary for maintaining normal nerve (and muscle) function. There is also transport so that the cell bodies are influenced by distal events. This system provides the conduit by which agents such as herpes virus may reach the nerve cell body. Given the complexity and length of the structures involved, it is not surprising that the normal functioning of the PNS is frequently disturbed.

ANATOMY

Except for the cranial nerves, peripheral nerves separate at the level of the roots. The dorsal roots contain afferent ("sensory") fibers that are located either pre- or postganglionic to the dorsal root ganglion on their way to the spinal cord. The ventral roots consist of efferent ("motor") fibers that originate from the lower motor neurons. The resultant mixed ("motor" and "sensory") nerves are the structures for providing information to and from the CNS throughout the body. In the thoracic and upper lumbar region, these nerves are joined by sympathetic fibers after these fibers have synapsed in the ganglionic chain adjacent to the vertebral column. The parasympathetic outflow originates either in the cranial region (cranial nerves III, VII, IX, and X) or in the sacral region passing distally as the pelvic splanchnic nerves (Fig. 13-1).

Individual muscles and areas of skin are supplied not only by particular nerves but also by fibers that originate in particular roots. This feature of the PNS

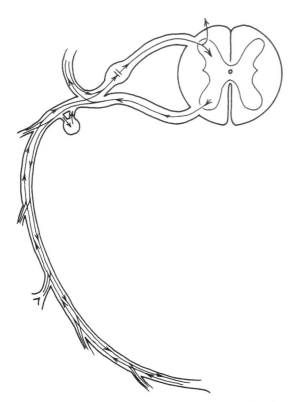

FIG. 13-1. Drawing of peripheral nerve originating from (1) ventral root with cells of origin in the anterior horn of the spinal cord and (2) dorsal root with a dorsal root ganglion. The postganglionic dorsal root fibers pass to the dorsal horn or more superiorly in the spinal cord. The posterior primary ramus extends dorsally, whereas the anterior primary ramus is the main extension of the peripheral nerve. Sympathetic fibers join the peripheral nerve by way of the sympathetic ganglion.

is important clinically, as will be discussed further on. The PNS distribution in the limbs is superficially complex because of the routing that occurs in the brachial and lumbosacral plexi involving the upper and lower limbs, respectively.

Individual nerves are composed of bundles of individual nerve fibers called *fascicles,* which, in turn, are surrounded by connective tissue. All of the motor fibers and many of the sensory fibers are surrounded by myelin. Myelin is formed by foldings of Schwann cell membranes. These supporting cells are ubiquitous throughout the PNS. In myelinated fibers, the junc-

tion of sheaths from two adjacent Schwann cells occurs at what are referred to as *nodes of Ranvier.* Most sensory fibers and all autonomic fibers are either poorly myelinated or nonmyelinated. It is important to emphasize, however, that all nerve fibers—even those that are unmyelinated—are ensheathed by Schwann cells.

Nerves are supplied by nutrient arteries that arise from adjacent blood vessels. The arterial supply is richly collateralized both to and within the nerves themselves. The result is a system remarkably resistant to large vessel ischemia.

INDICATIONS OF NEUROPATHIC INJURY

The symptoms and signs of neuropathic injury can be anticipated from the preceding discussion. If nerves to muscles are disrupted, weakness may be present, and atrophy of muscle fibers can occur. Cramping with fatigue is a common symptom. Reflexes may be decreased or lacking if the afferent or efferent nerves that subserve the reflex are disturbed.

A wide range of sensory disturbances are found. With complete loss of innervation, there may be total loss of feeling—anesthesia. This rarely happens because of the considerable overlap of sensory nerve supply. More commonly, alterations in sensation are found. A decrease in sensory perception is referred to as *hypoesthesia,* an increase in this perception is known as *hyperesthesia,* unusual feelings such as "pins and needles" are called *paresthesias,* and unpleasant sensations such as burning are called *dysesthesias.* A decrease in perception of position and vibration is attributed to dysfunction in the larger fibers, whereas diminished pinprick and temperature sensation is thought to indicate abnormalities in the smaller fibers.

Autonomic dysfunction may result in vasomotor disturbances as well as in alterations in sweating. Trophic changes of the skin and nails can be found, resulting from repeated injury and inadequate repair. The skin may become smooth and glossy, hair may decrease (or occasionally increase), and the nails may become thickened.

ANATOMIC DISTRIBUTION

Motor and sensory changes caused by PNS disease occur in the distribution of the roots, the plexi, or the peripheral nerves themselves. Charts are readily available that show these distributions. Although superficially complex, with even limited practice the information becomes readily usable. None of the motor or sensory charts are absolute. The information has been obtained indirectly based on root or nerve injury. Given the potential variability, particularly in sensory distribution, it is not surprising that there may be variations from patient to patient. It is hopeless to attempt to fit each patient into a circumscribed view of normal. General patterns of root and nerve distribution are reliable, and it is important to rely on these patterns (Fig. 13-2).

The muscles of the shoulder girdle are innervated mainly by the C5 root, those of the arm by C5 and C6 (triceps brachii, C7), those of the forearm by C7 and C8, and those of the hand by C8 and T1. In the lower extremity, the thigh muscles are supplied by the L2, L3, and L4 roots. Those muscles of the anterior leg are innervated mainly by L5, those of the posterior leg by S1, and the small muscles of the foot by S1 and S2.

The root sensory distribution can be visualized with the individual in the anatomic position. In general, C1–C4 innervate the back of the head, the neck,

and the shoulder region; C5 innervates the lateral aspect of the arm; C6 innervates the lateral portion of the forearm extending into the hand involving the thumb and index finger; C7 innervates the mid-portion of the hand and ring finger; and C8 innervates the more medial portion of the hand including the little finger. The posterior aspect of the upper extremity is then supplied by T1 and T2, and the torso is innervated sequentially by T2–L1, with T5 at about the level of the nipples and T10 at the umbilicus. The anterior thigh is supplied by L1, L2, and L3; the anterior leg and foot are supplied predominantly by L4 and L5; the posterior aspect of the lower extremity is supplied by S1 and S2; and the region of the anus is supplied by S3, S4, and S5.

The three main terminal nerves of the brachial plexus in the upper extremity are the radial, ulnar, and median nerves. The radial nerve innervates the extensor muscles as well as providing much of the cutaneous supply to the extensor surface of the arm, forearm, and hand. The median nerve is predominant in supplying the forearm flexors as well as the muscles of the thenar eminence controlling thumb movement. The remaining intrinsic hand muscles are innervated by the ulnar nerve. The median and ulnar nerves supply the cutaneous sensibility to the hand, with the ulnar territory encompassing the little finger, half of the ring finger, and the adjacent palmar surface, whereas the median nerve provides the remaining cutaneous innervation (Fig. 13-3).

In the lower extremity, the femoral nerve supplies the knee extensors in the thigh as well as the cutaneous branches for the anterior thigh and medial aspect of the leg and foot (by way of the saphenous nerve). The posterior thigh muscles controlling knee flexion, as well as all the muscles of the leg and foot, are innervated by the sciatic nerve. The anterior tibial (peroneal) branch of the sciatic nerve supplies the anterior compartment of the leg, that is, those muscles that affect dorsiflexion of the ankle and toes as well as foot eversion, whereas the posterior tibial portion of the sciatic nerve innervates those muscles affecting plantar flexion. The cutaneous distribution is comparable. The anterior leg and dorsum of the foot are supplied by branches of the anterior tibial nerve, whereas the posterior aspect of the leg and plantar aspect of the foot are innervated by branches of the posterior tibial nerve. The medial plantar aspect of the foot and toes is supplied by the medial plantar nerve, whereas their more lateral aspect is supplied by the lateral plantar nerve terminal equivalents of the upper extremity median and ulnar nerves, respectively.

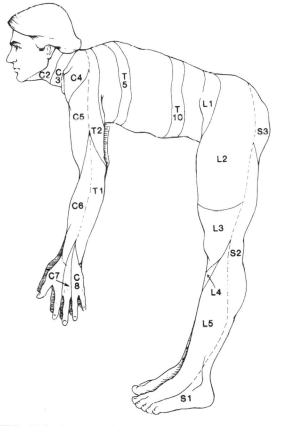

FIG. 13-2. Sequential nature of the cutaneous root distribution as shown with the individual in the quadruped position.

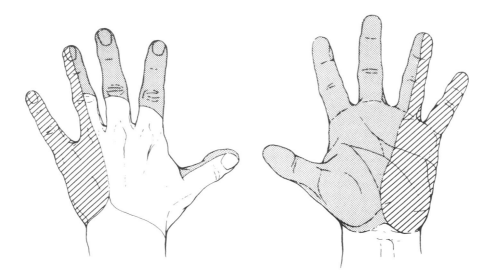

FIG. 13-3. Cutaneous innervation of the hand by the radial (*clear section*), median (*stippled section*), and ulnar (*diagonal lines*) nerves.

Table 13-1 indicates selected muscle movements with their innervation, and Table 13-2 shows a schema of the cutaneous innervation of the limbs. These tables and the preceding discussion are not meant to be a complete presentation of peripheral nerve distribution. Rather, it is hoped the information will provide a framework to allow clinical use of the material. Referral to more detailed charts can then be made in an active and meaningful manner.

PATTERNS OF ABNORMALITY

Derangements of motor, sensory, and autonomic function may be present with lesions at the level of the roots, plexi, or peripheral nerves. Sensory loss, for example, involving the lateral aspect of the leg combined with weakness of dorsiflexion of the toes would be consistent with a lesion of the L5 root; motor and sensory changes in the distribution of both the axillary and radial nerves would be compatible with injury to the posterior cord of the brachial plexus; and weakness as well as atrophy of intrinsic hand muscles combined with sensory loss involving the medial aspect of the palmar surface of the hand, the little finger, and adjacent half of the middle finger would indicate an ulnar nerve lesion.

There are four major categories of PNS disease, based on the anatomic distribution of the abnormality.

The most common type is the *symmetric polyneuropathy*, in which the distal extremities are primarily affected with decreased sensation and often abnormal uncomfortable sensations (dysesthesia). The signs and symptoms of neuropathy usually start in the feet, and clinical findings are present to the level of the mid legs often before they are found in the hands (glove and stocking neuropathy). Sensory signs and symptoms should be at comparable distances from the spinal cord (i.e., from C7 in the arms and T12–L1 in the legs). Diabetic polyneuropathy is a common example, although uremia and drug or toxic exposure are associated with the same pattern. One possible basis for this distribution of neurologic findings is related to the need to transport material along the entire length of the nerves. Even if the primary pathology then involves the nerve cell body, the manifestations of the disorder would be at the distal parts of the nerve.

The second type of neuropathy is *mononeuropathy*, in which a single nerve is damaged (wrist drop—radial nerve; foot drop—peroneal nerve). Compressive lesions are a frequent cause. *Mononeuropathy multiplex*, in which multiple single peripheral nerves are damaged, is particularly common in diabetes and polyarteritis nodosa. *Plexopathies* result from injury to the nerves in brachial, lumbar, or sacral plexi. Idiopathic brachial neuritis, traumatic injury to the brachial plexus, and retroperitoneal or apical lung tumors are

TABLE 13-1. Selected Muscle Movements and Their Innervation

JOINT	MOVEMENT	MUSCLES*	PERIPHERAL NERVES*	SPINAL SEGMENTS*
Upper Extremity				
Shoulder	Abduction	Deltoid	Axillary	C5
	Lateral (external) rotation	Infraspinatus	Suprascapular	C5
Elbow	Flexion	Brachialis	Musculocutaneous	C5, C6
		Biceps brachii		
	Extension	Triceps brachii	Radial	C7, C8
Radial-ulnar	Supination	Biceps brachii	Musculocutaneous	C6
		Supinator	Radial	
	Pronation	Pronator teres	Median	C7
Wrist	Dorsal flexion (extension)	Extensor carpi radialis longus and brevis	Radial	C7
	Palmar flexion	Flexor carpi radialis	Median	C7
		Flexor carpi ulnaris	Ulnar	
(Thumb)	Palmar adduction	Interossei	Ulnar	T1
	Palmar abduction	Abductor pollicis brevis	Median	C8
	Extension	Extensor pollicis longus et brevis	Radial	C7, C8
	Opposition	Opponens pollicis	Median	T1
(Finger) excluding thumb	Adduction	Palmar interossei	Ulnar	T1
	Abduction	Dorsal interossei	Ulnar	T1
	Extension (metacarpo-phalangeal joints)	Extensor digitorum Extensor indicis Extensor digiti minimi	Radial	C7, C8
Lower Extremity				
Hip	Flexion	Iliopsoas	Femoral	L2
	Extension	Gluteus maximus	Inferior gluteal	S1, S2
	Adduction	Adductor magnus Adductor brevis Adductor longus	Obturator	L2, L3
	Abduction	Gluteus medius	Superior gluteal	L4, L5
Knee	Extension	Quadriceps Femoris	Femoral	L3, L4
	Flexion	Biceps femoris Semitendinosus Semitendinosus	Sciatic	S1
Ankle	Dorsiflexion	Tibialis anterior	Peroneal	L4
	Plantar flexion	Gastrocnemius Soleus	Posterior tibial	S1, S2
	Inversion	Tibialis posterior	Posterior tibial	L4, L5
		Tibialis anterior	Peroneal	L4
	Eversion	Peroneus longus et brevis	Peroneal	L5
(Large toe)	Extension	Extensor hallucis longus	Peroneal	L5

*Only main controlling muscle, nerve, and roots listed.
Joint action listed because (1) it can be easily tested and (2) muscle, nerve, and root control is relatively simple. Parentheses indicate action at more than one joint.
Note: Terminal divisions of the brachial plexus can be tested at the thumb. Hip action controlled by muscles innervated by L2-S2 roots.

Table 13-2. Schematic Cutaneous Innervation of the Limbs

EXTREMITY*	LATERAL	ANTERIOR	MEDIAL	POSTERIOR
Upper				
Arm	C5 Axillary radial		Medial cutaneous nerve of arm T2	
Forearm	C6 Musculocutaneous		Medial cutaneous nerve of forearm T1	
Hand and fingers†	Thumb Index C6 C6		Middle Ring Little C7 C8 C8	
Lower				
Thigh	Lateral femoral cutaneous	Femoral L2, L3	Obturator	Posterior cutaneous nerve of the thigh S2
Leg	Peroneal L5		Saphenous L4	Sural S1, S2
Foot		Peroneal L5		Plantar nerves S1

*Portions of the posterior midline areas of the arm and forearm are supplied by branches of the radial nerve.
† For cutaneous distribution, see Figures 13-2 and 13-3.

common causes. More proximal injury produces root dysfunction. Motor or sensory loss is then in a dermatomal rather than peripheral nerve distribution. Disc and vertebral bone disease are among the conditions associated with these *radiculopathies*.

PATHOLOGY

The pathologic processes affecting nerves involve primarily myelin or axons, or both. In demyelinating processes, myelin is lost from individual nerve fibers. Characteristically, this occurs in a segmental fashion. There may be marked slowing and even block of conduction. The former is most pronounced in the inherited demyelinating neuropathies, whereas the latter is common in acquired, probably immunologically mediated, processes. Secondary axonal changes occur, but the axons are generally well preserved. As a result, clinical recovery in the acquired neuropathies can be both rapid and complete if remyelination occurs.

Primary axonal degeneration is associated with a large number of exogenous toxins and metabolic derangements. These processes may affect the nerve cell bodies as well as the axons and may be manifest as a dying back of the distal portion of the axon. Secondary demyelination occurs in those fibers with axonal damage. The disrupted myelin may be in the form of a ball or ovoids, but segmental demyelination may also be present. Recovery occurs by regeneration of axons, which often must then reinnervate denervated structures; as a result, recovery may be slow and incomplete.

With physical injury to nerves, the injury may be limited to paranodal demyelination with associated conduction block and rapid recovery (neuropraxia). If axons are interrupted (axonotmesis), total degeneration (Wallerian) of the axons and myelin occurs distal to the site of injury. Since the Schwann cell basal lamina and endoneurial tissue remain intact, axonal regeneration commences promptly after injury. If both the axon and surrounding connective tissue are disrupted (neurotmesis), Wallerian degeneration is inevitable and axon regeneration is limited by distorted connective tissue. Neuromas and aberrant regeneration may occur.

The potential pathologic processes that affect the PNS are similar to those that affect other systems. Metabolic or toxic derangements (e.g., vitamin deficiencies, uremia, alcoholism, heavy metals, industrial solvents, and certain medications) frequently result in nerve dysfunction. Vascular abnormalities affecting nerves usually involve the medium and small arteries, and these abnormalities may be found in rheumatoid arthritis, polyarteritis nodosa, and temporal arteritis. The polyneuropathy of diabetes mellitus may be metabolic in origin, whereas the mononeuropathies seen in this disease probably have a vascular etiology. Idiopathic polyneuritis (Landry–Guillain–Barré syndrome) is representative of an inflammatory process. This probably has an immunologic basis, as do the neuropathies seen in paraproteinemias and macroglobulinemia. Leprosy is a common infectious process affecting nerves. A genetic basis for PNS dysfunction such as peroneal muscular atrophy (Charcot–Marie–Tooth disease) is also not uncommon. Schwannomas and neurofibromas are representative tumors. Trauma is a frequent cause of nerve injury.

DIAGNOSIS

As in other areas of neurology, the physical examination remains a powerful tool for the evaluation of disorders of the PNS. The examination need not be subtle, but it must be accurate. Motor and sensory distributions of a polyneuropathy, mononeuropathy, or radiculopathy can often be appreciated.

The action of individual muscles should be tested and rated as normal strength, or mildly, moderately, or markedly decreased. One cannot test all muscles. Concentration must be in those areas that aid in the analysis of the particular problem. Frequently, an evaluation of total muscle strength acting at a joint is sufficient: for example, wrist flexion rather than the individual action of the flexor carpi radialis and ulnaris.

An accurate sensory examination need not be tedious. Again, concentration on areas relevant to the diagnostic question is important. A circumscribed area of sensory deficit often can be best outlined by the patient. This area can then be analyzed in more detail for light touch and pain sensations using a finger and a safety pin, respectively. (Separate pins should be used for each patient so as not to spread hepatitis.) A distal to proximal area of sensory change can be outlined in a similar fashion. Position sense can be tested by moving relevant joints. Slight movements of distal joints should be appreciated accurately. A 128-cycles-per-second (cps) tuning fork with the base placed on bony prominences is used for testing vibration. In neuropathies, vibration is characteristically more affected than position. The examination should start from the most distal area of potential abnormality. One need then test more proximal locations only if the patient does not perceive the duration of the vibration at the more distal site. A finger of the examiner touching the same bony region as the tuning fork can aid in evaluating the patient's sensitivity.

The most valuable ancillary study for analysis of PNS disorders is electromyography (EMG). This is best viewed as an extension of the neurologic examination. The data are consistently meaningful only if the study is approached in this framework. This is important because EMG, although harmless, does entail some discomfort. As a result, reliable information obtained in an efficient fashion is crucial, and this, in turn, must depend on the experience and skill of the electromyographer.

Electromyography consists of two basic parts. The first is an evaluation of the conduction in nerves. The second part involves analysis of the electrical activity in muscles—the EMG *per se*. The data can define the location of a lesion as well as aid in understanding the pathophysiology.

Conduction in motor fibers is determined by stimulating electrically and recording the resultant evoked motor response. Muscle fiber contraction is associated with electrical activity caused by the movement of charged ions across membranes, and this electrical activity can be recorded. Latency refers to the time from the stimulus to the onset of the electrical activity. The latency will be shorter if the stimulus is closer to the muscle than if it is more distant. The time difference between a distal and a more proximal latency divided by the distance between the two stimulating points enables a conduction velocity to be determined, that is, distance/time = conduction velocity (CV). When recording from muscle, a CV can be determined only if stimulation is performed at at least two points. The unknown time for transmission in slow-conducting terminal nerve fibers as well as across the junction between the nerve and the muscle is then "subtracted out" (Fig. 13-4).

Electrical responses from afferent (sensory) fibers may also be recorded. Since the amplitudes of these evoked afferent responses are several orders of magnitude less than the evoked motor responses, the sensory potentials are more difficult to record. At the same time, a meaningful CV can be obtained from a single latency because a CV may be calculated from the time taken to traverse a particular distance, since there is no unknown time across the region of the neuromuscular junction.

The amplitude of evoked motor or sensory responses is a less accurate indicator of normality than is the latency. Amplitude may be affected by the site of the recording as well as by the amount of tissue between the electrical-activity generator in the muscle or nerve and the recording electrodes. Nevertheless, the amplitudes of the evoked efferent or afferent responses reflect the amount of electrical-activity-generating tissue. Decreased amplitude responses, focal nerve injury, and side-to-side comparisons of response amplitudes can be particularly helpful.

The different fibers in a particular nerve conduct impulses at different rates. There is a linear relation between fiber size and conduction velocity, with the largest fibers conducting at the fastest velocities. If activity in the largest fibers is lost, then conduction will be slowed. The degree of slowing that may be

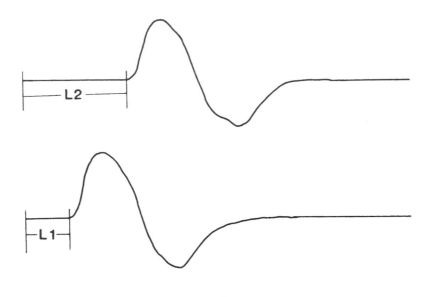

$$cv = d/L2-L1$$

FIG. 13-4. Evoked motor responses with the shorter-latency L1 resulting from stimulation closer to the recording site, in comparison with the latency L2 resulting from stimulation of the nerve at a more proximal site. The conduction velocity (CV) in the nerve is determined by dividing the distance (d) between the stimulating sites by the latency differences.

present with axon loss alone, however, is considerably less than that which may be found with demyelination.

In addition to slowed conduction and decreased amplitude, nerve injury can produce altered configuration and dispersion of evoked responses. These changes in evoked responses can define the location of focal nerve dysfunction. Temporal dispersion is characteristic of demyelinating injury, as is conduction block. In the latter, the size of the response is meaningfully decreased or even absent during stimulation proximal to the block. The result may be a striking picture in which nerve function is lost but conduction studies distal to the region of focal demyelination are entirely normal since those portions of the nerve distal to the block may be entirely normal.

Studies are available (i.e., H reflexes and F responses) which monitor conduction in nerve fibers to and from the spinal cord. These studies are important since proximal nerve injury may be present even in the absence of injury to the more distal nerves which are usually evaluated electrodiagnostically.

The electrical activity generated by muscles can be recorded from the muscle surface but is best appreciated by a needle electrode in the muscle itself. The resultant electrical activity can then be monitored, amplified, and displayed.

At rest, there is no electrical activity. Some activity is usually seen as a needle is moved through muscle ("insertional activity"), but these responses stop when needle movement stops. As a muscle contracts, there is increasing activity. This consists of the firing of motor units. A motor unit is composed of a lower motor neuron in the anterior horn of the spinal cord, its motor axon, and the muscle fibers innervated by that axon. Increasing force of contraction results primarily from the recruitment of more units, although an increased rate of firing also contributes to the increase in muscle tension. This increased muscle activity with increasing force of muscle contraction is readily appreciated during routine EMG. More electrical activity is seen; the amount of visible baseline without motor unit activity decreases; and the audio amplification of the muscle activity becomes increasingly prominent (Fig. 13-5).

Each motor unit is composed of muscle fibers scattered widely throughout a particular muscle. The number of muscle fibers in a motor unit varies with the fineness of control required. For example, there

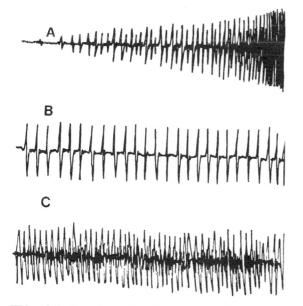

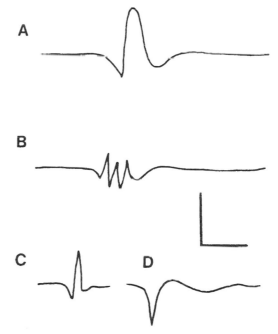

FIG. 13-5. Drawings of motor unit recruitment patterns. **A.** Normal pattern with increasing number and size of motor units with increasing force of muscle contraction. **B.** Repetitive firing of a single large motor unit characteristic of neuropathies. **C.** A "rich" pattern of many small motor units even at low levels of muscle tension seen in myopathies. Amplitude calibrations in the ratio of 1:5:0.5 for A:B:C.

FIG. 13-6. Tracings of **A.** normal triphasic motor unit potential, **B.** polyphasic potential, **C.** fibrillation, and **D.** positive sharp wave. Calibrations: vertical (microvolts)—*A* and *B*, 500; *C* and *D* 50; horizontal (milliseconds)—*A* and *B*, 5; *C* and *D*, 2.

may be only six muscle fibers per motor unit in the eye muscles, but up to several thousand in some of the large postural muscles. The simultaneous contraction of all the muscle fibers in a motor unit results in the usual integrated smooth, triphasic electrical response (Fig. 13-6). Motor unit size varies not only between muscles but also within muscles. The larger motor units have more muscle fibers, and, therefore, with discharge they will generate more electrical activity than smaller units. The larger units, therefore, will generally be of larger amplitude. During normal reflex or voluntary recruitment, motor units are activated sequentially according to size, with the smaller units discharging first. As a muscle contracts, not only are more units activated but they are also larger. In comparison to direct tension measurements, amplitude of a particular motor unit is a poor indicator of motor unit size because of (1) the potential variation of muscle fiber organization within a particular motor unit and (2) the relation of the

recording needle to those muscle fibers. Motor unit duration provides a better estimate of relative motor unit size, with the larger motor units having the larger motor unit durations.

When there is a disruption of the normal connection between nerve and muscle (i.e., denervation), abnormalities appear at rest 1 to 3 weeks after injury, and they can be detected by EMG. Individual muscle fibers may discharge at rest, and this type of electrical activity is referred to as *fibrillations* or *positive sharp waves*. This activity is not visible clinically. Other types of abnormal spontaneous activity may be present, such as runs of complex potentials (complex repetitive discharges). Particularly in disorders of the motor neuron itself, irregular contractions of entire motor units may appear; these contractions are called *fasciculations*. They are visible clinically and can be present in normal individuals, especially with fatigue.

Electrical activity from single muscle fibers can be recorded by EMG using special electrodes. This technique is particularly useful for defining abnormalities of the neuromuscular junction, which may be seen in rapidly progressive neuropathic injury or with reinnervation. This technique has also been used to define the physiologic characteristics of abnormal discharges as well as of normal and abnormal motor units.

In neuropathies, there is a loss of functioning axons. Fewer motor units than normal may be found on voluntary activation of a muscle. At its most extreme, only a single motor unit may be seen to discharge within the recording field of the electrode, even with maximum muscle contraction. In association with these changes, the motor units may be larger than normal. The muscle fibers that have been denervated may be reinnervated by the remaining viable axons of remaining motor units. As a result, these motor units may be larger than normal and also more complex in configuration. Small, complex (polyphasic)-appearing motor unit potentials, however, may also be found. Although these latter potentials are considered more characteristic of myopathies caused by a loss of functioning muscle fibers within motor units, they are seen in neuropathic injury during reinnervation. As motor axons grow into muscle that has lost its innervation, new motor units are formed, and these new units will initially be small and possibly polyphasic because they include a relatively limited number of muscle fibers. A reduced number of motor units, especially if they are large and associated with electrophysiologic evidence of denervation, would be characteristic of a neuropathic process.

These may be the only electrophysiologic findings in those neurogenic processes caused by loss of motoneurons such as amyotrophic lateral sclerosis (ALS). More commonly in neuropathies, slowing of conduction is present and provides evidence of nerve dysfunction. Prominent slowing with no or relatively little denervation and preserved response amplitudes would be consistent with a demyelinating process. Borderline to mildly slowed conductions associated with clear and relatively diffuse axonal injury would indicate predominant axonal injury. Low-amplitude evoked responses are most characteristic of axonal dysfunction because of loss of functioning nerve or muscle tissue.

Electromyographic studies can provide information not only about the severity and duration of a neuropathic process but also about the prognosis of nerve injury. The patient's symptoms may not correlate with the degree of nerve involvement. Dysesthesias may occur with relatively minor, partial nerve injury, whereas severe, diffuse nerve abnormalities may be accompanied by few complaints. Normal conduction and lack of denervation several weeks after the onset of nerve dysfunction would indicate a good prognosis because this pattern would indicate functional, but not necessarily structural, abnormalities of the nerve. This is a common clinical situation, for example, in Bell's palsy caused by disruption of facial nerve function.

Nerve biopsies can be performed, especially of the sural nerve. At times, the information may be pathognomonic, such as in infiltrative neuropathies (e.g., amyloidosis and metachromatic leukodystrophy). "Teased" fiber preparations allow an examination of individual fibers and thereby more accurate analysis of the pathology of nerve injury.

SPECIFIC PERIPHERAL NEUROPATHIES

The prime consideration in treating peripheral neuropathies is usually defining the underlying cause. The neuropathies associated with hypothyroidism, carcinoma, and vitamin deficiencies, for example, improve with treatment of these conditions. Uremic neuropathies can resolve after transplantation, and nerve dysfunction related to drugs [vincristine, heavy metals (lead), and industrial solvents (n-hexane, acrylamide)], can all improve by removing the offending agent. A representative list of systemic disorders and toxic causes associated with peripheral neuropathy is presented in Table 13-3. Disulfiram, dapsone, and vincristine can all cause peripheral neuropathies and yet are used to treat conditions in which peripheral neuropathy is a common presentation—alcoholism, leprosy, and carcinoma. Inherited neuropathies such as Charcot–Marie–Tooth disease are common. Three specific neuropathies are discussed in the following sections—inflammatory polyradicular neuropathy of the Guillain–Barré syndrome, idiopathic facial nerve paresis (Bell's palsy), and diabetic neuropathy.

ACUTE INFLAMMATORY POLYRADICULONEUROPATHY— THE GUILLAIN–BARRÉ SYNDROME

Of remitting polyneuropathies, acute inflammatory polyradiculoneuropathy (AIPN), also known as Guillain–Barré syndrome, is the most common, estimated to occur at a rate 1.5/100,000 persons. AIPN occurs most commonly in young adulthood and early middle age, preceded in almost half of patients by an

TABLE 13-3. **Disorders of the Peripheral Nervous System**

SYSTEMIC DISEASES	VITAMIN DEFICIENCY	EXOGENOUS TOXINS
Diabetes mellitus	Thiamine	Alcohol
Hypothyroidism	Pyridoxine	Chloramphenicol
Renal failure	Niacin	*Cis*-platinum
AIDS	Riboflavin	Dapsone
Intestinal malabsorption	Folic acid	Diphenylhydantoin
Acute intermittent porphyria	Vitamin B_{12}	Disulfiram
Amyloidosis		Ethionamide
Acromegaly		Glutethimide
Leprosy		Gold
Diphtheria		Hydralazine
Lyme disease		Isoniazid
Mycoplasma		Metronidazole
Rheumatoid arthritis		Nitrofurantoin
Systemic lupus erythematosus		Nitrous oxide
Polyarteritis nodosa		Perhexiline maleate
Wegener's granulomatosis		Pyridoxine
Carcinoma		Thalidomide
Waldenströms macroglobulinemia		Vincristine
Multiple myeloma		*Heavy Metals*
POEMS (polyneuropathy, organomegaly,		Arsenic
M protein, skin changes)		Lead
Cryoglobulinemia		Thallium
Paraproteinemia		*Industrial Agents*
(Monoclonal gammopathy of		Solvents
uncertain significance—MGUS)		*n*-Hexane
Sarcoidosis		Methyl-*n*-butyl-ketone
Whipple's disease		2,5 Hexanedione
		Carbon disulfide
		Trichlorethylene
		Acrylamide
		Dimethylaminopropionitrile
		Dichlorophenoxyacetic acid
		TOCP
		Organophosphorus compounds

antecedent infectious illness that usually clears before neurologic dysfunction begins. The hallmarks of the syndrome are progressive, often severe, ascending weakness, complete tendon areflexia, high spinal fluid protein, possible cranial nerve and respiratory compromise, and substantial or complete spontaneous recovery. Weakness develops over hours to days but should not progress longer than 4 weeks. The severe motor compromise, short duration of progression, and elevated cerebrospinal fluid (CSF) protein with few (<10 mononuclear cells/mm³) are features that distinguish this syndrome from others. Sensory loss may be mild but should be looked for carefully since abnormalities of sensation help differentiate this syndrome from other conditions that may appear similar, including hypokalemia, botulism, and poliomyelitis. Pathologically, there is widespread inflammatory segmental demyelination, most prominent proximally and presumably immunologically mediated. Prominent axonal injury and marked decrease in evoked motor response amplitudes argue for a slow recovery.

Although there are characteristic clinical features, the variability of clinical presentation in actual practice should be emphasized. These include ataxia, ophthalmoplegia, and hyporeflexia (Miller Fisher syndrome) and facial diplegia with cardiac arrhythmias. The CSF protein may not be initially elevated, and repeated lumbar punctures may be necessary to demonstrate an increased protein with the associated characteristic dissociation between protein and cells. EMG studies may reveal prominent slowing of nerve conduction, but evidence of conduction block associated with segmental demyelination and proximal conduction abnormalities may be the only findings. As indicated, an estimate of the degree of axonal injury on EMG examination has prognostic implications.

Acute inflammatory polyradiculoneuropathy is considered idiopathic in origin. Syndromes similar to AIPN, however, may be found in conditions such as acute intermittent porphyria and Hodgkin's disease, and less commonly with other neoplasms, hepatitis, infectious mononucleosis, Lyme disease, and recently acquired human immunodeficiency virus (HIV) infection. Certain toxic neuropathies such as with thallium may be similar.

Although recovery may be slow, the characteristic history of AIPN is one of almost complete improvement. As such, the most important treatment is symptomatic, particularly respiratory support and monitoring autonomic dysfunction. Steroids have been advocated, but they have not been beneficial and are possibly detrimental. Plasmapheresis can hasten recovery and appears particularly indicated for those with severe respiratory compromise and if used within 7 days of onset.

A syndrome similar to AIPN may sometimes occur in a chronic (CIP) or a chronic relapsing (CIRP) form. These forms are probably variants of the same condition. In comparison to AIPN, the onset is often more gradual; antecedent infections are less common; and sensory symptoms and signs are more frequent. As in AIPN, the basic pathologic process is an inflammatory segmental demyelination, but there is also a loss of myelinated fibers. Onion bulbs are found due to repeated episodes of demyelination with remyelination. The CSF again shows high protein and relatively few cells at some stage in the illness, but it may be normal at the time of a particular examination. EMG studies characteristically show slowed conduction. Nerve biopsy may be helpful for the diagnosis. The differential between the chronic inflammatory neuropathies and inherited demyelinative neuropathies may sometimes be difficult and

may only be resolved by examining family members. In contrast to AIPN, steroids are thought helpful in CIP and CIRP. Immunosuppressive agents have also been used, and plasmapheresis has produced a temporary improvement. Treatment with high-dose intravenous immunoglobulin has been reported effective in CIP and AIPN.

IDIOPATHIC FACIAL PARALYSIS (BELL'S PALSY)

Unilateral weakness of the facial muscles occurs when cranial nerve VII (the facial nerve) is damaged. Disease at the pontine nucleus of the nerve causes the same distribution of facial paresis but is uncommon when compared with the more peripherally placed lesions. Tumors, abscesses, vascular disease, or trauma can all cause this distribution of complete unilateral facial paresis, although these causes are rare. *Bell's palsy* is the term used to describe facial paralysis of undetermined origin that occurs acutely and has a usual natural history of good recovery. The popularized statement that Bell's palsy occurs in the United States every 13 minutes (20 persons per 100,000/year) emphasizes the frequency of this affliction. Because the facial nerve travels through the internal auditory meatus and later gives off branches for the stapedius muscle and for taste sensation on the tongue, patients with Bell's palsy may complain of ipsilateral hyperacusis and decreased taste sensibility in addition to weak facial muscles.

The cause of Bell's palsy remains obscure, but modern microsurgical techniques have permitted *in situ* examination of the nerve during paralysis. Marked edema with the nerve under tension is consistently seen during the acute phase. However, the cause of the edema and its relation, either causal or reactive, to the paralysis are unknown. However, pressure on cranial nerve VII can compromise its vascular supply and precipitate or aggravate weakness. An ischemic basis for neurologic dysfunction may underlie Bell's palsy. This could occur from direct vascular dysfunction and thrombosis of the vasonervora, the tiny vessels supplying the nerve itself. Alternatively, a primary inflammatory process, viral or immunologic, may induce edema with secondary vascular compromise. The result of both processes is anoxia to the nerve with resultant vasodilatation, transudation of fluid, and further pressure effects in the confined pathway of cranial nerve VII.

The clinical picture of Bell's palsy is a peripheral facial weakness occurring rapidly, occasionally attended by aching pain around the jaw or behind the ear. The specific constellation of signs and symptoms depends on the anatomic area of involvement. Although cranial nerve VII is predominantly a motor nerve to the muscles of the face, there are sensory components. As the facial nerve leaves the pons and enters the internal auditory meatus along with the acoustic nerve, it carries fibers for lacrimation, salivation, and taste. The nerve then descends through the petrous bone, at which point the fibers to the lacrimal glands branch off. The taste fibers depart in the chorditympani and cross the middle ear. Only motor fibers to the face emerge from the stylomastoid foramen. If the patient suffers with unilateral facial weakness that involves the forehead and lower face, cranial nerve VII has been damaged at or distal to the styloid mastoid foramen. If the same facial weakness is seen in association with decreased taste perception on the anterior part of the tongue on the ipsilateral side of the facial weakness, cranial nerve VII has been damaged more proximally before the chorditympani branches off. If cranial nerve VII is damaged in the internal auditory meatus, facial weakness, altered taste perception, and hyperacusis (related to paralysis of the stapedius muscle) will be encountered.

Recovery usually begins within a week, and 75% of patients fully recover over a period of several weeks. Some permanent motor deficit occasionally remains. In some patients, synkinetic or aberrant motor movements develop secondary to faulty and misguided reinnervation.

Steroids have been advocated, on the premise that they reduce swelling within the facial canal and thereby diminish vascular compression so that proper oxygenation occurs. This theoretically would interrupt the pathologic cycle. Adour and colleagues studied the effect of oral prednisone on 194 patients with Bell's palsy compared with 110 untreated patients. The steroid dose was 40 mg for 4 days, tapering within 8 days. They reported that the treated group recovered more fully and had fewer complications, although side effects related to drug treatment occurred in 4% of the patients. Unfortunately, the two groups were not entirely comparable because severely affected patients accounted for 42% of the original control group and only 30% of the steroid group. Furthermore, the investigators were so convinced that prednisone was superior to no treatment that they abandoned a double-blind format midway into the study. Complete facial recovery was seen in 89% of steroid-treated patients and in 64% of nontreated patients. Some investigators have suggested that the positive steroid effect is maximal if the treatment is started within the first few days of facial weak-

ness, whereas others have felt steroids benefit patients at all points of their illness.

However, not all investigators feel that steroids are selectively effective in Bell's palsy. In a small group of patients treated with vitamins, full recovery occurred in 65% of patients compared with 60% in the steroid group. In a large prospective and randomized study, 88% of steroid-treated and 80% of nontreated control patients recovered full strength. The incidence of residual autonomic synkinesis from probable regenerating neural fibers was less prominent in the steroid-treated group.

The overall excellent prognosis of Bell's palsy with or without steroid treatment is confirmed in all studies. Approximately 15% to 30% of Bell's palsy patients show some residual weakness, but severe weakness is usually seen in only 2% to 4%. The pharmacologic basis of steroid activity focuses on general anti-inflammatory or vasoactive properties with no presumed activity on neuronal function *per se*.

NEUROPATHY ASSOCIATED WITH DIABETES MELLITUS

Diabetes mellitus is common and is commonly associated with nerve dysfunction. The incidence of neuropathic abnormalities in diabetes has been estimated to range from about 5% to 95%. The wide discrepancy relates to differing criteria and techniques used to diagnose PNS injury in these patients. A balanced view would probably indicate a prevalence of 50% to 60% of some form of neuropathy in diabetic patients. The prevalence increases with the duration of the disease, but diabetic nerve dysfunction may be the initial sign of diabetes. Given the various presentations and probable pathogenesis, it is best to think in terms of diabetic neuropathies rather than a single entity.

Polyneuropathies, mononeuropathies, plexopathies, radiculopathies, and autonomic neuropathies are all found individually or in combination in diabetes, and diabetes can therefore be associated with abnormalities at any level of the PNS. Asymptomatic diabetics may show decreased nerve conductions that can normalize with improved control of blood sugar. A distal sensory or sensorimotor polyneuropathy is the commonest type of diabetic neuropathy. A "stocking–glove" sensory loss is characteristic. A loss of position, vibration, and light touch as well as decreased reflexes are prominent features of the "large fiber" pattern. Relatively pronounced loss of pain and temperature sensation, in association with pain, indicate predominant "small fiber" injury. The pain may have a dull, aching quality in the limbs and also a distal, burning discomfort most prominent at night. Rarely, there is a pattern of sensory ataxia, pain, and arthropathy (diabetic "pseudotabes"). The "small fiber" and "pseudotabetic" patterns may be associated with autonomic dysfunction including an involvement of the gastrointestinal, cardiovascular, and genitourinary systems. Autonomic dysfunction can also occur without other evidence for a neuropathy. Postural hypotension, diarrhea, impotence, urinary retention, and increased sweating are examples of symptoms that may be caused by a diabetic autonomic neuropathy. The painful, asymmetrical, proximal weakness of the legs found in diabetes (diabetic amyotrophy) is probably due to the involvement of the lumbar plexus. Clinical patterns of a polyradiculopathy may occur, particularly in association with a history of weight loss. Isolated peripheral nerve lesions are common. These mononeuropathies can affect almost every major peripheral nerve as well as the cranial nerves, particularly the extraocular muscles. The onset of symptoms is characteristically abrupt and frequently painful. Diabetes may present as peroneal palsies.

The pathogenesis of diabetic neuropathies is varied. Metabolic derangements are commonly considered the basis for the polyneuropathies. Accumulation of sorbitol or depletion of myoinositol in nerves are current theories. There is experimental evidence, however, that edema secondary to structural changes in endoneural blood vessels may be the primary cause. The abrupt onset of painful, focal lesions in the diabetic mononeuropathies is similar to that of other vascular neuropathies and has led to the concept that these neuropathies are due to occlusion of the small, nutrient blood vessels supplying nerves. This finding has not, however, been confirmed pathologically.

The natural history of diabetic mononeuropathies, amyotrophies, and polyradiculopathies is one of improvement, even if occasionally slow. The course of diabetic polyneuropathies varies: some diabetic neuropathies improve, many plateau, and some steadily progress. A severe disability is the exception; however, the pseudotabetic variety is generally progressive and more disabling. Pain, particularly the distal burning dysesthesias, can be a major problem in the polyneuropathies. The manifestations of the autonomic neuropathy may be subclinical but are not infrequently incapacitating. The prognosis for the autonomic neuropathy is among the worst of the diabetic neuropathies.

Good metabolic control is probably helpful for both preventing and ameliorating diabetic neuropathies, and good control of blood sugar should therefore be a goal in these patients. Other therapies are symptomatic. An eye patch is helpful in patients with the self-limited diabetic ophthalmoplegia, as may bracing in those with peroneal palsy. Diphenylhydantoin, carbamazepine, and tricyclic antidepressants have been helpful in the painful sensory neuropathies, and analgesics are reasonable for the acute pain associated with mononeuropathies. Trophic ulcers of the feet may require changes in shoe size, debridement, and antibiotics. Standard medical regimens should be tried for autonomic dysfunction. These regimens include codeine phosphate and diphenoxylate for diarrhea, support stockings and fluorocortisone for postural hypotension, and regular voidings assisted by suprapubic pressure in those with bladder atony. Nighttime lights can assist walking in those patients with sensory loss, by preserving visual cues.

FUTURE PERSPECTIVES

The potential for an increased understanding of peripheral neuropathies is exciting. Newer techniques of histopathologic evaluation, including electron microscopy, teased fiber preparations, and morphometric analysis of nerves, have already added meaningfully to our understanding of both normal and abnormal nerves. Similarly, more sophisticated forms of electrophysiologic analysis should allow for a better evaluation of nerve dysfunction. These techniques include recording from single muscle fibers (single fiber EMG); computer analysis of motor unit firing, which can relate the amount of electrical activity generated by a muscle to the force; and increasing routine study of a wider range of electrophysiologic responses. These responses allow for evaluation of conduction in the more proximal portions of nerves and possibly for analyzing the effect of peripheral nerve dysfunction on motor neuron firing. The recording of cortical responses evoked by peripheral nerve stimulation (somatosensory evoked responses) not only allows for a more detailed evaluation of certain peripheral nerve injuries but also provides a possible technique for evaluation at the interface between peripheral and CNS dysfunction.

Immunologic studies are becoming increasingly important for understanding the pathogenesis of nerve disorders and for providing guides to therapy. Patients with a clinical picture similar to ALS, but with conduction block on electrophysiologic examination and elevated titers to ganglioside GM_1, have been treated successfully with immunosuppressive agents. Finally, basic research in the physiology, biochemistry, immunobiology, and axonal transport of nerves provides a dynamism that makes an interest in peripheral nerves continually rewarding.

QUESTIONS AND DISCUSSION

1. A 64-year-old patient with a 10-year history of insulin-dependent diabetes mellitus complains of burning dysesthesias in the feet. Examination reveals a mild decrease in strength at the toes and ankles; absent Achilles' reflexes; decreased pinprick, touch, and vibration sensitivity to the knees; and decreased position sense in the toes. Electrodiagnostic studies indicate prolonged motor conduction velocities, no sensory potentials, and evidence of denervation distally in the lower extremities. Sensory conductions in the upper extremities are slowed.

Four weeks later, the same patient develops weakness in the left leg associated with some pain in the region of the left knee. An examination 3 weeks after onset reveals relatively more prominent decreased pinprick and touch sensation in the lateral aspect of the left leg and dorsum of the left foot, as well as lack of dorsiflexion and eversion of the left ankle. EMG examination shows no evoked motor response stimulating at the fibula head and denervation in the left tibialis anterior, peronei, and extensor digitorum brevis muscles.

Is the history in the first or second part of the first question indicative of a polyneuropathy, mononeuropathy, or radiculopathy?

Are both of these histories compatible with a diabetic etiology?

Answer: The description in the first part of the first question would be characteristic of a polyneuropathy. The clinical and electrodiagnostic examinations reveal a diffuse sensorimotor neuropathic process most prominent distally.

The history and findings in the second part, by contrast, would indicate a mononeuropathy of the left peroneal (anterior tibial) nerve. Clinically, there are sensory loss, motor weakness, and EMG abnormalities in the distribution of that nerve.

Diabetes mellitus can produce both a polyneuropathy and a mononeuropathy, not infrequently in the same patient. The polyneuropathy is probably secondary to the metabolic derangements of the illness, whereas the mononeuropathy may be vascular in origin.

A significant diabetic polyneuropathy is probably an argument for careful diabetic control. Diabetic mononeuropathies usually resolve with time because of the partial nature of the nerve injury secondary to the ischemic insult. A short leg brace to aid in dorsiflexion of the left ankle could be important for this patient during the recovery period.

2. A 50-year-old woman has a 6-month history of pain in her right wrist. A diagnosis of hypothyroidism has recently been made. This pain awakens her at night, usually within several hours of falling asleep. She has noticed clumsiness in the use of that hand and complains of paresthesias radiating into the thumb and index fingers. Recently, she has noted some discomfort in the left wrist. An examination reveals paresthesias and pain radiating to the fingers on tapping the wrists bilaterally (positive Tinel's signs), weakness of the right abductor pollicis brevis muscle, and numbness involving the right thumb, index finger, and middle finger as well as the adjacent one-half of the ring finger. There is also numbness involving the lateral half of the palmar surface of the right hand.

This history most likely represents mononeuropathy of which nerve? Where is the lesion located? Is the process probably unilateral or bilateral? EMG examination reveals a prolongation of the median distal motor latencies and a lack or slowing of median sensory potentials, more prominent on the right. Are these findings consistent with your diagnosis?

Answer: The case presentation would be compatible with a diagnosis of a carpal tunnel syndrome (CTS). This syndrome is a mononeuropathy caused by "entrapment" of the median nerve as it passes through the carpal tunnel at the wrist. A positive Tinel's sign is a common clinical finding in an area of partial nerve injury, and a progression of this sign distally can be used to follow regeneration after a nerve has been severed. Characteristic electrodiagnostic findings in the CTS are those that indicate median nerve dysfunction at the level of the wrist, that is, prolonged motor conduction stimulating the nerve at the wrist and recording from median-innervated thenar hand muscles as well as prolonged conduction when stimulating the digital nerves of median-innervated fingers and recording at the wrist. The history would suggest a bilateral process—an assumption confirmed by the electrodiagnostic studies. Bilateral involvement in the CTS is present in approximately 25% of the cases. This syndrome is frequently part of several systemic illnesses including hypothyroidism. A CTS may be the presenting complaint in a patient with abnormal thyroid function.

Initial treatment would consist of therapy for the hypothyroidism as well as splinting the wrists to limit movement. If these measures failed, the transverse carpal ligaments should probably be surgically sectioned. Steroid injections can produce symptomatic relief, but the long-term effectiveness and the possible harm of this therapy have been debated.

3. A 55-year-old patient on vincristine therapy has developed progressive weakness over several weeks, resulting in an inability to walk. An examination reveals a mild "stocking–glove" sensory loss to pinprick, with preserved position sense, absent reflexes in the legs, and moderate to marked weakness in the legs and mild to moderate weakness in the arms, most marked distally. Electrodiagnostic studies reveal borderline, slow motor conduction velocities with considerable evidence of denervation, again most prominent distally.

Does this polyneuropathy involve primarily axons or myelin, and what is the appropriate treatment?

Answer: The history and clinical findings would be typical for a polyneuropathy secondary to vincristine therapy. The prominent denervation indicates disruption of the normal connections between nerve and muscle. Combined with the borderline slowing of conduction velocities, the primary disease is of axons rather than of myelin—that is, an axonal type of neuropathy. The treatment, of course, is to stop the vincristine.

4. A 35-year-old man has a 6-month history of weakness in the hands that now involves the legs. An examination reveals atrophy and fasciculations in the intrinsic muscles of the hands, weakness that is distally more prominent in the upper than in the lower extremities, hyperactive reflexes, and extensor plantar responses bilaterally. Sensory testing is unremarkable. Electrodiagnostic examination reveals normal motor and sensory conduction studies in the presence of denervation and decreased activation of motor units in all four extremities. Many of the motor units are both large and polyphasic. A cervical myelogram has been unremarkable.

This would be characteristic of a neuropathic process at what level of the motor unit? What is the most likely diagnosis? Would a sural nerve biopsy be helpful for the evaluation of this neuropathy?

Answer: The history and findings are consistent with a diagnosis of ALS. The extensor plantar responses and hyperactive reflexes would indicate some involvement of the long motor system tracts in the CNS, but the atrophy and fasciculations would be consistent with involvement of the lower motor neurons. This is confirmed by the electrodiagnostic studies, which indicate a chronic motor neuropathic process not readily explained by a process primarily affecting peripheral nerves, plexi, or roots. The normal conduction velocities indicate preservation of at least some of the fast-conducting (i.e., largest) motor axons. Since the pathologic process involves strictly efferent (i.e., motor) fibers, a sural nerve biopsy would not be helpful. The sural is a sensory nerve and therefore contains only afferent fibers.

The important point is that nerve dysfunction may involve either motor or sensory fibers only. In ALS, the primary pathology is at the lower motor neuron level in the anterior horns of the spinal cord. It may be argued this is not an illness of the PNS. Conversely, since ALS involves the cell bodies of efferent fibers with resultant abnormalities in nerve and muscle, the illness might be considered a prototypical axonal neuropathy.

SUGGESTED READING

Adour K, Wingerd M, Bell D, et al: Prednisone treatment for idiopathic facial paralysis. N Engl J Med 287:1268, 1972

Asbury AK, Bolis L, Gibbs CJ Jr: Workshop on autoimmune neuropathies: Guillain-Barré syndrome. Neurology 40:381, 1990

Blume G, Pestronk A, Goodnough LT. Anti-MAG antibody-associated polyneuropathies: Improvement following immunotherapy with monthly plasma exchange and IV cyclophosamide. Neurology 45:1577, 1995

Donofrio PD, Alber JW: Polyneuropathy: Classification by nerve conduction studies and electromyography. Muscle Nerve 13:889, 1990

Dyck PJ, Thomas PK, Griffin JW, et al (eds): Peripheral Neuropathy, Vols 1 and 2. Philadelphia, WB Saunders, 1993

Gabriel J-M, Erne B, Mierscher GC, et al: Selective loss of myelin associated glycoprotein from myelin correlates with anti-MAG titre in demyelinating paraproteinaemic polyneuropathy. Brain 119:775, 1996

Kimura J: Electrodiagnosis in Diseases of Nerve and Muscle. Philadelphia, FA Davis, 1989

Latov N: Pathogenesis and therapy of neuropathies associated with monoclonal gammopathies. Ann Neurol 37(S1):S32, 1995

Notermans NC, Lokhurst JIM, Franssen H: Intermittent cyclophosphamide and prednisone treatment of polyneuropathy associated with monoclonal gammopathy of undetermined significance. Neurology 47:1227, 1996

Parry JG: Guillain-Barré Syndrome. New York, Thieme, 1993

Pestronk A: Motor neuropathies, motor neuron disorders, and antiglycolipid antibodies. Muscle Nerve 14:927, 1991

Schaumberg HH, Berger AR, Thomas PK: Disorders of Peripheral Nerves. Philadelphia, FA Davis, 1992

Stalberg E, Trontelj JE: Single Fiber Electromyography. Old Woking, England, Miravalle Press, 1994

Sumner AJ (ed): The Physiology of Peripheral Nerve Disease. Philadelphia, WB Saunders, 1980

Tuck RR, Schmelzer JD, Low PA: Endoneurial blood flow and oxygen tension in the sciatic nerves of rats with experimental diabetic neuropathy. Brain 107: 935, 1984

Neurology for the Non-Neurologist, Fourth Edition,
edited by William J. Weiner and
Christopher G. Goetz. Lippincott
Williams & Wilkins, Philadelphia © 1999.

C	H	A	P	T	E	R	1	4

Vertigo and Dizziness

Judd M. Jensen

Of all the reasons patients seek medical attention, few engender more frustration on the part of physicians and more anxiety on the part of patients than the complaint of dizziness. The physician's frustration seems to be rooted in the perceived difficulties of establishing an accurate diagnosis and providing effective therapy. The patient's fears are grounded in the significant discomfort associated with many of these syndromes and the subsequent assumption that whatever is wrong must be equally horrible. However, the majority of the syndromes discussed below are benign and not life-threatening. The explanation of this fact and the conveyance of an understanding of the disease process is the physician's first step in treating dizzy patients and, often, a very important one. This chapter will attempt to provide a logical approach to the evaluation of patients with vertigo and dizziness so that an accurate diagnosis and subsequent prognosis can be made. Effective therapies for some of these syndromes have been developed and these will be discussed in detail.

LET THE PATIENTS TELL THEIR STORY

In assessing patients with dizziness syndromes, it is important that physicians keep their questions open ended during history taking. Beginning the interview with direct questions alters the spontancity and character of the patient's replies and, thus, reduces their diagnostic value. The best approach is to coax the patient to first describe his symptom complex in his own words. An accurate diagnosis can often be made in the first few minutes of the encounter by using this method. Later, specific and important questions that were not addressed by the patient, such as symptom frequency and duration, precipitating body positions, and associated symptoms, can be asked. By using this approach, the history is diagnostic in the majority of cases. At the very least, the patient's symptom complex can be placed into one of the three following categories.

DEFINITIONS AND CATEGORIES

VERTIGO

Patients who have vertigo experience a false sensation of movement. Most commonly, they report that their environment is spinning around them. However, the sensations of tilting, swaying, and being impelled forward, backward, or to either side are also vertiginous. These patients have a disorder of either the peripheral or central vestibular system. They seek medical attention either with an acute episode of vertigo, usually associated with nausea, vomiting, and ataxia, or with a history of recurrent attacks of vertigo.

PRESYNCOPE

Patients who have presyncope describe their dizziness as "lightheadedness" or "feeling like I'm going to faint." This sensation is usually associated with generalized weakness, visual blurring or blackout, diaphoresis, shortness of breath, or palpitations. The patient usually looks pale to an observer. It should be noted that occasionally patients with presyncope report vertigo during their episodes, presumably because of inadequate perfusion in the brainstem vestibular nuclei. This can lead to diagnostic confusion with the primary vestibular syndromes, although the remainder of the clinical picture usually distinguishes the two types of dizziness. Presyncope is typically episodic and is caused by a transient reduction in global cerebral perfusion. Therefore, it is a primary cardiovascular problem rather than a neurologic one.

DISEQUILIBRIUM

Disequilibrium is a more complex category than the previous two. While patients with vertigo and presyncope tend to have episodic symptoms or attacks, patients with disequilibrium typically have more continuous symptoms. The key historical feature is that these patients are dizzy primarily when standing or walking and tend to improve when seated or supine. They often have difficulty describing what they feel. Responses such as "bad balance," "poor equilibrium," or "I'm just dizzy" are common. Disequilibrium is the result of dysfunction at one or more points in the complex system required for bipedal balance and ambulation. The causes of this dysfunction are many and varied, as will be discussed.

VERTIGO SYNDROMES

ANATOMY, PHYSIOLOGY, AND PATHOPHYSIOLOGY

Vertigo is a symptom of disease in the vestibular system. This system is usually divided into peripheral and central components. The peripheral vestibular apparatus includes the labyrinth, which is located in the petrous portion of the temporal bone, and the vestibular portion of the eighth cranial nerve, which connects the labyrinth to the brainstem and is located in the internal auditory canal and cerebellopontine angle. The labyrinth is divided into three semicircular canals that sense head rotation, and the otoliths (utricle and saccule) that sense head position relative to gravity. The central vestibular apparatus consists of vestibular nuclei at the pontomedullary junction in the brainstem. These nuclei receive impulses from the eighth cranial nerve and have rich connections with the nuclei controlling eye movements and the cerebellum. Normally, the paired labyrinths supply balanced tonic impulses to the central nervous system (CNS) regarding the position of the head and its movements. Vertigo occurs when a pathologic process acutely disrupts the input from one labyrinth. The remaining unbalanced contralateral input produces the false sensation of movement. With time, the CNS will adjust to unilateral input. Vertigo is thus typically acute and episodic. A pathologic process that slowly disrupts the input from one labyrinth either will be asymptomatic or will produce a disequilibrium syndrome such as those that follow.

NEIGHBORHOOD SIGNS

The physician must determine whether a patient's vertigo is of central or peripheral origin. The presence of one or more neighborhood signs and symptoms may be helpful in making this distinction. The most important neighborhood symptoms in peripheral vestibular lesions are hearing loss and tinnitus. These occur in diseases affecting the cochlea, the middle ear, and the acoustic portion of the eighth cranial nerve. Processes that disrupt the vestibular portion of the eighth nerve in the cerebellopontine angle or in the internal auditory canal usually also affect the acoustic portion. Likewise, labyrinthine processes may also affect the cochlea or middle ear. Central processes affecting the brainstem and cerebellum rarely cause hearing loss or tinnitus; thus, the presence of these symptoms almost excludes CNS disease.

Eighth cranial nerve and cerebellopontine angle mass lesions (i.e., acoustic neuroma) often present with progressive hearing loss and/or tinnitus and can have associated facial weakness, facial sensory loss, and/or a depressed corneal reflex. However, it is distinctly unusual for such lesions to produce either an acute vertigo syndrome or recurrent attacks of vertigo. When acoustic neuroma and other mass lesions of the eighth nerve and cerebellopontine angle produce dizziness, it is more commonly a disequilibrium syndrome related to slow destruction of the vestibular portion of the eighth cranial nerve or pressure on the brainstem vestibular nuclei.

The vertigo seen in central vestibular syndromes is frequently accompanied by one or more neighborhood symptoms and signs. It is important to note that it is often the presence of such additional findings that clearly defines the vertigo as central in origin. The list of possible neighborhood signs and symptoms includes diplopia, cortical blindness, homonymous hemianopsia, dysarthria, dysphagia, bilateral extremity weakness or sensory symptoms, and unilateral or bilateral facial weakness or numbness.

Gait ataxia is usually present during an acute attack of vertigo, whether the abnormality is in the peripheral or central vestibular apparatus. However, it tends to be more prominent in central vestibular disorders. In addition, prominent appendicular ataxia in the form of finger-to-nose or heel-to-shin dysmetria is suggestive of a central process, usually a cerebellar infarction or hemorrhage.

NYSTAGMUS

Nystagmus is present in virtually all patients during the acute experience of vertigo. It typically subsides as soon as the vertigo resolves in peripheral vestibular syndromes. However, the nystagmus may persist longer than the vertigo in central syndromes. Nystagmus is often difficult to appreciate in a vertigo syndrome of peripheral vestibular origin. Part of the reason for this has to do with the way physicians typically examine eye movements. By having the patient focus on the index finger while it moves side to side as well as up and down, the physician is requiring visual fixation. Such fixation tends to suppress nystagmus of peripheral vestibular origin. The optimal way to examine such patients is by watching their eye movements while fixation is prevented. This is ideally done with the use of Frenzel lenses. These are +30 diopter binocular lenses, which the patient wears during the examination. These lenses prevent visual fixation on the part of the patient but allow the examiner to see the eye movements. If such lenses are unavailable, there is a simple bedside technique that may be used to demonstrate nystagmus in peripheral vestibular lesions. While the examiner is performing a funduscopic examination on one eye with an ophthalmoscope, the contralateral eye is alternately covered and uncovered. When the eye is uncovered, the patient is asked to fixate on an object in the room. If the patient has a peripheral vestibular syndrome, the examiner should be able to detect an increase in the amplitude of the nystagmoid jerks (by watching the movement of the optic disk) when the contralateral eye is covered (fixation prevented) as opposed to when it is uncovered and the patient is able to fixate.

There are other ways of distinguishing central and peripheral nystagmus. Nystagmus of peripheral origin is unidirectional; that is, the fast component of the nystagmus always beats in the same direction, no matter which direction the patient is looking. For example, with a left peripheral vestibular lesion, the fast component of the nystagmus will be to the right

on left lateral gaze, right lateral gaze, or vertical gaze. Nystagmus of peripheral origin is also mixed; that is, it typically has both a horizontal and a rotatory or torsional component. Nystagmus of central origin is typically multidirectional (i.e., the fast component of the nystagmus changes with the direction of gaze). Pure horizontal, pure vertical, or pure rotatory nystagmus is almost always central. Unfortunately for diagnostic purposes, nystagmus of central origin can mimic peripheral nystagmus by being unidirectional or of a mixed form. Peripheral lesions, however, almost never produce multidirectional or pure forms of nystagmus. Perhaps the best means to distinguish central from peripheral nystagmus is by the response to fixation. Central nystagmus is not suppressed and is frequently enhanced by fixation. In general, the nystagmus of central vestibular disorders is more prominent and more persistent than the nystagmus of peripheral vestibular origin.

ELECTRONYSTAGMOGRAPHY

Electronystagmography (ENG) can be a useful test in evaluating patients with disorders of the vestibular system. The technique takes advantage of the rich connections between the vestibular and ocular motor nuclei. This examination requires skill and experience to perform and interpret. Unfortunately, the results do not always provide the clinician with definitive answers. At best, ENG can determine the presence of vestibular dysfunction, establish the unilateral or bilateral nature of the dysfunction, and distinguish central from peripheral vestibular dysfunction.

CAUSES OF RECURRENT EPISODES OF VERTIGO

BENIGN PAROXYSMAL POSITIONAL VERTIGO

Benign paroxysmal positional vertigo (BPPV) is the most common diagnosis in patients who seek medical evaluation for vertigo. It is also the most common cause of recurrent vertigo by a wide margin. The history is characteristic: The patients report that a few seconds after assumption of a certain head position (usually supine in bed), they experience the sudden onset of vertigo, which lasts 15 to 60 seconds and then resolves. The patients may also note that if they put their heads in the same position a second or a third time (within a relatively brief interval), the vertigo will be less intense each time. The key historical features are the characteristic head position (there can be more than one), the brief latency to onset of vertigo, and the fatigability of the vertigo with repeated trials.

The patient's symptom complex can frequently be reproduced in the office with the Dix-Hallpike maneuver (Fig. 14-1). This maneuver begins with the patient sitting on the examination table. His head is turned 45 degrees to the right and then he is quickly put in the supine position with his head hanging over the edge of the table and extended approximately 30 degrees. If the vertigo does not begin within 30 seconds, he is returned to the sitting position, his head is turned 45 degrees to the left, and the patient is again made supine with his head extended. If this

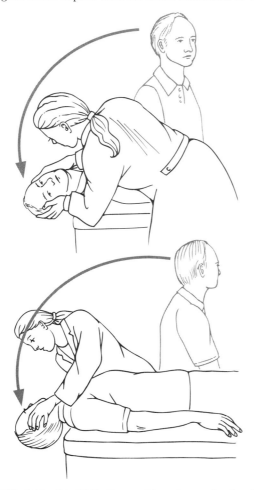

FIG. 14-1. Dix-Hallpike positional test for benign positional nystagmus. Patient is rapidly moved from the sitting to the head-hanging position. (Redrawn from, Baloh RW, Halmagyi GM (eds): Disorders of the Vestibular System. Copyright ©1996 by Oxford University Press, Inc. Used by permission.)

maneuver is performed during one of the patient's symptomatic periods, it almost always produces vertigo associated with nystagmus that has a prominent rotatory or torsional character.

This syndrome is most commonly idiopathic but can be seen after head trauma, an acute peripheral vestibulopathy, or, rarely, with a variety of other structural posterior fossa lesions. The pathophysiology of this syndrome is thought to be an accumulation of calcium carbonate crystals that form a plug, usually in the posterior semicircular canal. When the patient places his head in the recumbent position with the affected canal down, the calcium carbonate plug acts as a plunger and stimulates the labyrinth, thus producing the vertigo. The latency reflects the time required for the plunger to move in the canal and stimulate the system. The fatigability reflects dispersion of the calcium carbonate crystals in the canal with repeated movement. The treatment of this syndrome is directed at moving the calcium carbonate crystals from the posterior semicircular canal into the utricle by either a canal-particle-repositioning maneuver called the modified Epley maneuver (Fig. 14-2) or by a series of bedside exercises (see Brandt and Daroff: Physical Therapy for Benign Paroxysmal Positional Vertigo). The Epley maneuver should be performed until it no longer produces vertigo. This may require two to five repetitions of the maneuver at the time of initial treatment. The patient should then be instructed to sleep upright for the next two nights and to wear a soft cervical collar continuously for 72 hours. Both the Epley maneuver and the bedside exercises are effective treatments in the majority of patients. The natural history of this disorder is typically a waxing and waning course over months to years. The treatments will put most patients into a "remission," but the symptoms may recur at some point in the future. Most cases eventually resolve. Rare cases are unremitting, debilitating, and unresponsive to treatment. In such cases, surgical division of the posterior ampullary nerve or occlusion of the posterior semicircular canal can be considered.

In a clinically typical case of BPPV (with characteristic head position, latency, and fatigability) with a normal neurologic examination and a positive Dix-Hallpike maneuver, no brain imaging is necessary. The only workup required is a screening audiogram. Significantly asymmetric sensorineural hearing loss, especially high tone loss, would require that the patient have a magnetic resonance imaging (MRI) scan of the posterior fossa. This entity is not associated with hearing loss, tinnitus, or other vestibular system neighborhood signs. The presence of any of these should prompt a search for an alternate diagnosis, and such patients should have MRI of the brain and posterior fossa.

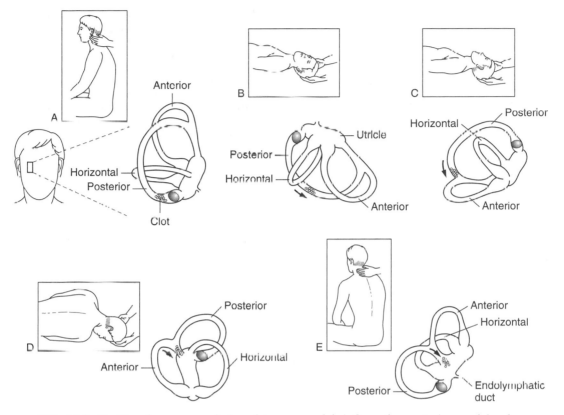

FIG. 14-2. Positional maneuver designed to remove debris from the posterior semicircular canal. **A.** In the sitting position the clot of calcium carbonate crystals lies at the bottommost position within the posterior canal. **B.** Movement to the head-hanging position causes the clot to move away from the cupula, producing an excitatory burst of activity in the ampullary nerve from the posterior canal (ampullofugal displacement of the cupula). **C.** Movement across to the other head-hanging position causes the clot to move further around the canal. **D.** The patient then rolls onto the side facing the floor, causing the clot to enter the common crus of the posterior and anterior semicircular canals. **E.** Finally, the patient sits up, and the clot disperses in the utricle. The maneuver is repeated until no nystagmus is induced, and the patient is then instructed not to lie flat for 48 hours (to prevent the debris from reentering the canal). (Redrawn from, Epley JM: The canalith repositioning procedure: for treatment of benign paroxysmal positional vertigo. Otolaryngol Head Surg 107:399, 1992)

A Word of Caution

Movement-related vertigo (MRV) can be a source of confusion and is occasionally misinterpreted as BPPV. MRV typically occurs after a patient has had a prolonged episode of vertigo (i.e., acute peripheral vestibulopathy, vertebrobasilar ischemia) but can occur *de novo*. In MRV, almost any head or body movement produces vertigo. In addition, there is no latency or fatigability as in BPPV. It is this lack of specificity of head movement and the absence of latency and fatigability that distinguish MRV from BPPV. MRV can be seen in any peripheral or central vestibular process.

MÉNIÈRE'S DISEASE

Ménière's disease is a syndrome characterized by recurrent attacks of vertigo, hearing loss, tinnitus, and aural fullness. Classically, the patient experiences the entire symptom complex with each episode. However, there is considerable variability and there are atypical cases of Ménière's that have only vestibular symptoms (i.e., vertigo) without cochlear symptoms (hearing loss and tinnitus), and others with cochlear symptoms and no vertigo. A typical attack of vertigo lasts 30 minutes to 24 hours. The hearing loss fluctuates and usually improves after the vertigo resolves. However, over time there is progressive loss of hearing. The pathologic findings associated with this syndrome are referred to as endolymphatic hydrops. However, the pathophysiology that leads to this pathologic endpoint is not understood. It is possible that there are multiple causes that lead to this common endpoint. Serial audiograms are very helpful in the diagnosis and management of these patients. As noted, fluctuating hearing loss is typical. Low frequency hearing is lost first but eventually there is a global loss of auditory function. All patients should have an MRI of the posterior fossa. Symptoms typically begin in one ear but ultimately become bilateral in nearly 50% of patients. Approximately 80% of patients go into remission within 5 years, although most of these will be left with significant hearing loss and some with a chronic disequilibrium syndrome.

Salt restriction has been shown in some studies to reduce the frequency of the attacks of vertigo and hearing loss. This treatment should be initiated with a restriction of 1–2 grams of sodium per day. If this level of restriction is ineffective, then sodium should be reduced to less than 1 gram per day. Thiazide diuretics and acetazolamide have also been reported to be helpful in some patients. Occasional patients have frequent, disabling attacks of vertigo. Historically, surgical ablative procedures, such as labyrinthectomy and vestibular neurectomy, have been offered in such patients. However, there has been increasing interest in the use of intratympanal gentamicin. This modality seems to prevent the recurring attacks of vertigo and often maintains some auditory function. Most authors feel that this is now the treatment of choice.

MIGRAINE

The vestibular nuclei in the brainstem receives its blood supply from branches of the basilar artery, so it is not surprising that migrainous vasospasm of the basilar artery can produce vertigo. Other neurologic symptoms such as scintillating scotoma, homonymous hemianopsia, cortical blindness, diplopia, dysarthria, ataxia, paresthesias, and quadriparesis may also be seen with vertigo in this syndrome. Hearing loss and tinnitus may also be associated with basilar artery migraine.

These patients are usually young and the history is typically dominated by the severe headache that follows the vertigo. In some patients, however, the headache may not be prominent, whereas in others the headache may not always follow the vasospastic component of the syndrome. This latter phenomenon is called a migraine equivalent and should be considered in a patient with isolated attacks of vertigo who also has a history of vertigo followed by headache. The treatment of basilar artery migraine is similar to the treatment of other migraine syndromes and is not discussed here.

PERILYMPH FISTULA

The perilymph fistula syndrome results from an abnormal communication between the perilymphatic space of the inner ear and the pneumatized middle ear. It is typically caused by head trauma or barotrauma. The latter can be obvious, as in the case of a deep sea diver, or quite subtle, as after straining at stool or a hard cough. The patients experience a variable symptom complex that can include episodic vertigo, fluctuating hearing loss, tinnitus, and a disequilibrium syndrome. The symptoms are typically triggered by valsalva, exertion, or further barotrauma. There is no completely satisfactory diagnostic test for this disorder. Findings on pneumatic otoscopy can be helpful but they are not specific or sensitive enough to be definitely diagnostic. The most reliable diagnostic method is the elicitation of a history of an appropriate inciting event and the reproduction of symptoms with valsalva or repeated barotrauma. Initial treatment should include at least 4 to 8 hours of strict bed rest with the head elevated and avoidance of any activity that would increase intra-abdominal pressure (i.e., bending, lifting, straining). If this fails to result in improvement, then surgical grafting of the oval and round windows can be considered.

TEMPORAL LOBE EPILEPSY

Rarely, vertigo can be experienced as part of a temporal lobe seizure, typically representing the aura of the seizure. However, the clinical picture is typically dominated by other manifestations of the seizure, including alteration of consciousness, automatisms, and postictal disorientation. On very rare occasions, the patient may experience frequent auras without the remainder of the seizure. In this circumstance, this syndrome could conceivably be confused with a vestibular disorder. However, an EEG is not considered part of the routine workup of patients with vertigo syndromes.

CAUSES OF A SINGLE ACUTE EPISODE OF VERTIGO

ACUTE PERIPHERAL VESTIBULOPATHY

This is the second most common cause of vertigo for which patients seek medical attention. *Vestibular neuritis, vestibular neuronitis,* and *labyrinthitis* are terms frequently used to refer to this syndrome, although the last should be used only when there is associated hearing loss. The pathophysiology of this disorder is incompletely understood. While it is thought to have a viral or postviral etiology, the proof of this pathogenesis is lacking. This syndrome is an acute disorder of the peripheral vestibular system and is benign in its prognosis. However, it must be distinguished from ischemic or hemorrhagic vertebrobasilar vascular disease, which will be discussed.

Despite the confusing nomenclature and uncertain pathophysiology, the clinical syndrome is well known to most clinicians. In the typical acute peripheral vestibulopathy, the vertigo is gradual in onset, peaks in several hours, and resolves by 24 to 48 hours. Patients remain fairly incapacitated during the experience of vertigo and usually have associated nausea, vomiting, and gait ataxia. They typically prefer to remain motionless during this time, as any head or body movement tends to exacerbate the vertigo. A disequilibrium syndrome often follows the resolution of the vertigo and may persist for days, weeks, or even months.

The neurologic examination during the vertigo phase is remarkable only for nystagmus of the type seen in peripheral vestibular lesions (as described above). There may be mild gait ataxia, with the patient tending to veer to the side of the affected vestibular apparatus. However, prominent gait ataxia, extremity ataxia, or other vestibular neighborhood signs should raise the question of a brainstem or cerebellar infarction or hemorrhage. During the period of disequilibrium, after the vertigo resolves, the neurologic examination may be quite normal despite the patient's complaints of persistent dizziness and imbalance.

A typical case in a young healthy adult requires no brain imaging. However, in older patients and in those with risk factors for vascular disease, an urgent noncontrast computed tomography (CT) scan of the brain is necessary to exclude a cerebellar hemorrhage. Ischemic disease of the cerebellum and brainstem is poorly imaged by CT. Therefore, MRI may be necessary in these patients (see below).

Therapy for acute vertigo consists of bed rest, intravenous fluids, phenothiazines, antihistamines, and benzodiazepines. Patients who develop a prolonged disequilibrium syndrome can be treated with vestibular exercises, discussed later.

VERTEBROBASILAR VASCULAR DISEASE

Vertigo is a cardinal symptom in several of the posterior circulation stroke syndromes. These diagnoses should be considered in any patient with persistent vertigo who has risk factors for vascular disease (hypertension, diabetes mellitus, heart disease, hyperlipidemia, tobacco abuse) or in any elderly patient regardless of the presence of risk factors. One recent study suggested that up to 25% of patients who present to the emergency room with isolated vertigo and who have risk factors for vascular disease may have inferior cerebellar infarctions.

The vertigo in these vascular syndromes is typically abrupt in onset and maximal at the beginning, unlike peripheral vestibular syndromes in which the vertigo typically worsens over several hours. Gait ataxia is usually a prominent feature in posterior circulation stroke, and many patients are unable to stand. Similarly, appendicular ataxia in the form of finger-to-nose or heel-to-shin dysmetria is often prominent. The most ominous posterior circulation disorder is cerebellar hemorrhage. This potentially fatal condition is important to recognize, as surgical decompression is often required and is life saving. These patients are usually identified by the presence of prominent headache and some degree of altered level of consciousness. However, headache and lethargy can be absent initially and then develop hours later when edema from the hemorrhage begins to produce brainstem compression. To complicate matters further, headache occurs in several of the posterior circulation ischemic strokes. Cerebellar hemorrhage can be accurately diagnosed by a noncontrast CT scan of the brain. Patients with this disorder require an urgent neurosurgical evaluation and intensive care unit monitoring.

The ischemic vertigo syndromes, in general, have a more benign prognosis. However, because of the increasing effectiveness of secondary or recurrent stroke prevention, these are important diagnoses to make. The most common ischemic syndromes are those of the vertebral artery (VA) and the posterior inferior cerebellar artery (PICA). After the VA enters the skull, it gives rise to the PICA and then supplies perforating branches to the lateral medulla before joining with the other vertebral artery to form the basilar artery. The PICA gives variable branches to the lateral medulla before supplying the inferior surface of the cerebellum. Occlusion of the VA typically produces a lateral medullary infarction. However, depending on the site of the occlusion, there may also be ischemia in the PICA distribution and, thus, an inferior cerebellar infarction. Similarly, primary occlusion of the PICA produces ischemia to the inferior cerebellum but may also cause infarction of the lateral medulla. Thus, there are many similarities in the vascular syndromes produced by disease of these two vessels.

Lateral medullary infarction is the most common brainstem ischemic stroke and is usually referred to as the Wallenberg syndrome. The vertigo in this syndrome can be associated with a wide variety of symptoms including dysarthria, dysphagia, hoarseness, hiccups, Horner's sign, diplopia, facial pain or numbness, and gait and limb ataxia. Most patients will have loss of pain and temperature sensation on the face ipsilateral to the infarction whether or not they complain of facial numbness. Most patients will also have loss of pain and temperature sensation on the contralateral side of the body. These patients are usually not aware of this deficit, so it must be sought by the examiner in all suspected cases of vertigo of ischemic origin. The typical Wallenberg syndrome has two or three of these symptoms and signs. The entire clinical picture is seen only rarely. In inferior cerebellar infarction, vertigo, ataxia, nausea, and vomiting are the only symptoms. A small percentage of these patients develop significant edema in the area of cerebellar infarction with resultant brainstem compression. This group of patients, like those with cerebellar hemorrhage, may require surgical decompression.

The anterior inferior cerebellar artery (AICA) supplies the lateral pons, the vestibular and cochlear structures via a branch called the internal auditory artery, and the anterior inferior portion of the cerebellum. Occlusion of the distal portion of this vessel can produce a cerebellar infarction that is clinically identical to that seen in the PICA syndrome. Occlusion of the internal auditory artery produces sudden, profound hearing loss and severe vertigo. Finally, occlusion of the more proximal portion of the AICA produces a brainstem syndrome with ipsilateral facial weakness, resembling a Bell's palsy. There may be associated hearing loss, and vertigo if the ischemia extends into the internal auditory artery.

The vertigo in these vascular syndromes tends to last longer than the vertigo seen with peripheral vestibular lesions. Moreover, the ataxia and nystagmus seen in central lesions tend to persist well beyond the resolution of the vertigo. This does not occur with peripheral vestibular disorders. Finally, the nystagmus seen with these posterior circulation vascular syndromes has the character of central nystagmus discussed previously.

Any of the ischemic stroke syndromes that can cause vertigo can also present as transient ischemic attacks. These episodes can be difficult to distinguish from a peripheral vestibular syndrome, as the patient is usually not examined until after the symptoms have resolved. As a general rule, any episode of vertigo lasting less than 30 minutes in a patient with risk factors for stroke should be considered a possible transient ischemic attack. Vertigo lasting seconds is unlikely to be ischemic in etiology and is probably related to a peripheral vestibular process.

Magnetic resonance imaging is the optimal diagnostic tool for evaluating patients with posterior circulation stroke syndromes. However, this examination is not required in all patients. As mentioned, any patient with persistent vertigo who is over age 60 or has risk factors for vascular disease should have a noncontrast CT scan of the brain to rule out a cerebellar hemorrhage. CT will not demonstrate most ischemic posterior circulation strokes. In patients with a vertigo syndrome where a clear distinction between a peripheral and a central etiology cannot be made, MRI should be performed. Evaluation for vertebrobasilar vascular stenosis can be done by either MR angiography (an imaging technique that does not require the injection of contrast material) or by transcranial Doppler ultrasonography (TCD). TCD is not available at many institutions. MR angiography is generally available wherever MRIs are performed. Both techniques have advantages and disadvantages. MR angiography produces a multidimensional image of the vessels being examined but often has a tendency to overestimate the degree of stenosis. TCD is very sensitive for the detection of significant stenosis in the vertebrobasilar system, but this technique can be limited by neck thickness and vessel tortuosity. These two noninvasive studies correlate best with standard angiography when they are in agreement.

As mentioned, neurosurgical decompression is required for many patients with cerebellar hemorrhage and some patients with large ischemic cerebellar infarctions. Otherwise, the acute management of posterior circulation stroke is similar to that of hemispheral stroke syndromes: avoidance of overaggressive blood pressure management, prevention of dehydration, swallowing evaluation when appropriate, deep vein thrombosis (DVT) prophylaxis, and antiplatelet agents. There is no proven role for anticoagulation in posterior circulation ischemia caused by atherosclerotic disease of the vertebrobasilar system. Patients with posterior circulation stroke due to cardiogenic embolism should be considered for anticoagulant therapy. If a cardiac or aortic cardiac source of embolism is suspected, transesophageal echocardiography is the diagnostic test of choice. Otherwise, risk-factor modification is the mainstay of secondary stroke prevention. Carotid endarterectomy is not indicated for secondary stroke prevention in posterior circulation ischemia.

MULTIPLE SCLEROSIS

Vertigo is one of the cardinal symptoms of multiple sclerosis. It can occur as the presenting symptom or in a patient with an established diagnosis. The clinical syndrome can mimic acute peripheral vestibulopathy. The character of the nystagmus may be the only distinguishing feature. Hearing loss is rare but does occur in this disease. Any young person who presents with an acute vertigo syndrome should be questioned about past neurologic symptoms. The long forgotten optic neuritis or the transient extremity paresthesias that were thought to reflect a pinched nerve may be a clue to the etiology of their vertigo syndrome. MRI is the diagnostic test of choice for multiple sclerosis. While it may not always demonstrate brainstem or cerebellar lesions, the periventricular white matter lesions are usually present. Therapy consists of pulse oral or intravenous corticosteroids.

PRESYNCOPE

After vertigo, the second category of dizziness is presyncope. Presyncope is a primary cardiovascular problem with neurologic symptoms. Lightheadedness, visual blurring or blackout, facial or extremity paresthesias, and generalized weakness are due to a global reduction in cerebral perfusion from either a drop in systemic arterial pressure, failure of cardiac output, or diffuse cerebral vasoconstriction. Diaphoresis, palpitations, and nausea are often present as the autonomic nervous system becomes activated in an attempt to restore cerebral perfusion. Most patients with presyncope will have their symptom complex reproduced by hyperventilation even if hyperventilation syndrome is not the cause of their symptoms. This can be useful in the bedside evaluation of patients with dizziness. Hyperventilation results in a drop in arterial PCO_2 with subsequent cerebral arterial vasoconstriction and global reduction in cerebral blood flow. The proce-

dure can be performed by holding a handkerchief or tissue 12 inches in front of the mouth and having the patient breath rapidly and deeply for up to 3 minutes. The handkerchief or tissue must be significantly displaced with each exhalation to ensure hyperventilation. If this procedure exactly reproduces the patient's dizziness, the physician can be confident of a presyncopal syndrome.

Presyncopy is caused by a global reduction in cerebral perfusion and, therefore, it is not a transient ischemic attack, which is always the result of a focal area of brain ischemia. While presyncope can occasionally be difficult to distinguish from a vertebrobasilar transient ischemic attack, this syndrome cannot be the result of carotid ischemia. Finally, presyncope is not a type of seizure and an electroencephalogram (EEG) is not a useful part of the diagnostic evaluation of patients with this syndrome.

CAUSES OF PRESYNCOPE

HYPERVENTILATION SYNDROME

Hyperventilation syndrome is a common cause of presyncope and occurs in two forms. The high-grade hyperventilator tends to have acute episodes of dizziness that are precipitated by stressful situations or panic attacks. These patients usually have the complete syndrome, including visual blurring, perioral and digital paresthesias, and generalized weakness. They are often aware of breathing rapidly or feeling short of breath. The low-grade hyperventilator has a more protracted and insidious form of dizziness. The symptoms tend to wax and wane over longer periods of time. Visual blurring, paresthesias, and generalized weakness are usually absent. Patients are almost never aware that they are overbreathing, and they do not feel short of breath. This syndrome occurs in anxious, pressured, driven individuals. They may exhibit frequent sighing during the office interview.

The symptom complex of both high-grade and low-grade hyperventilators can be reproduced easily by the technique of artificial hyperventilation, as described above. In fact, these patients tend to be very sensitive to even short periods of induced hyperventilation.

Reassurance regarding the etiology and benign nature of their symptom complex is the most important aspect of treatment for these patients. The high-grade hyperventilator may be helped by placement of a paper or plastic bag over the mouth during the attacks. Supportive psychotherapy or counseling may be helpful in some patients. Anxiolytic agents may be appropriate in selected patients.

ORTHOSTATIC HYPOTENSION

Orthostatic hypotension is also a common cause of presyncope, particularly in the elderly. The symptoms almost always occur when the patient is standing and are frequently maximal just after the patient rises from the sitting or supine position. Gravity decreases venous return to the heart, resulting in a decline in left heart filling. The autonomic nervous system is normally able to adjust peripheral resistance, cardiac rate, and contractility so that cardiac output and blood pressure are maintained. However, if the patient is hypovolemic from fluid loss or diuretic therapy, if he has been pharmacologically vasodilated, or if his compensatory autonomic responses are blunted by medication or disease, cardiac output and blood pressure may fall sufficiently to produce presyncopal symptoms. In these patients, a significant drop in blood pressure can usually be demonstrated at the bedside and this procedure will frequently reproduce the patient's symptom complex. The blood pressure should always be checked as the patient goes directly from the supine to the standing position. It is important to note that asymptomatic but demonstrable orthostatic blood pressure changes are common in the elderly. If the patient's history does not suggest orthostatic hypotension and the orthostatic maneuver does not reproduce the symptoms, then the observed fall in blood pressure may not be the cause of the dizziness.

The most common causes of orthostatic hypotension are diuretic and other antihypertensive medications. Other causes of this syndrome include autonomic neuropathy, primary orthostatic hypotension, and Shy–Drager syndrome. Symptomatic orthostatic hypotension from antihypertensive medications should be treated by adjusting the patient's medication regimen. The "neurologic" causes of chronic orthostatic hypotension have several possible treatments. Raising the head of the patient's bed by 30 degrees can be very helpful. Elastic stockings are another simple initial treatment. If these maneuvers do not provide adequate symptomatic relief, then sodium chloride tablets can be added judiciously if they are not contraindicated by hypertension, congestive heart failure, hepatic disease, or renal failure. The mineralocorticoid fludrocortisone acetate can be used in difficult cases. The initial dose is 0.05 mg (half a tablet) three times a week. This may be gradually increased as tolerated. Blood pressure and serum electrolytes must be monitored closely. The new alpha agonist midodrine can also be used in selected patients.

VASODEPRESSOR OR VASOVAGAL PRESYNCOPE

The patient's history is usually diagnostic. The episode of dizziness occurs either in a hot crowded room or in the setting of sudden pain or strong emotion. The patient is always standing and may have premonitory symptoms of yawning, diaphoresis, and pallor. The reduction in blood pressure and cerebral blood flow are caused by sudden, reflux dilation of the resistance arterioles. This syndrome usually occurs in young, otherwise healthy adults but can occur in the elderly. Hot, crowded rooms favor a vasodilation and could produce symptomatic hypotension in an elderly patient with otherwise compensated mild orthostatic hypotension. The only treatments for this syndrome are reassurance and avoidance of the precipitating circumstances.

CARDIAC PRESYNCOPE

Cardiac presyncope is usually caused by an arrhythmia that produces a sudden drop in cardiac output and a subsequent fall in cerebral perfusion. Common offending arrhythmias include sick sinus syndrome, paroxysmal supraventricular tachycardia, atrial fibrillation-flutter, complete heart block, and ventricular tachycardia. This diagnosis should be strongly considered in any patient whose presyncope occurs in the sitting or supine position. Workup includes an electrocardiogram (EKG) and Holter monitoring, although it sometimes requires repeated or prolonged monitoring to document the arrhythmia. Exercise-related presyncope may be caused by aortic stenosis or idiopathic hypertrophic subaortic stenosis (IHSS). An echocardiogram is used for the diagnosis of these conditions. Finally, paroxysmal episodes of lightheadedness and dizziness can be a manifestation of coronary ischemia. These episodes are sometimes called angina equivalents, as the patients may not experience chest pain. This diagnosis should be considered in any patient with unexplained episodes of presyncope and the appropriate risk factors.

CAROTID SINUS HYPERSENSITIVITY

Carotid sinus hypersensitivity is primarily a disorder of the elderly in which the carotid sinus in the neck becomes abnormally sensitive to pressure and produces episodes of bradycardia and reduced cardiac output. Classically, this syndrome was described in men who wore tight collars. However, such a history will not be present in most patients with this disease. It should be suspected in middle-aged or elderly patients with ongoing bouts of presyncope or syncope. The diagnosis is made by carotid massage under strictly controlled conditions (i.e., the presence of a crash cart and personnel skilled in cardiopulmonary resuscitation). The treatment is placement of a permanent pacemaker.

HYPOGLYCEMIA

Although this metabolic derangement does not cause a reduction in cerebral blood flow, its symptom complex is similar to that seen in presyncope, and thus, it should be considered in evaluating patients with episodic dizziness.

Most patients with symptomatic hypoglycemia are insulin-dependent diabetics who either did not consume an adequate caloric load for their insulin dose or took an excessive dose of insulin. Oral hypoglycemic agents are occasionally unpredictable in their action and can produce symptoms of hypoglycemia. Early diabetics who are not yet on therapy can have reactive hypoglycemia from surges of insulin. This typically occurs 2 to 5 hours after eating and is more often manifested by diaphoresis and palpitations than lightheadedness and other "neurologic" symptoms. The diagnosis is made by documenting serum hypoglycemia while the patient is symptomatic. In general, a serum glucose less than 50 mg/dl is necessary to produce CNS symptoms. Insulin-secreting tumors can present with repeated episodes of hypoglycemia.

DISEQUILIBRIUM

After vertigo and presyncope, disequilibrium is the third category of dizziness to consider. Disequilibrium is a common problem in the elderly but can be seen in younger patients after an acute vertigo syndrome or mild head trauma. Unlike the vertigo in presyncope syndromes, the dizziness tends to be more constant and is typically maximal with standing and ambulation. These patients often complain of feeling off balance and are insecure when walking. They tend to reach for walls or furniture when ambulating at home or in the office. They may feel even more uncomfortable when outside.

There are a number of etiologies of disequilibrium and some patients have more than one contributing cause. Before these causes are discussed, a review of the physiology of human balance mechanisms will be presented.

NORMAL MECHANISMS OF EQUILIBRIUM

Gravity and environmental stimuli are constant challenges to bipedal locomotion. Several coordinated events must occur to ensure proper maintenance of an upright posture and smooth ambulation. First, the CNS must get adequate sensory input regarding the position of the head and body in space relative to the earth and the pull of gravity. Second, the CNS must be able to correctly process the sensory input. Third, an appropriate motor response must be mounted to meet the gravitational and environmental challenge. Deficits in one or more of these physiologic functions result in imbalance or disequilibrium.

Four sensory inputs provide information regarding the position of the head and body in space. The most important of these inputs is vision. Visual loss alone (even complete blindness) does not usually produce disequilibrium. However, the visual system is an important compensatory mechanism when there are other sensory or motor deficits. Therefore, visual loss in the setting of such additional deficits can be very disabling for the patient and can produce significant balance difficulties. While visual loss alone does not usually produce disequilibrium, visual distortion often does. Such distortion typically occurs when the visual input from one eye is significantly different from the other.

The vestibular system is the second most important sensory input for balance. It provides information regarding movement and the relationship of the head to the pull of gravity. Acute, unilateral vestibular disturbances produce vertigo, but slowly progressive, bilateral, or healing vestibular lesions produce a disequilibrium syndrome. Position sense or proprioception in the joints and muscles of the lower extremities is the third input necessary for normal balance. Hearing is the fourth sensory modality necessary for normal equilibrium.

PROCESSES THAT DISTURB EQUILIBRIUM

A broad range of diseases can interfere with sensory input, central integration, or motor response and therefore produce disequilibrium. Some patients with this syndrome have disease at only one level. However, many patients have disease at multiple levels or with multiple facets of the same level (i.e., multiple sensory deficits).

ABNORMALITIES OF SENSORY INPUT

As mentioned, diseases that distort vision tend to cause disequilibrium more commonly than those that produce visual loss alone. Many patients with sudden ophthalmoplegia and resultant diplopia feel off balance during ambulation. Some corneal and retinal diseases that produce significant asymmetry of visual input can also produce disequilibrium.

A wide variety of diseases of the vestibular system can produce disequilibrium. As mentioned, many patients recovering from an acute peripheral vestibulopathy will have residual dizziness for as long as several weeks. Likewise, patients with recurrent peripheral vestibular dysfunction, as in Ménière's syndrome, may have persistent disequilibrium between their acute attacks of vertigo and hearing loss. A number of drugs are known vestibulotoxins. Anticonvulsants and benzodiazepines produce reversible vestibular dysfunction. Aminoglycoside antibiotics and cisplatin produce vestibular injury that is often not reversible. These drugs tend to produce a disequilibrium syndrome rather than acute vertigo. Slow-growing neoplasms of the posterior fossa (e.g., acoustic neuroma) may produce a feeling of imbalance as well as hearing loss, facial numbness, and facial weakness. There are a variety of congenital and hereditary vestibular disorders that can produce progressive disequilibrium. Finally, idiopathic degenerative vestibular dysfunction is a recognized cause of disequilibrium in elderly patients.

Peripheral neuropathy can produce proprioceptive loss in the lower extremities and subsequent disequilibrium. This is probably most commonly seen with diabetic polyneuropathy but can result from any cause of peripheral neuropathy. Spinal cord disease, particularly when involving the posterior columns, can produce significant proprioceptive loss in the lower extremities, and subsequent disequilibrium.

Hearing loss alone does not usually produce disequilibrium. However, in the presence of other deficits of sensory input, it can contribute to a patient's feeling of imbalance.

ABNORMALITIES OF CENTRAL INTEGRATION

Any process that produces a global impairment in CNS function can produce disequilibrium. Many patient's complain of dizziness after minor head trauma. This syndrome may be the result of mild, diffuse, cerebral dysfunction from the head injury. Medications, particularly those with sedative side effects, may impair central integration. Likewise, patients with metabolic encephalopathy of any etiology may have a disruption of central integrative processes and disequilibrium.

ABNORMALITIES OF MOTOR RESPONSE

There are three major elements in the human motor system: the pyramidal system, the extrapyramidal system, and the cerebellum. Disturbance in any one of these elements can produce a disequilibrium syn-

drome. Parkinson's disease, a degenerative disorder of the extrapyramidal system, produces bradykinesia, rigidity, flexed posture, and a loss of postural reflexes. Patients with Parkinson's disease occasionally complain of dizziness and feeling off balance because they are unable to mount a smooth motor response to their environmental challenges.

The pyramidal system can be involved with disease at multiple levels. Degenerative frontal lobe dysfunction can produce significant gait apraxia. Likewise, hydrocephalus and frontal lobe neoplasms can interfere with normal motor function. At the spinal level, cervical spondylitic myelopathy is a common cause of lower extremity stiffness and spasticity. All of these syndromes can significantly interfere with gait and cause a feeling of imbalance.

The cerebellum is significantly involved in the coordination of gait and can be affected by a wide variety of disease processes. These would include primary and alcoholic degenerative syndromes, cerebellar neoplasms, paraneoplastic syndromes, cerebellar infarction, and demyelinating disease. Any of these processes can produce a disequilibrium syndrome.

DIAGNOSTIC EVALUATION IN PATIENTS WITH DISEQUILIBRIUM

A review of the patient's medication regimen and a careful neurologic examination are the first steps in the evaluation of these patients. Medications that are vestibulotoxins should be discontinued if possible. Likewise, medications with significant sedative side effects should be reduced in dosage or discontinued.

If the patient offers complaints that suggest visual distortion, then an ophthalmologic evaluation should be obtained. A history of hearing loss or tinnitus should be sought. The unilateral presence of these symptoms should lead to a posterior fossa evaluation by MRI. Most patients who have had an acute peripheral vestibulopathy with vertigo will provide that history, but all patients with disequilibrium should be quizzed about past episodes of vertigo.

A careful and complete neurologic examination should be performed in all patients with disequilibrium. Proprioceptive function in the feet can be tested by having the patient close his eyes while the examiner moves the first toe of each foot up or down. The patient should be able to appreciate movements of 1 cm or less. The Romberg maneuver is a test of proprioceptive function in the lower extremities. However, this test can also be abnormal in patients with cerebellar or vestibular disease. Tone should be carefully tested in all extremities. The presence of cogwheel rigidity suggests the presence of an extrapyramidal syndrome. Spasticity in the lower extremities suggest either a spinal cord or frontal lobe dysfunction. These syndromes are usually associated with hyperactive deep tendon reflexes and bilateral Babinski signs. Observing the patient's gait is probably the most important part of the examination. Parkinson's disease produces a shuffling gait with a flexed posture and reduced movements in the upper extremities. Frontal lobe dysfunction produces a stiff gait with short steps. The patient may have difficulty initiating steps or getting through doorways. Feet may appear stuck to the floor. Spinal cord disorders tend to produce a spastic gait. Cerebellar disorders typically produce a wide-based, often staggering gait.

Patients with frontal lobe dysfunction will need either a CT or an MRI scan of the brain. Patients with cerebellar syndrome should be evaluated by MRI, as CT is not reliable for imaging of the posterior fossa. Patients with spinal cord syndromes require MRI scan of the cervical spine. All patients with frontal lobe or cerebellar dysfunction require a thyroid battery to rule out hypothyroidism.

THERAPY FOR DISEQUILIBRIUM

Patients with Parkinson's disease can be effectively treated with dopaminergic agents that can improve their gait and reduce the feeling of disequilibrium. There is no definitive therapy for the degenerative frontal lobe disorders. Patients with hydrocephalus can potentially be treated with ventricular shunting. Frontal lobe and cerebellar neoplasms can often be effectively treated with surgical excision. Alcohol cerebellar degeneration may improve somewhat with abstinence. Paraneoplastic cerebellar degeneration has been reported to improve after treatment of the underlying neoplasm. Cervical spondylitic myelopathy can potentially improve with surgical decompression.

Patients with peripheral neuropathy may improve with the use of a light cane, which can provide some adjunctive proprioceptive input through the hand. Patients with degenerative vestibular disorders sometimes benefit from the use of a soft cervical collar (best worn with the Velcro clasp in front). By reducing head movement, this modality dampens aberrant vestibular input.

Patients who are experiencing disequilibrium after an acute vestibular syndrome, with a chronic vestibular syndrome such as Ménière's disease, with drug-induced vestibular toxicity, or after an episode of minor head trauma, may experience benefit from vestibular exercises. These can be performed in the home or anywhere that a straight walkway 20 to 30 feet in length can be found. The patient begins the exercise by walking. The feet should be spread wide apart and the arms should be outstretched laterally and parallel to the floor. The patient should walk up and down the walkway, narrowing the distance between the feet with each pass until the balls of the feet touch with each step. The procedure is then repeated with the arms held tightly at the side. It is then performed a third time with the arms outstretched in front of the patient, parallel to the floor. When this procedure is completed the whole exercise is repeated with the eyes closed. The entire procedure should take 20 to 30 minutes and should be performed twice a day.

Finally, Meclizine is often used to treat patients with the various disequilibrium syndromes. With the exception of an occasional patient with a chronic vestibular disorder, this drug is ineffective and may actually exacerbate the disequilibrium for some patients by its sedative side effects.

QUESTIONS AND DISCUSSION

1. J. D. is a 42-year-old man who experienced the sudden onset of vertigo, nausea, vomiting, and ataxia 3 weeks ago. The vertigo, nausea, and vomiting resolved in 48 hours, but the patient still complains bitterly of "dizziness" and states that he cannot go back to work because "I walk like a drunk." When questioned, he admits that his dizziness is present only when he is standing or walking and seems to resolve when he is sitting or supine. He denies hearing loss and tinnitus. There is no associated visual blurring, diaphoresis, or pallor. His neurologic examination is normal except that he tends to veer to the right when walking. How would this patient's current symptom of dizziness be categorized?

A. Vertigo
B. Presyncope
C. Disequilibrium
D. Malingering
E. Not classifiable

The answer is (C). The patient's syndrome began with vertigo. However, it has converted to a disequilibrium syndrome. This is a common sequela to acute vestibulopathy, caused by a residual mismatch between the input from the paired vestibular systems. The symptoms usually resolve over several weeks and recovery is often hastened with the use of vestibular exercises.

2. S. T. is a 28-year-old woman who complains of a 2-week history of "everything is spinning around." The episodes are precipitated by any type of head movement in the horizontal or vertical plane. The vertigo begins immediately with each head movement. The patient denies hearing loss and tinnitus but does recall a 2-week episode of "numbness" below her waist about 3 months ago. When she was asked to follow the examiner's finger with her eyes, coarse horizontal nystagmus was noted on lateral gaze bilaterally and vertical nystagmus was present on upgaze. Her neurologic examination was otherwise remarkable only for questionable bilateral Babinski signs. The most likely diagnosis is:

A. Depression
B. Benign paroxysmal positional vertigo
C. Ménière's disease
D. Multiple sclerosis
E. Perilymph fistula

The answer is (D). This patient's symptoms are typical of movement-related vertigo, a nonspecific symptom that can be seen in any vestibular disorder. The multidirection, pure horizontal, or pure vertical nystagmus that is not suppressed by fixation is essentially diagnostic of a central vestibular disorder. The history of transient neurologic symptoms in the lower extremities would make multiple sclerosis a strong diagnostic consideration. The position-related vertigo of benign paroxysmal positional vertigo is usually produced by a single head position, there is a latency of several seconds to the onset of vertigo, and the vertigo tends to fatigue with repeated trials. Ménière's disease can be associated with movement-related vertigo, but there is also a history of hearing loss and tinnitus. Finally, in both benign paroxysmal positional vertigo and Ménière's disease, the nystagmus would have characteristics of peripheral vestibular disease (i.e., unidirectional, mixed, and suppressed by fixation).

3. H. L. is a 69-year-old man who complains of "dizzy spells." The patient describes 10 to 12 episodes in the last 6 weeks of sudden visual "blackout" and feeling "like I'm going to pass out." His wife notes that he breaks out in a cold sweat during the attacks and looks "glassy-eyed." The episodes last 30 to 60 seconds and the patient feels "fine" afterward. There is no history of vertigo, hearing loss, tinnitus, or other focal neurologic symptoms. The spells are not related to body position or exercise and have occurred in many different situations including watching TV and eating in a restaurant. The patient's neurologic examination is

normal, and 3 minutes of hyperventilation reproduces his symptom complex. The patient's dizziness should be categorized as:

A. Vertigo
B. Presyncope
C. Disequilibrium
D. Vertebrobasilar insufficiency
E. Hypoglycemia

The answer is (B). The patient's symptoms are typical of those caused by globally diminished cerebral perfusion. Vertebrobasilar insufficiency causes focal areas of ischemia and focal neurologic symptoms. The episodes are too brief and too discreet for hypoglycemic attacks.

What is the most likely etiology of this patient's presyncope?

A. Hyperventilation syndrome
B. Vasovagal attacks
C. Orthostatic hypotension
D. Cardiac arrhythmia
E. Aortic stenosis

The answer is (D). Hyperventilation should reproduce the symptom complex in all patients with presyncope so the diagnosis of hyperventilation syndrome must be made by other criteria (i.e., the situations of stress or anxiety in which it typically occurs). Vasovagal or vasodepressor attacks are also situational (i.e., hot, crowded room or sudden emotion) and always occur when the patient is upright. Likewise, orthostatic hypotension occurs only when the patient is standing. The aortic stenosis produces exercise-related presyncope. Most patients with type II symptoms that occur when sitting or supine have a cardiac arrhythmia.

4. Which of the following conditions can produce disequilibrium?

A. Chronic renal failure
B. Diabetes mellitus
C. Aminoglycoside antibiotic toxicity
D. Spondylitic cervical myelopathy
E. All are correct.

The answer is (E); all four conditions can produce disequilibrium. Chronic renal failure is associated with peripheral neuropathy that diminishes sensory input from the lower extremities. In addition, the metabolic encephalopathy of uremia may inhibit proper central integration of the sensory modalities required for balance and thus exacerbate the feeling of disequilibrium. Diabetes mellitus is also associated with a peripheral neuropathy. In addition, this disease is also frequently complicated by retinopathy, which decreases input from the most important sensory modality for balance. Aminoglycoside antibiotics can damage the vestibular portion of the eighth cranial nerve and produce a disequilibrium syndrome. Cervical spinal cord compression can decrease sensory input from the lower extremities and cause spasticity, which impedes the proper motor response for balance and ambulation. Parkinson's disease also prevents a smooth motor response and, therefore, can cause a disequilibrium syndrome.

SUGGESTED READING

Baloh RW: The Essentials of Neurology. Philadelphia, FA Davis, 1984

Baloh RW, Halmagyi GM: Disorders of the Vestibular System. New York, Oxford University Press, 1996

Baloh RW, Honrubia V: Clinical Neurophysiology of the Vestibular System, 2nd Edition. Philadelphia, FA Davis, 1990

Baloh RW, Honrubia V, Jacobson K: Benign positional vertigo: Clinical and oculographic features in 240 cases. Neurology 37:371, 1987

Brandt T: Vertigo and dizziness. In: Asbury AK, McKhann GM, McDonald WI (eds): Diseases of the Nervous System: Clinical Neurobiology, 561. Philadelphia, WB Saunders, 1986

Brandt T, Daroff RB: The multisensory physiological and pathological vertigo syndromes. Ann Neurol 7:195, 1980

Brandt T, Daroff RB: Physical therapy for benign paroxysmal positional vertigo. Arch Otolaryngol 106:484, 1980

Drachman DA, Hart CW: An approach to the dizzy patient. Neurology 22:323, 1972

Epley JM: The canalith repositioning procedure for treatment of benign paroxysmal positional vertigo. Otolaryngol Head Neck Surg 107:399, 1992

Epley JM: Particle repositioning for BPPV. Otolaryngol Clin North Am 29:323, 1996

Harner SG: Clinical findings in patients with acoustic neuroma. Mayo Clin Proc 58:721, 1983

Hotson JR, Baloh RW: Current concepts: Acute vestibular syndrome. N Engl J Med 339:680 1998

Jonas S, Klein I, Diment J: Importance of Holter monitoring in patients with periodic cerebral symptoms. Ann Neurol 1:470, 1977

Kaplan LR: Posterior circulation disease: Clinical findings, diagnosis and management. Boston, Blackwell Science, 1996

Lipsitz LA: Syncope in the elderly. Ann Intern Med 99:92, 1983

Nelson RL: Hypoglycemia: Fact or fiction? Mayo Clin Proc 60:844, 1985

Norrving B, Magnusson M, Holtas S: Isolated vertigo in the elderly: Vestibular or vascular disease? Acta Neurol Scand 91:43, 1995

Troost TB: Dizziness and vertigo in vertebrobasilar disease. Stroke 11:301, 1980

Zee DS: Vertigo. In: Johnson RT (ed): Current Therapy in Neurologic Disease, 8. St. Louis, CV Mosby, 1985

Neurology for the Non-Neurologist, Fourth Edition, edited by William J. Weiner and Christopher G. Goetz. Lippincott Williams & Wilkins, Philadelphia © 1999.

C H A P T E R 1 5

Behavioral Neurology

Christopher G. Goetz
Robert S. Wilson

Bizarre or altered behavioral patterns are traditionally felt to relate to psychiatric disorders or generalized delirium from drugs, toxins, or metabolic imbalances. However, some specific neurologic conditions present with remarkably consistent behavioral abnormalities. These conditions have equally consistent anatomic substrates and, when identified by an astute diagnostician, they suggest specific causes and treatments. In this chapter, five conditions are discussed, each with a prominent behavioral and seemingly psychiatric presentation, but with a pathologic basis related to a specific neurologic dysfunction. These conditions are temporal lobe epilepsy, fluent aphasia, Wernicke's encephalopathy, transient global amnesia, and herpes encephalitis.

These strange disorders are not rare, and their complexity often relates not to management problems but instead to accurate identification. The topic is thus particularly pertinent to the non-neurologist, who is most likely to be the first person to interview and evaluate these patients.

ANATOMIC BASIS—PAPEZ CIRCUIT

It is well recognized that the ability to recall and engender memories is intimately linked to the emotional makeup of such memories. Furthermore, several clinical conditions demonstrate combined and prominent memory–emotional alterations, suggest-

ing that the anatomic basis of these two functions may be linked. In 1937, the neuroanatomist Papez published a treatise describing an anatomic circuit that linked those nuclei and paths that appear important to many aspects of emotional–behavioral integration. This circuit, the *Papez circuit,* is probably the most important circuit for clinicians dealing with behavioral abnormalities; familiarity with it allows them to think systematically about the anatomic foundations of behavioral neurology.

The circuit is schematically diagrammed in Figure 15-1 **A**, with anatomic nuclei and paths identified in the sagittal brain section of Figure 15-1 **B**. As indicated, the pathway is circular, providing continual reintegration of information. The two focal cortical areas most prominently involved are the cingulate cortex and the hippocampus of the temporal lobe. Diffuse cortical impulses travel into the hippocampus, an area felt to be particularly important to memory and emotional expression. This information travels forward in the fornix path to the mammillary bodies of the hypothalamus and continues to the anterior lobe of the thalamus, and further to the midline cingulate cortex, which finally projects diffusely to cortical regions.

Familiarity with this circuit is useful, since disease anywhere along the pathway can be expected to result in aberrant emotional behaviors, although not necessarily the same patterns. This knowledge allows the clinician to focus immediately on a finite number

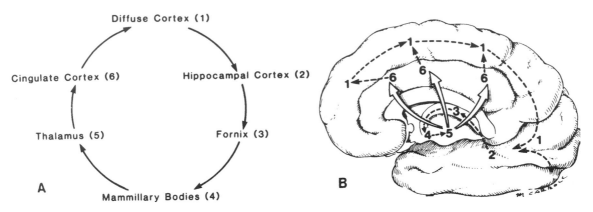

FIG. 15-1. Papez circuit. **A.** Schematic diagram of brain regions connected by the Papez circuit. **B.** Anatomic diagram of brain regions numbered in **A**, with *arrows* indicating the direction of general informational flow.

of nuclei and connecting paths to explain abnormal behavioral symptoms that may have a focal anatomic basis. The term *diffuse cortical input* is important, because toxic and metabolic encephalopathy often present with agitated behavior or a change in personality. The other areas, however, are focal, and identification of disease at these levels can lead to rapid intervention. Reference will be made to this circuit throughout this chapter.

TEMPORAL LOBE EPILEPSY

Also referred to as psychomotor epilepsy and partial complex seizure, psychomotor or psychosensory variety, temporal lobe epilepsy (TLE) may manifest itself with intermittent spells of bizarre behavior, including babbling nonsense and frank visual and auditory hallucinations, all related to organic disease of the central nervous system (CNS). Differentiation of this disorder from psychotic disorders such as schizophrenia can be difficult, and yet it is essential because their treatments are drastically different. Certain specific characteristics are helpful in establishing abnormal behavioral patterns as probable epilepsy, and they are the focus of this discussion.

Temporal lobe epilepsy represents an abnormal electrical discharge that begins in one temporal lobe and usually crosses rapidly to involve both sides of the brain. To recognize TLE in a patient, the clinician should attempt to elicit specific information in four

areas. If information in even one of these areas is characteristic of TLE, the diagnosis is suggested.

1. The distinctive temporal pattern of the spells
2. The presence of an aura
3. The presence of peculiar motor behaviors called *automatisms*
4. The specific type of loss of consciousness

The distinctive temporal pattern of TLE refers to repeated, but intermittent, and paroxysmal changes in behavior, not necessarily linked to any emotional provocation. The behavioral changes are brief, lasting seconds to minutes. Often, before any visible behavioral change can be appreciated by an observer, the patient experiences a stereotypic and fixed sensation, known as an *epileptic aura*. The aura represents the beginning of the seizure and can help in localizing the focus, or source, of the seizure activity. The aura may be olfactory, in which the patient suddenly smells a strange, often pungent odor, or it may be a gustatory sensation, or a strange abdominal "butterflies" feeling, also called *epigastric rising*. Emotional changes of sudden unfamiliarity with one's environment, "jamais vu," or sudden intense familiarity with the surroundings, "déjà vu," are seen, and there may be intense and vivid auditory or visual hallucinations. The aura and the area of the temporal lobe cortex that are felt to relate to the seizure focus are listed in Table 15-1. The presence of this stereotypic aura and sudden unprovoked change in behavior help to quickly identify a TLE patient. The aura is sensed by

TABLE 15-1. Temporal Lobe Foci and Related Auras

FOCUS	AURA
Uncus	Smell, taste
Cingulate cortex	Change in emotional perception—déjà vu, jamais vu, euphoria, sense of sudden doom
Insula	Epigastric rising sensation
Amygdala	Pupillary dilatation, photophobia, automatisms
Association temporal cortex	Auditory, visual hallucinations

the patient and is not identified by the clinician except by interview. The patient may not necessarily link the strange aura to his spells, so that information must be specifically solicited.

The presence of automatisms is also useful in the diagnosis of TLE. These activities appear as the seizure spreads in the amygdala region of the temporal lobe. The movements may range from rather primitive movements (lip smacking, eye blinking, or chewing motions) or may be highly complex (dressing and undressing, piling objects on top of one another). These are stereotypic and rather fixed from one spell to another, so a detailed record of two or more episodes helps to establish the pattern of behavior.

The peculiar characteristic of the loss of consciousness seen TLE is also helpful. After the aura, which the examiner cannot see unless it involves automatisms, there is a sudden loss of contact with the environment. Unlike patients who have other generalized seizures, these patients only rarely fall to the floor, shake all over, urinate, or bite their tongue. Instead, when they lose consciousness, they maintain body tone and may walk around, but "in a daze, out of contact" with the environment. When the spell is over, the patient is usually amnestic for the seizure, except that he may recall its beginning and be able to recount, if specifically asked, the details of the aura. Immediately after the spell, the patient is usually confused and sleepy. If restrained during this period, he may strike out randomly at people who try to assist. However, these patients are generally not violent in a goal-directed manner, either during or after their seizures. As strange as their behaviors may be, focused violence, such as tracking a person with a gun or retrieving a kitchen knife out of a drawer and stabbing a victim, is far outside the repertoire of TLE.

Two specific examples will help to delineate the methods used in diagnosing TLE.

Case 1 A quiet 34-year-old right-handed woman is admitted for observation after she suffered head trauma on a city bus. She was the cause of an unpro-

voked fist fight on the bus and reports, "They said I did it but I don't remember a thing."

The question is whether this patient suffers from (1) head trauma with retrograde amnesia, (2) socially deviant behavior, claiming ignorance to avoid responsibility, or (3) amnesia and bizarre behavior related to TLE. To differentiate TLE from the other two disorders, the interview focuses on the characteristics of TLE.

In discussing this event with the patient, it is found that this is only one of many violent episodes in this woman's life. The episodes are similar in that she cannot understand why she gets into fights, being a quiet, shy person, and she says that the events are never precipitated by an argument. She says she has no warning and that "that's all I remember." However, when specifically asked about smells, taste, sounds, and visions, she states that she usually starts thinking of a peculiar tune that always recurs in her head before a fight and makes her nervous for those last few seconds. It is important to note that this major clue is gleaned only with specific questioning.

When the victim of the fight, who is in the next hospital room, is interviewed, he comments that he and the patient were sitting quietly in the bus when suddenly the patient started fidgeting in her purse, picking at items, and smacking her lips loudly. She then started walking around the bus babbling noises and picking at her clothes. The bus was crowded and the patient bumped into several passengers. A minute later, she seemed to start swinging randomly at people. The man was hit in the head, fell over, and hit his face on the bus seat. As they were both taken to the hospital, this man noticed that the belligerent woman seemed now considerably confused and sleepy.

The characteristic aura, the paroxysmal quality of the repeated episodes by history, and the automatisms of lip smacking and clothes picking with amnesia all suggest TLE. An electroencephalogram (EEG) demonstrated epilepsy, and anticonvulsant medications have virtually abolished the episodes.

Case 2 A 16-year-old boy on the psychiatric unit with a diagnosis of schizophrenia and hallucinatory behavior is evaluated by the neurologist because of a single generalized seizure. On being interviewed, this patient says, "It's just like before, but this time much worse." Several times each week this patient sees "the man," a blurry but discernible bearded man who silently beckons him forward verbally. As this happens, everything in the patient's environment becomes suddenly more distinct, clearer, and more colorful, with a clear sense of familiarity and warmth. Then a strange feeling of dread and a "fog" come over the patient, who then appears to lose touch for approximately 5 minutes. He has no recollection of this period of losing touch, but the family says that he walks around in the house mumbling strange noises that are sometimes prayers, and at the same time he bows his head back and forth in a seemingly ritualistic manner. After this, he lies down and sleeps for approximately 2 hours. The same stereotypic pattern occurred immediately before the generalized seizure.

This patient again shows the stereotypic aura, which is hallucinatory this time, along with the sense of emotional familiarly with the environment. Stereotypic repetition of episodes and the automatisms with amnesia and sleepiness afterward strongly suggest TLE. In regard to this latter episode in which there was a generalized motor seizure with bilateral shaking, this pattern can be seen with TLE when the seizure activity spreads throughout both sides of the brain. An EEG study with nasopharyngeal recordings demonstrated abnormal epileptiform activity. On medication the patient has shown remarkable improvement. This case demonstrates the important interface between psychiatric symptoms and clear focal neurologic disease.

Table 15-2 serves as a summary and outlines additional guidelines for differentiating TLE episodes from psychotic bizarre behaviors of schizophrenia.

These patterns are clinically useful, although no absolute rules hold true.

ANATOMY AND CLINICAL FINDINGS

The anatomic lesions of TLE naturally relate to the temporal lobe and, depending on the area damaged, will give rise to different auras (see Table 15-1). As can be seen, some of these nuclei are primary portions of the Papez circuit, and the others have direct input into the circuit.

In examining a patient with TLE, static findings may include a homonymous hemianopia, or a homonymous quadrantanopsia, especially in the superior fields (Fig. 15-2). Because these fibers pass through the temporal lobe *en route* to the occipital cortex, the superior quadrantanopsia should be specifically sought.

Much has been written about psychopathology in TLE patients. Although the seizures and bizarre behavior are intermittent, interictal or between-seizure abnormalities are often attributed to TLE. Problems such as sedation, inattention, and depressed mood may be seen as dose-related side effects of antiepileptic medications. If toxicity can be ruled out, the most common psychiatric problem in epilepsy is depression. Although not specific to TLE, research suggests rates of depression as high as 75% in some clinical samples. Paradoxically, depression may appear after seizure control is accomplished, suggesting that seizures, like electroconvulsive therapy (ECT), may serve to elevate mood, possibly through opioid mechanisms.

Aggressive behavior is often attributed to TLE. There is, however, no good evidence of a disproportionate level of aggressive or violent behavior in TLE or epilepsy. Aggressive behavior may be seen following a seizure, but it is typically nondirected and random, occurring when the patient is aroused or restrained. The hypothesis that TLE is characterized by a distinct personality profile has not been sup-

TABLE 15-2. Clinical Distinctions between TLE Behavior and Schizophrenia

	TLE	SCHIZOPHRENIA
Environmental precipitants	Rare	Frequent
Duration of attack	0.5–5 min	May be days
Aura	Usual	Lacking
Injury to others	Rare and undirected	Unpredictable—may be directed or undirected
Disturbance of consciousness	Present	Lacking or only mind-clouding
Symptoms and signs after attack	Sleepy, confused	Lacking

TLE = temporal lobe epilepsy.

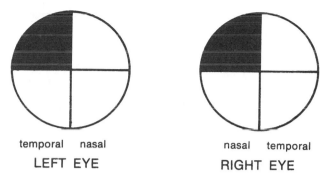

temporal nasal

LEFT EYE

nasal temporal

RIGHT EYE

FIG. 15-2. Visual field defect associated with right temporal lobe disease, termed *left superior quadrantanopsia.*

ported by recent research. On the other hand, psychiatric signs and symptoms in general are more commonly seen in TLE than in other forms of epilepsy, particularly in patients with severe, uncontrolled TLE.

ETIOLOGY

Temporal lobe epilepsy is often seen in patients with a history of birth trauma. Brain tumors, both primary and metastatic, may also involve the temporal lobe and present early with characteristic TLE. Subacute onset of TLE with fever should suggest encephalitis, specifically resulting from herpes simplex, which has a predilection for the temporal lobes. EEG findings are discussed in Chapter 8. Drugs useful in the control of TLE are listed in Table 15-3, along with usual doses, plasma levels, and common side effects.

FLUENT APHASIA

Aphasia is a specific language deficit that occurs without weakness of the articulatory muscles, and it is caused by cortical brain disease. The two basic types of aphasia are subfluent and fluent. The former group is not difficult to diagnose and would not be confused with psychiatric disease, since in most cases an obvious right hemiparesis accompanies the change in speech pattern. The fluent aphasias, however, are not associated with motor problems, so that these patients present with behavioral alterations in the form of strange speech. The adage taught to young neurologists, that when evaluating an acute behavioral change, one must always rule out fluent aphasia, is applicable to all clinicians.

Aphasic problems occur with focal dominant hemisphere disorders. For most people, the left hemi-

TABLE 15-3. Drugs Used in the Control of TLE: Dosages, Therapeutic Plasma Levels, and Common or Important Side Effects

DRUG	USUAL DAILY ADULT DOSAGE (mg)	PLASMA LEVEL (μ/mL)	TOXICITY
Carbamazepine*	600–1200	4–10	Agranulocytosis, nausea, vomiting, sedation, ataxia
Phenytoin	300	10–20	Lymphadenopathy, nausea, vomiting, sedation, vitamin K and folate deficiency, ataxia
Valproic acid*	750–1500	50–150	Nausea, vomiting, sedation, elevated liver enzymes, ataxia
Lamotrigine	300–700	2–15	Dizziness, diplopia, headache, ataxia
Phenobarbitol	90–180	15–40	Sedation, hyperactivity in children, vitamin K deficiency, ataxia
Gabapentin	750–1000	4–8	Somnolence, dizziness, ataxia
Primidone*	20–60	7–15 primidone 20–40 phenobarbital	Lymphadenopathy, nausea, vomiting, sedation, ataxia

* Indicates drug preferentially recommended for TLE as opposed to other forms of seizures.

sphere is dominant for speech, although in a small percentage of left-handed persons the right hemisphere may be dominant. Subfluent aphasias relate to frontal lobe disease, and fluent aphasias relate usually to dominant temporal or temporoparietal damage. Since the temporal lobe is involved in the Papez circuit, behavioral alterations in fluent aphasias are expected and characteristic.

In contrast to the frustration and depressed affect common in subfluent aphasia, fluent aphasics are often seemingly unaware of their deficit and unconcerned. Patients may not realize that their speech is incomprehensible to others. In extreme cases, these patients may blame their inability to communicate on others to the point of frank paranoia. Impulsivity is also observed. The combination of such behaviors can result in serious management problems.

The evaluation of aphasia is usually rapid and requires no unusual implements. Table 15-4 outlines the manner of examination, which has three focal points. First, by listening to the patient's spontaneous speech, the clinician decides whether the speech is subfluent, slow, and sparse, or fluent, rapid, and free flowing. This evaluation makes no judgment on content of speech but instead on rhythm and ease of word production. Second, the examiner asks the patient to follow a verbal command—"Show me a spoon," "Raise your left hand," and so forth, testing his ability to comprehend. This integration of auditory information helps to distinguish various aphasias and localizes the disease. The command must be verbal, and the investigator must discipline himself not to use nonverbal communication during this task. Third, the patient is asked to repeat a sentence—first a reasonable phrase, such as "Today is Tuesday; tomorrow I will phone Bill," and then a nonsense phrase such as "No ifs, ands, or buts." These three simple maneuvers can be performed by confused or intoxicated patients and by patients with short atten-

tion spans. However, they are not performed by aphasics. Furthermore, the pattern of disability in the three tasks isolates the specific areas of dominant cortical dysfunction.

The patient who is usually diagnosed as confused, agitated, and often schizophrenic is the patient with a Wernicke's aphasia (not to be confused with Wernicke's encephalopathy, which is discussed in the next section).

The following case history helps to typify this syndrome, and it emphasizes the common confusion between this condition and the word salad of schizophrenia.

Case 3 A 65-year-old hypertensive right-handed woman was well until 3 hours before an evaluation in the emergency room. Her family lived with her and reported that after lunch the patient took a 40-minute nap; upon awaking, she "began speaking nonsense—crazy talk." Her past medical and psychiatric history was negative, and no similar events had ever occurred.

The patient is alert and talkative, but her speech has no discernible sense. Phrases such as "oh, me, why not, should we, what now, amen Moses" are spoken rapidly and spontaneously. She can follow no verbal commands nor will she repeat simple phrases. The family feels she may be poisoned or has gone crazy.

The highlights of this case are the patient's age, the acute onset, the characteristic speech pattern, and the easily retrieved results of an accurate aphasia testing screen. Importantly, in a patient who is 65 years old without prior psychiatric history, the new onset of schizophrenia, regardless of how bizarre the behavior or speech may be, would be exceptional.

ETIOLOGY

Wernicke's fluent aphasia is usually seen with dominant temporal lobe disease in the form of cere-

TABLE 15-4. Major Types of Aphasia with Guides to Their Rapid Identification

NAMES	FLUENCY	FOLLOW COMMANDS	REPEAT	FOCAL DAMAGE	ASSOCIATIVE PROBLEMS
Broca's	Subfluent	Yes	No	Dominant frontal lobe	Right hemiparesis
Wernicke's	Fluent	No	No	Dominant temporal lobe	Visual field abnormalities, no weakness
Conductive	Fluent	Yes	Yes for short phrases; cannot repeat "no-ifs, ands, or buts"	Dominant connecting fibers between Broca's and Wernicke's area	Visual field abnormalities or mild weakness, decreased sensation on right side of body and face

brovascular accidents or sometimes tumors. The rapid onset in an elderly individual suggests the former, whereas a more indolent course can be seen with tumors. When this speech pattern is encountered, the clinician should immediately focus attention on the dominant temporal lobe. Associated findings often include the superior quadrantanopsia (see Fig. 15-2), and temporal lobe seizures may be an associated phenomenon.

The other fluent aphasia, conduction aphasia, does not appear to be a psychiatric illness; thus it will not be discussed in detail. These patients speak fluently and usually make sense, except that they mix up words or make new words (paraphasic errors). Although they can repeat simple sentences, they have trouble with nonsense phrases like "no ifs, ands, or buts." This disease localizes to the arcuate fasciculus of the parietal lobe connecting the temporal and frontal speech areas. Strokes and tumors are again the likely causes, although sometimes Wernicke's aphasia, as it resolves, tends to become a conduction aphasia. Anomic aphasia, in which the patient is fluent and behaviorally appropriate but has trouble finding the proper word, is seen as other forms of aphasia resolve.

WERNICKE–KORSAKOFF'S SYNDROME

Wernicke–Korsakoff's syndrome, also known as Wernicke's encephalopathy–Korsakoff's psychosis, represents a neurologic emergency. The important triad of Wernicke's encephalopathy is behavioral alterations, extraocular movement abnormalities, and ataxia. These symptoms occur to a greater or lesser extent with a selective memory impairment, and when this memory impairment is marked, the syndrome is called Korsakoff's psychosis. The two diseases are the same but are referred to with different terms depending on the degree of memory deficit. The pathogenesis of this syndrome relates to vitamin deficiency in the form of vitamin B_1, or thiamine. Patients at high risk for this syndrome are, first, alcoholics who obtain calories through the alcohol but do not receive essential vitamins. Patients with prolonged emesis or with gastric bowel resection can also suffer with thiamine deficiency. Occasionally, voluntary starvation in the form of political protest, psychotic disturbances, or unsupervised treatment of obesity can also induce this syndrome. Finally, and important to surgical patients, hyperalimentation can be associated with Wernicke's encephalopathy when water-soluble B vitamins are not included in the formula.

The behavioral picture of Wernicke's encephalopathy–Korsakoff's psychosis ranges among three different presentations. The patient with acute Wernicke's encephalopathy shows global confusion and his demeanor is usually quiet and apathetic. He is alert and responsive, but inattentive, and he appears fatigued. Occasionally, a patient may be more agitated, especially if he is undergoing delirium tremens associated with alcohol withdrawal. The usual presentation, however, is one of an affable but dull affect.

In the partially treated patient or in the early stages of chronic disease, the affect becomes more bright, and the patient becomes more loquacious. The memory deficits become more apparent as the patient is less globally confused. He is nonhesitant in his speech, and it is at this point that the famed confabulatory aspects of Korsakoff's psychosis may be seen. Confabulation is not an essential component of Korsakoff's psychosis; the characteristic trait of this condition is the preferential loss of recent memory.

The patient with chronic Wernicke–Korsakoff's syndrome is typically alert and oriented but displays characteristic deficiencies in recent and remote memory. The recent memory deficit is usually profound and consists of an inability to make an enduring record of daily experiences. The remote memory deficit is temporally graded such that more remote events are relatively more accessible to recall. Thus, a patient asked to name presidents since World War II may recall Truman and Eisenhower but not their successors. Confabulation is not typically seen in chronic patients. Behaviorally, such patients are usually apathetic and indifferent, with occasional outbursts of irritability.

In diagnosing this syndrome, the neurologic signs of extraocular muscle palsy or nystagmus and ataxia are important features to recognize. In many ways, the patient with acute Wernicke's encephalopathy looks like a drunkard, in that he has trouble walking; he may have nystagmus from the alcohol itself; and he has an altered affect. Because of the similarity, it is a common adage that a patient seen in the emergency room who is drunk should be given an injection of thiamine (1) to treat possible Wernicke's encephalopathy and (2) to prevent a future episode of the condition. The chronic patient is difficult to manage because, although the extraocular movements improve quickly with thiamine therapy and the ataxia improves to a moderate extent, the memory problems are least abated by thiamine therapy. There has been new interest in the treatment of memory deficits with presumed cholinergic precursors such as lecithin or choline chloride, but these agents have not been tested extensively. The dose of thiamine given is usually 50 mg intravenously (IV) and 50 mg intramuscularly (IM) or 100 mg IM. B vitamins should be continued orally until the patient resumes a normal diet.

ANATOMIC BASIS

The unifying basis for this disorder involves the Papez circuit where there is capillary proliferation at the level of the mammillary bodies. In some cases in which the mammillary bodies are spared, the anterior lobe of the thalamus is involved. Additional pathologic findings may involve cerebellar and diffuse cortical degeneration. Although the clinical picture of Korsakoff's psychosis should immediately suggest vitamin deficiency and disease that at least includes the mammillary bodies, it can be seen in diseases that involve other aspects of the Papez circuit. The same syndrome has been reported in patients who recover from a viral encephalitis with prominent hippocampus involvement. Such clinical overlap again emphasizes the importance of the Papez circuit in localizing diseases that involve both memory and affective disorders.

TRANSIENT GLOBAL AMNESIA

The syndrome of transient global amnesia occurs in middle-aged or elderly patients who usually have diabetes or hypertension, or who are at high risk for cerebrovascular disease. Physical or emotional stress often precedes the amnestic episode.

When the spell has begun, the patient is unable to learn new information until it is over. His memory for events that day and the preceding day are almost always poor. Memory for prior events will be better, although memory losses will sometimes be detectable even for events that took place years before the amnestic spell. The syndrome is transient and clears completely within 24 hours, except for a permanent amnesia for the episode itself. Significantly, the patient's affect is often bland during the episode, although family members are distressed.

These patients are often brought to medical attention when the family notes that they repeatedly ask the same questions and seem unable to remember the answer and sometimes deny that an answer has been given. At the same time, these patients may perform complex tasks during an episode without difficulty, as long as these tasks were learned prior to the event.

These patients are not globally confused. In testing orientation, however, they may report the wrong answer because they cannot integrate changes in place and time. When asked to do arithmetic calculations or use logical processing, they respond appropriately.

Memory testing during an attack demonstrates a marked inability to establish new memories despite preserved attention, language, and higher cognitive functioning. If the physician leaves the room of a patient with this disorder, he will have to reintroduce himself when he returns. Recent memory function is deficient in such patients regardless of which sensory system is employed in the memory tasks, so that visual, tactile, and auditory memories are disturbed. The retrograde amnesia is such that the activities of the previous days may be only dimly recollected during the episode. The retrograde amnesia is occasionally more extensive, affecting memories formed years before the episode. Confabulation is notably lacking in these patients. Upon recovery, there is no recollection of the episode itself, and there is typically a permanent retrograde amnesia for events occurring in the hour or so prior to the episode.

This syndrome with its peculiar constellation of memory and behavioral features can be highly confusing unless it is recognized.

The anatomic basis for transient global amnesia is felt to relate to poor vascular perfusion to the posterior and undersurfaces of the temporal lobes by the vertebral basilar vessels. In this sense, it is a transient ischemic attack in almost all instances, although the prognosis for these patients has been said to be better than for those with other forms of transient ischemic attacks. Associated vertebral basilar symptoms, such as vertigo, nausea, and mild ataxia, may accompany this syndrome, but they clear quickly. Because this syndrome is so often a single episode without recurrence, it is important to identify it as such.

On the other hand, the additional features of impaired cognition (orientation, language, judgment), other focal neurologic signs or symptoms observed during or following the episode, or epileptic features or visual symptoms such as flashing lights or a homonymous hemianopsia should prompt consideration of an alternate diagnosis and further evaluation.

In patients whose amnesic episodes are brief (e.g., less than 1 hour) and/or recurrent, TLE should be considered, and treatment with anticonvulsant medications can be successful. In patients with focal neurologic signs or symptoms during or subsequent to the amnesic episode, tumors and cerebrovascular disease should be considered, and the prognosis may be more guarded. If the amnesia includes additional disorientation and/or inattention, drug ingestion, especially of anticholinergic or sedative drugs, may be the cause.

Transient global amnesia is most often confused with psychogenic amnestic states. Hysterical amnesia may occur abruptly but is frequently associated with a specific precipitating event, with retention of memory for other events within the time interval. One does not see the profound yet selective deficit in recent memory, nor the temporally graded retrograde amnesia.

In the more severe hysterical amnesia, such as in fugue states, there is the characteristic dissociative behavior with an additional loss of personal identity, a feature not seen in transient global amnesia. In contrast to the transient global amnesia patient, the hysterical patient will often acknowledge that the memory is poor, but will have an inappropriate affect, "*la belle indifférence.*"

Because the episodes tend not to recur, no pathologic studies have been performed on patients with typical transient global amnesia. The anatomic basis of this syndrome, however, is felt to relate to temporal lobe disease of the area involved in the Papez circuit. The combination of memory problems and bland affect helps to direct the clinician to focus on the Papez circuitry in the differential diagnosis.

The unifying points of this chapter have been that abnormal behavior can be a manifestation of focal neurologic disease, and the lesions responsible for such behaviors are, mainly, predictably located somewhere in or near the Papez circuit. Using the Papez circuit as the foundation provides two major diagnostic advantages. First, behavior can be analyzed with a systematic, rigorous discipline provided by neuroanatomy. Second, because this is an anatomic circuit, there is the plasticity to integrate diseases that may be of different etiologies, that may affect different nuclei in the brain, and yet that present with similar clinical presentations.

HERPES SIMPLEX ENCEPHALITIS

Herpes encephalitis affects primarily the temporal lobes and leads to necrosis and hemorrhagic destruction of brain tissue. The mortality rate in herpes simplex encephalitis has been reduced, but the prevalence of neurologic deficits among survivors remains high. These deficits are almost exclusively in the behavioral realm. Temporal lobe seizures already described are a common presenting feature of this disease. The most common sequela is an amnesia that can be isolated, with sparing of other cognitive functions. The amnesia consists of an inability to form enduring memories. In more severe cases, the deficit in recent memory is accompanied by alterations in language, perception, and intelligence such that global dementia is seen. This linguistic disorder typically resembles a fluent aphasia with poor comprehension and paraphasic or nonsensical speech. Profound perceptual problems may also be seen: patients may be unable to recognize family members or friends (prosopagnosia) or common objects (visual agnosia).

The most striking sequelae of herpes simplex encephalitis, however, are the often bizarre behavioral and emotional changes that, in the extreme, resemble those reported by Kluver and Bucy in primates after bilateral removal of the temporal lobes. In humans, the syndrome is sometimes referred to as a *limbic dementia* and consists of (in addition to the visual agnosia) emotional placidity, distractibility, and alterations in sexual behavior. Thus, patients are often apathetic with flat affect and may show childlike compliance. In humans, the hypermetamorphosis consists of manual and oral exploration of the environment with placement of objects in the mouth. Episodes of bulimia may be seen along with ingestion of inappropriate material. The sexual changes consist primarily of inappropriate comments and overtures. The Kluver–Bucy syndrome is not diagnostically specific: the symptom complex may also be seen with head trauma, Alzheimer's disease, and Pick's disease. The behavioral alterations in herpes simplex encephalitis are typically less extreme than the full Kluver–Bucy syndrome and they consist of episodically inappropriate behavior, personality changes, delusions, and hyposexuality. Such behavioral sequelae are frequently viewed as psychogenic by the family and may be resistant to traditional forms of psychiatric treatment.

QUESTIONS AND DISCUSSION

1. Patients at high risk for developing Wernicke's encephalopathy include:

A. Patients with posthepatitis cirrhosis
B. Hospitalized patients receiving intravenous hyperalimentation

C. Alcoholics

D. Health food advocates who consume large quantities of B vitamins

The answers are (B) and (C). Wernicke's encephalopathy relates to thiamine deficiency. Patients who do not receive vitamins in hyperalimentation will eventually become depleted, as will patients whose dietary caloric intake involves only alcohol. Cirrhosis *per se* is not associated with water-soluble vitamin problems, and patients ingesting megavitamins may develop many other problems, but certainly not Wernicke's encephalopathy.

2. A patient says he has a seizure disorder. He is under arrest for having destroyed his friend's apartment and beaten up his girlfriend. He says, "I didn't mean to. I don't remember a thing." This behavior could represent TLE or could alternatively be antisocial behavior by a patient trying to plead ignorance. Along with an EEG, what facts will help you decide that the patient's behavior is probably related to a seizure?

A. After an argument, the patient raced after his girlfriend, caught her in the parking lot, and beat her up.

B. He was observed to exhibit picking movements of his hands and lip smacking before any belligerent behavior began.

C. The fighting and destructive behavior occurred when the girlfriend tried to restrain the patient from rising out of his chair.

D. The patient says this happened three times before: "I know when I'm going into a spell because I hear a strange buzz in my ears. That's all I remember, everything else is a complete blank."

The answers are (B), (C), and (D). Automatisms like those described in (B) are common in TLE; the aura of primitive auditory sensation is helpful, since the primary auditory cortex is in the temporal lobe. The destructive combative behavior should be *non-directed*—the patient will not chase after someone, but instead will be *combative* only if restrained or somehow confined. Running after his girlfriend in the midst of an argument and searching for her in a dark parking lot is a highly directed violent activity.

3. Transient global amnesia is felt to relate to vascular insufficiency in the distribution of which cerebral vessel or vessels?

A. Frontal lobe anterior cerebral arteries

B. Parietal lobe middle cerebral arteries

C. Hippocampal posterior cerebral arteries

D. Carotid arteries

The answer is (C). The vertebrobasilar system provides the vascular supply to the hippocampus, specifically by the posterior cerebral artery.

4. Other conditions, besides transient global amnesia, that are part of the differential diagnosis of amnestic syndromes include:

A. Anticholinergic drug effect

B. Psychomotor epilepsy

C. Head trauma

D. Migraine headaches

The answers are (A), (B), (C), and (D). It is important to consider clinically the differential diagnosis of amnestic syndromes.

5. Match the anatomic area of disease most consistently related to each clinical condition.

A. Bilateral hippocampal regions	**1.**	Psychomotor epilepsy
B. Temporal lobe	**2.**	Transient global amnesia
C. Mammillary bodies	**3.**	Wernicke's encephalopathy
D. Dominant temporoparietal lobe	**4.**	Fluent aphasia

The correct matches are (A) and (2); (B) and (1); (C) and (3); and (D) and (4).

6. During or after herpes encephalitis, which of the following occur?

A. Temporal lobe seizures

B. Aphasia

C. Amnesia

D. Childlike affect and hypersexual behavior

The answers are (A), (B), (C), and (D). During the encephalitis, and as a residual, seizures may occur and they may be difficult to control. Because there may not be generalized shaking, tongue biting, or incontinence associated with the spells, they may not be appreciated as epileptic aphasia. Especially fluent forms can occur, since the dominant temporal lobe may be diseased, and when both temporal lobes are affected, amnesia and the Kluver–Bucy syndrome may occur.

7. In regards to language recovery from Wernicke's aphasia, which of the following are true:

1. The outcome is better than seen with Broca's aphasia

2. Patients are usually highly frustrated and depressed during rehabilitation

3. Paranoid ideations are common

4. Patients are often unaware of their deficit

A. 1 and 2
B. 2 and 3
C. 3 and 4
D. 1 and 4

The answer is (C). Patients with Wernicke's aphasia pose major management problems for rehabilitation specialists. In contrast to patients with Broca's aphasis, who are depressed and frustrated over how poorly they communicate, the Wernicke's aphasia patient is often unaware of the deficit. In addition, there can be thought disorders, including paranoia. For these reasons, the outcome for Wernicke's aphasia is much worse than Broca's asphasia.

8. Transient global amnesia is characterized by:

A. Severe retrograde amnesia that overshadows anterograde amnesia
B. Quiet affect, patient only speaking when prompted
C. Usually lasting only minutes
D. Causes that include atherosclerotic vascular disease, seizures and migraine

The answer is (D). Transient global amnesia is primarily anterograde amnesia, and the extent of retrograde amnesia is variable and less pronounced. The patient is usually quite distressed and confused, asking repeatedly "Where am I?" and "What is this?" Typically, the amnesia lasts for hours, not minutes, but it can be short or long, lasting up to several days.

SUGGESTED READING

Benson DF: Aphasia, Alexia, and Agraphia. New York, Churchill Livingstone, 1979

Benson DF, Ardila A: Aphasia: A Clinical Perspective. New York, Oxford University Press, 1996

Bogen JE: Wernicke's region—Where is it? Ann NY Acad Sci 280:834, 1976

Engel J, Caldecott–Hazard S, Bandler R: Neurobiology of behavior: Anatomic and physiological implications related to epilepsy. Epilepsia 27(Suppl 2):53, 1986

Flor-Henry P: Lateralized temporal-limbic dysfunction and psychopathology. Ann NY Acad Sci 280:777, 1976

Gabrieli JDE: Memory systems analyses in aging and age-related diseases. Proc Nat Head Sci 93:13534, 1996

Geschwind N: Aphasia. N Engl J Med 284:654, 1971

Greenwood R, Bhalla A, Gordon A et al: Behaviour disturbance during recovery from herpes simplex encephalitis. J Neurol Neurosurg Psychiatry 46:809, 1983

Hanibert G: Emotional disturbance and temporal lobe injury. Compr Psychiatry 19:441, 1978

Hodges JR, Warlow CP: The aetiology of transient global amnesia: A case-control study of 114 cases with prospective follow-up. Brain 113:639, 1990

Luria AR, Hutton JT: Modern assessment of the basic forms of aphasia. Brain Lang 4:190, 1977

Miller JW, Peterson RC, Metter EJ: Transient global America: clinical characteristics and prognosis. Neurology 37:733, 1987

Papez JW: A proposed mechanism of emotion. Arch Neurol Psychiatry 38:725, 1937

Pincus JH, Tucker GJ: Behavioral Neurology. New York, Oxford University Press, 1974

Pritchard PB, Lombroso CT, McIntyre M: Psychological complications of temporal lobe epilepsy. Neurology 30:227, 1980

Victor M, Adams RD, Collins GH: Wernicke–Korsakoff's syndrome—A clinical and pathological study of 245 patients. Contemp Neurol Sci 1:1, 1971

Wyllie E: The Treatment of Epilepsy. Baltimore, Williams and Wilkins, 1997

Neurology for the Non-Neurologist, Fourth Edition, edited by William J. Weiner and Christopher G. Goetz. Lippincott Williams & Wilkins, Philadelphia © 1999.

C H A P T E R 1 6

Alzheimer's Disease and Other Dementias

David A. Bennett

Loss of cognitive function associated with age was recognized in antiquity. The concept of acquired dementia occurring prior to old age, however, developed more slowly. By the middle of the 19th century, neurosyphilis was recognized as a major cause of dementia in young and middle-aged persons; reports subsequently appeared describing cases of dementia associated only with cerebral atrophy. In the early 20th century, Dr. Alzheimer presented the clinical history and detailed postmortem findings of a 51-year-old woman with progressive dementia. For the next 60 years, the term *Alzheimer's disease* referred to an uncommon progressive dementia in young or middle-aged persons. The much more common dementia of older persons was attributed to the effects of cerebral atherosclerosis ("hardening of the arteries") or the inevitable manifestations of aging. In the past 25 years, however, it has become apparent that most of these elderly persons have Alzheimer's disease.

Many persons with dementia are cared for by their primary care physician; only a small proportion are managed in specialized dementia centers. Unfortunately, because physicians often do not look for or recognize dementia, many others are not recognized as having the condition. A recent survey found that many physicians do not take advantage of formal, published diagnostic criteria for dementia, and many do not perform structured mental status tests. Dementia often develops over many years. For much of this time, the patient is not totally disabled and is more functional in a familiar and stable environment. Further, many families are determined to care for demented relatives. Therefore, increased awareness of dementia offers the physician an opportunity to greatly improve the lives of patients and of their caregivers.

DEMENTIA

Dementia refers to acquired intellectual deterioration in an adult. Evaluating a person for dementia involves determining whether there has been a loss of cognitive function relative to a previous level of performance. Typically, evidence is obtained through the clinical history from a knowledgeable surrogate and is documented by mental status testing. In some situations, when the clinical history is not adequate, test results from a single evaluation can be contrasted with the estimated premorbid level of ability. In cases of progressive dementia, formal neuropsychological performance testing on two or more occasions over a period of 6 to 12 months may be necessary to document decline.

Criteria for dementia have been developed by the National Institute of Neurological and Communicative Disorders and Stroke (NINCDS) and the Alzheimer's Disease and Related Disorders Association

(ADRDA). The NINCDS–ADRDA criteria require unmistakable deterioration in at least two cognitive domains relative to the patient's previous level of function. This is determined by a history of intellectual decline and must be documented by formal mental status testing. The NINCDS–ADRDA criteria for dementia do not require that the loss of cognitive function be severe enough to interfere with impaired social and occupational functioning, as dictated by some other criteria.

The terms *benign senescent forgetfulness* and *age-associated memory impairment* have been proposed to refer to some persons with evidence of cognitive impairment who do not meet present clinical criteria for dementia. Some of these persons will, as seen at follow-up evaluation, develop dementia. At present, there is no way to make this prediction. When effective drug therapy to prevent dementia becomes available, this issue will assume greater importance.

ALZHEIMER'S DISEASE

EPIDEMIOLOGY

Prevalence estimates suggest that Alzheimer's disease affects about 10% of persons over the age of 65, making it one of the most common chronic diseases of older persons. The occurrence of Alzheimer's disease is strongly related to age. Therefore, the rapid growth of the oldest population age groups is expected to have a profound effect on the public health problem posed by this disease, as Alzheimer's disease is associated with an increased risk of death and institutionalization.

Other than age, there are few well-documented risk factors for Alzheimer's disease. The presence of one apolipoprotein E ε4 allele approximately doubles an individual's risk of developing Alzheimer's disease, and the risk is even higher among those homozygous for the allele. The mechanism whereby this allele causes the disease is unknown. Fewer years of formal education has also been linked to risk of Alzheimer's disease, but it is not known whether this association is the result of early life or late life experiences, or to bias due to the association of education with cognitive performance testing. Head trauma and high blood pressure have also been implicated as possible risk factors. Possible protective factors under investigation include postmenopausal estrogen use, use of nonsteroidal anti-inflammatories, and cigarette smoking.

CLINICAL FEATURES

The clinical evaluation of persons for Alzheimer's disease has four objectives: (1) to determine if the person has dementia; (2) if dementia is present, to determine whether its presentation and course are consistent with Alzheimer's disease; (3) to assess evidence for any alternate diagnoses, especially if the presentation and course are atypical for Alzheimer's disease; and (4) to evaluate evidence of other, co-existing, diseases that may contribute to the dementia, especially conditions that might respond to treatment. The clinical history should focus on the temporal relationship between the loss of different cognitive functions and the development of behavioral disturbances and impairment of physical function.

The most common initial symptom of Alzheimer's diseases is difficulty with memory. The family will report that the patient has left important tasks undone, such as bills unpaid and appointments not kept. At the onset, this disease may be almost imperceptible, but it will typically progress to become a more serious problem in a few years' time. The family members will no longer feel comfortable leaving messages with the patient, and they will have to remind him about the same things innumerable times. After the memory disorder becomes apparent, the family will notice other disorders of cognition. Difficulty in balancing a checkbook is a common early complaint. Difficulty in carrying out normal occupational duties may also be seen if the patient is still employed. Confusion in following directions can also be a common earlier symptom, and if the patient is driving a car, he may become lost (an event that frequently precipitates the first evaluation by a physician). Frightening lapses of memory, such as leaving on a gas stove, may also occur.

As the disease progresses, difficulty in communication becomes more apparent. The patient may have difficulty in remembering simple words or names and may be unable to participate in normal conversation. Reading and writing will also be impaired, as will simple activities of daily living, such as bathing and dressing. The patient may not recognize family members, which causes the family great distress and dismay. The family will become afraid to leave the patient alone, and the patient will require constant attention.

Agitation, hallucination, delusions, and even violent outbursts may be seen at any time during the course of the illness. Previous personality traits may be exaggerated or may be obscured completely by new behavior patterns. Changes in sleep–wake patterns may also disrupt normal living patterns. These types of symptoms are particularly difficult for the family and place a great burden on the caregiver.

A general physical decline is not seen until the latest stages of the illness. Incontinence may be seen at any time and may initially reflect the patient's inability to find the bathroom. As the illness progresses, there seems to be a true loss of bladder control and ultimately even bowel function. The loss of the ability to walk is also a common occurrence seen at the late stages of the illness. This may be due to excessive restraining and tranquilization in an institutional setting, but it is also part of the natural history of the illness. Some patients with even the most profound dementia seem to maintain the ability to walk until some type of medical or orthopedic disaster occurs, however. Seizures and an inability or unwillingness to eat may also occur in the later stages of Alzheimer's disease.

Atypical presentations can be seen in Alzheimer's disease. Patients with progressive aphasia, apraxia, and lengthy periods of isolated memory disorders may ultimately be found to have Alzheimer's disease. The clinical diagnosis is less certain in these patients, and a neurologic consultation is appropriate.

The typical history in Alzheimer's disease is a gradually progressive dementia over several years. The average patient with Alzheimer's disease survives about a decade from the time of diagnosis, although the variation may be from a few years to 20 years. There may be plateau periods during which a deterioration is not obvious; however, a lengthy plateau would be unusual. There is no clear evidence that the age of onset determines the natural history. Younger patients generally tend to have more speech disorders as the illness progresses, but longevity does not seem to vary significantly with the age of onset. Obviously, the older the patient, the more prone he is to other medical problems that might cause an early death. One question that is asked frequently by the family is whether the physician can predict the course of the illness. No proven methods are yet available to make predictions, although the presence of parkinsonian signs (slowness, unstable gait, rigidity or tremor) appear to portend a worse prognosis. Alzheimer's disease is associated with increased risk of death, especially among patients in institutions. In the community, persons with Alzheimer's disease who have mild or moderate cognitive impairment have survival comparable to that of persons without the disease. By contrast, those with more severe cognitive impairment, cachexia, or parkinsonian signs have a much greater risk of dying.

DIAGNOSIS

Formal, standardized assessment of cognition is required to make a diagnosis of dementia and Alzheimer's disease. A wide range of measures are available for this purpose. Several brief measures (e.g., the Mini–Mental Status Examination and the Blessed Orientation, Memory Concentration Test) are suitable for use at the bedside or in the physician's office. Although they may help distinguish persons with dementia from persons without dementia, they are less effective in distinguishing Alzheimer's disease from other dementias.

In the office or hospital, routine mental status testing should include checking the patient's orientation by asking for his full name, the day of the week, the day of the month, the month and the year, where he is, and also his age and date of birth. Show the patient four or five objects and then ask him to name them twice (e.g., a coin, a safety pin, keys, and a comb). Tell the patient that you will ask him to recall the objects in a few minutes. Then check the patient's knowledge of common events by asking him for the names of well-known public figures (e.g., the president, governor, or mayor). Ask the patient to repeat some numbers (the typical patient can remember six numbers forward and three or four backward). Then ask him to do some simple calculations (e.g., multiplication, addition, and "serial sevens"). Ask the patient to repeat a simple phrase; to follow a two-step direction (e.g., "point to the ceiling, then point to the floor"); and to do something with his right hand and then his left hand (e.g., "make a fist with your left hand," followed by "salute with your right hand"). Ask the patient to write his name; to write a brief phrase to dictation (e.g., "Today is Monday"); and then to draw something (usually a clock). Also ask the patient to read a simple phrase. Finally, ask him to recall the four or five objects that you showed him previously.

This mental status test can be administered in a few minutes and should be part of the routine clinical evaluation of all older persons. In a busy office practice, the physician may want to ask an assistant (e. g., a nurse) to administer a formal mental status test. For example, recommended education-adjusted cut-offs have been developed for the Mini-Mental Status Examination. The results can serve as guidelines to direct further evaluation, and they also provide valuable screening information. To make a diagnosis of dementia, a deficit should exist in more than one area of cognition. Patients with early Alzheimer's disease may have profound memory problems with only mild deficits in other aspects of cognition. As the disease progresses, however, language and other aspects of cognitive dysfunction typically become more obvious.

PHYSICAL EXAMINATION

The most important function of the neurologic examination in evaluating persons with dementia is in diagnosing conditions other than Alzheimer's disease. The general physical examination is usually normal in Alzheimer's disease. The neurologic examination (excluding the mental status testing) is also usually normal. Minor parkinsonian features, myoclonic jerks, frontal lobe signs (grasp reflex, snout and glabellar signs), and similar abnormalities may occasionally be seen on examination, especially later in the course of the illness. Any other significant abnormality of the neurologic examination should alert the physician to the possibility of a diagnosis other than, or in addition to, Alzheimer's disease.

GENETICS

As with many other common chronic diseases of older persons, first-degree relatives appear to have a slightly greater risk of disease. In rare families, however, Alzheimer's disease is inherited as an autosomal dominant disease in which half of the family members are affected. In these families, the disease has been linked to mutations on one of three different chromosomes: 21, 14, and 1. Chromosome 21 was examined because it was known that nearly all persons with Down's syndrome developed Alzheimer's disease. The mutations on chromosome 21 are in the region that codes for the precursor of the amyloid protein that is deposited in the brains of people with Alzheimer's disease. (This site is adjacent to, but not within, the obligate Down's syndrome region.) The other two genes are called presenilin 1 (chromosome 14) and presenilin 2 (chromosome 1). How these mutations lead to Alzheimer's disease is unknown. Chromosome 19 is also related to Alzheimer's disease, because it codes for the apolipoprotein E alleles. Additional mutations and susceptibility genes will be found in the future. It is likely that environmental factors interact with genetics to cause the disease, because, although the concordance rate for monozygotic twins greatly exceeds that for dizygotic twins, it is substantially less than 100%. Further, even when both monozygotic twins develop the disease, it is not necessarily at the same age nor do they follow the same course.

LABORATORY INVESTIGATION

There is no reliable antemortem diagnostic test for Alzheimer's disease. The purpose of laboratory testing is to identify other conditions that might cause or exacerbate dementia. These tests routinely include a brain scan and blood tests (see Table 16-1).

The purpose of morphologic imaging with magnetic resonance imaging (MRI) or computed tomography (CT) is to look for evidence of another disease process that can cause or contribute to cognitive impairment, including stroke, tumor, or hydrocephalus. MRI is superior to CT because it is subject to less artifact; it provides greater contrast between gray and white matter; and coronal images, which provide excellent views of the mesial temporal lobes, can easily be obtained. With agitated patients, however, CT is often preferred because the image can be obtained more quickly. There is also strong research interest in using morphologic imaging as a direct diagnostic tool for Alzheimer's disease. At present, these are not at the stage of being suitable for wide clinical use.

Several diagnostic tests for Alzheimer's disease are currently under investigation. Although the apolipoprotein E ε4 allele is not a test for Alzheimer's disease, the presence of the allele in a person with dementia of uncertain etiology slightly increases the likelihood that the dementia is due to Alzheimer's disease. Fragments of amyloid or tau proteins in the cerebrospinal fluid are also being studied as diagnostic tests, but neither have proven to be of diagnostic value. Volume of the hippocampus (a structure in the medial temporal lobe important for memory) on brain MRI is also being investigated as a diagnostic aid; although the technique is widely available, it has not been shown to improve diagnostic accuracy. However, brain MRI should still be used as an adjunct to identify conditions other than Alzheimer's disease that may be causing or contributing to disease. Finally, examining cerebral blood flow, oxygen consumption, and the integrity of neural systems using positron emission tomography (PET) or single photon emission computed tomography (SPECT) are under evaluation. Currently, it is both more worthwhile and less expensive, to refer the patient to the nearest Alzheimer's disease specialist if the diagnosis of dementia is uncertain.

DIFFERENTIAL DIAGNOSIS

The differential diagnosis of dementia should emphasize potentially treatable disorders that may cause, or exacerbate, dementia. Although reversible disorders are uncommon, their importance justifies a thorough evaluation of each patient.

TABLE 16-1. Laboratory Aids in the Differential Diagnosis of Dementia

ROUTINE TESTS	CONDITIONS
Vitamin B_{12}	B_{12} deficiency
T_4 or TSH	Hypothyroidism
RPR, FTA, MHA-TP	Syphilis
Brain scan (CT or MR)	Vascular disease (MR more sensitive but less specific), mass lesions, hydrocephalus, demyelinating diseases and leukodystrophies (MR superior)

OTHER TESTS	CONDITIONS
Lumbar puncture	Chronic meningitis, syphilis, inflammatory disease(s)
Electroencephalography	Creutzfeld–Jacob disease, epilepsy
Single photon emission computed tomography	Pick's disease and frontal lobe dementias
Drug screen/levels	Delirium due to drug toxicity
Heavy metal screen	Lead, mercury, arsenic, copper poisoning
Sedimentation rate autoimmune profile	Inflammatory disease(s)
Angiography	Inflammatory disease(s)
Cerebral biopsy	Inflammatory disease(s)
Chemistry profile	Chronic metabolic disturbances, endocrinopathies
Complete blood count	Chronic infections, anemia
Human immunodeficiency virus	HIV encephalopathy
Ceruloplasmin	Wilson's disease
Long-chain fatty acids	Adrenoleukodystrophy
Arylsulfatase A	Metachromatic leukodystrophy
Chest x-ray	Cardiopulmonary disease, lung tumors
Electrocardiogram	Cardiopulmonary disease

TOXIC/METABOLIC CONDITIONS

Many toxic/metabolic conditions produce a delirium, and rarely dementia. Delirium differs from dementia by the onset and duration of cognitive impairment, and by the level of consciousness. The onset of cognitive impairment in delirium is typically hours or days, and it lasts days to weeks; in addition, patients are either hyper- or hypoalert.

Drug toxicity is a common reversible cause of delirium in the elderly. Older persons may be more susceptible than younger persons to drug side effects on cognition. This is the result of many factors, including altered drug kinetics and use of multiple medications in older persons with several illnesses or complaints ("polypharmacy"). Clinicians should also be alert to the possibility of drug side effects further impairing cognition in persons with preexisting cognitive impairment. A typical presentation is the rapid worsening of dementia following the administration of a new drug (or following the reinstitution of a previous medication that the patient has not taken for some time), with or without altered level of consciousness. Psychotropics such as neuroleptics and sedative–hypnotics, and cardiovascular medications, especially antihypertensives, are common offending agents.

METABOLIC AND HEMATOLOGIC DISORDERS

Hypothyroidism has been recognized for many years as being associated with an organic brain syndrome. Although clinical manifestations of myxedema are usually seen, a patient may occasionally present with dementia without other manifestations of hypothyroidism. Similar cases are seen with disorders of calcium metabolism, especially hypercalcemia, and also with an electrolyte imbalance.

Chronic liver and renal disease are frequently associated with an organic brain syndrome. However, it is unusual for these diseases to be present without prominent manifestations of the primary illnesses. Repeated episodes of hypoglycemia can cause dementia, although in this case, the history is usually clearly episodic rather than gradual.

Pernicious anemia can cause an organic brain syndrome even without hematologic or other neurologic findings. Whether this is also true for folate deficiency is unclear. Various types of neurologic dysfunction have been reported with folate deficiency, including organic brain syndromes. There are some cases in the literature of organic brain syndromes, without any other findings, that did reverse with folic acid treatment. This deficiency syndrome, however, is not as clearly described as that of B$_{12}$.

Korsakoff's syndrome, due to thiamine deficiency, presents with an anterograde amnesia in which the patient is unable to learn new information. Classically, it develops in the wake of an acute Wernicke's encephalopathy with confusion, ophthalmoplegia, and ataxia. However, many patients with Korsakoff's syndrome do not present with a Wernicke's encephalopathy. Although alcoholism is the most frequent setting for this syndrome in developed countries, it may also be associated with other conditions leading to nutritional deficiency, including starvation, malnutrition, protracted vomiting, and gastric resection. It can also be precipitated by administration of carbohydrates to patients with marginal thiamine stores.

The possibility of any of these conditions coexisting with and exacerbating an underlying dementia due to Alzheimer's disease must be considered.

VASCULAR DEMENTIA

Vascular dementia includes all dementia syndromes resulting from ischemic, anoxic, or hypoxic brain damage. It is, therefore, a markedly heterogeneous group of conditions. The concept of multi-infarct dementia (MID) suggests that vascular dementia is caused by the combined effect of multiple, discrete cerebral infarctions. However, currently, the classification of the vascular dementia syndromes is unsettled, and MID is now considered one of many vascular dementia syndromes.

A history of multiple strokes, an abnormal physical examination with focal neurologic findings, and the presence of vascular risk factors in a person with dementia are suggestive of vascular disease but do not prove that the dementia is related to cerebrovascular disease. Both Alzheimer's disease and stroke are common among older persons. They often occur in the same individual by chance alone. Therefore, it is important that an attempt be made to temporally relate the onset, or worsening, of cognitive impairment to a stroke. There is no typical neuropsychological profile of persons with vascular dementia, as the behavioral manifestations are dependent on the vascular territory involved, and this may differ widely among patients. However, persons with vascular dementia rarely present with the insidious onset of memory loss characteristic of early Alzheimer's disease.

White matter lesions are commonly found on MRI or CT in elderly persons, but their etiology and significance remain controversial. Many demented persons with white matter lesions on MRI or CT have Alzheimer's disease at autopsy. Therefore, although the presence of vascular dementia should be supported by evidence of vascular disease on CT or MRI, the presence of these lesions does not necessarily indicate that the dementia is of vascular origin.

Careful control of vascular risk factors such as hypertension and cigarette smoking may alter the natural history of this illness. The value of drugs such as aspirin in preventing the progression of MID is still unknown.

Vasculitides can also cause cognitive dysfunction and psychiatric symptoms, often associated with focal motor signs and seizures. An elevated Westergren erythrocyte sedimentation rate often suggests that further evaluation for a specific immunologic disease is warranted. Further evaluation may require electroencephalography, cerebrospinal fluid studies, and/or angiography. In some cases, meningeal and cerebral artery biopsy are necessary for definitive diagnosis.

SYMPTOMATIC HYDROCEPHALIC DEMENTIA

No other syndrome causing dementia has generated such intense interest (and frustration) among neurologists as normal pressure hydrocephalus. The syndrome consists of gait disturbance, dementia, and incontinence. The onset usually occurs over several months, although the disease may present more acutely. As opposed to Alzheimer's disease, the dementia is mild compared with the gait disturbances, although some cases have been associated with prominent dementia without major gait abnormalities.

Brain scans typically demonstrate hydrocephalus with enlargement of ventricles out of proportion to sulci. Several studies have attempted to determine predictors of improvement following ventricular shunting. Useful clinical indices include motor signs preceding cognitive dysfunction, short duration of dementia prior to surgery, and the presence of a known cause, such as traumatic or spontaneous subarachnoid hemorrhage, meningitis, or partial obstruction.

Some patients with gait problems or dementia improve with CSF shunting procedures; however, the insertion of a shunt is not a benign procedure, especially in geriatric patients. Although the diagnosis of normal pressure hydrocephalus can rarely, if ever, be made with complete confidence, an etiology for the hydrocephalus should be sought prior to recommending shunting. Reasons for hydrocephalus include a history of meningitis or subarachnoid hemorrhage from either a ruptured aneurysm or, more commonly, a previous traumatic head injury.

DEPRESSION

Loss of interest in hobbies and community activities, apathy, weight loss, and sleep disorders may be interpreted by the family as depression, although they actually may result only from dementia. In some cases, depression coexists with dementia. It is useful to ask the caregiver about symptoms suggesting dysphoric mood such as crying, complaining, or even suicidal ideation. Depression may contribute to impairment of activities of daily living, and rarely to the cognitive deficits. If impairment in activities of daily living exceeds what is expected for the severity of cognitive dysfunction, the possibility of a coexisting depression should be considered. Pseudodementia, a syndrome of depression with impaired cognition in which treatment of the depression relieves the cognitive deficit, has been described but is probably rare.

INFECTIONS

Cognitive impairment is the most common neurologic manifestation of acquired immunodeficiency syndrome (AIDS) and may precede the development of other signs of infection with the human immunodeficiency virus (HIV). Patients with the AIDS dementia complex present with forgetfulness and poor attention, typically over several months. The memory impairment is typically less striking than that seen in Alzheimer's disease. Other signs of AIDS should be sought, and, if found, a high index of suspicion for other infections should be maintained.

Chronic meningitis, especially cryptococcal meningitis, can present as dementia, although there are almost always other associated signs and symptoms. The same can be said for neurosyphilis. Brain abscesses, like brain tumors, can present solely with dementia, although focal findings are usually also present. Creutzfeldt–Jakob disease has been shown to be caused by a slow virus. Its onset is subacute rather than chronic, and there are other neurologic abnormalities such as myoclonic jerks, extrapyramidal findings, and visual disturbances, as well as the organic brain syndrome. Its significance far outweighs its frequency, in that similar causes are being suggested for some of the other illnesses.

MASS LESIONS

Brain tumors are frequently associated with organic brain syndromes. Classically, there are also major focal findings and signs of increased intracranial pressure. However, it is well recognized that brain tumors, especially in the "silent" areas of the brain, may present exclusively as a change of personality and intellectual decline. Subtle focal findings can

usually be demonstrated on the neurologic examination, but they are occasionally lacking. Similar comments may be applied to subdural hematomas, especially in the geriatric age group.

PARKINSON'S DISEASE

Dementia is common among persons with Parkinson's disease. It is unclear at this time to what extent this reflects the coincidental occurrence of two diseases of the elderly. Clearly, however, many persons with Parkinson's disease with dementia do not have concomitant Alzheimer's disease. The dementia of Parkinson's disease has been referred to as "subcortical" dementia, characterized by forgetfulness, slowing of thought processes, apathy or depression, and an inability to manipulate acquired knowledge. The term, however, is controversial and should be considered a syndrome or symptom complex. Whether it serves as a useful construct remains a matter of debate.

PICK'S DISEASE

Pick's disease is a degenerative dementia of unknown etiology. Clinically similar cases, often called *lobar dementia* or *dementia of the frontal lobe type,* may have the same pathogenesis. Classically, personality changes precede intellectual decline. When cognitive changes begin, language may be affected before memory. MRI or CT scans may reveal predominantly frontal and temporal lobe atrophy.

PATHOLOGY

The general pathologic features of Alzheimer's disease have been described. Grossly, there is atrophy and dilatation of the ventricles. Microscopically, there are large numbers of neuritic plaques and neurofibrillary tangles. Although both of these lesions can be seen in the brains of older persons without dementia, they are found in greater numbers in the neocortex, hippocampus, and amygdala in persons with Alzheimer's disease. The current pathologic criteria for Alzheimer's disease, in fact, are based on the demonstration of a sufficient number of neuritic plaques and neurofibrillary tangles on microscopic examination.

Plaques are composed of a central extracellular proteinaceous amyloid core, surrounded by dystrophic axon terminals. Some evidence suggests that amyloid is neurotoxic and that its deposition is the initial event in plaque formation. By contrast, others propose that it accumulates after the neurites degenerate. Of interest is the fact that the amyloid comes from a larger precursor protein coded on chromosome 21, and a point mutation in this gene has been reported in some families with Alzheimer's disease.

The major constituents of neurofibrillary tangles are paired helical filaments. Evidence suggests that these tangles are composed of abnormally phosphorylated tau proteins. The mechanism of this process is currently under intense investigation.

Cerebrovascular amyloid (amyloid angiopathy) is also a common finding in persons with Alzheimer's disease, as are granulovacuolar degeneration and Hirano bodies.

TREATMENT

There are many areas in which intervention can improve quality of life for both the patient and the caregiver. Successful intervention requires that the physician work effectively with providers of many other medical and nonmedical services. In general, four areas should be discussed with the family: (1) community resources, (2) advocacy, (3) pharmacotherapy, (4) behavior management, and (5) experimental therapies and procedures.

COMMUNITY RESOURCES

Most major cities now have a local chapter of the Alzheimer Association (AA). The address and phone number of the local chapter can be obtained from the national headquarters at 919 North Michigan, Chicago, Illinois, 60611-1676; phone: (800) 272-3900; fax: (312) 335-1110; Web site: http://www.alz.org/. The association provides information regarding local support services for both the patient and the caregiver from other persons facing similar problems. Community services include adult day-care programs, inpatient and outpatient respite care programs, nursing home special care units, and hospice services.

Most patients with Alzheimer's disease in the mild to moderate stage can be cared for at home, assuming a caregiver is available and willing to assume this responsibility. This decision can be made only by the family. It is not appropriate for the physician (or others not involved in daily care) to insist on home care when the family finds this objectionable. Many patients do well in the day-care setting, and this greatly alleviates the burden on the caregiver. Family support groups, usually sponsored by the Alzheimer Association, are also helpful. The caregiver's mental and physical health must be maintained. This ultimately benefits the patient, since a sane, healthy caregiver can manage a patient with Alzheimer's disease longer and better than one who is overwrought and

exhausted. The caregiver must have rest, and other family members should be urged to take turns in caring for the patient. Nursing home placement, however, is ultimately chosen by most families at the later stages of the illness. The family should be advised to seek out a nursing home where activities and exercise are stressed and where tranquilizers and restraints are minimized.

Last, it must be stressed that Alzheimer's disease places a tremendous social, economic, physical, and psychological burden on the family. The psychological stress on the family is frequently not dealt with adequately. Stress is placed on the family in general, and particularly on the caregiver. Informal counseling through family self-help groups and formal psychological counseling may be necessary. The physician should be available and supportive throughout the course of the illness.

When the patient's death is drawing near, an open discussion of the family's desire for intervention should be initiated. A family occasionally feels that aggressive intervention is mandatory to the very end. Most families, however, are against resuscitation and life-support equipment. Patients with Alzheimer's disease may end up intubated and on respirators because the physician has never discussed the question of resuscitation with the family. The physician's role is to be supportive and informative. Most families have a clear feeling of what the patient would have wanted and they need only be asked in advance.

ADVOCACY

Because patients with Alzheimer's disease may eventually lose all decision-making capabilities, it is important that, at the time of the initial diagnosis, the physician alert the patient and family of the need to make decisions regarding living wills and trusts, power of attorney, and guardianship. The determination of power of attorney or guardianship is fundamental to making economic or ethical decisions regarding the care of the patient. Many patients with mild cognitive impairment are legally competent to execute a valid power of attorney, placing in the hands of another person decisions regarding his health and estate. Guardianship must be imposed on a patient who has become incompetent to render informed consent. Advice in legal matters by a competent and sympathetic attorney is often of great value.

Dementia appears to be a risk factor for unsafe motor vehicle operation. Although most demented persons stop driving on their own, or after encouragement from family members, many others continue to drive after disease onset. This can be a particular problem in this age group, in which many of the women do not drive.

PHARMACOTHERAPY

Two agents have recently been approved by the U.S. Food and Drug Administration for the symptomatic treatment of Alzheimer's disease of mild to moderate severity: tacrine (Cognex) and donepezil (Aricept). Both drugs work to enhance cholinergic transmission in the brain by reducing the degradation of acetylcholine, and they have similar efficacy, although donepezil is better tolerated and easier to use. Both drugs cause peripheral side effects, including nausea and vomiting, although this appears to be less prominent with donepezil. Patients taking tacrine need liver-enzyme monitoring weekly for 6 weeks, and about a third will need to discontinue the drug because of elevated transaminases. Tacrine needs to be increased gradually from 10 mg four times daily to 40 mg four times daily. By contrast, donepezil administration is only once a day, in the evening, starting at 5 mg and increasing to 10 mg. Neither drug, to date, has been shown to slow the progression of the underlying disease. Thus, patients should be monitored for improvement with both formal mental status testing and discussions with the patient's family and/or caregiver. In addition, neither medication, to date, has proven efficacy among persons with mild memory problems who do not have Alzheimer's disease, or among persons with dementia caused by conditions other than Alzheimer's disease.

One study suggested that a high dose vitamin E (2,000 IU/day) delayed overall time to one of the following outcomes: death, institutionalization, loss of the ability to perform basic activities of daily living, or severe dementia. The mechanism of this effect, and its specificity, remains to be elucidated since vitamin E did not appear to have an effect on cognitive function.

BEHAVIORAL MANAGEMENT

The course of Alzheimer's disease is often punctuated by neuropsychiatric disturbances. Among these, depression, alterations of sleep–wake cycles, and aggressiveness may respond to pharmacologic intervention. Few controlled studies exist from which to guide the dose and duration of pharmacotherapy. In persons with dementia and depression, studies of imipramine, L-deprenyl, and methylphenidate have demonstrated marginal efficacy. In persons with disturbances of sleep, a low-dose, sedating neuroleptic may be preferable to hypnotics for the nondepressed Alzheimer's disease patient with a significant sleep disorder. Persons with coexistent depression should be treated with an antidepressant.

Physical aggression may have the most severe consequences for the family, eventually leading to institutionalization of the patient. Numerous studies have addressed the pharmacologic management of behavioral disturbances among patients with Alzheimer's disease. The majority of studies, focusing on neuroleptics such as thioridazine, haloperidol, and loxapine, have shown small benefits. Thioridazine, starting at 10 mg in the evening, can be tried. It can be gradually (e.g., each week) increased. The more potent neuroleptics should be reserved for the acutely and uncontrollably agitated patient. It is important to be aware of side effects such as increased confusion and extrapyramidal signs.

EXPERIMENTAL TREATMENT

Several neurotransmitter systems affected in Alzheimer's disease may contribute to the cognitive dysfunction and provide the basis of neurotransmitter replacement therapy. Dysfunction of the cholinergic system in Alzheimer's disease and evidence that this system is involved in human cognition spawned numerous clinical trials of cholinergic agents, ultimately leading to approval of the acetylcholinesterase inhibitors tacrine and donepezil. Several other neurotransmitter systems and peptidergic systems are also affected in Alzheimer's disease. Agents affecting these systems, however, have had disappointing results. In 1991, the National Institute on Aging funded the Alzheimer's Disease Cooperative Study, clinical trials conducted by a multicenter consortium of Alzheimer's disease centers. This consortium conducted the trial of vitamin E (mentioned previously) and is currently studying estrogen and prednisone. Numerous other agents are under active investigation in most major cities. The local AAs should have information about studies being conducted across the country.

QUESTIONS AND DISCUSSION

1. A 75-year-old man with a 2-year history of gradually declining cognitive function presents with an acute worsening of mental status, hallucinations, and a decreased level of consciousness. What may be going on?

A. Alzheimer's disease
B. Chronic tubercular meningitis

C. Alzheimer's disease with a new superimposed infection

D. Alzheimer's disease and a change in the patient's living environment

The answers are (C) and (D). The 2-year history of declining cognitive function resembles Alzheimer's disease, but the acute deterioration suggests more of a "toxic encephalopathy" in the context of preexisting Alzheimer's disease. Major diagnostic considerations would include the recent use of drugs that may impair cognition, some type of febrile illness, or a metabolic disturbance. The work-up would usually consist of drug screen and systemic blood work. Occasionally, a new focal process can also cause this, such as a cerebral infarct or hemorrhage in one of the "silent" areas of the brain. If a careful examination reveals no focal abnormalities and the diagnosis remains dubious, a CT scan or MRI scan should be done. A patient who has recently moved to a new environment may also decompensate suddenly, since he no longer has the social cues and references that aided him previously.

2. What is the current status of treatment for Alzheimer's disease?

A. Ergoloid mesylates (Hydergine) and Gingko biloba are widely advocated for reversing memory loss.

B. Agitation often can be ameliorated with low-dose neuroleptics such as thiordizine.

C. Tacrine (Cognex) is known to slow the progression of Alzheimer's disease.

D. Donepezil (Aricept) is currently the treatment of choice for the symptomatic improvement of Alzheimer's disease.

The answers are (B) and (D). Hydergine and Gingko biloba, although widely used in Europe, are not popular in the United States. There may be a small benefit of Hydergine; however, the results of recent trials have been negative. Several studies have reported small benefits of the Gingko biloba. High rates of dropout and loss to follow-up in the largest and most recent study precludes a definitive conclusion. Agitation frequently responds to low dose neuroleptics, although the newer atypical neuroleptics such as risperidone (Risperdal) are rapidly becoming much more popular. Neither tacrine nor donepezil are known to slow the progression of disease; by contrast, data suggest that high dose vitamin E might.

Tacrine and donepezil are equally efficacious. However, because of the once a day dosing and the lower frequency of side effects, donepezil is now the drug of choice. Other cholinesterase inhibitors, such as metrifonate, are likely to be on the market within the next year or two.

3. What is the clinical difference between Alzheimer's disease and multi-infarct dementia?

A. CT scanning will detect differences.

B. Multi-infarct dementia is more rapidly progressive and is associated with depression.

C. Multi-infarct dementia is usually accompanied by other focal signs in addition to the mental decline.

D. The two terms are synonymous.

The answer is (C). There is no absolute way to differentiate between these two clinical syndromes. The history in Alzheimer's disease is generally that of a gradual progressive dementia with a normal general neurologic examination and an imaging procedure that shows atrophy. The medical history is also usually negative. The more characteristic picture of multi-infarct dementia is that of a stepwise deterioration in neurologic function with a background of risk factors for cerebrovascular disease, particularly hypertension. Minor focal abnormalities might be found in the neurologic examination, although not always, and imaging procedures, particularly MR scanning, may show signs of numerous small infarcts. A significant number of patients, particularly elderly ones, have elements of both syndromes and, therefore, complete differentiation is sometimes impossible.

SUGGESTED READING

Bennett DA, Beckett LA, Wilson RS et al: Parkinsonian signs and mortality from Alzheimer's disease. The Lancet 351:1631, 1998

Bennett DA, Gilley DW, Wilson RS et al: Clinical correlates of high signal lesions on magnetic resonance imaging in Alzheimer's disease. J Neurol 239:186, 1992

Callahan CM, Hendrie HC, Tierney WM: Documentation and evaluation of cognitive impairment in elderly primary care patients. Ann Intern Med 122:422, 1995

Corey-Bloom J, Thal LJ, Galasko D et al: Diagnosis and evaluation of dementia. Neurology 45:211, 1995

Cronin-Stubbs D, Beckett LA, Scherr PA et al: Weight loss in people with Alzheimer's disease: a prospective population based analysis. British Medical Journal 314:178, 1997

Evans D, Beckett L, Field T et al: Apolipoprotein E ε4 and incidence of Alzheimer's disease in a community population of older persons. JAMA 277:822, 1997

Evans DA, Scherr PA, Cook NR et al: Estimated prevalence of Alzheimer's disease in the United States. Milbank Mem Fund Q 68:267, 1990

Gilley DW, Wilson RS, Beckett LA et al: Psychotic symptoms and physically aggressive behavior in Alzheimer's disease. J Am Geriatr Soc 45:1074, 1997

Gilley DW, Wilson RS, Bennett DA et al: Cessation of driving and unsafe motor vehicle operation by dementia patients. Arch Intern Med 151:941, 1991

Inouye SK, Charpentier PA: Precipitating factors for delirium in hospitalized elderly persons: predictive model and interrelationship with baseline vulnerability. JAMA 275:852, 1996

Lendon CL, Ashall F, Goate AM: Exploring the etiology of Alzheimer disease using molecular genetics. JAMA 277:825, 1997

McKhann G, Drachman D, Folstein M et al: Clinical diagnosis of Alzheimer's disease. Report of the NINCDS-ADRDA Work Group under the auspices of the Department of Public Health and Human Services Task Force on Alzheimer's Disease. Neurology 34:939, 1984

Mittelman MS, Ferris SH, Shulman E et al: A family intervention to delay nursing home placement of patients with Alzheimer disease: a randomized controlled trial. JAMA 276:1725, 1996

Morris JC, Cyrus PA, Orazem J et al: Metrifonate benefits cognitive, behavioral, and global function in patients with Alzheimer's disease. Neurology 50:1222, 1998

Morris MC, Beckett LA, Scherr PA et al: Vitamin E and vitamin C supplement use and risk of incident Alzheimer's disease. Alzheimer's Disease and Associated Disorders 12:121, 1998

Post SG, Whitehouse PJ, Binstock RH et al: The clinical introduction of genetic testing for Alzheimer disease: an ethical perspective. JAMA 277:832, 1997

Qizilbash N, Whitehead A, Higgins J et al: Cholinesterase inhibition for Alzheimer disease: a meta-analysis of the tacrine trials. Dementia Trialists' Collaboration. JAMA 280:1777, 1998

Quality Standards Subcommittee, American Academy of Neurology: Practice parameter for diagnosis and evaluation of dementia (summary statement). Neurology 44:2203, 1994

Rogers SL, Farlow MR, Doody RS et al: A 24-week, double-blind, placebo-controlled trial of donepezil in patients with Alzheimer's disease. Donepezil Study Group. Neurology 50:136, 1998

Roman GC, Tatemichi TK, Erkinjuntti T et al: Vascular dementia: Diagnostic criteria for research studies. Report of the NINDS-AIREN International Work Group. Neurology 43:250, 1993

Sano M, Ernesto C, Thomas RG et al: A controlled trial of Selegiline, aipha-tocopherol, or both as treatment for Alzheimer's disease. N Engl J Med 336:1216, 1997

Schneider LS, Pollock VE, Lyness SA: A metaanalysis of controlled trials of neuroleptic treatment in dementia. J Am Geriatr Soc 38:553, 1990

Small GW, Rabins PV, Barry PP et al: Diagnosis and treatment of Alzheimer disease and related disorders: consensus statement of the American Association for Geriatric Psychiatry, the Alzheimer's Association, and the American Geriatrics Society. JAMA 278:1363, 1997

Stern Y, Gurland B, Tatemichi T et al: Influence of education and occupation on the incidence of Alzheimer's disease. JAMA 271:1004, 1994

Stern Y, Tang M, Albert M et al: Predicting time to nursing home care and death in individuals with Alzheimer's disease. JAMA 277:806, 1997

Tangalos EG, Smith GE, Ivnik RJ et al: The Mini-Mental State Examination in general medical practice: Clinical utility and acceptance. Mayo Clin Proc 71: 829, 1996

Yaffe K, Sawaya G, Lieberburg I et al: Estrogen therapy in postmenopausal women: effects on cognitive function and dementia. JAMA 279:688, 1998

Neurology for the Non-Neurologist, Fourth Edition, edited by William J. Weiner and Christopher G. Goetz. Lippincott Williams & Wilkins, Philadelphia © 1999.

C H A P T E R   1 7

Neurotoxic Effects of Drugs Prescribed by Non-Neurologists

Christopher G. Goetz

Cynthia L. Comella

Neurotoxicology is a growing field of clinical interest, and physicians are increasingly required to evaluate and treat patients with numerous complications of toxic exposure. The usual compounds discussed in a chapter on neurotoxicology would include metals (e.g., lead, mercury, and arsenic), industrial toxins (e.g., organic solvents, gases, pesticides, and other environmental toxins), and biologic toxins (e.g., bacterial exotoxins, animal poisons, venoms, and botanical poisons). Syndromes associated with these toxins, however, are not frequently encountered by the non-neurologist. On the other hand, many drugs that are commonly prescribed by treating physicians may precipitate neurotoxic signs or exacerbate underlying neurologic disease. The neurologic complications of drugs commonly prescribed for the medical management of ambulatory adults are discussed in this chapter.

ANTIBIOTICS

PENICILLINS

Penicillin and related agents rarely cause nervous system toxic effects, although seizures and myoclonic jerks have been reported with high intravenous (IV) doses. Such effects appear more commonly in elderly patients with compromised renal function. Meningitic inflammation may enhance neurotoxic effects by promoting the penetration of these drugs into the central nervous system (CNS) and decreasing their egress. Polyneuritis, with paresthesias, paralysis, and loss of tendon reflexes, has also been reported.

AMINOGLYCOSIDES

The toxicities of all aminoglycoside antibiotics, *neomycin, kanamycin, streptomycin, gentamycin, tobramycin,* and *amikacin,* are similar. The two major adverse effects are (1) damage of the eighth cranial nerve and hearing apparatus, and (2) a potentiation of neuromuscular blockade. Cochlear and vestibular damage is the result of direct toxicity of these drugs. Auditory toxicity is more common with the use of amikacin and kanamycin, whereas vestibular toxicity predominates following gentamycin and streptomycin therapy. Tobramycin is associated equally with vestibular and auditory damage. The incidence of clinical ototoxicity due to these drugs ranges from 5% to 25% depending on whether audiometry is used to detect hearing deficits. Aminoglycoside hearing loss is usually irreversible and may even progress after the discontinuation of drug therapy.

A potentially fatal neurotoxic effect of all aminoglycosides is a neuromuscular blockade. The aminoglycosides act similarly to curare, blocking the neuromuscular junction. Aminoglycosides also possibly potentiate ether and other anesthetics during surgery. Sudden or prolonged respiratory paralysis due to aminoglycosides may be reversed by the administration of calcium or neostigmine.

ANTIFUNGAL AGENTS

The *polymyxins* are related closely to the aminoglycosides in structure and neurotoxicity. The incidence of neurotoxic reaction has been estimated at 7%, and syndromes other than neuromuscular blockade include paresthesias, peripheral neuropathy, dizziness, and seizures. Respiratory paralysis, however, is the most serious neurotoxic reaction. An underlying renal dysfunction predisposes to the neuromuscular blockade induced by this drug group. Signs of neuromuscular blockade include diplopia, dysphagia, and weakness.

Amphotericin B is widely used against systemic fungal infection. When the drug is used intrathecally, seizures, pain along the lumbar nerves, mononeuropathies (including foot drop), and chemical meningitis have occurred.

ANTITUBERCULOUS DRUGS

Isoniazid (INH) has been associated with neurotoxic effects felt to be related to drug binding of pyridoxine and resultant excessive vitamin excretion. A prominent polyneuropathy is associated with chronic INH administration, and symptoms include paresthesias; diminished pain, touch, and temperature discrimination; and eventual weakness. Seizures, emotional irritability, euphoria, depression, headache, and psychosis may rarely occur. The neurotoxic reactions due to INH are dose related and are more common in "slow inactivators." In these patients, neurotoxic reactions can be prevented or diminished by the administration of pyridoxine at a dose of 50 mg daily. Patients who intentionally or inadvertently overdose acutely with INH may develop severe ataxia, generalized seizures, and coma. Supportive measures, anticonvulsants, and pyridoxine should be administered to these patients.

Rifamycin is frequently administered with INH. Neurologic side effects are uncommon but may include headache, dizziness, inability to concentrate, and confusion. Less commonly, signs of peripheral neuropathy may develop. *Ethambutol* precipitates a reversible optic neuritis, as well as a more generalized peripheral neuropathy. A metallic taste in the oral cavity is frequently associated with ethambutol therapy and may be due to an impairment of receptor activity.

ANTIVIRAL DRUGS

The treatment of selected viral infections in non-HIV-positive individuals (HIV, human immunodeficiency virus) has become possible over the past few years. The neurologic complications of HIV and the drugs used to treat it will be discussed elsewhere.

Acyclovir can be administered either intravenously or orally. Acyclovir is used orally for the treatment of localized or ophthalmic varicella zoster, treatment of minor herpes simplex virus, and reducing the severity of varicella. Neurologic side effects are rarely associated with oral acyclovir. However, seizures, encephalopathy, hallucinations, and coma have been described, as has tremor.

Amantadine has been used to prevent influenza A infections. This agent appears to have, in addition to its antiviral action, anticholinergic and dopaminergic effects, which has led to its use in mild Parkinson's disease. The neurologic side effects associated with amantadine include sedation, confusion, myoclonus, hallucinations, delirium, and seizures. As amantadine is excreted through the kidney, the presence of renal impairment may reduce its clearance, causing it to accumulate in the body and resulting in amantadine toxicity.

OTHER COMMONLY PRESCRIBED ANTIBIOTICS

Sulfonamide, pyrimethamine, and *trimethoprim* are used mainly in the treatment of urinary tract infections (UTIs). They are generally considered safe drugs and are not associated with marked neurotoxicity. They may, however, cause headache, fatigue, tinnitus, and acute psychosis. Some signs may mimic meningitis. On the second or third day of therapy, patients may complain of difficulty in concentrating and impaired judgment. *Nitrofurantoin* is also used commonly in the treatment of UTIs. A polyneuropathy is the major toxic syndrome with this drug. Like the Guillain–Barré syndrome, this neuropathy is usually subacute and begins in the distal extremities, often with sensory complaints of paresthesias and numbness. The neuropathy ascends and involves the motor system, with progressive weakness and areflexia. Discontinuation of the drug is essential, and not all patients will recover. The prognosis appears to relate most significantly to the extent of the neuropathy at the time of drug withdrawal.

Chloramphenicol has been associated with toxic encephalopathy and symptoms of confusion and delirium when high doses were used. Underlying neoplastic disease and liver and renal dysfunction may predispose to excessive drug accumulation and toxic encephalopathy. A reversible optic neuritis has been associated with prolonged therapy with high doses (>2 g/kg). The optic neuropathy is sudden in onset and is associated with decreased visual acuity and ocular pain. Ototoxicity has been associated with chloramphenicol installation into the middle ear, although patients had multiple drug therapy in most cases. Finally, a peripheral neuropathy may occur, and this complication often accompanies the optic neuropathy. The neuropathy is predominantly sensory, so that patients complain of numbness and paresthesias. In patients who are receiving phenytoin or phenobarbital, chloramphenicol will inhibit the metabolism of these drugs so that there will be a marked elevation in anticonvulsant blood levels in these patients. This effect occurs quickly, and therefore immediate adjustment of the anticonvulsant dose must be effected to avoid toxicity. The practical management of seizure patients who require chloramphenicol must include the careful monitoring of the blood level of the anticonvulsants.

Tetracycline can be associated with pseudotumor cerebri or increased intracranial pressure. The syndrome is characterized by headache, papilledema, elevated spinal fluid pressure, and, in babies, bulging fontanels. Significant vestibular toxicity has also been associated with a tetracycline derivative, minocycline.

Erythromycin is probably the least toxic of the commonly used antibiotics from a neurologic perspective. An uncommon side effect is temporary hearing loss. Erythromycin interacts with carbamazepine, thus the anticonvulsant levels increase rapidly when erythromycin is introduced.

Nitrofurantoin therapy has been associated with polyneuropathy. Generally seen with prolonged therapy, neuropathy can occur as early as the first week of treatment. It is usually subacute, begins in the distal extremities with paresthesias, and tends to progressively ascend to involve the motor system with weakness and areflexia. Although this polyneuropathy clinically resembles Guillain–Barré syndrome, the spinal fluid is usually normal, except that 25% of patients have a slight increase in protein without pleocytosis. When polyneuropathy is recognized, drug withdrawal is essential, although 10% to 15% of patients will not improve and 15% will have only partial recovery. The

prognosis appears to correlate with the extent of the neuropathy at the time of drug withdrawal, but not to the total dose exposure or the duration of therapy.

CARDIAC DRUGS

GLYCOSIDES

Digitalis and related agents are the mainstay of treatment for congestive heart failure. Neurologic complications of digitalis therapy have been recognized for almost 200 years and are characterized by nausea, vomiting, visual disturbances, seizures, and syncope. Adverse effects on the CNS reportedly occur in 40% to 50% of patients with clinical digitalis toxicity and may occur before, simultaneously with, or after the signs of cardiac toxicity develop.

The most frequent and often the first sign of clinical intoxication is nausea, which appears to be due to central mechanisms rather than gastrointestinal irritation. The incidence of digitalis-related visual disturbances has been estimated at 40%, and although these symptoms may occur as an isolated symptom, they usually occur concomitantly with other toxic signs. Blurred vision, reversible scotomas, diplopia, defects of color vision, and total amaurosis represent the spectrum of optic side effects.

Seizures are most commonly seen in pediatric patients. The incidence of digitalis-related seizures is difficult to estimate since other seizure etiologies (e.g., arrhythmia) are so high in cardiac patients. Transient mental aberrations felt to be caused by intermittent cerebral hypoperfusion resemble transient global amnesia. Syncope, probably due to conduction delay or hyperactivity of baroreceptors, has also occurred in digitalis toxicity. Other neurotoxic reactions include facial neuralgia, paresthesias, headache, weakness, and fatigue. Cerebral symptoms consisting of confusion, delirium, mania, and hallucinosis have been reported in as many as 15% of patients with digitalis toxicity. Although the mechanism for the symptoms is unknown, it is felt that they are not the result of altered cardiac function.

ANTIANGINAL AGENTS

Nitroglycerine and nitrate therapy is frequently associated with headache. According to currently proposed mechanisms, nitric oxide is the common mediator in experimental vascular headaches. Nitroglycerin produces a throbbing or pulsating sensation in many patients and an overt headache in many others. Often, the headaches attenuate or disappear with time, but 15% to 20% of patients will not be able to tolerate long-acting nitrates because of headache. Patients should be encouraged to use analgesics during the initial days or weeks of nitrate therapy and should be educated as to the nature of this problem and its probable resolution with time.

Nitroglycerin therapy can cause dose-related increases in intracranial pressure, which in rare cases can result in a clinically overt syndrome. Furthermore, the hypotensive effects of nitroglycerin can result in dizziness and light-headedness, or even syncope.

ANTIARRHYTHMICS

Quinidine is used mainly to treat auricular fibrillation. Nervous system manifestations are usually not significant, but with overdosage or in susceptible individuals the following may occur: headache, nausea, vomiting, blurring of vision, ringing of the ears, flushing, palpitations, and even convulsions. A precipitous drop in blood pressure related to vagal influences can cause syncope, vertigo, and respiratory arrest (on rare occasions).

Lidocaine-induced CNS toxicity occurs commonly and may relate to its rapid absorption across the blood–brain barrier. The syndrome appears to relate to a diffuse excitement of neuronal systems, with an early prodrome of altered behavior. Garrulousness and loss of inhibitions may be the prominent feature, as may agitation or psychosis. Circumoral numbness, diplopia, and tinnitus may also occur, with progressive muscle twitches and tremors. Generalized myoclonic seizures and finally CNS and respiratory depression are seen with higher doses. In both cardiac and surgical patients, hypoxia and acidosis develop rapidly if the lidocaine syndrome is not reversed. Treatment focuses on adequate oxygenation and support, because the half-life of bolus lidocaine given acutely is 6 to 8 minutes. Since repeated injections, however, change the kinetics of lidocaine and prolong its half-life to approximately 90 minutes, more long-lasting effects can be seen.

Procainamide may cause light-headedness and even syncope because of the hypotensive action. Additionally, a lupus erythematosus syndrome can develop in patients on procainamide, and 80% of patients receiving the drug for 6 months have antinuclear antibodies; these antibodies clear with the withdrawal of the agent. During lupus-like syndrome, encephalopathy with confusion and agitation can develop. Procainamide also has a curare-like effect at the neuro-

muscular junction and hence can precipitate myasthenia gravis or exacerbate it.

Tocainide hydrochloride is an antiarrhythmic agent that is structurally and pharmacologically similar to lidocaine, except that it is well absorbed when given orally. Tocainide has been proven effective in managing various ventricular arrhythmias; however, because it crosses the blood–brain barrier, it frequently causes several neurologic side effects, which include light-headedness, dizziness, tremor, twitching, paresthesias, sweating, hot flashes, blurred vision, diplopia, and mood changes. Peak plasma concentrations of tocainide occur within 1 to 2 hours of ingestion; the plasma half-life is 12 to 15 hours in patients with unimpaired renal and hepatic systems. CNS side effects appear to be linearly related to the dose.

Bretylium is a parenteral antiarrhythmic drug used in the prophylaxis and treatment of ventricular fibrillation and life-threatening ventricular arrhythmias that do not respond to first-line agents such as lidocaine. The antiarrhythmic mechanisms of bretylium in humans are not clearly defined, but in animals it increases the ventricular fibrillatory threshold and also the action potential duration and effective refractory period. It induces a state of chemical sympathectomy.

The most significant side effect of this drug is severe supine and orthostatic hypotension. Patients report dizziness, light-headedness, vertigo, and faintness. Bretylium may also rarely cause flushing, hyperthermia, confusion, paranoid psychosis, mood changes, anxiety, lethargy, and nasal stuffiness.

Amiodarone is an orally effective antiarrhythmic drug that, like bretylium, slows repolarization in various myocardial fibers and raises the threshold for ventricular fibrillation. Early reports of adverse effects include corneal microdeposits, thyroid dysfunction, and cutaneous photosensitivity. Recently, however, toxic neurologic side effects have been described and, in a series of 54 patients studied, these side effects were the most common reason for either altering or discontinuing amiodarone therapy.

A reversible syndrome of tremor, ataxia, and peripheral neuropathy without nystagmus, dizziness, encephalopathy, or long-tract signs developed in 54% of these patients. Tremor occurred earliest and most frequently (29%). The 6- to 10-Hz flexion–extension movements in the fingers, wrists, and elbows were indistinguishable from essential tremor. Thirty-seven percent of the patients reported ataxia associated with falls, staggering, and difficulty in dressing the lower limbs. The ability to walk was seriously impaired in 18% of the patients. None of these patients had preexisting gait problems and none had sensory or long-tract abnormalities on examination. Peripheral neuropathy associated with this drug was first reported in 1974 and continues to account for a significant portion of the neurologic toxicity reported today. The neuropathy is sensorimotor in type and generally causes numbness and tingling of all four extremities. Proximal weakness occasionally accompanies the paresthesias. Sural nerve biopsies have been examined and have revealed demyelination with mild axonal loss in some cases. Lamellated inclusions of lysosomal origin were found in all cell types in the nerves and are a characteristic finding of this neuropathy.

DIURETICS

Diuretics are divided into three principal groups: thiazide, loop, and potassium sparing. Diuretics most frequently cause extracardiac side effects as a direct result of the electrolytes lost or retained in the renal system. Each group can, however, cause adverse effects that are indirectly linked to electrolyte and water balance.

The *thiazide* diuretics have been reported to cause syncope, acute muscle cramps and pain, hyporeflexia, weakness, flaccid paralysis, and epileptiform movements. The deterioration of mental function, including the development of coma, can be precipitated with thiazide administration in patients being treated for cirrhosis. Thiazides given concomitantly with triamterene and amantadine can increase the likelihood of neurotoxicity from the amantadine.

If loop diuretics, particularly *furosemide,* are given quickly and in high doses, they can cause deafness and paresthesias. If they are given to a patient who is also receiving lithium chronically, loop diuretics can alter the renal clearance of lithium and increase the risk of lithium toxicity and fluid electrolyte abnormalities. Loop diuretics can also potentially increase the success with which succinylcholine blocks the neuromuscular junction in anesthetized patients.

Potassium sparing diuretics, including spironolactone and triamterene, have been reported to cause confusion, drowsiness, muscle weakness, paresthesias, dizziness (although this may be a result of cardiac rhythm changes), and headache.

SYMPATHOLYTICS

Methyldopa can cause sedation, which is usually transient in nature but may persist in as many as 5% of patients. Mood alterations including depression are not uncommon, although most patients who develop behavioral changes usually have a prior history of affective illness. The depressive state is reversible on withdrawal of the drug. Parkinsonism, resulting from dopamine antagonism, has been reported several times; however, considering the widespread use of this agent, this is probably rare. Other minor neurologic complaints associated with methyldopa include confusion, dizziness, headaches, and syncope.

Clonidine is an alpha$_2$-noradrenergic agonist, and some people have suggested that this drug induces an overall decrease in norepinephrine release, possibly through a presynaptic mechanism. Sedation is the most common adverse neurologic effect of clonidine. Other less common neurotoxic reactions include depression, nightmares, and reversible dementia syndrome.

Reserpine was historically a popular drug in the treatment of hypertension, but disabling neuropsychiatric side effects have limited its current use. Drug-induced parkinsonism can occur and is felt to relate directly to the depletion of central dopaminergic stores by reserpine. This effect may occur in patients with no prior neurologic deficits or can be seen as a marked and sudden exacerbation of already present, but mild, Parkinson's disease. Psychiatric depression with early morning awakening, melancholy, loss of appetite, and diminished self-confidence are also seen with reserpine therapy and may also relate to central neurotransmitter depletion. This effect is more common with higher dosage and in patients with a history of prior affective disturbance. Drug withdrawal does not always result in immediate reversal, and early symptoms of depression should alert the physician to discontinue therapy.

Propranolol is one of many beta-adrenergic receptor blockers currently in clinical usage in the United States. Propranolol is used mainly in the medical management of angina pectoris, hypertension, and certain cardiac arrhythmias. Propranolol seems to promote hypotension by reducing cardiac output and by reducing renin synthesis, possibly by CNS effects not yet elucidated.

Neuropsychiatric symptoms occur frequently during treatment with propranolol. Lassitude or insomnia and depression are the most common reactions, although vivid nightmares, hypnagogic hallucinations, and psychotic behavior have been reported with high-dose (more than 500 mg/day) propranolol therapy. The nighttime behavioral problems can often be avoided by eliminating doses after 8. More recently, psychotic symptoms and confusion have been seen even with low-dose therapy and especially in two classes of high-risk patients—those with prior histories of major psychiatric illness and those with hyperthyroidism. This toxic psychosis clears promptly after the withdrawal of the drug. The pharmacology of propranolol-induced psychosis is unclear, although pre- and postsynaptic noradrenergic inhibition has been implicated (as has serotonergic antagonism). Orthostatic light-headedness, mild unsteadiness of gait, and dizziness may also be seen and may relate to the hypotensive effect of the drug. Paresthesias and slurred vision also occur. Sexual impotency, which is reversible with the withdrawal of the drug, can be particularly troublesome, and the physician must often ask the patient specifically about the problem to learn of it. This side effect can often be overlooked or misinterpreted by the patient, family, and physician in a rehabilitation setting after a myocardial infarction or after cardiovascular surgery. Propranolol has also been reported to unmask signs of hypoglycemia in predisposed individuals. Finally, propranolol has been reported to exacerbate or precipitate myasthenia gravis in susceptible individuals because of its curare-like depolarization blockade of nicotinic receptors. A long-acting propranolol preparation is now available and may be associated with fewer neurologic side effects. To avert side effects of nonselective beta blockage, selective β_1 antagonists have been developed. Neurologically, however, these drugs have the same types of side effects a seen with propranolol and its derivatives.

Prazosin competitively blocks the vascular postsynaptic alpha-adrenergic receptors and is the first of a class of similar antagonists derived from quinazoline. The selective affinity of prazosin for alpha-receptors allows it to block the contractile response of vascular smooth muscle to norepinephrine, consequently lowering mean arterial pressure and peripheral resistance. Like other antihypertensives that cause vasodilatation, prazosin causes hypotension: dizziness and faintness have been reported in up to 50% of patients receiving this drug. These are most pronounced after the first dose(s) or in patients who have had a hiatus from the drug and are reinstituting treatment. Hypotension can be minimized if the initial dose is small and is given at bedtime. Other CNS side effects include headache, dry mouth, nasal stuffiness, lassitude, hallucinations, depression, paresthesias, nervousness, and priapism.

VASODILATORS

Hydralazine is the only direct-acting vasodilator generally available for the treatment of chronic hypertension. The neurologic side effects of hydralazine are few and uncommon in clinical practice. Periph-

eral neuropathy characterized by diffuse numbness and tingling is the only consistent neurotoxic reaction and is felt to be due to a direct toxic effect of the drug.

Verapamil, nifedipine, and *diltiazem* are calcium-entry blocking agents that decrease coronary vascular resistance and increase coronary blood flow. Each of these drugs selectively inhibits the transport of slow-channel calcium ions in cardiac tissue. These slow-channel ions link myocardial excitation to contraction and help control energy storage and use. Verapamil is used primarily to treat or prevent supraventricular tachyarrhythmias; nifedipine and diltiazem are used primarily to treat angina. These agents all have antihypertensive properties.

The extracardiac side-effect profile is similar for all three drugs. The most prominent symptoms of toxicity are associated with excessive vasodilatation: patients complain of dizziness, light-headedness, flushing, headache, and increased fatigue. Adverse neurologic effects may also include confusion, tremor, paresthesias, insomnia, sedation, equilibrium changes, blurred vision, weakness, and nervousness. The calcium-entry blocking agents should generally be used cautiously with beta-adrenergic blocking agents because the risk of severe hypotensive side effects is compounded. In addition, both verapamil and nifedipine can increase serum digoxin levels, thus compounding the potential risk of digitalis toxicity. Flecainide has been associated with tremor and dystonia. Mexiletine has been associated with an action tremor that increases in incidence as blood levels increase.

ANGIOTENSIN-CONVERTING ENZYME INHIBITORS

Captopril has been used in the United States to treat moderate to severe hypertension, based on its effect on the renin–angiotensin–aldosterone (RAA) axis. This cascading hormonal axis simultaneously maintains systemic arterial pressure and sodium balance by detecting and correcting even small changes in renal perfusion. Alongside the increased understanding of the RAA axis has come the discovery of drugs that specifically and selectively inhibit the RAA cascade.

Few neurologic side effects have been reported; however, in a large multinational study, 5% of the participating patients reported symptoms of hypotension, including dizziness, light-headedness, and vertigo. These symptoms were generally transient and mild and most frequently occurred in patients who were sodium or water depleted. Dysgeusia occurred in 2% to 4% of patients participating in this small trial. The incidence of taste change or loss increased in patients with impaired renal function.

GASTROINTESTINAL AGENTS

Common gastrointestinal problems include the hypermotility disorders with vomiting and/or diarrhea; hypomotility disorders, with constipation; or excessive acid secretion leading to "heartburn" or ulcerations. A wide variety of drugs are commonly recommended for these disorders. Fortunately, neurologic complications from these frequently prescribed agents are infrequent.

LAXATIVES

There are only a few neurologic complications associated with the drugs used to treat constipation. *Docusate sodium* (Colace) is a stool softener that occasionally causes nausea or a bitter taste. The long-term use of nonprescription laxatives may cause neurologic complications arising secondary to depletion of electrolytes. Profound muscle weakness may occur from the potassium depletion following chronic laxative intake. The irritant purgatives, such as cascara, may damage the myenteric plexus of the colon, leading to a reduction of intestinal motility and a worsening of constipation.

ANTIEMETICS

Of the antiemetic drugs, several commonly prescribed agents act as dopamine-receptor blockers in similar fashion to the neuroleptic drugs described later. *Metoclopramide* (Reglan), *prochlorperazine* (Compazine), and *promethazine* (Phenergan) are three widely used antiemetics with neuroleptic properties. Sedation may occur as an early complaint with the introduction of these agents. In addition, acute dystonia, with distressing involuntary spasms of head, neck, eyes, facial, and trunk muscles, may occur, particularly in children treated with prochlorperazine. If not recognized by the clinician, these acute, sometimes bizarre symptoms may be inaccurately thought to have a psychogenic etiology. The treatment of the acute dystonia from the dopamine-receptor blocking antiemetics is the administration of anticholinergic agents.

In addition to acute dystonia, these dopamine-receptor antagonist, antiemetic agents may cause a parkinsonian syndrome, clinically indistinguishable from idiopathic Parkinson's disease. Those of more advanced age appear to be more susceptible to this neurologic complication and may even be treated with antidopaminergic agents if the symptoms are not recognized as being associated with the medication. Akathisia may also occur as a side effect of these medications. If these agents are used on a long-term basis, as in the treatment of chronic esophageal reflux, the potentially irreversible symptoms of tardive dyskinesia may even occur.

A different type of agent with predominantly anticholinergic effect, *scopolamine*, is prescribed for the treatment of motion-induced nausea and vomiting. Recently, scopolamine has become available in a long-acting, transdermal patch preparation. The neurologic side effects of scopolamine are those associated with blockade of muscarinic receptors. The most frequent is xerostomia. The reduction in saliva production, if severe, can lead to mucosal ulcerations and dental problems. Other peripheral effects of scopolamine include blurred near vision resulting from alterations in accommodation, reduced sweating, and urinary retention from effects on bladder muscles. A potentially irreversible effect of the anticholinergic agents is the exacerbation of closed-angle glaucoma with the potential for causing blindness.

The CNS side effects of these drugs include sedation and confusion. Losses in recent and immediate memory can occur at high doses. Finally, with toxicity, delirium and hallucinations have been described.

ANTIDIARRHEALS

Drugs used to symptomatically alleviate diarrhea frequently contain morphine or morphine derivatives. These compounds act to reduce the propulsive contractions of the small bowel and colon. The neurologic adverse effects from these agents include sedation, respiratory depression, and coma, typically with pupillary constriction.

Anticholinergic agents have also been used to treat symptoms of diarrhea. *Diphenoxylate–atropine* (Lomotil) is a widely prescribed antidiarrheal agent. Overdoses of this agent most frequently cause a predominantly opioid intoxication.

Some antidiarrheal compounds, for example Donnatal, are combinations of morphine derivatives and from one to three different anticholinergic agents. Donnatal contains phenobarbital, hyoscyamine, atropine, and scopolamine. Although each component is present only in small amounts, patients taking several tablets a day or elderly persons may experience significant side effects.

Bismuth compounds, as found in the nonprescription *bismuth subsalicylate* (Pepto-Bismol), have been recommended for the treatment of "traveler's diarrhea." The neurologic sequelae of these agents are rare. There have been reports of an acute reversible psychotic reaction following excessive use of these compounds as a result of acute bismuth toxicity. More commonly, tinnitus is noted with large doses, arising from the salicylate component in this compound.

ANTIACIDITY AGENTS

The magnesium and aluminum antacids, if taken in large quantities or with renal impairment, may cause neurologic symptoms secondary to alteration in electrolytes. Sucralfate is an aluminum compound that coats the gastric mucosa. Although little of this agent is absorbed directly, sulcrafate may reduce the absorption of phenytoin and, in those taking this anticonvulsant, may result in a drop in phenytoin levels below the therapeutic range.

The H_2-receptor antagonists inhibit acid secretion from the parietal cells. Currently, four H_2-receptor antagonists are approved for use in the United States. *Cimetidine* (Tagamet) is the first to be developed. More recently developed H_2-receptor antagonists include *ranitidine* (Zantac), *nizatidine* (Axid), and *famotidine* (Pepcid). The neurologic complications of these medications include lethargy, confusion, depression, hallucinations, and headache. Individuals developing unexplained encephalopathic symptoms who are treated with these drugs may improve with the discontinuation of these agents. Additionally, the effect of cimetidine and, to a lesser degree, the other H_2 blockers, on the cytochrome P-450 enzymes in the liver may alter the pharmacokinetic profile of other drugs undergoing hepatic degradation, including warfarin and phenytoin.

RESPIRATORY AGENTS

ADRENERGIC DRUGS

Of the three types of adrenergic receptors (alpha, β_1, β_2), it is the β_2 receptor that mediates bronchodilation. The first sympathomimetics available for the treatment of asthma were not β_2 selective (*metaproterenol, isoproterenol, epinephrine, ephedrine*); therefore, in addition to dilating the bronchioli, they also produced significant cardiac and CNS effects. The introduction of β_2-selective agents (albuterol, terbutaline) resulted in a reduction in the number of adverse effects. These agents are most efficiently administered by inhalation, resulting in benefit with minimal side effects. When these agents are administered parenterally, there may be nausea, vomiting, headache, and a variable-amplitude postural and action tremor associated with these agents.

XANTHINE BRONCHODILATORS

The xanthine compounds include *aminophylline* and *theophylline*. These agents are now prescribed only for those patients suffering with chronic rather than intermittent symptoms of bronchoconstriction. Theophylline is metabolized primarily in the liver, and drugs that affect hepatic enzymes, including tobacco, may alter the metabolism of theophylline. Liver disease, heart failure, and pulmonary disease tend to slow the metabolism of theophylline, sometimes resulting in toxicity even at low dosages. The therapeutic serum concentration of theophylline is 10–20 µg/ml. The side effects from theophylline tend to be dose related. However, even in the therapeutic range, neurologic side effects may occur. These include nausea, nervousness, insomnia, and headache. Although usually associated with toxic levels of theophylline, seizures may also occur in the high therapeutic range, particularly in the elderly or those with a history of previous brain injury. This latter group is likely to develop prolonged seizures with a poor outcome. The mechanism of theophylline-induced seizures is not clearly understood. In otherwise healthy asthmatics, the seizures are typically short-lived with a good outcome. A recently described neurologic side effect observed in children is the occurrence of acquired stuttering, which resolves with the discontinuation of this drug.

PSYCHIATRIC DRUGS

NEUROLEPTICS

Phenothiazine drugs and *haloperidol* are antipsychotic agents with the common property of dopaminergic receptor blockade. As a class, they are associated with various important neurologic complications, which include sedative effects, autonomic dysfunction, acute dystonic reactions, akathisia, parkinsonism, and the late complication of tardive dyskinesia. The sedation and encephalopathy associated with these drugs may relate primarily to their anticholinergic properties. Although these drugs can reduce agitation in young patients, the anticholinergic effects may lead to confusion in elderly patients and may induce paradoxical agitation rather than sedation. These drugs may lower the seizure threshold and have been associated occasionally with exacerbation of preexisting epilepsy. The management of acute encephalopathy caused by neuroleptics involves the general maintenance of life systems. Physostigmine 1–2 mg IV may reverse anti cholinergic toxicity.

A curious neurotoxic sign associated with neuroleptic management is neuroleptic malignant syndrome, which includes extrapyramidal signs and severe hyperthermia. Laboratory findings usually include transient elevations of serum aldolase or creatine kinase. The treatment of neuroleptic malignancy syndrome involves, first, the patient's removal from heat sources. The neuroleptic should be stopped and the patient should be placed in a cool environment. Ice packs about the body and ice-water stomach lavage may be instituted. When the rectal temperature drops to 38°C, these dramatic efforts at cooling can be stopped, since patients have been reported to experience seizures when temperatures drop too rapidly. Dantrolene, an agent that acts at the muscle, can be used to decrease rigidity and lower body temperature. Doses range from 1 mg to 10 mg/kg IV in four divided doses. Levodopa can also be used, and bromocriptine has been tried with success.

Neuroleptics may also induce dystonias early in the course of neuroleptic treatment or after a new dosage increase in chronically treated patients. The manifestations are diverse and may include oculogyric crises, painful postures of the head and neck, and forced tongue protrusion. Acute management involves IV or intramuscular (IM) injection of an anticholinergic agent. This treatment will ameliorate the dystonia within minutes, but since the anticholinergic effect is short-lived, oral anticholinergic agents should be prescribed for the next 24 to 48 hours.

Drug-induced parkinsonism occurs usually after weeks of therapy and will respond to low doses of anticholinergic drugs. Since most parkinsonian signs are self-limited, the need for anticholinergic drugs should be reevaluated every 2 months.

Tardive dyskinesia is an abnormal involuntary movement disorder that occurs after chronic exposure to neuroleptics. The movements are usually stereotypic or choreic and involve predominantly the linguofaciobuccal muscles. In patients on neuroleptics who develop this syndrome, an attempt to remove the neuroleptics should be made if the patient's psychiatric condition permits. If the movements do not resolve after neuroleptics have been removed, reserpine may be used, usually between 1 and 2 mg/day. Side effects of reserpine, however, include hypotension and drug-induced depression as well as parkinsonism.

ANXIOLYTICS

Benzodiazepines are commonly prescribed anxiolytic agents. The therapeutic index of these agents is 10 to 30 times that of the barbiturates and, hence, their absolute toxicity is less. However, since these agents are so widely used, adverse reactions are frequently reported. The predominant toxic symptom is drowsiness or paradoxical excitation. Withdrawal seizures have also been reported. Dry mouth, tachycardia, dilated pupils, and depressed bowel sounds may occur early after the introduction of benzodiazepines because of possible anticholinergic effects. Withdrawal symptoms include excessive apprehension, anorexia, nausea, postural tremulousness, insomnia, and confusion. Withdrawal symptoms are best handled in the hospital, and barbiturates are usually substituted.

Meprobamate is widely used to treat anxiety, and the major toxicity of this drug relates to sedation and ataxia. Sedation is enhanced when meprobamate is consumed along with other drugs, including tricyclic antidepressants (TCAs), monoamine oxidase inhibitors, and possibly ethanol.

ANTIDEPRESSANT AGENTS

Tricyclic antidepressants induce an acute encephalopathy that is characterized by agitation, confusion, mydriasis, and sometimes convulsions. Tremor and myoclonus may be prominent motor features of this syndrome. Medical complications of these drugs include complex cardiac arrhythmias and heart block. Generalized support measures should be instituted for the patient who takes an overdose of TCAs. *Physostigmine,* a centrally active cholinesterase inhibitor, 1 to 2 mg given IV, will often awaken a patient from coma. This finding suggests that much of the toxic mental alteration relates directly to central anticholinergic toxicity.

Tricyclic antidepressants may also precipitate a more chronic neurotoxic syndrome in which tremor and sedation or insomnia are the prominent features. The tremor is usually postural or intentional and resembles that seen with amphetamine intoxication or use of lithium. Currently, most TCAs can be monitored with plasma levels, so that intoxication can be detected at early stages.

Newer-generation antidepressants have been developed to be more selective for the noradrenergic or serotonergic systems. Many of these agents (e.g., *trimipramine, amoxapine,* or *maprotiline*), however, still have significant anticholinergic side effects, including blurred vision, urinary retention, and confusion. Trazodone can cause priapism.

Selective serotonin reuptake inhibitors (SSRIs) are potent and selective inhibitors of serotonin reuptake at the presynaptic terminal. They are currently considered first-line therapy for depression because of their prescribing ease and superior side-effect/safety profile. SSRI-induced side effects are usually transient and rarely result in discontinuation of the medication. In addition, they appear to be safer than TCAs in overdose.

The major CNS side effects of the SSRIs include nausea, headache, dry mouth, insomnia/somnolence, agitation, nervousness, sweating, dizziness, tremor, and sexual dysfunction. Fluoxetine is often associated with anxiety, nervousness, insomnia, and anorexia. Paroxetine, fluvoxamine, and nefazodone are associated with sedation. Sexual dysfunction manifests itself as ejaculatory delay in men and anorgasmia in women. There have been reports suggesting that fluoxetine can induce or exacerbate suicidal tendencies, and several mechanisms have been proposed. However, since suicide is an important feature of depression, it is difficult to draw conclusions, while, on the other hand, it is difficult to exclude the possibility that suicidal ideation occurs as a rare adverse reaction with some drugs.

Selective serotonin reuptake inhibitors have been shown *in vitro* and *in vivo* to inhibit the P-450 system and therefore to result in increased levels of drugs that are substrates of P-450 as well (e.g., TCAs). There has been debate over whether the combination of SSRIs and monoamino-oxidase inhibitors or TCAs can lead to the serotonin syndrome characterized by hyperpyrexia, myoclonus, rigidity, hyperreflexia, shivering, confusion, agitation, restlessness, coma, autonomic instability, nausea, diarrhea, diaphoresis, flushing, and, rarely, rhabdomyolysis and death. This occurrence is probably very uncommon but should be watched for and handled immediately with supportive care and drug withdrawal if it occurs. Several case reports in the literature suggest that SSRIs can produce extrapyramidal symptoms in the form of akathisia, dyskinesia, acute dystonia, and deterioration in Parkinson's disease, but controlled clinical studies are needed to determine the validity of these observations.

Monoamine oxidase (MAO) inhibitors are drugs that have been used for decades in the treatment of depression. The characteristic of acute MAO inhibitor intoxication is hyperpyrexia, with fevers as high as 108°F. Coma, tachycardia, tachypnea, dilated pupils, and profuse sweating occur. Rapid recovery after hemodialysis suggests that this means of therapy is effective. A second cataclysmic syndrome is the hypertensive crisis associated with combined use of MAO inhibitors and tyramine products or other centrally active agents. Cheese, chicken livers, chocolate, wine, and some forms of herring have been associated with this syndrome in patients ingesting MAO inhibitors. Much less dramatic and also more common are mild side effects, such as mild dizziness, a generalized weakness, dysarthria, and confusion, which can occur in patients receiving therapeutic doses of these agents.

Lithium carbonate is well established as an effective agent in the treatment of manic–depressive illness. Neurotoxic effects are not rare, and the most common and annoying effect is a fine postural intention tremor, which may be seen even in therapeutic doses. A reduction of the dosage will usually either eliminate the tremor or significantly reduce its intensity. The β-adrenergic blocker propranolol may prove beneficial. Toxic confusional states may also occur with lithium and, if this develops, lithium blood levels should be checked. Ataxia, seizures, and coma can occur in high doses (serum levels exceeding 2.0 mEq/l). There is no specific antidote for severe lithium intoxication. After severe intoxication, residual symptoms including ataxia, nystagmus, choreoathetoid movements, and hyperactive deep tendon reflexes have been reported.

HYPNOSEDATIVE AND OTHER AGENTS

Barbiturates are usually used to manage seizure disorders but are still used to calm patients and facilitate sleep. Drowsiness is a common complaint associated with their use, and ataxia (often without nystagmus) can develop when the plasma level rises above 50 μg/ml. In higher doses, severe ataxia, nausea, vomiting, and nystagmus predominate. A second encephalopathic syndrome occurs in children on phenobarbital and is highly distinctive. Instead of somnolence, these children develop remarkable agitation and hyperactivity. This can give the picture of attentional deficit disorder (ADD), or childhood hyperactivity. Patients with chronic toxic exposure to barbiturates show ataxic gait, slurred speech, and periods of intermittent agitation. Tremors and confusion, as well as diplopia and nystagmus, are characteristic.

Ethchlorvynol has a rapid onset and a short duration of action. The common side effects associated with its use are a strange mintlike aftertaste, dizziness, nausea, vomiting, and facial paresthesias. Idiosyncratic reactions characterized by marked excitation and histrionic behavior have also occurred. Chronic abuse of this drug results in both tolerance and physical dependence. Withdrawal symptoms resemble those seen with delirium tremens and may be especially severe in elderly patients.

Methaqualone may induce transient and persistent paresthesias and other signs of peripheral neuropathy. Paradoxical restlessness and anxiety instead of sedation and sleep are also reported with this drug. As with many of the drugs already mentioned, methaqualone with alcohol may have addictive sedating effects. Other drug interactions include enhanced effect of MAO inhibitors and TCAs. Delirium and marked myoclonus may also occur in patients who acutely overdose with these drugs.

Disulfiram is used in the rehabilitation of alcoholics, since high levels of acetaldehyde accumulate when alcohol is ingested with the drug. Chronic disulfiram therapy is associated with two distinct neurotoxic syndromes, an encephalopathy and a neuropathy. The encephalopathy is usually acute or subacute in onset, characterized by delirium and paranoid and psychotic behavior, and it is often confused with the diagnosis of schizophrenic reaction. The behavioral response to neuroleptics or other psychotropic drugs is generally not marked, a finding that should suggest a toxic cause; withdrawal of disulfiram and mild sedation with supportive care (but without neuroleptic therapy) are recommended in the treatment of disulfiram encephalopathy.

Disulfiram is also associated with a rare, axonal distal sensory/motor polyneuropathy. The recovery after drug withdrawal both clinically and pathologically suggests a dying-back or distal axonopathy rather than new degeneration secondary to the loss of nerve cells. It is not known whether disulfiram is the responsible agent or whether a toxic metabolite induces the neuropathy. Disulfiram is possibly metabolized to carbon disulfide, a compound capable of causing an axonal neuropathy in humans and animals.

ANTI-INFLAMMATORY AGENTS

SALICYLATE COMPOUNDS

Because of their ready availability in most households, *salicylates* represent a common source of intoxication, accounting for the largest yearly number of serious childhood poisonings. In acute intoxication, the prominent neurologic and respiratory signs may immediately suggest the correct diagnosis and direct prompt and appropriate intervention. The neurologic manifestations of salicylate toxicity include a rapid and dramatic alteration in consciousness and global function with convulsions and coma. Confu-

sion and restlessness are seen early, leading within a few hours to excitability, tremor, incoherent speech, and often delirium or hallucinosis. This phase has been referred to as a "salicylate jag" to indicate its similarity to alcoholic inebriation, although euphoria and elation are conspicuously absent with salicylates. After this phase, a gradual depression in the level of consciousness occurs with a rapid lapse into coma. Seizures are especially common in children and are usually generalized. The pathophysiology of the convulsions appears to relate to combined effects of metabolic and respiratory disturbances. In infants, salicylate intoxication induces a marked hypoglycemia, and seizure activity is especially hazardous in this young age-group. Diplopia, dizziness, and decreased visual acuity can also be seen with salicylate intoxication. Involvement of the audiovestibular (eighth cranial) nerve can lead to tinnitus, vertigo, and complete deafness. This complication is more common with chronic salicylate intoxication and is seen especially in elderly patients treated for arthritic or headache conditions where aspirin or salicylate compounds are ingested daily. The treatment of salicylate toxicity involves minimizing drug absorption, hastening drug elimination, correcting acid–base disturbance, and treating existing neurologic or medical complications. Induced emesis in the awake patient is the most effective means of emptying the stomach. Enhanced elimination is affected by alkalinization of the urine or by peritoneal dialysis or hemodialysis. Careful fluid and electrolyte management is tantamount and depends on the age of the patient and the stage of intoxication. The complications of hypoglycemia in infants must be anticipated and thereby prevented. Seizures are usually treated with phenytoin and phenobarbital.

There is a poor correlation between the serum salicylate levels and the clinical severity of intoxication. Despite apparently adequate treatment and progressive lowering of toxic plasma salicylate levels, sudden and unexplained deaths are not rare.

STEROIDS

Steroids induce three neurotoxic syndromes: increased intracranial pressure (pseudomotor cerebri), toxic encephalopathy, and myopathy. Infants are more likely than adults to develop steroid-related, increased intracranial pressure, hydrocephalus, and papilledema. This syndrome may occur while patients are receiving steroids or after withdrawal. The pathophysiology of this syndrome is unknown, although it may relate to water intoxication. When it occurs, patients have been treated for weeks or months with steroid compounds.

In contrast, steroid-induced toxic encephalopathy may occur within days of steroid introduction. The behavior is varied and fluctuant, ranging over 24 hours from momentary euphoria to depression to fully developed psychosis. Depersonalization and motor retardation may make these patients difficult to manage during the intoxication phase. Paranoia with visual and auditory hallucination and markedly delusional thinking may predominate. Although this syndrome typically occurs early in the course of steroid therapy, cases exist where mental decline developed after more than 3 months of treatment. Doses of medication do not clearly correlate with symptoms, although the encephalopathy is generally more frequent in high-dose treatment groups. Patients with a prior history of psychiatric care or depression may be at higher risk for encephalopathy than other patients. Suicides have occurred, making this encephalopathy a significant source of potential morbidity. Treatment focuses on withdrawal of the steroid and medical and psychiatric support. Steroids can sometimes be reintroduced later without the reappearance of the problem.

Steroid myopathy, characterized by proximal weakness and atrophy, appears unrelated to the actual duration of drug treatment, and type II fibers appear to be selectively affected. Patients complain of progressive weakness that focuses primarily on the proximal muscles (shoulders and thighs).

Because the steroid compounds alter coagulation factors, secondary hypercoagulable states can occur, resulting in cerebrovascular disease. Rapid withdrawal of steroids induces the behavioral manifestations seen clinically in Addison's disease. These manifestations are secondary phenomena and are not related directly to drug neurotoxicity.

NONSTEROIDALS

The nonsteroidal anti-inflammatory agents account for approximately 4% of the prescription market. There are a variety of types currently available, and ibuprofen is even available in low doses as a nonprescription drug. Despite widespread use, these agents infrequently cause significant neurologic adverse effects. The most common neurologic side effect is headache. Other rare but serious central disturbances include confusion, hallucinations, and overt psychosis. Although these agents have not been evaluated well in controlled studies, it has been suggested that there may be subtle, associated cognitive and memory changes, particularly in more elderly patients. Another infrequent yet important side effect

described is the occurrence of aseptic meningitis. Initially reported in 1978, there have been subsequent case reports in which *ibuprofen* was the most commonly associated drug, although *sulindac, naproxen,* and *tolmetin* have also been implicated. From these case reports, it appears that young women with connective tissue disorders are the most likely to develop this side effect. The clinical picture is that of aseptic meningitis, with fever, chills, and meningismus. The cerebrospinal fluid has an elevated protein content, a pleocytosis of granulocytes, and a normal or reduced glucose level. The underlying mechanism for this syndrome is felt to be a hypersensitivity reaction to the drugs. Although an infectious source for meningitis must be sought, no communicable agent has been isolated. The meningeal syndrome resolves with the discontinuation of the nonsteroidal, only to recur, sometimes more rapidly and severely, if treatment is reinitiated.

Indomethacin has proved to be a potent anti-inflammatory drug but appears less efficacious than salicylates in the treatment of arthritis and rheumatoid variants. Its mode of action is still uncertain, but it may act by way of inhibition of prostaglandin synthesis. CNS toxicity is one of the most frequent dose-limiting factors, precluding the use of indomethacin in 30% to 50% of patients. Neurotoxic effects consist of headaches, depression, agitation, and, rarely, hallucinations. Ataxia, clumsiness, and impaired postural reflexes may also occur, although slow increases in dosage may prevent their development.

Phenylbutazone, used in the treatment of ankylosing spondylitis, is not associated with marked neurotoxic effects. An alteration in the sensation of taste is the most frequently reported neurologic side effect. Phenylbutazone alters the metabolism of phenytoin and, in seizure patients, may be associated with anticonvulsant toxicity or increased seizure activity.

Naproxen has been associated with adverse neurologic reactions in approximately 8% of patients. These effects include headache, drowsiness, vertigo, inability to concentrate, and depression. Because of its protein-binding affinity, naproxen can be associated with phenytoin toxicity in seizure patients. By displacing phenytoin from proteins, naproxen causes higher levels of unbound phenytoin to circulate, so that toxic signs develop even though the total serum phenytoin level remains in the therapeutic range.

Sulindac is another recently marketed nonsteroidal anti-inflammatory agent recommended for use in various types of arthritis. Its mode of action may be the inhibition of prostaglandin synthesis by one of its metabolites, a sulfide. The neurotoxicity of sulindac has been estimated to be between 1% and 10%, with headache and dizziness being most common. Vertigo, tinnitus, and decreased hearing occur in less than 1% of reported patients. Paresthesias, peripheral neuropathy, and transient blurring of vision are rare, but more clinical experience is needed to confirm the true incidence of these reactions.

HORMONES

Oral contraceptives have become widely prescribed, and related neurotoxic syndromes have emerged with disturbing frequency. The most alarming side effect is cerebrovascular disease. The risk of cerebrovascular accidents in young women taking oral contraceptives is increased, and stroke syndromes are 3 to 8 times more frequent, than in those who are not taking oral contraceptives. The symptoms of transient ischemic attacks and stroke syndromes may be varied. In hemispheric strokes, dominant hemispheric lesions provoke aphasias and right hemiparesis. Left hemiparesis with hemisensory loss in the face and body follow a right middle cerebral artery occlusion. Brainstem cerebrovascular accidents presenting with "crossed-syndrome" (e.g., decreased sensation on the right face with decreased sensation on the left body, or decreased strength of the right face with decreased strength of the left body) follow vertebrobasilar disease of the brainstem circulation. The treatment for such strokes involves the removal of the oral contraceptives and the general rehabilitation efforts used in other forms of cerebrovascular disease. Angiographic findings more typical of embolic disease are usually seen with oral contraceptive–induced strokes, although thrombotic disease also occurs. High estrogen–containing oral contraceptives are associated with more cerebrovascular disease than are other contraceptive products.

Chorea is another serious problem related to oral contraceptives. The involuntary movements appear days or weeks after starting birth control pills and may be more frequent in patients with prior history of Sydenham's (rheumatic) chorea. The chorea usually starts abruptly and may involve only one side of the body (hemichorea). Theoretically, the early childhood chorea of rheumatic fever relates to striatal vasculopathy, and estrogens during adult life may precipitate a chemical alteration that unveils the long quiescent lesion. A similar phenomenon occurs occasionally during pregnancy when a woman develops severe involuntary movements that terminate when the pregnancy ends (chorea gravidarum). Birth control chorea may disappear within 48 hours after medication is stopped, although the abatement may take longer.

Neuro-ophthalmologic signs also occur with patients who are taking oral contraceptives. Pseudotumor cerebri may occur in patients who are often not the typically obese women with pseudotumor cerebri in other settings. Vascular headaches (migraines) may also appear for the first time or suddenly change in pattern when oral contraceptives are started. Common migraine (without an aura) may become classic migraine, with patients beginning their headache syndrome with symptoms or signs of focal cerebral dysfunction. In cases where migraines appear for the first time, increase in frequency, or become focal, a cessation of oral contraceptives is suggested.

Various other neurologic disorders are occasionally associated with the use of oral contraceptives. Seizures may change in pattern of frequency. Carpal tunnel syndrome of median nerve neuropathy or other pressure neuropathies may occur related to the increased fluid retention associated with oral contraceptives. Drug-induced and reversible myasthenia gravis has also rarely been reported.

VITAMINS AND ADDITIVES

Caffeine and other xanthine derivatives, including aminophylline, are CNS stimulants that excite all levels of the central nervous system, the cortex being the most sensitive. Caffeine increases energy metabolism throughout the brain but decreases cerebral blood flow, inducing a relative brain hypoperfusion. The drug activates noradrenaline neurons and may act as a second messenger at dopamine receptors to effect the local release of dopamine. Mobilization of intracellular calcium and inhibition of specific phosphodiesterases occurs at high, nonphysiological concentrations of caffeine. The most likely mechanism of action of methylxanthine is the antagonism at the level of adenosine receptors.

Caffeine's psychostimulant action on humans is often subtle and difficult to detect. Its effects on learning, memory, performance, and coordination are related to methylxanthine-induced arousal, vigilance, and fatigue. An increased awareness of the environment or hyperesthesia may be an unpleasant experience for some patients. The patient becomes loquacious and restless and often complains of ringing in the ears and giddiness. In high doses, xanthines affect the spinal cord, resulting in increased reflex excitability, tremulous extremities, and tense muscles. Caffeine clearly alters sleep patterns, and if taken within 1 hour of attempted sleep, it increases sleep latency, decreases total sleep time, and worsens the subject's estimate of sleep quality. Less time is spent in stages three and four and more in stage two. Xanthine-associated seizures are seen as a complication of aminophylline therapy, especially when the drug is administered intravenously. They are usually generalized but can be focal. Cessation of the use of products containing caffeine can cause a withdrawal syndrome of headaches, drowsiness, fatigue, decreased performance, and, in some instances, nausea and vomiting. These symptoms begin within 12 to 24 hours after the last use, peak at 20 to 48 hours, and last approximately 1 week.

Nicotine increases circulating levels of norepinephrine and epinephrine and stimulates the release of striatal dopamine. It exerts stimulant effects through specific nicotinic receptors, whose activation may facilitate dopaminergic transmission centrally. Nicotine has been reported to affect a number of neurologic diseases, such as spinocerebellar degeneration, multiple system atrophy, multiple sclerosis, tic disorders, parkinsonism, and myoclonic epilepsy.

Nicotine, despite being a powerful stimulant, has no major therapeutic application. Its high toxicity and presence in tobacco smoke give nicotine a considerable medical importance, however. Clinically, tremors and convulsions are major neurologic signs of nicotine intoxication. Respiration is stimulated and vomiting is induced. Nicotine also has marked antidiuretic activity resulting from direct hypothalamic stimulation. If acutely ingested, nicotine can be fatal at a level of approximately 60 mg of the base product. Autonomic overactivity with dilated pupils, irregular pulse, sweating, and muscle twitching are characteristic signs of nicotine toxicity. Coma may rapidly supervene, although convulsions are usually not present. If death occurs, it is caused by paralysis of respiratory muscles. Cardiac arrhythmias are significant and are other potential sources for demise. Chronic intoxication due to nicotine occurs among tobacco pickers, or "croppers," consisting of nausea, vomiting, dizziness, and prostration. The illness is intermittent and lasts between 12 and 14 hours; it then clears, only to recur with return to work. There are no mortalities or long-term sequelae, however. During the 1973 harvesting season, an estimated 9% of the 60,000 tobacco growers in North Carolina reported illnesses.

Vitamins are vital trace substances, and neurologic syndromes are generally associated with deficiency syndromes. However, since health enthusiasm has reached passionate proportions for many individuals, especially Americans, clinicians are encountering neurotoxic syndromes associated with these seemingly safe agents. Of the fat-soluble vitamins, vitamin A is directly associated with neurotoxicity, and vitamin D can alter bone and renal metabolism, causing secondary neurologic dysfunction. Of the water-soluble vitamins, only pyridoxine (B_6) is established to provoke neurologic complications.

Vitamin A, required for normal growth, vision, reproduction, and maintenance of epithelium, in high doses accumulates and can induce the syndrome of increased intracranial pressure (pseudotumor cerebri). Foods high in vitamin A include broccoli, cabbage, and liver, although dietary hypervitaminosis A is most unusual. Medically, vitamin A is used in the treatment of acne vulgaris and other dermatologic illnesses. Whereas the generally recommended daily allowance is 5,000 IU, individual capsules can contain 5 times that value, with subjects often ingesting 100,000 IU daily. At these doses, intoxication will develop over several months; at 200,000 IU daily, intoxication may develop within weeks. Recent publicity about the cancer preventive properties of vitamin A may increase the number of people who expose themselves to this product.

Early signs of increased intracranial pressure include headaches, blurred vision, transient obscuration of vision, and sixth cranial nerve paresis. On funduscopic examination, gradual papilledema develops without further signs of focal neurologic deficit. No neurologic clue exists to establish the etiology, but the skin changes, organomegaly, and history of vitamin ingestion will establish the diagnosis. Since vitamin zealots are often "antimedication," these patients must be specifically questioned about vitamins.

Vitamin D, when given in massive amounts, mobilizes bone calcium and phosphorus. When there is bone demineralization and degeneration, nerve root and spinal cord compression can occur. Alterations in the calcium balance can produce generalized weakness, muscle aches, cramps, and mild metabolic encephalopathy. Meningeal symptoms and trigeminal neuralgia are two additional reported findings without clear pathogenesis. The latter may relate to bony foraminal alterations. When renal impairment occurs, progressive secondary encephalopathy, not directly related to the vitamin, develops, and coma may result.

Pyridoxine, or *vitamin B_6,* has been implicated in a highly selective toxic syndrome provoking a sensory ataxia and dorsal root gangliar dysfunction. Widely used, especially by women to treat premenstrual tension and edema, pyridoxine induces this neurotoxic syndrome in occasional patients consuming chronic daily doses of 2 g or more. Gradually, the patient notes difficulty walking, with lightning-like dysesthesias in the back. Numbness of the extremities occurs and, importantly, facial dysesthesias, so uncommon with most toxic neuropathies other than trichloroethane, quickly develop. Areflexia, stocking–glove sensory loss, and profound sensory ataxia with preserved strength are typical. On electromyography, marked slowing of the sensory nerve conduction is seen with normal motor conduction.

Tryptophan is an amino acid that has become popular for management of insomnia and behavioral changes related to the menstrual cycle (premenstrual syndrome). Myalgia and eosinophilia have been reported in numerous patients, as well as a progressive neuropathy affecting primarily the lower extremities with aching weakness. In some instances, patients are so disabled that they are wheelchair bound and need ventilatory assistance. Cessation of exposure to tryptophan and plasma exchange have been associated with clinical improvement in some cases.

QUESTIONS AND DISCUSSION

1. Match the cardiac drug with a prominent side effect:

A.	Propranolol	**1.** Visual disturbance in as many as 40% of patients
B.	Digitalis	**2.** Depression and impotency
C.	Alpha methyldopa	**3.** Garrulous, uninhibited behavior
D.	Lidocaine	**4.** Parkinsonism
		5. Peripheral neuropathy in 25%

The correct matches are (A) and (2); (B) and (1); (C) and (4); and (D) and (3). Propranolol and other beta-antagonists can cause depression and impotency that can be obscured in the rehabilitative setting after a myocardial infarction or surgery. Digitalis has prominent visual side effects, and patients often complain of halos around everything. Alpha methyldopa can cause or aggravate parkinsonism, and lidocaine is often associated with a bizarre and alarming change in behavior.

2. Factors that contribute to the acid–base abnormality of salicylate intoxication include the following:

A. Salicylates initially depress medullary breathing activation.

B. Salicylates are acids that displace bicarbonate and can also lead to ketosis.

C. Myoglobinuria usually precipitates renal shutdown and metabolic acidosis.

D. All of the above

The answer is (B). Salicylates initially activate the medullary breathing center and cause respiratory alkalosis. Later, at high doses, the medullary breathing center can be inhibited. In addition, salicylates induce and enhance the chemosensitive response and are acids as described in (B). The net response is a metabolic acidosis with either a respiratory acidosis or alkalosis. Myoglobinuria is not a feature of salicylate intoxication.

3. True statements regarding birth control pills and neurologic disability include:

A. Peripheral neuropathy of the axonal type can mimic multiple sclerosis.

B. Cerebrovascular accidents usually relate to cardiac valvular vegetations.

C. Chorea often resolves within days or weeks of drug cessation and is rarely a permanent sequela of oral contraceptive ingestion.

D. Papilledema, when it occurs, is caused by the steroid-induced hypervitaminosis A.

The answer is (C). Birth control pills are not associated with a peripheral neuropathy, but instead their toxicity relates predominantly to a CNS function. Cerebrovascular accidents are an alarming complication of these drugs in young women and may be of embolic or thrombotic origin. They do not relate specifically to valvular vegetations. Chorea often occurs within days of the first ingestion of birth control pills and may promptly stop after drug cessation. Only in rare instances (usually a hemiballistic syndrome) will the chorea be long-standing after drug cessation. In such cases, a static cerebrovascular accident is hypothesized to underlie the chorea as opposed to the transient chorea, which probably relates to a hormonally induced functional alteration in dopaminergic sensitivity at the striatum. Papilledema, when it occurs in patients on birth control pills, may have multiple etiologies, including venous thrombosis and pseudotumor cerebri. It does not appear to relate to hypervitaminosis A.

4. Five neurologic complications of neuroleptic therapy are listed (1) through (5). Match them with their usual characteristics using the (A) through (C) list.

1.	Dystonia	**A.** Acute, occurring minutes or hours or, at most, days after starting the drug

2. Parkinsonism

3. Chorea

4. Tremor
5. Oculogyric crises

B. Subacute, occurring days, weeks, or a few months after starting the drug
C. Chronic, occurring after several months or years of drug treatment

The correct matches are (A) and (1) or (5); (B) and (2) or (4); (C) and (3). The acute neurologic side effects related to neuroleptic drugs are dystonia and akathisia. The contorted posture of dystonia is frightening to see or experience. An oculogyric crisis, with the eyes thrown back and the neck usually hyperextended, is only one example of a dystonic complication of neuroleptics. Recently, a late-onset dystonia has been described as within the realm of tardive dyskinesia, but this is probably uncommon. Tardive dyskinesia should be mainly considered a choreic or stereotypic disorder and is the major chronic side effect of neuroleptic drugs. The subacute problem associated with neuroleptic medication is parkinsonism, which may include any of the following: tremor, bradykinesia, rigidity, or postural reflex compromise.

5. True statements regarding the use of antiemetic drugs include:

A. Metoclopramide is particularly useful in Parkinson disease patients with nausea secondary to their dopaminergic medication.
B. Children receiving prochlorperazine for gastrointestinal distress are least likely to have neurologic complications.
C. In a patient using a scopolamine patch who reports acute right eye pain, an emergency visit to an ophthalmologist and removal of the patch should be recommended.
D. Scopolamine may cause drug-induced parkinsonism by a mechanism similar to that of neuroleptics.

The answer is (C). Scopolamine is an anticholinergic agent that may exacerbate narrow-angle glaucoma, with painful symptoms in the eyes. If not recognized and treated emergently, this may result in blindness. Both metoclopramide and prochlorperazine are dopamine-receptor blockers, similar to the neuroleptics. Hence, both agents may cause drug-induced parkinsonism or worsen preexisting Parkinson's disease. Children treated with these drugs are at more risk for developing acute dystonic reactions. In contrast, scopolamine, being an anticholinergic agent, does not cause drug-induced parkinsonism.

6. In patients receiving theophylline, which of the following is true?

A. Seizures occur only if serum levels are in the toxic range.
B. Theophylline is a useful agent in an elderly patient with congestive heart failure and a previous stroke with a history of intermittent asthma.
C. A child receiving IV infusions of theophylline is at increased risk for developing acute dystonic reactions.
D. The pharmacokinetics of drugs metabolized in the liver may affect the metabolism and serum levels of theophylline.

The answer is (D). Theophylline is metabolized by the hepatic enzymes. Other drugs metabolized in the liver may alter theophylline metabolism, affecting the serum levels. The seizures associated with theophylline may occur in the therapeutic range. In particular, patients with previous brain injury are at increased risk. Congestive heart failure may increase theophylline levels even when the drug is administered at recommended doses. Theophylline is a xanthine, compound without dopamine receptor activity, and it is not known to cause acute dystonic reactions.

7. Which of the following antibiotics is associated with a high incidence of neurotoxicity?

A. Penicillin
B. Trimethoprim
C. Minocycline
D. Erythromycin

The answer is (C). Minocycline provokes ototoxicity, and women are more susceptible to these effects than men. The remaining agents are associated with neurotoxic syndromes only on occasion, unless they are given by unusual routes or in unusual doses.

8. Which condition is associated with vitamin excess?

A. Clinical findings of Guillain–Barré syndrome
B. Increased intracranial pressure
C. Myasthenia gravis
D. Wernicke-Korsakoff syndrome

The answer is (B). Excess vitamin A and B_6 are known to cause neurotoxic syndrome. B_6 provokes a sensory neuropathy with loss of reflexes, but it should not be confused with Guillain–Barré, which predominantly affects the motor system. Vitamin A causes the syndrome of pseudotumor cerebri, with increased intracranial pressure, often associated with headache and other nonfocal neurologic findings. (Sixth-nerve paresis, unlike other cranial neuropathies is a "false-localizing" sign. Because of the long trajectory of the nerve along bony surfaces, a sixth-nerve paresis does not locate the level or side of neurologic damage.) Vitamin D, when given in high doses chronically, affects calcium and phosphorus balance, which may clinically provoke global weakness. The classical neuromuscular fatigue typical of myasthenia and the response to edrophonium are not seen. Wernicke–Korsakoff syndrome is related to vitamin deprivation and not to intoxication.

SUGGESTED READING

Bahls FH, Ma KK, Bird TD: Theophylline-associated seizures with "therapeutic" or low toxic serum concentrations: Risk factors for serious outcome in adults. Neurology 41:1309, 1991

Giménez-Roldàn S, Mateo D: Cinnarizine-induced parkinsonism. Clin Neuropharmacol 14:156, 1991

Goetz CG: Neurotoxins in Clinical Practice. New York, SP Medical and Scientific Books, 1985

Goetz CG, Kompoliti K, Washburn KR: Neurotoxic Agents. In: Joynt RJ, Griggs RC (eds): Clinical Neurology, p 1. Philadelphia, Lippincott-Raven, 1997

Heiman-Patterson TD, Bird SJ, Parry GJ et al: Peripheral neuropathy associated with eosinophilia–myalgia syndrome. Ann Neurol 28:522, 1991

Hoppmann RA, Peden JG, Ober SK: Central nervous system side effects of nonsteroidal anti-inflammatory drugs. Arch Intern Med 151:1309, 1991

Lipsy RJ, Fennerty B, Fagan TC: Clinical review of the histamine-2 receptor antagonists. Arch Intern Med 150:745, 1990

Miller LG, Jankovic J: Persistent dystonia possibly induced by flecainide. Mov Disord 7:62, 1992

Pappert EJ: Neuroleptic-induced movement disorders: Acute and subacute syndromes. In: de Wolff FA (ed): Intoxication of the Nervous System, Part II, Amsterdam, Elsevier Science BV, 1994

Sacristan JA, Soto JA, de Cos MA: Erythromycin-induced hypoacusis: 11 new cases and literature review. Ann Pharmacother 27:950, 1993

Silverstein A (ed): Neurological Complications of Therapy: Selected Topics. Mt. Kisco, NY, Futura, 1982

Spencer PS, Schaumburg HH (eds): Experimental and Clinical Neurotoxicology. Baltimore, Williams & Wilkins, 1980

Vinken PJ, Bruyn GW, Cohen MM et al (eds): Handbook of Clinical Neurology, Vols 36 and 37: Intoxications of the Nervous System. Amsterdam, North Holland, 1979

Yokota T, Kagamihara Y, Hayashi H et al: Nicotine-sensitive paresis. Neurology 42:382, 1992

Neurology for the Non-Neurologist, Fourth Edition, edited by William J. Weiner and Christopher G. Goetz. Lippincott Williams & Wilkins, Philadelphia © 1999.

CHAPTER 18

Sequelae of Minor Closed Head Injuries

Charles M. D'Angelo

Richard W. Byrne

The National Center for Health Statistics, a branch of the United States Department of Health, Education and Welfare, records almost 8 million head injuries yearly. Of these, 1.5 million are classified as major head injuries, including severe cerebral concussion, cerebral contusion, and intracranial hemorrhage. Fortunately, over 6 million cases are classified as minor head injuries. Many excellent textbooks deal with the diagnosis and treatment of the severe head injury patient. This chapter deals with the patient who has a minor head injury: typically, this patient sustains a head injury, is evaluated in an emergency facility, and is sent home soon after the injury or after 24 to 48 hours' observation. This chapter is a discussion of dire possibilities, of suspicions that should arise when confronted by a patient who complains of a headache or mild neurologic deficit after a head injury.

SCALP INJURIES

The scalp has five layers: skin, subcutaneous tissue, galea aponeurotica, loose areolar tissue, and periosteum. Superficial contusions, abrasions, or lacerations of the scalp seldom pose a problem for the patient. A delayed wound infection occasionally necessitates a consultation with the family doctor. Local wound care results in good healing, because the scalp is well vascularized.

Three conditions can be a problem: subgaleal hematoma, subgaleal infection, and subperiosteal hematoma. The galea aponeurotica has abundant blood vessels. Injuries that lacerate the galea can be associated with excessive bleeding. An improper closure of the wound that does not tightly approximate the galea can result in arterial bleeding into the loose areolar layer, a *subgaleal hematoma*. The hemorrhage can extend throughout the loose areolar space, confined by the superior eyelids, the zygomatic arch, and the superior nuchal line. The patient returns a few hours to a few days after skin closure with a "pumpkin head." The loose areolar layer may be contaminated by bacteria during injury or wound closure. The resultant *subgaleal infection* is associated with fever, headache, and marked scalp tenderness.

Injuries that tear the periosteum cause subperiosteal bleeding. This bleeding further separates the periosteum from the underlying calvarium, a *subperiosteal hematoma*. The mass of a subperiosteal hematoma, which can be large and disfiguring, slowly recedes without treatment. Since the soft center is surrounded by a ring of firm periosteum, a subperiosteal hematoma can be misdiagnosed as a depressed skull fracture. A tangential view skull roentgenogram differentiates the two possibilities. The elevated periosteum incites new bone formation. The resultant bony lump can cause undue anxiety but resolves without treatment.

SKULL FRACTURES

Skull fractures, like fractures elsewhere in the body, are classified as simple, compound, or comminuted. The skull fracture itself has little clinical significance: It indicates that the intracranial contents have been subjected to significant rotational force and could be damaged. A skull fracture alerts the physician to possible impending intracranial complications. The site and course of a fracture are important. A linear fracture traversing the middle meningeal groove or a major venous sinus can cause an epidural hematoma or subdural hematoma, respectively. Linear fractures approaching the foramen magnum are associated with posterior fossa subdural hematomas: Such fractures are termed *complicated fractures.*

Skull fractures with a break in the scalp are called *compound fractures.* Fractures that enter the various skull sinuses (e.g., mastoid sinus, sphenoid sinus, or frontal sinus) also communicate with the external environment and are compound fractures. Such fractures may herald the development of pneumocephalus, cerebrospinal fluid (CSF) fistula, or meningitis. A sinus air–fluid level or the presence of intracranial air seen on a skull roentgenogram indicates a compound skull fracture.

Fractures of the skull base, *basilar fractures,* are seldom seen on routine roentgenograms. The most common sites of basilar fractures are the cribriform plate and petrous bone. Cribriform plate fractures should be suspected in patients with periorbital ecchymoses (raccoon sign), anosmia, or CSF rhinorrhea. Petrous bone fractures are often accompanied by mastoid ecchymosis (Battle's sign), hemotympanum, CSF otorrhea, and cranial nerve (CN) VII dysfunction. Basilar skull fractures can traverse neural foramina with injury to cranial nerves. The suspicion of a basilar skull fracture should alert the treating physician to the possibility of impending CSF fistula and meningitis.

At the time of impact, a fracture edge may lacerate the dural and subarachnoid membranes, trapping the membranes in the fracture line. CSF flows into the trapped membranes and cannot exit. The expanding, trapped CSF forms a cyst, known as a *leptomeningeal cyst,* that erodes or expands the fracture line. Such cysts are not uncommon in children and cause the so-called *growing* or *spreading fracture.*

CEREBROSPINAL FLUID FISTULA

All CSF fistulae have a defect in the dura-arachnoid membranes, which allows CSF to escape from the subarachnoid space. CSF fistulae commonly present clinically as CSF rhinorrhea or otorrhea. Traumatic CSF fistulae occur in 2% to 3% of patients with head injuries. There is little correlation between the severity of the head injury and the development of a CSF fistula. Almost 50% of patients who had a traumatic CSF fistula had no loss of consciousness or only a brief loss of consciousness at the time of injury.

A CSF fistula may be immediate or delayed. Immediate CSF rhinorrhea ceases spontaneously within 1 week in 85% of patients; immediate otorrhea ceases within 1 week in nearly all cases. Delayed CSF rhinorrhea usually occurs within 3 months of the head injury.

The most common cause of CSF rhinorrhea is a basilar fracture involving the cribriform plate of the frontal fossa. Basilar fractures entering the frontal, ethmoid, or sphenoid sinuses may also cause CSF rhinorrhea. Otorrhea is caused by fractures of the petrous bone involving the mastoid air cells. It is interesting that a petrous bone fracture can cause CSF rhinorrhea. In such cases, the tympanic membrane is intact and the communication with the nasal cavity is by way of the eustachian tube.

A CSF fistula should be suspected in any patient who develops signs or symptoms of meningitis after a head injury. A headache that increases in intensity in the erect position is a suspicious symptom. Occasionally, a patient describes an intracranial "swooshing" sensation (pneumocephalus) with inhalation. The appearance of clear, watery fluid draining from the nose is highly suspicious. The fluid often "pours out" in the head-dependent position. CSF may often be seen behind the eardrum.

The diagnosis can be confirmed if collected nasal fluid, uncontaminated by blood, contains greater than 30 mg glucose per 100 ml. CSF glucose may be less than 30 mg/100 ml if meningitis is present. Dextrostix testing is unreliable because the tape often turns positive as a result of sugar in normal nasal mucus. The diagnosis of a CSF fistula can be suspected if a routine skull roentgenogram reveals pneumocephalus. A definitive diagnosis may require the extraarachnoid detection of radioimmunosorbent assay (RISA) or 99m-technetium (^{99m}Tc) serum albumin injected into the lumbar subarachnoid space. Detection of radioactivity in the nasal cavity or auditory canal confirms the diagnosis of CSF fistula but does not always indicate the site of the leak. Often, a contrast-enhanced computed tomography (CT) scan will reveal a collection of contrast material, "puddling," at the site of the fistula.

POST-TRAUMATIC MENINGITIS ABSCESS

Head trauma as the leading cause of meningitis in adults highlights the clinical importance of CSF fistulae. Meningitis occurs in 3% to 50% of patients who have traumatic dural fistulae. The infection rate tends to be high if the CSF leak persists for 7 days or longer. In 85% of the patients with meningitis, the etiologic organism is *Pneumococcus*. Unlike pneumococcal meningitis in the general population, the mortality rate in patients with CSF fistulae is less than 10%. Meningitis due to CSF fistulae should be treated aggressively with antibiotics determined by CSF sensitivity studies.

The question of whether prophylactic antibiotics should be used in patients with CSF fistulae is controversial. Some centers in which prophylactic antibiotics were employed reported the development of meningitis due to highly resistant strains of organisms. Many centers, therefore, do not use routine prophylactic antibiotics. We, however, obtain a nasal and pharyngeal culture on all patients with a CSF fistula. If signs of meningitis occur, we institute antibiotic therapy based on the "predominate growth" in the cultures until CSF sensitivity studies are complete.

Because of the proximity of the undersurface of the frontal lobes of the brain to the cribriform plate, a frontal lobe abscess can develop in a patient with a CSF fistula. Symptoms may be nonspecific, such as a headache and mild obtundation. Spinal fluid may be normal. The diagnosis is confirmed by using brain scan techniques.

INTRACRANIAL EXTRA-AXIAL LESIONS

EPIDURAL HEMATOMA

Epidural hematoma, a mass of clotted blood between the inner skull table and the dura, is the best known neurosurgical emergency, yet the diagnosis is often delayed, resulting in mortality rates exceeding 90% in some series. The classic description of an acute epidural hematoma progresses as follows: a blow to the head causing a linear fracture crossing the middle meningeal groove of the temporal bone; brief loss of consciousness; a regaining of consciousness ("lucid interval"); arterial bleeding with an expanding epidural mass; increasing intracranial pressure with obtundation; tentorial herniation with contralateral hemiparesis and ipsilateral pupillary dilatation; decerebrate rigidity; respiratory irregularity; and death. This classic presentation occurs in less than 10% of cases of epidural hematomas.

In many cases, there is no loss of consciousness or the patient never regains consciousness. Up to 60% of epidural hematomas form in patients with minimal underlying brain damage and no loss of consciousness, or a brief period of being "dazed." Furthermore, although most epidural hematomas are associated with fractures crossing the middle meningeal groove, the middle meningeal vein, not the artery, is often lacerated. The evaluation of cerebral compression is, therefore, slower, extending over several hours or days, or occasionally weeks. Likewise, about 30% of epidural hematomas do not occur in the temporal area but are located in the frontal or occipital areas or posterior fossa. An epidural hematoma should be suspected in any patient sustaining a skull fracture.

SUBDURAL HEMATOMA

Bleeding into the subdural space commonly occurs by two mechanisms: (1) During a rotational injury of the brain, the frontal or temporal poles are severely contused or lacerated; bleeding from the contused brain extends into the subdural space; and (2) during a rotational injury of the brain, veins bridging the subdural space from the cerebral cortex to the dura are torn, with venous bleeding directly into the subdural space. The second mechanism is more common in patients with cerebral atrophy (i.e., the elderly and alcoholics).

Subdural hematomas are classified arbitrarily according to the time interval between the head injury and the development of clinical manifestations. Acute subdural hematomas occur within 4 days of trauma, subacute subdural hematomas occur between 4 and 14 days, and chronic subdural hematomas occur after 14 days.

Unlike the acute subdural hematoma, the *chronic subdural hematoma* initially forms in the absence of underlying brain injury. Indeed, the initial injury is often trivial or forgotten altogether. The venous hemorrhage is encapsulated by a membrane. The atrophic brain allows the development of a large mass that shifts the cerebral structures initially without a significant increase in intracranial pressure. Patients present with a headache and obtundation. The depressed level of alertness or awareness overshadows the neurologic deficit.

SUBARACHNOID HEMORRHAGE

Trauma is the most common cause of subarachnoid hemorrhage, and subarachnoid bleeding is the most common hemorrhage following trauma. Abrasions, contusions, and lacerations of the cortical surface produce bleeding into the subarachnoid space. The blood can cause meningeal irritation with headache, nuchal rigidity, and photophobia in an otherwise normal patient.

Blood in the subarachnoid space can incite fibrosis within the basal CSF cisterns, impeding normal CSF flow. Patients may develop hydrocephalus several days to several weeks after a head injury. The clinical picture is similar to so-called normal-pressure hydrocephalus with the development of mental deterioration, urinary incontinence, and gait dysfunction. Ventriculomegaly is seen on CT or magnetic resonance imaging (MRI) scans of the brain.

INTRACRANIAL INTRA-AXIAL LESIONS

At the moment of impact, the skull and the intracranial contents are suddenly accelerated or decelerated. The intracranial structures are subjected to severe rotational stresses during acceleration or deceleration. During rotation, cortical surfaces may be damaged by bony protuberances of the cranial vault; or white matter–gray matter junctions may shear from one another. Such shearing rotational injuries include concussion, contusion, and intercerebral hemorrhage.

CONCUSSION

Cerebral concussion denotes the loss of consciousness without significant anatomic damage to the brain. This brief loss of awareness may be due to rotational stress that temporarily blunts neural activity in the reticular activating system (RAS) of the brainstem. The membrane potential may change because of a breakdown of "tight junctions." The severity of the concussion is quantified by the duration of amnesia. The duration of amnesia is the length of amnesia following impact (retrograde amnesia) plus the length of amnesia prior to impact (anterograde amnesia). The duration of unconsciousness is usually overestimated by observers. Therefore, it is helpful to record the time interval between "the first thing and the last thing remembered" after and before the accident. A cerebral concussion itself is of little clinical significance; its importance is in the fact that it may be the first warning of more severe neurologic injuries. Patients who sustain a cerebral concussion should consequently be observed for a progressive neurologic deficit. This observation may be done by hospital personnel or reliable family members.

CONTUSION

Cerebral contusions occur usually on the undersurface or the poles of the frontal lobes, or on the poles of the temporal lobes. The frontotemporal poles are the common sites damaged by bony prominences during rotation. Subpial hemorrhage and edema formation occur at the site of the contusion. The swelling may not be significant or maximal for 2 to 4 days after impact. The patient is awake and alert after the initial concussion. Increasing intracranial pressure, decreased level of consciousness, and focal neurologic deficit may develop later as the contusion mass increases in bulk.

HEMATOMA OR HEMORRHAGE

If the cerebral contusion is severe, the cerebral tissue can be disrupted with intracerebral bleeding. The site of bleeding, like cerebral contusion, is most common in the frontotemporal region. The development of a neurologic dysfunction may be delayed because the hemorrhage is delayed. The initial hemorrhage may be small, and signs develop only when surrounding edema increases the mass effect.

CRANIAL NERVE INJURIES

A dysfunction of any cranial nerve may be seen following closed head injury. A cranial nerve can be sheared, stretched, contused, or lacerated as it transverses bony protuberances or through bony canals. Cranial nerves may be involved directly in fractures of the skull base. The olfactory nerve (CN I) is most often injured.

OLFACTORY NERVE

The loss of smell (anosmia) or the perversion of smell (parosmia) occurs in 5% of patients who sustain a head injury. Anosmia is reported in 40% of patients exhibiting CSF rhinorrhea after a head injury. The olfactory filaments can be sheared from the olfactory bulb during the rotation of the brain, or the filaments can be injured by fractures through the cribriform plate. Because CN I is often not evaluated in an emergency situation, the dysfunction may not be detected until weeks after the head injury when the patient complains of changes in the sense of taste or smell. Many patients regain the sense of smell within 2 years but are annoyed by parosmia during the recovery period. This condition cannot be treated effectively.

FACIAL NERVE

An injury to the facial nerve (CN VII) is next in frequency; however, it is only one third as common as an injury to CN I. Because of the proximity of the facial and vestibuloacoustic nerve (CN VIII) as it courses through the petrous bone, either one or both of these nerves can be injured by transverse fractures of the petrous bone. Fractures near the internal auditory meatus usually involve CN VII and CN VIII with ipsilateral peripheral facial weakness (i.e., the forehead musculature is involved as well as the face), ageusia in the anterior two thirds of the tongue, and ipsilateral deafness. Fortunately, such injuries are less common than trauma to the facial nerve further along its course, which results in ipsilateral facial paresis or paralysis. The onset of facial weakness 4 to 5 days after an injury, especially in patients with hemotympanum, suggests a swelling of the nerve in the facial canal. Such patients should be started on a course of corticosteroids and should be evaluated for possible facial nerve decompression. Computerized visual field testing aids in discovering small scotomata.

TRIGEMINAL NERVE

The gasserian ganglion of the trigeminal nerve (CN V) is occasionally traumatized when fractures of the petrous bone involve Meckel's cave. A complete dysfunction of the ganglion is rare. A spotty decrease in facial sensation usually occurs. Corneal sensation may be decreased, resulting in corneal laceration or conjunctival inflammation.

OPTIC NERVE

The optic nerve (CN II) is rarely injured by basilar skull fractures. A delayed discovery of scotomata is noted occasionally during a visual field examination. Such scotomata are probably the result of a contusion of the optic nerve in the optic foramen.

OCULOMOTOR NERVE AND ABDUCENS NERVE

A dysfunction of the oculomotor nerve (CN III) and the abducens nerve (CN VI) are usually caused by an increased intracranial pressure with uncal herniation. Consequently, pupil inequality and diplopia are noted more often in acute head injury. Residual dysfunctions such as ptosis, pupillary dilation, and paresis of outward gaze may be noted by an examining physician on a future occasion.

CAROTID CAVERNOUS FISTULA

Sixty percent of carotid cavernous fistulae, or pulsating exophthalmus, result from a head injury. A traumatic tear in the intracavernous portion of the carotid artery, or one of its small branches, forms an arteriovenous communication in the cavernous sinus. The unrestricted flow of arterial blood into the cavernous sinus increases venous pressure within the cavernous sinus as well as in the superior and inferior orbital veins that drain the orbit. Almost all clinical signs and symptoms are caused by the increased pressure within the cavernous sinus and orbital venous system. The force required to produce a tear in the intracavernous arterial structures is not known, but it is generally assumed to be severe enough to cause a basilar skull fracture. The signs and symptoms of the fistula occur usually ipsilateral to the site of the fistula. Bilateral findings can occur in patients with severe bilateral basilar skull fracture, with large patent intercavernous veins, and in patients with elastic-collagen disorders, such as the Ehlers–Danlos syndrome.

The most common clinical features are pain, intracranial bruit, pulsating exophthalmus, chemosis, ophthalmoplegia, and diminished visual acuity. A *headache,* usually described as a steady or pulsating "fullness," occurs in the ipsilateral supraorbital region: It is increased in the head-dependent position. The *intracranial bruit* is ipsilateral and incessant, and it is the patient's most annoying symptom. The machinery-like bruit can also be heard by the physician using a stethoscope, which is pressed lightly over the orbit. The bruit is diminished by compression of the ipsilateral carotid artery in the neck. *Exophthalmus* usually averages 8 mm but may reach 24 mm, with consequent restriction of globe movements. Decreased orbital venous drainage results in increased interstitial fluid of the conjunctiva, or *chemosis.* Severe chemosis causes eyelid eversion with further inflammation of the conjunctiva. *Diplopia* is most often the result of compression of CN VI in the cavernous sinus. The diplopia is most marked with lateral gaze. Paresis of CN III or trochlear nerve (CN IV) also occurs, but it is only half as common as an abducens dysfunction. Venous stasis within the orbit causes retinal ischemia and *decreased visual acuity* or blindness.

The diagnosis of carotid cavernous fistula should be suspected in any patient presenting with signs of a basilar skull fracture, such as CSF rhinorrhea and periorbital or mastoid ecchymoses. The diagnosis is confirmed by cerebral angiography.

POST-TRAUMATIC EPILEPSY

The incidence of chronic seizures following nonpenetrating, closed head injuries is approximately 5%. The causal relationship between the occurrence of a head injury and the development of chronic seizures is controversial. Multiple factors determine the likelihood of developing chronic seizures following a closed head injury. They include the patient's age, focal brain injury, diffuse brain injury, the site of brain injury, and the time of the first seizure.

AGE

The development of a chronic seizure disorder is influenced by the age of the patient at the time of injury. Children under 5 years of age, and particularly under 1 year of age, frequently have a seizure immediately following a head injury; however, few children develop a chronic seizure disorder. Patients who are 16 years of age or older and who have an early post-traumatic seizure are more likely to have chronic seizures than their counterparts who are under 16 years of age.

FOCAL BRAIN INJURY

Focal cortical lacerations, such as those that occur with depressed skull fractures, may be associated with chronic seizures in 60% of patients. Likewise, 40% of patients with deeper cerebral lesions, as seen with intracerebral hematomas, develop chronic seizures. The likelihood of developing a chronic seizure disorder appears to be related to the severity of the focal cerebral lesion.

DIFFUSE BRAIN INJURY

The degree and duration of cerebral hypoxia influence the onset of chronic seizures. The more severe the ischemic brain damage, the greater the likelihood of developing seizures. In this regard, the presence of post-traumatic amnesia that lasts for more than 24 hours increases the likelihood of developing a chronic seizure disorder.

SITE OF BRAIN INJURY

Chronic seizures more commonly follow injuries near the central sulcus of the brain than injuries to frontal or occipital poles.

TIME OF FIRST SEIZURE

Seizures that occur within 24 hours of a head injury probably have no prognostic implications for further seizures. Chronic seizures have been reported in only 3% of patients who had a seizure during the first week following a head injury but in 25% of patients who had a seizure during the first week.

The development of chronic seizures following a head injury is problematic. For example, in one series of 265 patients, 8% "developed" their first seizure 10 years or more after their head injury. Furthermore, 50% of patients who develop post-traumatic seizures will cease seizing spontaneously with the use of anticonvulsant therapy.

POST-TRAUMATIC SYNDROME

The post-traumatic or postconcussion syndrome often receives little attention. The problem is not life threatening, yet it can disable a patient for weeks to months. Symptoms include headache, dizziness or giddiness, memory loss, poor concentration, nervousness, disturbed sleep, and decreased libido. The etiology is still unknown; however, a loss of neuron membrane "tight junctions" may play a role in these vague "psychogenic complaints." The result of the neurologic examination is usually normal. The symptoms last for 2 to 6 weeks in most cases but can be present for 1 to 2 years. The occurrence of the syndrome is more likely in patients who sustain a mild head trauma (i.e., a short duration of amnesia following cerebral concussion). It is more common in women, in people of average intelligence, and in assembly line workers. The diagnosis is made by the multiplicity of symptoms and the exclusion of a significant structural lesion. CT and MR scanning can exclude mass lesions. Labyrinthine testing of auditory evoked potentials helps evaluate the complaint of dizziness. The treatment consists of reassurance, rest, and analgesics.

Although the patient usually has many bothersome complaints that interfere with his usual work routine, it is important that he return to work as soon as possible. If a patient with the post-traumatic syndrome is initially disabled because of his headache or inability to concentrate, it is difficult to discontinue his disability 2 months later when he may still complain of his original symptoms. The physician should indicate to the patient's employer, if necessary, that the patient's symptoms may persist for a long time. Every effort should be made to have him return to work, even at a reduced work load if necessary. The granting of disability can be the greatest problem area for the treating physician.

NECK INJURIES

Following a head injury, an examination of the neck is often cursory or omitted. Injuries of the cervical vertebrae and carotid arteries can consequently be overlooked. The cervical spine is flexed, extended, and rotated in almost all head injuries. Roentgenograms of the cervical spine, including views from the odontoid process to the C7–T1 interspace, should be obtained in patients sustaining a significant head injury and in patients complaining of neck, upper extremity, or suboccipital pain.

Bruises on the neck should alert the examining physician to the possibility of carotid artery injury. Intimal tears of the carotid artery result in clot formation and possible cerebrovascular accident (CVA). Auscultation for carotid artery bruits should be part of the post-traumatic examination.

PITUITARY INJURY

At the time of impact, small hemorrhages may occur in the pituitary stalk or anterior lobe of the pituitary gland. Disorders of water retention and menstrual cycle are not uncommon after head injuries. Damage to the pituitary stalk can decrease the release of antidiuretic hormone (ADH), resulting in increased thirst, polyurea, dehydration, and hypernatremia (diabetes insipidus). Injuries to the hypothalamic–pituitary axis may cause an unphysiologic increase in ADH production, with water retention and hyponatremia (inappropriate ADH syndrome). Cerebral edema may occur.

Menstrual irregularity may occur for 2 to 3 months following a head injury. The cause is probably damage to the anterior lobe of the pituitary gland.

QUESTIONS AND DISCUSSION

1. A 23-year-old man sustains a severe closed head injury during a motorcycle accident. He regains almost all neurologic function and is discharged from the hospital 5½ weeks after injury. Ten weeks after injury, his parents took him to their physician and stated that he was "getting worse." Specifically, he is incontinent of urine, intermittently confused, and "clumsy." The most likely diagnosis is:

A. Meningitis
B. Hydrocephalus
C. Brainstem CVA
D. Cervical myelopathy
E. Subdural hematoma

The answer is (B). Subarachnoid hemorrhage is common during any head injury. The subarachnoid blood may obstruct normal CSF channels, causing ventricular dilation. The enlarged ventricles compress white matter tracts and cause changes in mentation, gait, and urination.

2. A 37-year-old woman was discharged from the hospital 5 days after admission for a "cerebral concussion" incurred in an automobile accident. The discharge summary reads: "cerebral concussion—no neuro deficit." Two weeks after discharge, she complains to her physician that she cannot smell. Her examination is normal except for periorbital ecchymosis. Which diagnosis is possible?

A. CSF fistula
B. Basilar skull fracture
C. Brain abscess
D. All of the above
E. None of the above

The answer is (D). Anosmia indicates a possible fracture of the cribriform plate. Such basilar fractures can communicate with the 'outside world,' resulting in a CSF fistula and secondary infection.

3. Intracranial air seen on 'routine' post-traumatic skull roentgenograms may indicate:

A. CSF fistula
B. Depressed skull fracture
C. Epidural hematoma
D. Subdural hematoma
E. Intracerebral hematoma

The answer is (A). Pneumocephalus is an indicator of a rent in the cranial vault. CSF may exit; bacteria may enter.

4. A 72-year-old man is sent home from an outpatient emergency facility after being seen following a fall in his garage. He has no neurologic deficit. He is seen again 9 days later because "he sleeps all the time." The neurologic examination is normal. The most likely diagnosis is:

A. Subclinical meningitis
B. Hyponatremia secondary to pituitary injury
C. Impending CVA
D. Subdural hematoma
E. Post-traumatic seizures

The answer is (D). Subdural hematomas are more common in patients with cerebral atrophy, such as the elderly and chronic alcoholics.

5. The post-traumatic syndrome occurs most frequently following:

A. Acute subdural hematoma
B. Craniotomy for cerebral aneurysm
C. Closed head injury with severe temporal lobe contusion
D. Minor closed head injury
E. Traumatic CSF fistula and meningitis

The answer is (D). The post-traumatic syndrome occurs more frequently following a minor head injury. Indeed, among individuals sustaining a minor head injury, post-traumatic headache is more common in patients who were dazed than in those experiencing 30 minutes of amnesia.

SUGGESTED READING

Annegers JF, Grabow JD, Groover RV et al: Seizures after head trauma: A population study. Neurology 30:683, 1980

Brown FD, Mullan S, Duda EE: Delayed traumatic intracerebral hematomas. J Neurosurg 48:1019, 1978

Clark CT, Apuzzo MJ: The Evaluation and Management of Trauma to the Odontoid Process, Management of Post-Traumatic Spinal Instability, Chap. 6, pp. 77–97, American Association of Neurological Surgeons Publication, 1990

Cooper PR: Head Injury, 3rd Edition, Baltimore, Williams and Wilkins, 1993

Evans RW: Neurology and Trauma. Philadelphia, WB Saunders, 1996

Feeney DM, Walker AE: A prediction of post-traumatic epilepsy: A mathematical approach. Arch Neurol 36:8, 1979

Fleischer AS, Patton JM, Tindall GT: Cerebral aneurysms of traumatic origin. Surg Neurol 4:233, 1975

Friedman WA: Head injuries. Ciba Clin Symp 35:1, 1983

Grossman RG, Gildenberg PL: Head Injury: Basic and Clinical Aspects. New York, Raven Press, 1982

Gurdjian ES, Webster JE: Head Injuries. Boston, Little, Brown, 1958

Guthkelch AN: Benign post-traumatic encephalopathy in young people and its relation to migraine. Neurosurgery 1:101, 1977

Hall S, Bornstein RA: The relationship between intelligence and memory following minor or mild closed-head injury: Greater impairment in memory than intelligence. J Neurosurg 75:378, 1991

Healy CB: Hearing loss and vertigo secondary to head injury. N Engl J Med 306: 1029, 1982

Jeret JS, Mandell MA, Anziska B et al: Clinical predictors of abnormality disclosed by computed tomography after mild head trauma. Neurosurgery 32:9, 1993

Kihlberg JK: Head injury in automobile accidents. In: Caveness WF, Walker AE (eds): Head Injury, pp 27–36. Conference Proceedings. Philadelphia, JB Lippincott, 1966

Kline DG, Hudson AR: Nerve Injuries. Philadelphia, WB Saunders, 1996

Leech PJ, Paterson A: Conservative and operative management for cerebrospinal fluid leakage after closed head injury. Lancet 1:1013, 1973

Lende RA, Erickson TC: Growing skull fractures of childhood. J Neurosurg 18:479, 1961

Levin HS, Goldstein FC, High WMJN et al: Disproportionately severe memory deficit in relation to normal intellectual functioning after closed head injury. J Neurol Neurosurg Psychiatry 51:1294, 1988

Lobato RD, Rivas JJ, Gomez PA et al: Head-injured patients who talk and deteriorate into coma. J Neurosurg 75:256, 1991

Markwalder TM: Chronic subdural hematomas: A review. J Neurosurg 54:637, 1981

Masters SJ: Evaluation of head trauma: Efficacy of skull films. Am J Neuroradiol 1:329, 1980

Narayan RK, Wilberger JE, Povlishock JT (eds): Neuro-trauma. New York, McGraw Hill, 1996

Rizzo M, Tranel D (eds): Head Injury and Post-concussive Syndrome. New York, Churchill Living-stone, 1996

Schechter PJ, Henkin RI: Abnormalities of taste and smell after head trauma. J Neurol Psychiatry 37:802, 1974

Walker AE, Caveness W, Critchley M: The Late Effects of Head Injury. Springfield, IL, Charles C. Thomas, 1969

Wilkins RH, Rengachary SS: Trauma. In: Wilkins RH, Rengachary SS (eds): *Neurosurgery*, pp 1531–1688. New York, McGraw-Hill, 1985

Wrightson P, Gronwall D: Time off work and symp-toms after minor head injury. Injury 12:445, 1981

Youmans JR. Neurological Surgery. 4th Ed. Philadel-phia, WB Saunders, 1996

Neurology for the Non-Neurologist, Fourth Edition, edited by William J. Weiner and Christopher G. Goetz. Lippincott Williams & Wilkins, Philadelphia © 1999.

| C | H | A | P | T | E | R | 1 | 9 |

Neuromuscular Diseases

Hans E. Neville

Steven P. Ringel

Neuromuscular diseases involve primarily the anterior horn motor neuron, the peripheral nerve (see Chapter 13), the neuromuscular junction, or the muscle. Weakness is a common symptom, but unlike disorders of the central nervous system (CNS), neuromuscular diseases may be accompanied by striking muscular atrophy and diminished muscle tone. Patients may also present with muscle pain, stiffness, cramps, twitching, limb deformities, or myoglobinuria.

This chapter discusses the clinical presentations of neuromuscular diseases and their diagnostic evaluation. Following the classification of disorders (Table 19-1), individual diseases will be described in detail and principles of management covered.

Since the original publication of this book, there have been significant developments in the genetics of neuromuscular disorders. Accordingly, we have added the latest information on chromosome localization, gene determination (when known), and the DNA diagnostic testing available to the clinician for genetic counseling (Table 19-2).

CLINICAL PRESENTATIONS

WEAKNESS

The mode of onset, location, and progression of weakness are important diagnostic features. The rapid onset of weakness is characteristic of most diseases of the neuromuscular junction, the Guillain-Barré syndrome, and acute electrolyte disturbances. Remissions and relapses suggest myasthenia gravis, periodic paralysis, or channelopathies. Insidious and slowly progressive weakness occurs in many diseases. Three patterns of weakness frequently encountered are proximal, distal, and cranial. Each pattern is associated with typical symptoms that are mentioned frequently by the patient, and with signs that are easily observed even before individual muscles are tested. These features are usually absent in patients with non organic complaints, who may have vague symptoms and demonstrate normal strength.

Proximal weakness is characteristic of myopathies and the spinal muscular atrophies. These patients report difficulty in climbing stairs or arising from low chairs because of weakness of the hip and knee extensors. When standing from a chair, they will lean forward and push with their hands on the armrests. In arising from the floor or a squatting position, they may require one or more supports with the hands on the floor, knees, and thighs (Gowers' maneuver, Fig. 19-1). Their gait has a waddling appearance because of weakness of the hip fixators. Knee extensor weakness may cause the leg to "give out." The knee is kept locked, gradually leading to hyperextension (back-kneeing), which in turn produces an exaggeration of the lumbar lordosis. Shoulder–girdle weakness produces difficulty in elevating the arms and may be accompanied by scapular winging (Fig. 19-2). With the arms hanging at

TABLE 19-1. Classification of Neuromuscular Disorders

DISORDERS OF THE ANTERIOR HORN CELL (MOTOR NEURON)

Spinal muscular atrophies (SMAs)
  TYPE I: Infantile SMA (Werdnig-Hoffmann disease)
  TYPE II: Intermediate SMA
  TYPE III: Juvenile SMA (Kugelberg-Welander disease)
  TYPE IV: Adult SMA
X-linked spinal and bulbar muscle atrophy
  (Kennedy's syndrome)
Amyotrophic lateral sclerosis (ALS)
Poliomyelitis and postpolio syndrome

DISORDERS OF THE PERIPHERAL NERVE (SEE CHAP. 13)

Radiculopathy
Plexopathy
Mononeuropathy
Polyneuropathy

DISORDERS OF MUSCLE

Dystrophies
  Duchenne/Becker dystrophy
  Facioscapulohumeral dystrophy
  Limb–girdle dystrophy
  Congenital dystrophy
  Oculopharygeal dystrophy
Myotonic disorders
  Myotonia congenita
  Myotonic dystrophy
Inflammatory Myopathies
  Polymyositis
  Dermatomyositis
  Inclusion body myositis
  Sarcoidosis
  Polymyalgia rheumatica
Metabolic myopathies
  Glycogen storage diseases
    Myophosphorylase deficiency (McArdle's)
    Acid maltase deficiency and others
  Disorders of lipid metabolism
    Carnitine deficiency
    Carnitine palmitoyl transferase deficiency
  Mitochondrial myopathies
  Malignant hyperthermia
Toxic myopathies
  Alcoholic myopathy
Endocrine myopathies
  Thyroid dysfunction
  Parathyroid dysfunction
  Adrenal dysfunction
  Pituitary dysfunction
Congenital myopathies
  Central core disease
  Nemaline myopathy
  Myotubular myopathy
Periodic paralysis and paramyotonia congenita

the sides, there is an inward rotation of the shoulders with the backs of the hands facing forward, producing an oblique axillary crease. The high-riding scapulae produce a conspicuous "trapezius hump"; the clavicles slope downward and stand out prominently from the atrophic neck musculature (Fig. 19-3).

Distal weakness accompanied by sensory loss is characteristic of neuropathies. When sensation is normal in the presence of atrophy and weakness, one should suspect amyotrophic lateral sclerosis (ALS) (Fig. 19-4), inclusion body myositis, or myotonic dystrophy. These patients find it difficult to manipulate small objects including buttons, and they also have difficulty when eating or using writing utensils. They may complain of "dragging" their legs because of a foot drop, or of frequent tripping on uneven ground. The knees are raised high in walking, while the feet flap limply and the soles are scuffed.

Cranial weakness affects the extraocular, facial, and oropharyngeal muscles and is an important differential feature in diagnosis (Figs. 19-5 and 19-6). Ptosis and ophthalmoparesis occur in disorders of the neuromuscular junction, myotonic dystrophy, and the syndrome of progressive external ophthalmoplegia. Dysphagia and dysphonia may occur in these disorders and also in ALS.

ATROPHY AND HYPERTROPHY

The disuse of a limb will produce a modest degree of muscle atrophy, which is seen after the casting of a fracture or in the hemiplegic limb of a stroke patient. The muscle retains much of its strength in disuse atrophy, and the shrunken-appearing limbs of the elderly may similarly be surprisingly strong. In contrast, patients with neuromuscular disease may have striking muscular atrophy and obvious weakness.

Atrophy of the muscles around the shoulder reveals the underlying bony prominences. The knee or elbow may be greater in circumference than the thigh or arm, respectively. Flattening of the thenar eminence and guttering of the interossei produce a wasted, claw-like deformity of the hand (see Fig. 19-4). Several disorders produce characteristic appearances. Examples include "Popeye arms" in facioscapulohumeral dystrophy, "stork legs" in Charcot-Marie-Tooth neuropathy, and the "hatchet-face" appearance in myotonic dystrophy (see Figs. 19-5 and 19-6).

Pseudohypertrophy of the gastrocnemius occurs in Duchenne muscular dystrophy and occasionally in limb–girdle dystrophy and juvenile spinal muscular atrophy (Fig. 19-7). Diffuse hypertrophy suggests myotonia congenita, hypothyroidism, or amyloidosis.

(*text continues on page 280*)

TABLE 19-2. Gene Abnormalities in Neuromuscular Diseases

DISORDER	CHROMO-SOME	RECESSIVE (R) DOMINANT (D)	GENE PRODUCT	ABNORMAL GENE DETECTION BY:	SPECIAL FEATURES
ANTERIOR HORN CELL					
1. Spinal muscular atrophy			1a. Motor Neuron Survival Protein (SMN) and/or Neuronal Apoptotic Inhibiting Protein (NAIP)	1a. Linkage analysis, PCR	1a. Disease produced by defect of one or both gene products
1a. Childhood type I, II, and III SMA	5	(R)			
1b. Adult type IV	Unknown	(R)&(D)	1b. Unknown	1b. Not available	1b. 30% of cases autosomal dominant
2. Spinal and bulbar muscular atrophy (Kennedy's Disease)	X		2. Androgen receptor	2. PCR	2. Androgen receptor gene enlarged (multiple CAG repeats in first exon)
3. Amyotrophic lateral sclerosis					
3a. Sporadic (90–95%)	No known defect		3a. None	3a. Not applicable	
3b. Familial (5–10%) (FALS)	2,21,22	(D)	3b. Superoxide dismutase (SOD-1) mutation	3b. Linkage analysis, PCR	3b. SOD-1 mutation demonstrable in only 20% of cases. Gene defect unknown for 80% of FALS
PERIPHERAL NERVE (See Chapter 13)					
NEUROMUSCULAR JUNCTION DISORDERS	No known genetic defects		N.A.	N.A.	
MUSCULAR DYSTROPHIES					
1. Duchenne/Becker dystrophy	X	(R)	1. Dystrophin	1. PCR; Western blot	1. Gene deletion (30–70%); point mutation in rest
2. Facioscapulohumeral dystrophy	4	(D)	2. Unknown	2. Linkage analysis, PCR	2. Specific deletions on chromosome 4 can be detected—gene still unknown
3. Limb–girdle dystrophy (recessive) LGMD 2A, 2B, 2C, 2D, 2E, 2F	2,4,5,13, 15,17	(R)	3. Four sarcoglycans, & one calpain, identified so far	3. Linkage analysis	3. LGMD 2A and 2B have mild phenotype—others very severe
4. Limb–girdle dystrophy (dominant) LGMD1A	5	(D)	4. Unknown	4. Linkage analysis	4. Disease termed LGMD 1A

(continued)

TABLE 19-2. Gene Abnormalities in Neuromuscular Diseases (*Continued*)

DISORDER	CHROMO-SOME	RECESSIVE (R) DOMINANT (D)	GENE PRODUCT	ABNORMAL GENE DETECTION BY:	SPECIAL FEATURES
5. Congenital muscular dystrophy	5a. 6 5b. 9	(R) (R)	5a. Laminin in some 5b. Unknown for Fukuyama	5a. Linkage analysis 5b. Linkage analysis	5b. Has severe CNS changes
6. Oculopharyngeal dystrophy	14	(D)	6. Cardiac myosin heavy chain	6. Linkage analysis, PCR	
MYOTONIAS					
1. Myotonia congenita	7	(D) & (R)	1. Muscle chloride channel	1. Linkage analysis	1. Autosomal dominant forms (Thompson's disease) account for bulk of cases.
2. Myotonic dystrophy	19	(D)	2. Myotonin (protein kinase)	2. PCR; Southern blot	2. Gene enlarged (CTG repeats)
GLYCOGEN STORAGE DISEASES					
1. Phosphorylase deficiency (McArdle's)	11	(R) & (D)	1. Phosphorylase	1.–6. Linkage analysis possible for each of the glycogen storage disorders but no testing commercially available yet	1.–6. Diagnosis best confirmed by biopsy, muscle enzyme assay and glycogen content
2. Acid maltase deficiency	17	(R)	2. Acid maltase		
3. Phosphofructokinase deficiency	1	(R)	3. Phosphofructokinase		
4. Phosphoglycerate mutase deficiency	7	(R)	4. Phosphoglycerate mutase		
5. Phosphoglycerate kinase deficiency	X	(R)	5. Phosphoglycerate kinase		
6. Lactic dehydrogenase deficiency	11	(R)	6. Lactic dehydrogenase		
LIPID STORAGE DISORDERS					
1. Carnitine palmitoyl transferase deficiency (CPT)	1	(R)	1. Carnitine palmitoyl transferase	1. Linkage analysis	1. Diagnosis by muscle biopsy and CPT enzyme assay
2. Carnitine deficiency	Unknown	(D)	2. Unknown	2. Not yet described	2. Diagnosis by muscle biopsy and carnitine assay

TABLE 19-2. Gene Abnormalities in Neuromuscular Diseases (*Continued*)

DISORDER	CHROMOSOME	RECESSIVE (R) DOMINANT (D)	GENE PRODUCT	ABNORMAL GENE DETECTION BY:	SPECIAL FEATURES
MITOCHONDRIAL MYOPATHIES					
1. Kearns–Sayres	Disorders 1, 2, 3, 4a result from errors in mitochondrial DNA; inheritance by maternal DNA		1. Various mitochondrial proteins	1. Southern blot	1. Single mitochondrial DNA deletion
2. MELAS			2. Mitochondrial tRNA	2. PCR	2. Mitochondrial tRNA point mutation causes defective protein production during translation
3. MERFF			3. Mitochondrial tRNA	3. PCR	3. Mitochondrial tRNA point mutation causes defective protein production during translation
4a. Familial PEO syndrome			4a. Unknown mitochondrial protein	4a. Southern blot	4a. No mitochondrial deletions detected to date
4b. Familial PEO syndrome	4b. Unknown nuclear DNA mutation	(D)	4b. Nuclear protein that controls mitochondrial DNA replication	4b. Southern blot	4b. Unique autosomal dominant transmission
CONGENITAL MYOPATHIES					
1. Myotubular myopathy					1–3 Diagnosis best confirmed by muscle biopsy structural changes
1a. Neonatal	X		1a. Unknown	1a. Linkage analysis	1a. Carrier identification possible
1b. Late infantile	Unknown	(R)	1b. Unknown	1b. Not known	
1c. Late childhood/adult	Unknown	(R)	1c. Unknown	1c. Not known	
2. Central core disease	19	(D)	2. Unknown	2. Linkage analysis	2. Same gene as for malignant hyperthermia (ryanodine receptor)
3. Nemaline (rod) myopathy	1	(D) and (R)	3. Unknown	3. Linkage analysis	
PERIODIC PARALYSIS					
1. Hypokalemic form	1	(D)	1. Muscle calcium channel	1. PCR, Southern blot	
2. Hyperkalemic periodic paralysis/paramyotonia congenita	17	(D)	2. Muscle sodium channel	2. PCR, Southern blot	2. Variable mutations of sodium channel gene define clinical features

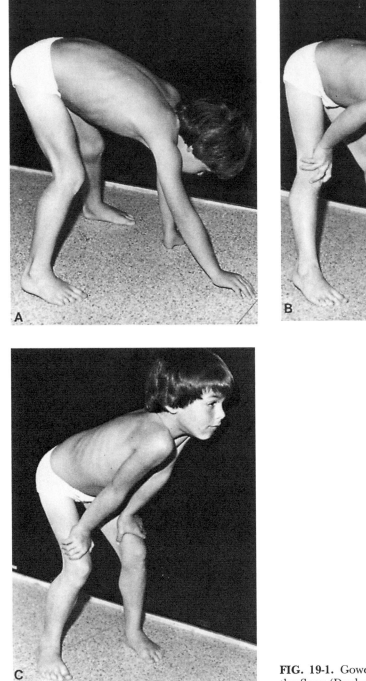

FIG. 19-1. Gowers' maneuver displayed in arising from the floor (Duchenne muscular dystrophy).

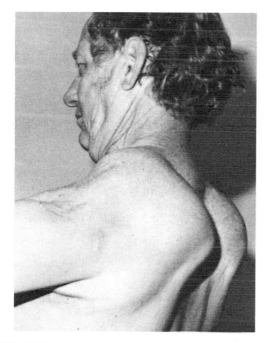

FIG. 10-2. Winging of the scapulae when the arms are elevated (Fascioscapulohumeral dystrophy [FSH]).

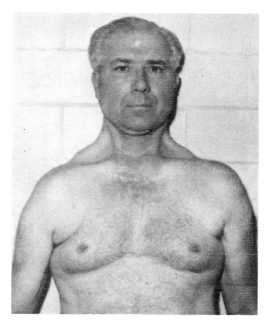

FIG. 19-3. Shoulder–girdle weakness with "trapezius hump," "step-sign" with prominent down-sloping clavicles, and an oblique anterior axillary crease (LGD).

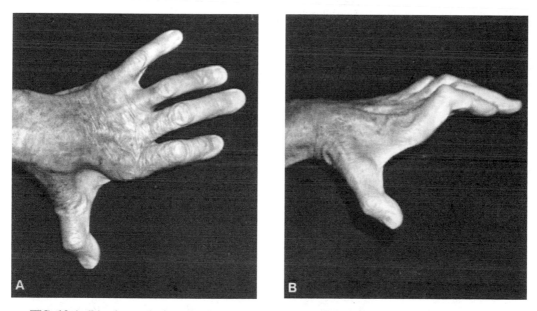

FIG. 19-4. Distal atrophy in motor neuron disease. **A.** Loss of first dorsal interosseus produces a prominent depression. **B.** Guttering of the back of the hand (ALS).

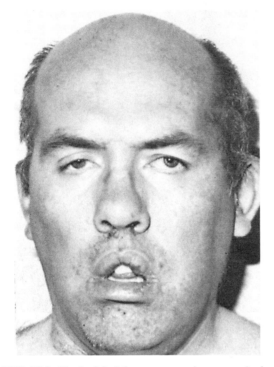

FIG. 19-5. Typical facial appearance in myotonic dystrophy with frontal balding, temporalis and masseter atrophy, ptosis, and protuberant lower lip.

PAIN, STIFFNESS, AND CRAMPS

Inflammatory myopathies and other collagen-vascular diseases may produce muscle pain and tenderness, but the absence of these symptoms does not exclude the diagnosis. Rarely, similar discomfort is present with trichinosis, influenza, or an acute denervating disorder. In older patients, pain, aching, and stiffness in the shoulder and hip-girdle muscles should suggest polymyalgia rheumatica. Most patients with limb aching and pain without weakness do not have a neuromuscular disease. The diagnosis of fibrositis or fibromyositis is often evoked, particularly in otherwise healthy middle-aged women who have diffuse aches and pains; however, this purported entity has no pathologic foundation.

Stiffness may be a nonspecific symptom, or it may be a symptom of *myotonia*, a phenomenon consisting of a delayed relaxation of the muscle following voluntary contraction or percussion. This produces a difficulty in releasing the grip or initiating movements after a period of rest.

Muscle *cramp*, a prolonged involuntary contraction, is a universal and benign symptom that occurs with increased frequency during unaccustomed exercise, "body building," pregnancy, or electrolyte disturbance. It may also occur in hypothyroidism, partial denervation (especially in ALS), tetany (with hypocalcemia, hypomagnesemia, or alkalosis), and certain metabolic myopathies.

MUSCLE TWITCHING

Fasciculations (the tiny twitches with the terrible reputation) are contractions of muscle fibers in a single motor unit. Fasciculations appearing in a strong muscle are usually benign and are exacerbated by many factors, including fatigue and caffeine. When they occur in a weak muscle, they are most frequently associated with ALS, but they also occur after root or peripheral nerve injury. Fasciculations differ from *myokymia,* which consists of brief tetanic contractions of independent small bands of muscle. Myokymia may be benign (upper eyelid twitching) but has been reported with thyrotoxicosis, uremia, tetany, and rare motor unit hyperactivity states. Myokymia occurring in facial muscles suggests multiple sclerosis or a pontine glioma.

HYPOTONIA

Various unrelated disorders present with infantile hypotonia. The most frequent abnormality in the "floppy baby" is a CNS disease, such as perinatal asphyxia. The hypotonic infant may exhibit normal muscle strength, with the ability to lift its head or limbs against gravity. In the absence of other abnormalities, the prognosis for normal development may be excellent. In infants with obvious weakness, the underlying disorder may be spinal muscle atrophy or a congenital myopathy. Weaknesses of sucking and respiration are serious concomitants, but the prognosis in these disorders varies widely.

DEFORMITIES

Neuromuscular disorders are often associated with skeletal deformities and should be suspected in the patient with unexplained hip dislocation, scoliosis (Fig. 19-8), contracture, or malformation of the feet (e.g., club foot, equinovarus, or pes cavus deformity). Arthrogryposis or multiple congenital limb deformities may occur with various diseases affecting any part of the motor unit (see Fig. 19-6).

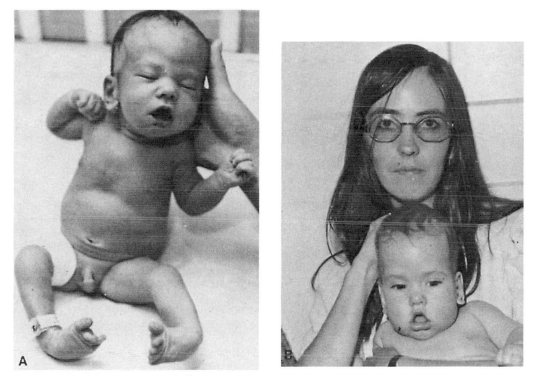

FIG. 19-6. A. Congenital myotonic dystrophy with typical "shark mouth" and club feet. **B.** Same infant whose evaluation led to the diagnosis of myotonic dystrophy in the mother.

MYOGLOBINURIA

The syndrome of myoglobinuria consists of weakness and painful swelling of affected muscles in association with headaches, nausea, and vomiting. The urine turns reddish brown within 24 hours and is positive for benzidine and Hemastix. Most episodes are not associated with an underlying neuromuscular disease but are related to unusual circumstances that produce acute muscle necrosis, including vigorous exercise (particularly in someone deconditioned), mechanical trauma, burns, electrical shock, recurrent seizures, viral infections, gram-negative sepsis, and low potassium or low phosphate syndromes. Certain myotoxic agents such as alcohol, cocaine, amphetamines, heroin, neuroleptics, and halothane in susceptible individuals may also induce myoglobinuria.

A patient with recurrent myoglobinuria should be evaluated for an underlying neuromuscular disease. Any of the glycogen storage disorders, but most commonly McArdle's disease, carnitine palmitoyl deficiency, and polymyositis, are among the possibilities.

The major complication of myoglobinuria is acute renal failure. Affected patients should be hydrated to maintain a high urine output, and serum electrolytes should be closely monitored. Hyperkalemia may require correction.

CLINICAL INVESTIGATION

ENZYME ELEVATION

Muscle necrosis results in elevated levels of "muscle enzymes," including serum creatine phosphokinase (CPK). The highest levels occur in the syndrome of myoglobinuria, Duchenne muscular dystrophy, and polymyositis. Normal or slightly elevated values occur in most of the chronic muscular dystrophies and motor neuron disorders.

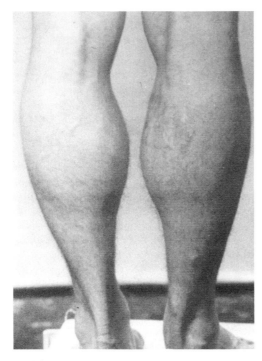

FIG. 19-7. Pseudohypertrophy of the calves (Duchenne dystrophy).

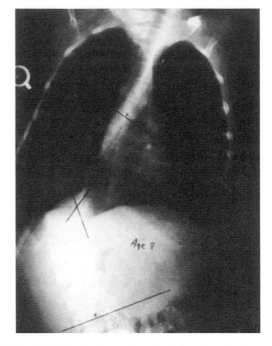

FIG. 19-8. Scoliosis in chronic infantile muscular atrophy. The angle of curvature is measured and followed closely (55 degrees in this patient).

ELECTROMYOGRAPHY

Electrophysiologic investigation includes nerve conduction velocity studies, needle electromyography (EMG) examination, and evaluation of neuromuscular transmission. A description of these tests is provided in Chapter 13.

Electromyography is useful in differentiating *neuropathic* (anterior horn cell and peripheral nerve) from *myopathic* disorders (Fig. 19-9). *Neuropathic* disorders are associated with spontaneous electrical activity of individual muscle fibers, detected as *fibrillation* potentials. Fewer motor units are available for voluntary recruitment, producing a decrease in the electrical interference pattern. Following chronic denervation, surviving motor axons develop collateral sprouts that reinnervate muscle fibers. This results in abnormally large polyphasic motor unit potentials.

In *myopathic* disorders, the random loss of individual muscle fibers results in a decreased size of the motor unit potentials. Many units are recruited simultaneously during voluntary contraction, producing an increased interference pattern.

In disorders of the *neuromuscular junction,* repetitive stimulation of a peripheral nerve may produce a characteristic change in the amplitude of the muscle twitch. Single-fiber EMG may reveal increased "jitter," a measure of the synchrony of depolarization occurring in muscle fibers nearby.

MUSCLE AND NERVE BIOPSY

Muscle biopsy is performed easily under local anesthesia as an outpatient procedure, allowing histologic, histochemical, ultrastructural, and biochemical studies.

Normal muscle stained for enzyme activity shows a checkerboard distribution of two muscle fiber types (Fig. 19-10A); type 1 or slow-twitch oxidative fibers (lightly stained with *p*H 9.4 myofibrillar ATPase), and type 2 or fast-twitch, glycolytic fibers (darkly stained with 9.4 ATPase). With chronic denervation and reinnervation, as in anterior horn cell disorders and neuropathies, fiber-type grouping is seen (Fig. 19-10B). In contrast, most myopathies are characterized by the destruction of individual fibers (Fig. 19-10C,D).

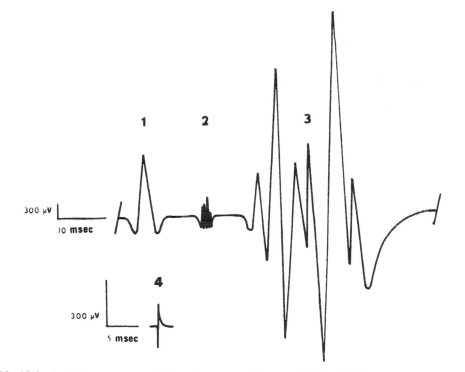

300 μV

10 msec

300 μV

5 msec

FIG. 19-9. 1–4. Single motor unit action potentials recorded by EMG in a voluntarily contracting skeletal muscle. **1.** Normal motor unit action potential. **2.** The *myopathic* potential is brief, small amplitude, and polyphasic. **3.** The *neuropathic* potential is prolonged, high amplitude, and polyphasic. **4.** A fibrillation potential is *spontaneously* produced by a denervated muscle fiber at rest.

Abnormal storage products or an enzyme deficiency can be characterized biochemically. Disorders of the neuromuscular junction are generally associated with a normal muscle biopsy.

The muscle biopsy is useful in the evaluation of patients suspected of having a myopathy, anterior horn cell disease, "paralytic" hypotonia, or a collagen-vascular disorder associated with neuromuscular symptoms. It is particularly valuable in the dystrophies and spinal muscular atrophies, where genetic counseling requires a confident diagnosis, and in polymyositis, where intensive immunosuppression may be recommended. Muscle histochemistry (particularly fiber typing) is essential whenever a biopsy is performed.

Nerve biopsy is used less frequently because routine histologic sections are rarely of diagnostic use except with vasculitis, amyloidosis, granulomatous disorders, and in the inherited neuropathy HMSN type I (Hereditary Motor Sensory Neuropathy, Type I or Charcot-Marie-Tooth disease).

GENETICS AND GENETIC TESTING OF NEUROMUSCULAR DISEASE

Molecular biology techniques have produced a torrent of information concerning gene abnormalities that form the underlying basis of many neuromuscular disorders. In this section, the authors will define some basic terms and concepts designed to facilitate understanding the progress made to date in genetically determined neuromuscular disorders.

DNA

The bulk of the cell's DNA is contained in the nucleus and consists of alternating sugar and phosphate molecules to which are attached individual nucleotides. The numbers and sequence of these nucleotides define portions of the DNA termed genes, which transfer the necessary information to RNA by tran-

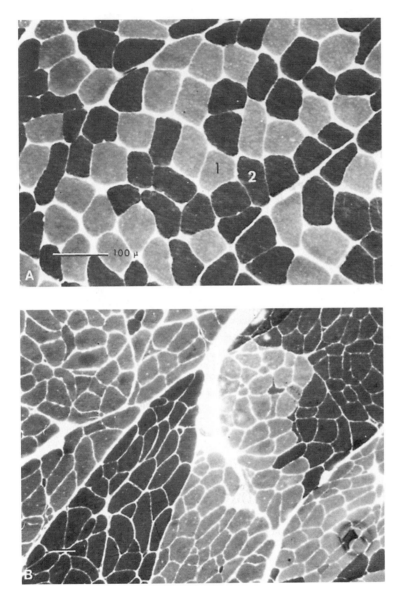

FIG. 19-10. Muscle biopsy. **A.** Histochemical fiber typing with pH 9.4 myofibrillar ATPase shows the checkerboard distribution of type 1 (oxidative) light reacting and type 2 (glycolytic) dark reacting fibers in normal muscle. **B.** Fiber-type grouping in chronic denervation (pH 9.4 ATPase).

scription. Individual mitochondria also possess short DNA strands that are necessary for the production of mitochondrial proteins. Although the bulk of mitochondrial protein is coded for by mitochondrial DNA, several key proteins do receive subunit coding from nuclear DNA that passes by messenger RNA into the mitochondria for final translation and protein assembly.

RNA

Ribonucleic acid is essential in transferring the gene information of the DNA from the nucleus into the cytoplasm where protein assembly can take place. Messenger RNA brings the information to the cytoplasm and transfer RNA brings individual amino acids to the messenger RNA template so that protein translation can occur.

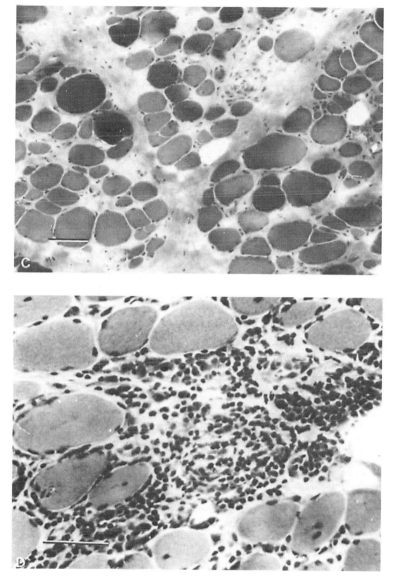

FIG. 19-10. (*continued*).
C. Histologic stains reveal characteristic features of Duchenne dystrophy, including necrotic and opaque fibers, marked variation in fiber size, and proliferation of connective tissue (Trichrome stain). D. Mononuclear cell infiltrate around muscle fibers and vessels in polymyositis (H + E Stain). Bar = 100 μ.

GENE DEFECT

An error in the nucleotide sequence of DNA can result in an abnormality of protein synthesis. The gene error can take the form of a missing segment of the gene nucleotide sequence (deletion), be a segment of reduplicated gene nucleotide sequences, or be a single nucleotide substitution (point mutation). The result-ing mutant protein may have no effect on the cell or produce a specific disease state.

POLYMERASE CHAIN REACTION

If a known gene contains a sizable deletion, it can be detected by the polymerase chain reaction (PCR). This technique can be carried out on blood or muscle specimens. The DNA is first isolated and the segment of DNA to be studied is reproduced in large quantities using the standard PCR technique commonly available in research and commercial laboratories. The resulting amplified DNA fragment is then run on an electrophoresis gel and its size compared to known standards of the segment being studied. In this way, the segment of interest may be found to be normal, smaller (if there are deletions), or larger (if there are excess triplet repeats).

SOUTHERN BLOT

Some DNA analyses that cannot be carried out by PCR may utilize this technique. Large quantities of cellular DNA are cut into smaller pieces by special restriction enzymes, and separated by gel electrophoresis. The fragment of interest can be identified by first flooding the gel with a solution containing radiolabeled complementary DNA (which binds to the fragment of interest), followed by exposure of the gel to radiographic film to find the location of the fragment identified. The molecular weight of the fragment will determine whether or not it is normal.

WESTERN BLOT

In this technique, the tissue, usually muscle, is solubilized and individual proteins are separated by electrophoresis. The gel is then exposed to a radiolabeled antibody to the specific protein of interest. Binding of the antibody to the protein can be detected by exposure of the gel to radiographic film, and from that the size of the protein can be calculated and compared to known normals.

LINKAGE ANALYSIS

For some disorders, the actual gene segment may not have been isolated, so direct detection of an abnormality is not possible. Certain DNA segments, however, are known to travel in close proximity to certain genes, even if the precise gene location is not known. By analyzing the presence of these closely associated DNA segments (i.e., by linkage analysis), geneticists may make inferences as to the probability of abnormal genes being transferred to progeny.

DISORDERS OF THE ANTERIOR HORN CELL (MOTOR NEURON)

SPINAL MUSCULAR ATROPHIES

The spinal muscular atrophies (SMA) constitute a group of hereditary disorders characterized by a loss of spinal and cranial motor neurons. Virtually all cases are based on autosomal recessive inheritance.

TYPE I SMA (WERDNIG-HOFFMANN DISEASE)

In patients with type I SMA, symptoms of hypotonia, poor feeding, weak cry, and respiratory distress may be present at birth or may develop by age 6 months. Examination reveals flaccid, areflexive extremities, fasciculations of the tongue, pooling of saliva in the posterior pharynx, and paradoxical respiration. Many patients die of respiratory failure by 2 years of age.

TYPE II SMA (INTERMEDIATE SMA)

Type II SMA presents during the first 18 months of life with delay of motor milestones as a common initial observation. On examination there is limb hypotonia and weakness as well as tongue fasciculations. These children often learn to sit independently but are rarely able to stand or walk. Sensation is normal. Progressive limb weakness, if untreated, will lead to skeletal deformities, including contractures at the hips and knees, hip dislocation, and scoliosis (see Fig. 19-8). Many patients survive into adolescence or adulthood but ultimately succumb to respiratory insufficiency. Good pulmonary management, including spinal fusion to prevent progressive kyphoscoliosis with its attendant restrictive pulmonary disease, can increase the life expectancy of these patients by many years.

TYPE III SMA (KUGELBERG-WELANDER)

Type III SMA presents with insidious proximal weakness beginning in late childhood or early adolescence. The clinical picture often mimics that of limb–girdle dystrophy with proximal arm and leg weakness. The appearance of tongue fasciculations and severe limb atrophy should the alert the clinician to the possibility of a motor neuron disorder. Progression is slow, but because of leg weakness many patients require a wheel chair by their mid thirties. The prevention of contractures and scoliosis, and good respiratory care are important.

TYPE IV SMA

Type IV SMA presents in patients who are normal until their twenties, when they develop slowly progressive weakness and atrophy of proximal leg muscles with spread to involve arms as well. The deep tendon reflexes are hypoactive or absent, and sensation is normal. In about one third of patients, inheritance is autosomal dominant. In the remaining two thirds, when several siblings are affected, transmission is considered to be autosomal recessive. In the absence of such a family history, these isolated patients are considered to have progressive muscular atrophy (PMA), which is essentially a lower motor neuron disorder sharing many of the clinical findings of type IV SMA. One extremely rare condition that can mimic both type IV SMA and PMA is that occurring in young adults having hexosaminidase A deficiency. This is an autosomal recessive disorder that can initially present with wasting and weakness in an asymmetric pattern in arms and legs, mimicking spinal muscular atrophy. Reflexes are generally reduced or absent, but the appearance of frank psychosis should suggest the possibility of this disorder, which is based on accumulation of GMI gangliosides in neurons. The adult form is caused by a gene mutation on chromosome 15, resulting in a partial deficiency of hexosaminidase A activity.

Genetics Types I, II, and III SMA are inherited as an autosomal recessive trait due to a defect of one or two genes located in chromosome 5. One of these has been called the Motor Neuron Survival (SMN) gene and the other the Neuronal Apoptotic Inhibitory (NAIP) gene. A defect in one or both of these genes is involved to produce these disorders and accounts for their variable presentations at different ages. Linkage analysis can provide useful information to parents wishing advice on the probability of affected children in future pregnancies.

X-LINKED SPINAL AND BULBAR MUSCULAR ATROPHY (KENNEDY'S DISEASE)

Kennedy's disease is an unusual disorder that can be confused with ALS. Patients in their thirties and forties present with swallowing dysfunction, slurred speech, perioral and tongue fasciculations, facial weakness, mild limb weakness, hand tremor, gynecomastia, and impotence. The disorder is very slowly progressive but, unlike ALS, rarely is fatal. Some link to an androgen abnormality had been suspected, but only recently has the precise genetic abnormality been identified.

Genetics This familial disorder results from a gene abnormality on the X chromosome. Thus, only males are affected, there is never male-to-male transmission, and females, although unaffected clinically, are carriers. In this respect, the genetics of the disorder are identical to that seen in Duchenne and Becker dystrophy. The disease is caused by multiple CAG trinucleotide repeats on the first exon of the androgen receptor gene. As numbers of CAG repeats increase, the age of disease onset is earlier but there is no correlation with disease severity. Since androgen receptors are present in motor neuron cell membranes, a defect of receptor structure is somehow involved in premature cell death. Recent works suggests this may be related to an unexpected gain of receptor function that is deleterious to motor neurons.

AMYOTROPHIC LATERAL SCLEROSIS

Amyotrophic lateral sclerosis is characterized by progressive muscle wasting and weakness resulting from degeneration of brainstem and spinal cord lower motor neurons and accompanied by varying degrees of spasticity and hyperreflexia caused by degeneration of upper motor neurons. The vast majority of cases are sporadic, although between 5% and 10% are familial. Initial clinical symptoms may be limited to asymmetrical limb weakness in the presence of fasciculations. A foot drop or marked hand deformity due to interosseus wasting (see Fig. 19-4) can be seen. In addition, there is hyperreflexia (usually generalized), pathological reflexes such as a Hoffman's response and crossed adductor responses, and in some cases extensor plantar responses. The sensory examination is entirely normal. Speech may develop a slurred or spastic quality. The rate of spread and involvement of other muscles is quite unpredictable. Though facial weakness may be seen late in the disease, eye muscle movement is never affected. Diaphragm weakness often leads to a critical time in the disease, as vital capacity drops progressively. On average, 50% of patients will still be alive at 4 years, and 10% survival at 10 years, although unusual, has been reported.

Diseases to be excluded include spinal cord compression from tumors or cervical spondylosis, hyperparathyroidism and hyperthyroidism, blood cell dyscrasia, hexosaminidase A deficiency, and multifocal motor neuropathy. Diagnosis is generally confirmed by the finding of acute and chronic denervation on needle EMG studies in the presence of normal nerve conduction velocities.

The treatment of this progressive disorder is symptomatic since the cause remains unknown. There are encouraging results of recent treatment including the finding that the oral agent riluzole prolongs survival. Several other neurotrophic factors have been tried in large human trials but are not beneficial (Brain Derived Neurotropic Factor [BDNF] and Ciliary Neutrotrophic Factor [CNTF]), or are of questionable value (Insulin-Like Growth Factor-1 [IGF-1]). Symptomatic treatment includes exercise, stretching, use of adaptive equipment and bracing, attention to swallowing dysfunction with consideration of G-tube placement, and for cramps the use of quinine or baclofen. Family counseling and end-of-life decisions are critical to the care of a patient with ALS.

Genetics The vast majority of ALS cases are sporadic and have no known genetic defect, but in 5% to 10% there is a familial form with autosomal dominant inheritance. Approximately 20% of these patients have been shown to have an abnormality on chromosome 21 for the gene coding for superoxide dismutase (SOD-1). To date, over 50 point mutations have been described for SOD-1, but the disease is not necessarily a result of loss of SOD-1 function in removing intracellular free radicals. The presence of the defective SOD-1 protein itself may exert a deleterious effect to produce premature neuronal death (apoptosis).

POLIOMYELITIS AND POSTPOLIO SYNDROME

Acute poliovirus infection in nonimmunized individuals leads to a nonspecific febrile illness, followed by paralytic symptoms in a minority. Although the widespread use of immunization has reduced the frequency of new cases in developed countries, many adult patients still have residual weakness.

Unpredictably, progressive weakness may develop after many years of static deficit. In some cases, this results from unrecognized nerve compression that can easily occur in a weakened extremity. In other patients, the progression of weakness may result from a dysfunction of surviving motor neurons. There is no evidence for viral reactivation.

DIAGNOSIS OF ANTERIOR HORN CELL DISEASES

The diagnostic confirmation of any of the motor neuron diseases relies heavily on accurate electrical studies, which will show acute and chronic denervation in multiple arm and leg muscles in the presence of normal motor and sensory conduction velocity. Since EMG and nerve conduction velocity (NCV) are difficult to do accurately in infants and children, a muscle biopsy is a reasonable alternative for types I, II, and III SMA. For these types, the biopsy abnormalities consist of group atrophy and type grouping. In all the motor neuron disorders, serum creatine kinase is only modestly elevated (rarely reaching greater than 1,000).

DISORDERS OF THE PERIPHERAL NERVES

This topic is discussed in Chapter 13.

DISORDERS OF THE NEUROMUSCULAR JUNCTION

MYASTHENIA GRAVIS

Myasthenia gravis (MG) is an autoimmune disorder that is associated with a postjunctional defect of the acetylcholine receptor. It may occur at any age but is most frequent in women in the third decade and men in the fifth decade of life. Fluctuating weakness and fatigue in cranial, limb, or trunk musculature are characteristic. Ocular symptoms, including alternating ptosis, diplopia, and blurred vision, are present initially in more than 50% of patients and eventually in 90%. Facial muscles are often weak, producing a snarling appearance when laughing. Speech becomes increasingly slurred, nasal, or hoarse as the patient continues to talk, and progressive dysphagia with choking and aspiration of food may occur. Neck muscle weakness may be so prominent that the patient uses his hand to prop up his head. Generalized MG frequently involves the respiratory muscles, and sudden respiratory collapse was a serious complication before the advent of modern immunosuppressive therapy.

The clinical course is occasionally fulminating but is characterized more commonly by a gradual progression of symptoms with frequent remissions and relapses. Sudden worsening may occur with an overdose of anticholinesterase medication, superimposed infection, electrolyte disturbance (especially hypokalemia), pregnancy, emotional stress, or the development of hyperthyroidism.

The diagnosis of MG should be considered in any patient who has an unexplained acute weakness, and in patients who demonstrate objective signs of fatigue such as ptosis or diplopia following sustained upward gaze. A possible diagnosis of MG may be strengthened by three tests, any of which may be negative. An intravenous (IV) injection of edrophonium (Tensilon) may briefly correct ptosis, ophthalmoparesis, or limb weakness. Repetitive stimulation of a peripheral nerve may produce a decremental response in the train of muscle twitches. Antibodies to the acetylcholine receptor (AChR) are present in the serum of almost 90% of patients with generalized MG, and they have been shown to produce both a transmission blockade and the destruction of the postsynaptic receptor site of the neuromuscular junction.

The treatment of MG has changed considerably in the last two decades, with increasing recognition of the primary autoimmune disturbance. Anticholinesterase drugs such as pyridostigmine (Mestinon) and neostigmine are still used for symptomatic relief but are no longer the mainstay of treatment. Patients frequently become refractory to these medications during exacerbations of the disease, leading to overdosage and a paradoxical increase in weakness. An overdosage is suggested by signs of cholinergic excess, including abdominal cramping, diarrhea (which may lead to hypokalemia and further weakness), profuse salivation and lacrimation (with increased risk of aspiration), miosis, fasciculations, or cramps. If early signs of ventilatory failure develop, anticholinesterases should be discontinued and intubation should be considered.

Corticosteroids are effective in the treatment of MG. When given initially, a transient exacerbation of weakness may occur in the first 2 weeks with a potential for respiratory failure. Azathioprine is also used, alone or in combination. Intensive immunosuppression is continued for 6 months to 1 year and is then tapered slowly providing the patient regains full strength.

Thymectomy has been recommended for all patients with generalized MG, except the very young and very old. Ten percent of patients harbor a thymoma, but all patients are believed to benefit from surgery.

Plasmapheresis is a mainstay for MG patients with acutely worsening symptoms of weakness, problems with secretions, or respiratory distress. A minority of patients may require intravenous immune globulin as well if pheresis is insufficient. Both modalities confer only transient benefit so that immunosuppressive therapy must be continued.

Other ancillary measures include the use of ephedrine and potassium and the avoidance of medications known to potentiate neuromuscular blockade, including aminoglycoside antibiotics, propranolol, procainamide, phenytoin, quinine, and curare.

Patients with isolated ocular symptoms (ocular MG) may develop generalized MG, but the risk is low after 2 years. These patients may not require surgery or intensive immunosuppression. MG in childhood differs little from the adult form but is treated conservatively because aggressive treatment may retard growth.

Fifteen percent of infants born to affected mothers develop transient myasthenic symptoms such as hypotonia and feeding difficulties, probably due to the transplacental passage of maternal AChR antibodies. These newborns usually respond to anticholinesterase medication with symptom resolution over 6 to 12 weeks.

A reversible myasthenic syndrome may develop following chronic use of d-penicillamine in adults.

EATON-LAMBERT SYNDROME

This rare autoimmune disease of the neuromuscular junction results from antibodies against voltage-gated calcium channels. The antibodies are produced in patients by a small-cell lung carcinoma.

Unlike in MG, cranial muscles are usually spared, patients may have distal paresthesias or dry mouth, and a repetitive stimulation produces an incremental response. The diagnosis mandates a search for malignancy. Symptoms may improve with the removal of the malignancy, immunosuppression, and intravenous immune globulin.

BOTULISM

Improperly canned food may contain the toxin of *Clostridium botulinum,* which also impairs the release of acetylcholine. A sudden onset of blurred vision, diplopia, dysphagia, and dysphonia is rapidly followed by a generalized weakness. Patients frequently require respiratory support, but recovery, though prolonged, may be complete. The diagnosis rests on the isolation of the toxin from stool, gastric contents, or contaminated food, and there is a characteristic electromyographic abnormality.

In infants, honey has been implicated as a source of botulinum spores that germinate in the intestine and produce the toxin, leading to hypotonia and severe constipation.

DISORDERS OF MUSCLE

DYSTROPHIES

DUCHENNE AND BECKER DYSTROPHY

Duchenne muscular dystrophy is an X-linked recessive disorder in which new spontaneous mutations may account for about one third of cases. From the time they first walk, boys who are affected with this disorder have a clumsy waddling gait. An examination reveals a protuberant abdomen resulting from an accentuation of the lumbar lordosis, pseudohypertrophy of the calves (see Fig. 19-7), and tight heel cords with a tendency toward toe walking. In arising from the floor, these children adopt a characteristic four-point stance with hands planted first on the ground, then on the knees and thighs as they come to a stand (see Fig. 19-1). Mental retardation is common, whereas eye movements, swallowing, and sensation are unaffected. When the child is 9 to 12 years of age, increasing proximal weakness makes independent walking impossible. Once in a wheelchair, these children develop progressive kyphoscoliosis, contractures in all joints, and equinovarus deformity of the feet. In subsequent years, these children become virtually immobile and require complete care. The combination of weak respiratory muscles and kyphoscoliosis drastically reduces pulmonary reserve, and they generally succumb by the late teens or early twenties.

Becker dystrophy differs from Duchenne only in that onset is usually later, the course more benign, and survival is seen into the thirties and forties. Mental impairment is less often seen.

The CPK is markedly elevated (20 to 100 times normal) even before the disease is clinically evident. Muscle biopsy is characteristic, with increased fibrosis, grouped basophilic fibers, large round opaque fibers, and scattered necrosis (see Fig. 19-10C). Steroids for treatment of Duchenne's dystrophy have shown to slow disease progression, but their use is tempered by the problems of long-term corticosteroid complications.

Although no specific treatment is available, a competent rehabilitative team can improve the quality of life for these patients. The prevention of contractures, particularly of the Achilles tendon and iliotibial band, is important early in the disease. A surgical release of contractures along with the use of long leg braces can prolong independent walking for several years. When the patient becomes confined to a wheelchair, the development of kyphoscoliosis can be slowed with proper upright positioning and, in selected cases, spinal fusion. Unfortunately, hip and knee contractures are accelerated by the constant sitting position, so that these children can sleep only on their side and require numerous pads for comfort. Respiratory management and a host of devices that are useful to patients with chronic disability are described in the section on treatment.

Genetics Duchenne and Becker dystrophy are two of the most thoroughly studied genetically determined diseases. For many years, clinicians and geneticists knew that the disease was transmitted by a gene defect on the X chromosome. Females were known to be asymptomatic carriers, and males would manifest the disease. Duchenne patients were always the most seriously affected, usually dying in their teens or early twenties. Becker patients were considered by many to have a more slowly progressive form of Duchenne dystrophy. In some patients diagnosed as having facioscapulohumeral or even limb–girdle dystrophy, the latest DNA work has shown them to have, in actuality, Becker dystrophy.

Investigation of the X chromosome has shown a wide variety of deletions and point mutations that may lead to a total absence of the muscle membrane protein dystrophin (Duchenne dystrophy) or the production of a smaller-molecular-weight dystrophin present in diminished quantity in the cell (Becker dystrophy). The test for dystrophin gene abnormalities is now done in many medical centers and is commercially available.

For children suspected of having the disease, a blood specimen should be screened first, since 60% to 70% of cases will demonstrate a deletion or duplication. The abnormality detected in these may be specific for either the Duchenne or Becker form of the disease. For the remaining 20% to 30% where no deletion or duplication is found, or where the differentiation between Becker and Duchenne is necessary, a small specimen of skeletal muscle obtained by biopsy should be analyzed by Western blot for determination of dystrophin quantity and quality.

The carrier status of females can be done using PCR and Southern blot techniques to detect DNA deletions or duplications in the dystrophin gene. The results of these analyses are best discussed with the carrier suspect and her family by a physician or genetic counselor who is fully acquainted with the techniques and the diseases. Counseling on carrier status is sometimes less than a perfect statistical proposition and requires great care in presentation to a family.

Finally, for the carrier suspect who is already pregnant and wishes to know whether the fetus is affected with Becker or Duchenne dystrophy, prenatal diagnosis may be achieved using cells obtained at amniocentesis or chorionic villus biopsy. By PCR techniques as described, major deletions or duplications may be detected. If none are found and point mutations are suspected, a linkage analysis of the fetal DNA is possible if sufficient numbers of affected and unaffected relatives are available for study.

FACIOSCAPULOHUMERAL DYSTROPHY (FSH)

This disorder is characterized by a slowly progressive weakness with predominant involvement of the shoulder girdle muscles and variable degrees of facial and peroneal muscle weakness. Most cases are autosomal dominant. Symptoms may begin insidiously in the first two decades of life and progress slowly or not be noted until later decades. Common symptoms include difficulty whistling, blowing up a balloon, or drinking through a straw. The lips are often pouting (bouché de tapir), and the smile is transverse. During sleep the eyes may remain slightly open. The clavicles are prominent and downsloping (see Fig. 19-3). The shoulders droop and are rotated forward, producing an oblique axillary crease. The scapulae wing out when the patient attempts to elevate the arms (see Fig. 19-2) and the trapezius muscles are pushed up prominently. Atrophy of the triceps and biceps contrasts with preserved forearm muscles, producing a "Popeye" appearance. Peroneal muscle weakness with foot drop occurs in some patients, but hip muscles are generally spared and patients retain the ability to walk. Surgical fixation of the scapula to the posterior thoracic wall has occasionally been performed, because many are able to abduct the arm fully when the scapula is forcibly held in place; unfortunately, the scapula may tear loose. General guidelines for treatment are outlined at the end of this chapter.

The characteristic clinical findings in a patient with a positive family history makes diagnosis fairly straightforward. Muscle biopsy will usually show mild chronic myopathic changes but there are no findings specific to facioscapulohumeral dystrophy.

Genetics A mutation in the gene localized to chromosome 4 is thought to cause this disorder. The gene has not been identified, but the presence of deletions near the telomeric end of chromosome 4 provide diagnostic confirmation.

LIMB–GIRDLE MUSCULAR DYSTROPHY (LGMD)

Limb–girdle dystrophy is associated with a progressive proximal muscle weakness in childhood or adult life. A variety of molecular defects in muscle membrane-associated proteins have now been described but the clinical features in the commonest forms (LGMD 2A, 2B) are similar. Weakness usually begins in proximal leg muscles and later is seen in the arms, along with scapular winging.

Facial, tongue, and pharyngeal weaknesses are usually lacking. The shoulder weakness differs from that of facioscapulohumeral dystrophy in that the deltoid is affected and winging is usually less prominent. An anterior axillary fold and neck flexor weakness is usual (see Fig. 19-3). Respiratory muscle involvement may occur in some patients. General supportive measures for these patients are outlined at the end of this chapter. Rare forms of LGMD (2C, 2D, 2E, 2F) has severe, early symptoms resembling Duchenne dystrophy.

Progressive proximal weakness is a common complaint in the neuromuscular clinic. Many patients with a limb–girdle syndrome are now recognized as having a specific entity such as adult spinal muscular atrophy or polymyositis, which might previously have been classified on clinical grounds as limb–girdle dystrophy.

Genetics Symptoms of limb severe girdle dystrophy have now been linked to four chromosomes producing abnormal sarcoglycans— muscle membrane proteins

closely associated with dystrophin (LGMD, 2C, 2D, 2E, 2F). Milder LGD is due to a muscle calpain defect (LGMD 2A). Transmission in all of these is by autosomal recessive inheritance. A rare autosomal dominant form of the disease (LGMD 1A) is caused by a mutation on chromosome 5, but the defective protein product is unknown.

CONGENITAL MUSCULAR DYSTROPHY

This rare disorder is characterized by hypotonia and weakness at birth. Limb contractures may be pres-ent from the beginning and restrict movement of already weakened muscles. Despite severe pathological changes in muscle on biopsy, there seems to be little progression in the weakness and a few patients actually may walk eventually. The creatine kinase levels are modestly elevated and muscle biopsy shows nonspecific dystrophic changes. A variant of this disease, the Fukuyama form, seen primarily in Japan, is associated with severe CNS abnormalities, including mental retardation, seizures, enlarged ventricles, and microcephaly.

Genetics Transmission is by autosomal recessive inheritance. The first type is associated with mutation of a gene on chromosome 6 that codes for laminin, a muscle membrane protein associated with dystrophin and the sarcoglycans. The defective gene for the Fukuyama form is located on chromosome 9, but the specific protein product is unknown.

OCULOPHARYNGEAL DYSTROPHY

Patients are normal until their forties or fifties, when symptoms begin, usually with progressive ptosis developing over several years accompanied by increasingly restricted eye movements without diplopia. Swallowing difficulties usually develop and aspiration can be a serious problem in a minority of patients. Limb weakness occurs rarely. Invariably, these patients will recall similarly afflicted family members and the pattern of an autosomal dominant disease will emerge. Diagnosis is confirmed by the finding of a relatively normal appearing muscle biopsy except for the appearance of scattered small angular fibers containing red-rimmed vacuoles. Treatment is directed to the surgical correction of ptosis and the prevention of aspiration. A gastrostomy feeding tube is occasionally needed.

Genetics The gene mutation, located on chromosome 14, is known to code for cardiac myosin heavy chains, but why this should lead to this syndrome where there are no cardiac symptoms is still unexplained.

MYOTONIC DISORDERS

MYOTONIA CONGENITA

Impaired muscle relaxation is encountered in both autosomal dominant and autosomal recessive varieties of myotonia congenita. Patients complain of difficulty in releasing their hand grip, stiffness of muscles, and difficulty in initiating activity after a prolonged rest. They may report subjective weakness if normal exertion is opposed by myotonia in antagonistic muscles. Muscle hypertrophy is frequent and occasionally produces a herculean appearance. EMG is useful in establishing the diagnosis, because muscle biopsy is nonspecific. Several medications are helpful in reducing myotonia, including phenytoin, procainamide, quinine, and mexiletine.

Genetics Recently, a defect of the chloride channel in skeletal muscle has been defined in both the autosomal dominant form (Thompson's disease) and recessive forms of myotonia congenita. The gene abnormality is caused by a point mutation within the chloride channel gene on chromosome 7. At present, linkage analysis may be done on family members in the autosomal dominant form, but the techniques are still not commercially available to clinicians.

MYOTONIC DYSTROPHY

A predominantly *distal* weakness, in contrast to most myopathies, is encountered in adults with myotonic dystrophy. Advanced cases have a characteristic facial appearance with ptosis, temporalis and masseter wasting, protuberant lower lip, and thinning of the sternocleidomastoid muscle, producing a typical "hatchet face" appearance (see Figs. 19-5 and 19-6). The speech is often dysarthric and nasal, and the patient may complain of dysphagia. As in other autosomal dominant disorders, mild and severe cases may appear in the same family; however, a unique, commonly observed feature is patient denial of a familial disorder, even in obvious cases (see Fig. 19-6B).

Other organ systems are involved in this disorder, leading to cataract formation, impairment of gastrointestinal motility, and endocrine abnormalities. Patients are frequently noted to have low intelligence, no goal orientation, poor work histories, and bizarre personalities. Progressive cardiac conduction abnormalities may lead to sudden death. Serial electrocardiograms (EKGs) are recommended, and a pacemaker should be considered in patients with progressive conduction disturbance. A reduced ventilatory drive may produce symptoms of alveolar hypoventilation including disturbed sleep. General anesthesia should be given cautiously because patients are unduly sensitive to barbiturates and other medications that depress ventilatory drive. The myotonia is generally asymptomatic and does not require treatment. Weakness of the ankles may be improved with polypropylene splints. Proximal weakness is rarely severe enough to prevent walking.

Genetics This disorder is based on autosomal dominant inheritance with strong penetrance in each generation. The gene defect on chromosome 19 has been well described as an unstable expansion of CTG trinucleotide repeats resulting in a critical error of the gene product protein kinase. The gene region for these repeats is particularly unstable during meiosis, resulting in further amplification of the numbers of repeats. With increased repeats, the severity of the disease is increased. This is thought to explain the phenomenon of "anticipation" in which successive generations of affected individuals seem to express the disorder with increasing severity. Such anticipation is particularly severe in mothers carrying the myotonic dystrophy gene. Although they themselves may show only moderate symptoms, their children at birth, if affected, show severe clinical changes of limb and facial weakness and will exhibit slow milestones and mental retardation. Testing for this gene defect is now available and can be given to patients and their relatives who may wish to know their disease status.

INFLAMMATORY MYOPATHIES

An autoimmune disturbance underlies polymyositis (PM) and dermatomyositis (DM), whereas other syndromes may be caused by Coxsackievirus, pyogenic bacteria, trichinosis, sarcoid, or tuberculous granuloma. In polymyalgia rheumatica, an inflammatory process may involve fascia rather than muscle, although patients complain of muscular pain and weakness.

Dermatomyositis and polymyositis have similar clinical symptoms and signs, with the exception of the characteristic rash of DM. The latter disorder may be a paraneoplastic syndrome in adults. In patients with an associated collagen-vascular disease (i.e., systemic lupus erythematosis, rheumatoid arthritis, Sjögren's syndrome), the inflammatory myopathy may be a minor or major manifestation of the disease. Patients with juvenile DM may have a systemic vasculitis with pulmonary fibrosis, myocarditis, gastrointestinal ulcers, cerebral vasculitis, skin ulceration, and calcification.

Although PM may develop at any age, most cases occur in childhood and in the fifth and sixth decades of life. The disease often begins insidiously with systemic features such as fever, arthralgias, myalgias, and Raynaud's phenomenon. Weakness may begin relatively suddenly and may become profound, but more commonly there is a subacute progression of proximal weakness that is not readily distinguishable from other limb–girdle syndromes. Muscle tenderness may be absent. The rash of DM may take several forms, appearing before, after, or in association with the onset of weakness. The upper eyelids often have a lavender or *heliotrope* discoloration, and periorbital edema and flushing of the cheeks occurs in advanced cases. The chest and neck may become reddened and develop telangiectasia. *Gottran's* papules are thickened erythematous patches that occur over the knuckles and other joint extensor surfaces. Skin nodules may break down and exude calcium.

The disease often has a variable course. Some patients have an acute episode with complete recovery, even without treatment. Other patients demonstrate a relapsing, remitting course with incomplete recovery between episodes, or a chronic progressive course that responds poorly to treatment. The serum CPK is elevated in most cases, particularly those with acute onset. A muscle biopsy shows necrosis of muscle fibers, perivascular inflammatory infiltrate, and perifascicular atrophy (see Fig. 19-10D).

Corticosteroids are generally prescribed, although some patients may not respond despite the addition of azathioprine or other immunosuppressants. Adult patients who have DM should be screened for an occult malignancy.

Inclusion body myositis (IBM) is a disorder predominantly seen in men over 50 with asymmetric symptoms of hand grip and shoulder–girdle weakness along with proximal leg weakness. The creatine kinase level is only modestly elevated. Electrical studies in such patients, some of whom may be suspected of having motor neuron disease, shows a mixed neurogenic and myopathic pattern. On muscle biopsy there are distinctive findings of increased connective tissue, variation in fiber size, isolated patches of inflammatory cells, and small red-rimmed vacuoles containing amyloid within individual muscle fibers. No specific drug therapy is useful in these patients and treatment is directed to rehabilitation measures discussed later.

Genetics The vast majority of IBM cases are sporadic, but in recent years reports describe similar biopsy findings in members of several large kindreds in which clinical patterns resembling limb–girdle dystrophy, distal myopathy, fascioscapulohumeral dystrophy, and, in some, CNS white matter disease, are seen. Inheritance is autosomal recessive with the candidate gene probably on chromosome 9. Several small kindreds of individuals appearing as typical sporadic IBM but with affected family members in multiple generations, indicate that IBM may also be inherited as an autosomal dominant trait, but to date no candidate gene has been identified.

Polymyalgia rheumatica (PMR) is characterized by muscle pain and stiffness, which is most severe in the morning and has a predilection for the shoulders. It rarely occurs before 55 years of age and is most frequent in women. Other constitutional symptoms may be present, including anorexia, fever, and night sweats. Temporal arteritis (TA), which is manifested by scalp tenderness, temporal headaches, or visual obscuration, is associated with PMR in 20% to 50% of cases and can produce a sudden, permanent blindness. With the exception of the erythrocyte sedimentation rate, which is markedly elevated, all tests are usually normal. PMR responds dramatically to low doses of prednisone. High doses are used if TA is suspected or documented by temporal artery biopsy.

METABOLIC MYOPATHIES

GLYCOGEN STORAGE DISEASES

These rare autosomal recessive disorders exhibit the common finding of excess glycogen in skeletal muscle and sometimes other organ systems.

McArdle's disease is the commonest of those listed in Table 19-2 and presents in childhood or early adulthood with symptoms of exercise intolerance due to cramping and myoglobinuria. All of the disorders can exhibit fixed muscle weakness but it is unusual except for McArdle's and acid maltase deficiency. Such fixed proximal weakness rather than exercise-induced cramping is a particular feature of acid maltase deficiency, in which early diaphragm involvement in adults may bring the patient to medical attention because of breathing difficulty. Infantile acid maltase deficiency is rare, severe, and usually rapidly fatal.

Diagnosis of these disorders can be made only by muscle biopsy, which will show distinctive glycogen storage and abundant lysosomal material. Assays for specific enzyme deficits are available commercially.

Genetics Gene loci for all of these disorders are known and all are inherited on an autosomal recessive basis (see Table 19-2). McArdle's disease can occur as an autosomal dominant as well, but this is uncommon.

DISORDERS OF LIPID METABOLISM

Carnitine palmitoyl transferase deficiency mimics the glycogen storage diseases in that patients develop stiffness and pain (though no cramping) with exercise, and then myoglobinuria. The disorder is the commonest cause of recurrent myoglobinuria. Other precipitating causes include general anesthesia, infection, and a diet low in carbohydrate and high in fat. The major risk to the patient is renal failure related to the myoglobinuria for which hospitalization, treatment with fluids, and dialysis is needed for some patients. Diagnosis of this disorder is not always obvious since the muscle biopsy may be surprisingly normal (except after myoglobinuria when extensive, although nonspecific, necrosis may be seen). The specific enzyme defect of either CPT I or CPT II can be detected in muscle specimens submitted to commercial laboratories.

Genetics The gene locus for this autosomal recessive disorder is on chromosome 1. The reason for male preponderance is not known.

Carnitine deficiency presents either as a myopathic disease with limb weakness or as more serious systemic illness. The myopathic form usually begins in childhood with painless proximal weakness and in rare instances a cardiomyopathy. In the more severe systemic form, onset is earlier, encephalopathy common, and sometimes severe cardiomyopathy and rapid death occur. The disorder results from reduced or absent carnitine, a carrier protein vital to the transport of fatty acids into mitochondria. On biopsy, the major change is a massive accumulation of fat within the skeletal muscle and biochemical assay can detect low or absent carnitine levels.

Genetics It is likely that autosomal recessive inheritance is involved although the majority of cases appear sporadic.

MITOCHONDRIAL MYOPATHIES

All of these disorders share the common feature of excessive numbers of abnormal mitochondria in skeletal muscle and, often, in other tissues. Building on these morphologic observations, the nature of the multiple underlying metabolic defects and the genetic errors responsible for each disorder is now known.

The first of these to be described, the *Kearns-Sayre syndrome* (KSS), is characterized by extraocular muscle weakness, pigmentary retinal degeneration, and cardiac conduction block. These abnormalities define the syndrome, although some patients may demonstrate, as well, ptosis, short stature, hearing loss, mental retardation/dementia, ataxia, peripheral neuropathy, ele-

vated CSF protein, depressed ventilatory drive, delay of secondary sexual characteristics, and rarely hypofunctioning thyroid and parathyroid glands. Symptoms usually are noted in childhood and characteristic EKG findings of heart block may require urgent pacemaker placement to prevent sudden death.

Closely resembling the KSS group are those with the *familial progressive external ophthalmoplegia (PEO) syndrome.* These patients demonstrate progressive external ophthalmoplegia, ptosis, and limb weakness as major symptoms, varying degrees of tremor, ataxia, hearing loss, and peripheral neuropathy, but no cardiac conduction defects. Differentiating this syndrome from KSS and other mitochondrial myopathies requires special DNA tests described later.

Two rare mitochondrial myopathy syndromes have been described. The first, termed Myoclonus Epilepsy with Ragged Red fibers on muscle biopsy (MERRF) is characterized by limb weakness, both myoclonus and generalized seizures, progressive dementia, ataxia, and hearing loss. A second disorder, Mitochondrial Myopathy, Encephalopathy, Lactic Acidosis, and Stroke (MELAS), begins in childhood and is characterized by retarded growth, recurrent strokes, progressive mental deterioration, and death by age 20. Neither of these disorders has any impairment of extraocular muscles or retinal abnormalities.

Several very rare syndromes involving mitochondrial complex II deficiency and cytochrome c oxidase deficiency with diagnosis by muscle biopsy are detailed in Evaluation and Treatment of Myopathies by Griggs, Mendell, and Miller (1995).

With the exception of KSS, where pacemaker placement may be lifesaving, treatment of these disorders is symptomatic. Muscle biopsy will demonstrate excessive numbers of mitochondria (the ragged red fibers) and this in turn should prompt the ordering of mitochondrial DNA assays on blood and skeletal muscle.

Genetics For the majority of these maternally inherited disorders, the diagnosis can be confirmed by analysis of mitochondrial DNA using Southern blot and PCR techniques. The KSS typically has a single mitochondrial deletion; MERFF and MELAS result from a variety of single point mutations that can be detected by PCR; some of the familial PEO group can result from multiple nuclear DNA deletions which cause a primary defect of a mitochondrial protein and transmission as an autosomal dominant trait.

MALIGNANT HYPERTHERMIA

Patients with malignant hyperthermia are free of symptoms unless exposed to certain anesthetic agents, particularly halothane and succinylcholine. The full syndrome includes an elevation in temperature up to 43°C, muscular rigidity, tachycardia, marked lactic acidosis, myoglobinuria, and refractory cardiac arrhythmias. Untreated cases are uniformly fatal. Anesthesia and the surgical procedure must be terminated immediately, while dantrolene sodium is administered with cooling measures.

The disease is autosomal dominant in many patients, and there may be subtle evidence of an underlying myopathy. There is no reliable confirmatory test, so patients with a previous episode and their relatives should not receive these agents.

Genetics The latest work suggests that a genetic mutation closely associated with the gene defect for central core disease on chromosome 19 may be causative for malignant hyperthermia. No DNA testing is available to the clinician at present.

TOXIC MYOPATHIES

A wide variety of medications and toxic compounds can produce either acute muscle necrosis or a slowly progressive chronic myopathy. Alcohol can produce both of these syndromes in the same patient and is the most common myotoxin. The acute myopathy usually follows a binge of drinking and may be accompanied by myoglobinuria. Other drugs and toxins associated with acute myopathy include ipecac, amiodarone, clofibrate, other cholesterol-lowering agents, heroin, aminocaproic acid, chlorthalidone, vincristine (where a sensorimotor neuropathy is usually superimposed), and any substance that produces hypokalemia including diuretics, purgatives, licorice, carbenoxolone, or amphotericin B.

A chronic proximal myopathy is associated with prolonged corticosteroid therapy, particularly with dexamethasone and fluorinated steroids. A discontinuation leads to a slow recovery. The aforementioned drugs associated with acute myopathy may also produce a chronic myopathy.

ENDOCRINE MYOPATHIES

Hypothyroidism is associated with cramps, mild weakness, and "hung-up" reflexes. Hyperthyroidism may produce mild weakness, whereas ophthalmoplegia occurs in Graves' disease.

Hypoparathyroidism may lead to a carpopedal spasm or tetany. Hyperparathyroidism may combine weakness with brisk reflexes, which are reminiscent of ALS.

Acromegaly is associated with a chronic myopathy and the carpal tunnel syndrome. The weakness in Addison's disease and hyperaldosteronism is probably caused by electrolyte disturbances. Cushing's disease may produce the same myopathy as exogenous steroids.

CONGENITAL MYOPATHIES

The three most common congenital myopathies are summarized in Table 19-2.

Myotubular myopathy, sometimes termed *centronuclear myopathy*, can present in several ways. The neonatal form presents at birth with hypotonia, respiratory distress, extraocular muscle weakness, and early death. In the early childhood form, milestones are delayed, limb weakness is prominent, scoliosis and a high arched palate, ptosis and extraocular muscle weakness are major features. In the adult form, mild limb weakness with onset in the thirties is the only problem. In all forms, the muscle biopsy shows typical chains of nuclei running centrally within muscle fibers.

Genetics The neonatal form is caused by a mutation on the X chromosome, which aids in prenatal and carrier diagnosis. The early childhood form is autosomal recessive and the adult form is autosomal dominant but the chromosome and gene location are still unknown.

Patients with *central core disease* are hypotonic at birth and show delayed milestones but usually walk normally and show no progression of weakness. Hip dislocation, scoliosis, and pes cavus may be seen. Diagnosis is by muscle biopsy, which shows prominent areas of noncontractile protein in the center of type I muscle fibers.

Genetics Inheritance is in an autosomal dominant pattern due to a point mutation for the ryanodine gene located on chromosome 19. Other mutations of this gene are associated with inherited malignant hyperthermia.

Nemaline myopathy presents in a severe neonatal form with early death or, more commonly, in childhood with delay of milestones, generalized weakness, high arched palate, and scoliosis. Diagnosis is by muscle biopsy, which shows distinctive, thin threadlike inclusions throughout the muscle fiber.

Genetics Inheritance is as an autosomal recessive or dominant pattern due to a gene mutation on chromosome 1.

PERIODIC PARALYSIS

Hypokalemic periodic paralysis is characterized by bouts of extreme weakness separated by periods of normal strength. Although limb weakness is profound, the diaphragm is spared so that the weakness is virtually never fatal. Meals high in carbohydrate or sodium may precipitate an attack which can last hours. Diagnosis is confirmed by the finding of a low serum potassium during an attack of weakness. Fixed weakness can develop with multiple attacks and muscle biopsy in these cases will demonstrate prominent vacuoles within muscle fibers. Treatment is by avoidance of precipitating factors such as high carbohydrate meals. Acetazolamide prophylactically may be helpful.

Genetics A mutation of the gene coding for the muscle calcium channel on chromosome 1 accounts for this autosomal dominant disorder.

Hyperkalemic periodic paralysis (HPP) and paramyotonia congenita (PMC) are discussed together since they seem to be variants of the same general class of disorders with mutations of the muscle sodium channel. In uncomplicated HPP, patients become weak, sometimes for hours, and particularly after high potassium intake. PMC presents with episodes of weakness that are provoked by cold exposure. In either of these, normal or elevated serum potassium may be seen. Treatment of the weakness is by oral intake of carbohydrates. Prophylaxis from episodes may be obtained by oral acetazolamide.

Genetics These disorders are caused by several point mutations of the muscle sodium channel gene located on chromosome 17.

TREATMENT OF NEUROMUSCULAR DISEASES

The initial reaction of the patient and family to the diagnosis of a neuromuscular disease is often one of despondency and hopelessness. In time, with support and understanding, they may understand that the future is less bleak and that a well-balanced rehabilitative approach will maximize their function, prolong ambulation, deter complications, and create an optimistic environment. The problems that these patients face depend more on the degree of the disability than on the disease that produces it. The treatment of the ambulatory patient is discussed in this section, and an approach to the problems of the weaker wheelchair-bound patient is provided.

All patients are encouraged to maintain a normal range of motion through a program of stretching, while avoiding overexertion. The frozen shoulder is a painful complication particularly in ALS, but it is easily avoided. In children, contractures at the hips and ankles may impair walking long before a muscle weakness becomes critical, and this must be prevented. A foot drop may be remedied by a lightweight posterior polypropylene splint that is molded to the shape of the foot and fits into the shoe. An arthrodesis may be necessary for a marked ankle instability. Painful calloses that accompany foot deformities may be treated by a podiatrist. In patients with hip weakness, raising the height of seats with a toilet seat elevator or electric lift chair makes standing without assistance easier. Patients rely heavily on hand supports for getting up from the toilet, getting out of a tub, or going up stairs. Supports must, therefore, be securely anchored. A cane, crutches, or a walker is necessary as the weakness increases. Long leg braces that allow locking of the knee joint may prevent precipitous knee buckling. If a patient becomes temporarily bedridden due to an intercurrent illness, early ambulation is imperative to prevent further atrophy and contracture. In Duchenne dystrophy, the percutaneous release of contractures at the Achilles tendons, iliotibial bands, and hamstrings combined with the use of long leg braces may prolong ambulation for several years.

Weakness of the hands impairs the fine dexterity required for eating, writing, and dressing. Various pieces of adaptive equipment are designed to splint the hand and allow easier grasping. Large-handled utensils, a buttonholer, or a pencil attached to the hand with a Velcro strap may be useful. The patient who has a shoulder weakness can use a long-handled reacher to get objects from cabinets or high shelves.

Visual obstruction due to ptosis may be relieved by lid crutches attached to eyeglasses or by surgery. Head instability due to neck weakness may be improved by wearing a neck collar. Patients who have severe dysarthria can develop alternate means of communication with the help of a speech therapist and devices.

Patients who have dysphagia may benefit from an evaluation including a modified barium swallow and a consultation with a nutritionist and a therapist with experience in swallowing disorders. Occasionally, symptoms are temporarily ameliorated by an inferior constrictor myotomy; however, in advanced cases, the patient may require diversion by gastrostomy feeding tube (PEG). Salivary secretions that cannot be swallowed may be decreased with amitriptyline or they may be removed with a portable suction unit. Families should be instructed in the Heimlich maneuver.

Palpitations or unexplained syncope due to a heart block can occur with various neuromuscular disorders, particularly myotonic dystrophy and Kearns-Sayre syndrome. These patients may require periodic ECGs or Holter monitoring, and a pacemaker may be indicated. With acute generalized weakness, pulmonary and swallowing function should be monitored in an intensive care unit because respiratory failure or aspiration can develop rapidly, particularly in myasthenia and the Guillain-Barré syndrome.

Respiratory failure is the most serious complication of the nonambulatory patient and is produced by a combination of respiratory muscle weakness, atelectasis, recurrent aspiration, poor cough reflex, and decreased lung volume from progressive kyphoscoliosis. The usual physical signs of pneumonia are often difficult to detect in a patient who has a baseline tachy-pnea because of small tidal volumes. The patient's family should therefore seek an early medical evaluation if any new respiratory symptoms develop. Daily postural drainage with chest percussion can be performed at home by the family, and immunization should be considered.

Kyphoscoliosis in preadolescent patients (see Fig. 19-8) is minimized by a properly fitting wheelchair and polypropylene jackets or braces that restrict lateral movement. Spinal fusion may be suggested if the curve progresses despite conservative therapy. Segmental spinal instrumentation allows early postoperative ambulation and has replaced the use of Harrington rods.

A great deal of mobility and comfort is possible for the patient who is confined to a wheelchair if the wheelchair is properly designed and fitted. Detachable arm rests and swing-away elevating leg rests facilitate transferring and prevent lower extremity contractures and edema that develop if the legs are constantly dependent. Ball-bearing feeders and a lap tray make independent eating possible for the patient who cannot elevate his arms to his mouth, and a thick foam cushion prevents decubiti. A motor-powered wheelchair is useful for patients who lack the upper limb strength or the attendance of another person necessary to propel the chair.

The transfer of an overweight patient in and out of a wheelchair can be difficult even with a hoist, thus reduction diets should be encouraged. A patient with total paralysis will often sleep more comfortably on an air or water mattress that distributes weight evenly, preventing unrelenting pressure and decubiti. A frequent change of position in both the wheelchair and bed as well as padding to support the limbs prevent nerve compression palsies.

Apart from minimizing the physical handicap, the physician must be aware of the patient's social, emotional, and sexual needs. A severely handicapped patient who relies on others for eating, hygiene, and elimination will understandably become depressed over this extreme dependency. Active counseling of the patient and family should be directed toward solutions to the various problems in "personal space" and independence that arise.

The patient in the final stage of a neuromuscular disease will succumb to respiratory failure unless ventilatory support is provided. Noninvasive positive pressure devices (BIPAP) are helpful in the early stages and are useful, particularly at night, in keeping carbon dioxide levels low. With increasing bulbar weakness and difficulty with secretions, a tracheostomy is usually needed if aspiration is to be prevented and adequate ventilation ensured. The thought of prolonging life on a respirator is unacceptable for many patients, but for others considerable satisfaction can still be gained if the environment is supportive. The physician, patient, and family should discuss these options well in advance.

The treatment of patients with chronic neuromuscular weakness requires the services of the primary physician; physical, occupational, and respiratory therapists; an orthotist; a podiatrist; an orthopedist; a nutritionist; a social worker; and a psychiatrist. With proper management, the patient can be educated to compete in a world that is inherently easier for those who are able-bodied.

QUESTIONS AND DISCUSSION

1. A 61-year-old woman is admitted to the hospital with a 4-day history of progressive weakness. Her medical history is unremarkable except for congestive heart failure that is being treated. She had been constipated for several days and she then had diarrhea after taking laxatives. Her examination was remarkable for generalized mild weakness, hypoactive reflexes, and flexor plantar responses. Cognition, cranial nerves, and sensation were normal.

Discussion: A quadriparesis with intact cognition, a lack of sensory disturbances, and flexor plantar responses are most likely caused by a disorder of the peripheral nervous system.

The differential diagnosis includes the Guillain-Barré syndrome (reflexes are more likely to be absent than diminished), botulism poisoning (lack of cranial nerve dysfunction, especially ocular, is atypical), myasthenia gravis (cranial nerve involvement would also be expected), acute polymyositis, and an electrolyte disturbance.

Useful studies include an electrolyte and serum CPK determination and a sedimentation rate. An EMG-nerve conduction study would be helpful early on, when the physician is looking for decrement with repetitive stimulation (seen in myasthenia and botulism).

This patient's potassium level was 1 mEq/dl due to diuretics and diarrhea, and her strength returned to normal with treatment.

2. A 19-year-old pregnant woman reports that two maternal uncles died of muscular dystrophy at the ages of 15 and 16. She wants to know if her fetus or her 1-year-old daughter may be affected.

Discussion: Some cases of muscular dystrophy may have actually been spinal muscular atrophy. This is usually an autosomal recessive disorder, and the risk of the woman developing muscular dystrophy would be low.

Death occurring in the teenage years is characteristic of Duchenne dystrophy. This illness in two male siblings would not be due to a spontaneous mutation, and it indicates that their mother was a carrier. Genetic linkage analysis requires blood samples from the affected uncles but is not an option in this case.

Blood samples on mother and daughter as well as fetal cells obtained by amniocentesis can be screened for 70% of patients carrying the abnormal gene. If no deletion is found, linkage analysis can be carried out on all specimens to determine the probabilities of all three having the identical X chromosome. Since there is no linkage information from the two deceased brothers of the pregnant mother, no accurate probability can be given concerning her being a carrier or having passed the abnormal gene on to her fetus. The situation might be clarified if the mother's CPK is significantly elevated, which would argue for her being a carrier. Since CPK levels usually decrease during pregnancy, the finding of normal values would not be helpful. In such a complex situation the assistance of an experienced genetic counselor is advised.

3. A 51-year-old woman is admitted to the hospital because of symptomatic bradycardia. She reports frequent "dizzy spells" for about 1 year, but she has never fainted. She has also had a lifelong stiffness in her hands and a nasal voice, and she trips frequently.

Discussion: Myotonic dystrophy is suggested by the history of grip myotonia and systemic complaints. Recurrent abdominal pain, gallstones, chronic diarrhea, dyspepsia, and dysphagia are common symptoms. Cardiac conduction disturbances may present with dizziness or may be discovered on a routine ECG. A careful examination for clinical myotonia, as well as for the characteristic facial features, supported the diagnosis in this case. Myotonic dystrophy is a common disorder, although it is frequently overlooked.

An ECG demonstrated a complete heart block, and a pacemaker was implanted during the patient's stay in the hospital. Bilateral foot drop was relieved with polypropylene ankle bracing.

All relatives of this patient should be evaluated clinically for signs and symptoms of this autosomal dominant disorder. Symptomatic relatives can be counseled and followed for the disorder. Asymptomatic individuals can be given information regarding the disease. Should they wish to know their carrier status with certainty, a DNA analysis of blood would provide definite information regarding the presence or absence of trinucleotide repeat sequences. This information would be of use particularly to unaffected individuals planning families.

SUGGESTED READING

Dyck PJ, Thomas PK, Griffin JW et al: Peripheral Neuropathy. Philadelphia, WB Saunders, 1993

Emery AEH, Rimoin DL: Principles and Practice of Medical Genetics, Vols. 1 and 2. New York, Churchill Livingstone, 1990

Engel AG, Banker BQ: Myology, Vols. 1 and 2. New York, McGraw-Hill, 1986

Evans RW, Baskin DS, Yatsu FM: Prognosis of Neurological Disorders, Second Edition. New York, Oxford University Press, 1999

Griggs RC, Mendell JR, Miller RG: Evaluation and Treatment of Myopathies. Philadelphia, FA Davis, 1995

Mitsumoto H, Chad DA, Pioro EP: Amyotrophic Lateral Sclerosis. Philadelphia, FA Davis, 1998

Nickel VL, Botte MJ: Orthopedic Rehabilitation. New York, Churchill Livingstone, 1992

Neurology for the Non-Neurologist, Fourth Edition,
edited by William J. Weiner and
Christopher G. Goetz. Lippincott
Williams & Wilkins, Philadelphia © 1999.

C H A P T E R   2 0

Neurologic Aspects of Cancer

Deborah Olin Heros

Cancer and cancer treatment may affect the peripheral and central nervous system in many ways. Cancer is the second leading cause of death in the United States, with an incidence of more than 1 million cases of cancer each year and resulting in more than 1 million cancer-related deaths per year. Over 17,500 new cases of primary brain tumors were diagnosed in 1997 in the United States. Primary central nervous system (CNS) tumors occur in people of all ages; they are the third leading cause of cancer deaths between the ages of 15 and 34 years. Statistical data suggest that the incidence of primary CNS tumors is on the rise. Autopsy studies identify metastatic tumors to the brain in 24% of patients with systemic cancer. Each year, more than 125,000 patients with systemic cancer develop intracranial metastatic tumors, the majority of which are symptomatic. Furthermore, systemic cancer may affect the peripheral and central nervous system as a result of metastatic involvement of the dura and leptomeninges, bony metastases resulting in epidural spinal cord compression, and peripheral involvement to the brachial and lumbosacral plexi. Cancer may also result in nonmetastatic complications to the CNS, including various vascular disorders, metabolic and nutritional disorders, infection, and neurologic complications from cancer treatment. Indirect, or paraneoplastic, syndromes have been recognized as the result of systemic cancer. More than 80% of cancer patients will develop neurologic complications, and the resultant impact on their quality of life and survival is significant.

The medical specialty of neuro-oncology addresses the diagnosis and treatment of primary CNS neoplasms and the metastatic and nonmetastatic neurologic complications of systemic cancer. In addition, as pain is a significant component of cancer, the neuro-oncologist is often actively involved with cancer pain management. Neurologic complications of cancer are common and often serious. Unfortunately, the incidence of neurologic complications is increasing as a result of improved survival of cancer patients. Identification and treatment of neurologic complications may improve the quality of life and survival of the cancer patient. Often the problems associated with these neurologic complications are unique and may even present clinically before the systemic cancer has been identified. Therefore, it is very important for the physician involved in the care of cancer patients to be aware of the neurologic aspects of cancer.

This chapter addresses some of the more common problems in neuro-oncology. It is divided into four sections to address primary CNS tumors, CNS complications of systemic cancer from direct involvement, indirect neurologic complications of systemic cancer (paraneoplastic syndromes), and complications of cancer therapy.

PRIMARY CNS TUMORS

Primary CNS tumors are classified by the cell of origin. The incidence of primary intracranial tumors is between 2 and 19 per 100,000 persons per year and is dependent on age. In adults, supratentorial tumors are more common, whereas the majority of primary intracranial tumors of childhood occur in the posterior fossa. The most common primary brain tumors are glial in origin and include astrocytomas, oligodendrogliomas, and ependymomas.

ASTROCYTOMA

The most common glial tumor is the astrocytoma, which stains positive for glial fibrillary acidic protein (GFAP) and is classified or graded according to histologic characteristics reflecting aggressiveness and survival. The majority of pathologists continue to use the classic Kernohan grading system of astrocytoma, based on the pathologic characteristics of cellularity, pleomorphism, proliferation, and necrosis. Kernohan grades I and II represent the "well-differentiated astrocytoma," Kernohan grade III represents the intermediate or anaplastic astrocytoma, and grade IV astrocytoma is synonymous with a glioblastoma multiforme. In an attempt to improve the correlation between prognosis and grade of the tumor, the World Health Organization (WHO) in 1993 suggested a descriptive, three-tiered system that includes the well-differentiated astrocytoma, anaplastic astrocytoma, and glioblastoma multiforme. Because there is a slight difference between the pathologic characteristics described by the two systems, the physician must know which system is being used. The three-tiered system emphasizes cellular pleomorphism and vascular proliferation. Necrosis, the pathologic hallmark of the glioblastoma in the Kernohan system, is not necessary for the diagnosis of glioblastoma in the WHO classification system. The physician must also be aware that there are several subtypes of gliomas, with different treatment and prognostic implications. Treatment decisions for the subtypes must be appropriate to avoid causing iatrogenic complications. Furthermore, subtypes vary in their sensitivities to treatment modalities (e.g., oligodendrogliomas are sensitive to chemotherapy).

The pilocytic astrocytoma, often located in the cerebellum, is a low-grade neoplasm occurring in a younger population. Surgical resection may offer a complete cure. The majority of astrocytomas are of the fibrillary type. The pleomorphic xanthoplasmic astrocytoma (PXA) may appear histologically bizarre and similar to a glioblastoma, but, like a low-grade tumor, it may actually carry a more favorable prognosis. It is thought that this particular subtype of glioma may have been previously misdiagnosed as a glioblastoma multiforme and may account for some of the long-term survivors of glioblastoma in the literature. More recently, the pathologic entity of dysembryoplastic neuroepithelial tumor (DNT) has been recognized as a very well circumscribed, often cortical lesion causing seizure activity. The DNT may behave in a very "benign" manner and may even represent a hamartoma rather than a true neoplasm. Often, this is treatable by surgery alone. A high-grade gemistocytic astrocytoma may portend a particularly poor prognosis.

The most important factors that determine the prognosis of a patient with an astrocytoma include histology, age of the patient, and the Karnofsky Performance Status (KPS) of the patient. Age appears to be very important. Patients younger than 40 with a glioblastoma have a 50% chance of surviving 18 months, whereas those between the ages of 40 and 60 have a 20% chance, and those patients older than 60 have a 10% chance. Patients with an anaplastic astrocytoma have a significantly better prognosis than patients with a glioblastoma, with median survivals of 36 months and 10 months, respectively. Patients with a KPS of greater than 70 have a 34% survival at 18 months compared to 13% for those patients with a KPS less than 60. Less significant prognostic factors may include a long duration of symptoms prior to diagnosis, presence of seizures, location of tumor, and degree of surgical resection. In general, younger patients have a higher chance of responding to chemotherapy than older patients. Furthermore, the extremes of age tolerate radiation therapy less well.

Risk factors for the development of an astrocytoma are poorly understood. This tumor most often occurs sporadically. Previous epidemiologic studies have suggested a slight increase in risk of developing astrocytomas with exposure to certain industrial chemicals. Recent developments in molecular biology have allowed researchers to identify various abnormalities of growth factors that play a role in tumor oncogenesis. Autocrine stimulation of growth factors and their receptors have been identified in glioblastomas. The oncogene c-sis, which encodes for part of the platelet-derived growth factor (PDGF), has been found in the glioblastoma, and the level of autostimulation has been correlated with the degree of malignancy in tumor cells. The degree of expression of PDGF and its receptor has been associated with the transformation of cells from benign to malignant. Experimental therapy using biotherapeutic agents for the treatment of malignant gliomas is addressing this observation by utilizing inhibitors of growth factors and their receptors that regulate cell growth and differentiation.

Chromosomal analysis of glioblastoma cells has identified multiple gene abnormalities involving chromosomes 10, 17, and 22. Chromosome 17 abnormalities have been found in all grades of astrocytoma and therefore may be an early change in tumorogenesis. Abnormalities of chromosome 10 are seen in the more anaplastic tumors. Interestingly, the hereditary neurofibromatosis syndrome type I has been associated with abnormalities of chromosome 17, and neurofibromatosis syndrome type II with abnormalities of chromosome 22. The heterogeneity of the glioblastoma multiforme and the array of abnormalities of the chromosomes observed makes it quite difficult to simplify the key abnormality that induces tumorogenesis in the astrocytoma. Abnormalities of the tumor suppressor gene p53 are found in tumors of the familial Li-Fraumeni syndrome. Patients with this syndrome are at risk for developing malignant astrocytomas as well as a variety of systemic malignancies. Recently, the presence of p53 mutations in glioma has been identified in a younger patient population and may be predictive of treatment response and prognosis. In the future, genetic markers may offer a new dimension to the classification system of brain tumors.

CLINICAL PRESENTATION

The clinical presentation of astrocytoma is determined by tumor location, pathology, and age of the patient. The majority of astrocytomas in adults occur in the supratentorial compartment. Presenting symptoms may include headache, seizure, focal neurologic deficits, and personality change. The increasing availability of neuroimaging studies with improved resolution has resulted in earlier discovery of brain tumors. Unexplained first seizures in adults, atypical neurologic symptoms, or an unexplained change in personality or mood should be investigated by either computed tomography (CT) or magnetic resonance imaging (MRI). Contrast for the appropriate neuroimaging studies is important if a primary brain tumor is in the differential diagnosis. A brainstem glioma is less common and may present with sensorimotor abnormalities, coordination difficulties, or cranial nerve dysfunction. The tumor grade correlates somewhat with the abnormalities on the neuroimaging study. Low-grade tumors usually do not enhance, and they appear hypodense on a CT scan and have abnormalities on MRI T2-weighted images. Increasing tumor grade results in increasing contrast enhancement. Central necrosis, with surrounding en-

hancement and peritumoral edema, is typical for a glioblastoma.

TREATMENT

Treatment options for astrocytoma are determined by pathology, location, clinical presentation, and age of the patient. Often, the patient is clinically symptomatic from cerebral edema; therefore, corticosteroids (usually dexamethasone) are started prior to surgery, and they often offer improvement of symptoms. Caution should be used if a primary CNS lymphoma is in the differential diagnosis, because the use of corticosteroid therapy prior to biopsy may decrease the chance of obtaining a positive biopsy. An anticonvulsant to prevent seizures for supratentorial lesions is also often started prior to surgery.

A definitive diagnosis is obtained by pathologic examination of the surgical specimen. The primary goals of tumor surgery for astrocytoma include (1) to determine pathology, (2) to identify tumor grade, and (3) to identify any subtype of glioma that may affect prognosis and treatment options. Surgical debulking is preferred over a biopsy, when possible, to reduce the tumor burden, provide an adequate pathology specimen, and improve symptomatic relief from mass effect. Theoretically, tumor debulking may also improve the chance to respond to adjuvant therapy. Stereotactic biopsy is most often reserved for patients whose poor medical condition precludes a craniotomy, and for those with deep-seated lesions or lesions in neurologically eloquent locations. The use of neuronavigational systems and intraoperative neuroimaging studies have improved the ability of the neurosurgeon to attain maximal resection with minimal morbidity. Survival benefit has been correlated with good tumor resection, but the infiltrative nature of astrocytomas prohibits a complete resection.

Postoperative radiation therapy has been shown to increase the median survival of patients with an anaplastic astrocytoma and glioblastoma. Limited-field brain irradiation with a "radiation boost" to the most active central portion of the tumor is generally performed over a course of 5 to 6 weeks. Recently developed techniques to deliver radiation therapy to astrocytomas include radiosurgery, three-dimensional conformal radiation therapy, boron neutron capture therapy, and the use of radiosensitizers. The role of these techniques for the treatment of high-grade astrocytomas has yet to be defined.

The role of radiation therapy for low-grade astrocytomas is even less clear. Statistically, patients with low-grade astrocytomas who have received radiation therapy have improved survival over those patients not so treated. However, the timing is controversial. It is not clear whether radiation therapy should be administered at the time of diagnosis (e.g., when the neoplasm has been identified after a single seizure, or perhaps as an incidental finding by a neuroimaging study) or delayed until the tumor is more symptomatic from tumor transformation. Recent studies suggest that the timing is not a major prognostic determiner.

Various techniques of administering radiation therapy have been used in an attempt to increase its effectiveness and reduce its toxicity. Hyperfractionation (delivering radiation in more frequent but smaller doses) has been used for various primary brain tumors, but without consistent benefit. Neurologic toxicity from radiation therapy may be a significant problem for patients with gliomas, in particular when additional forms of radiation therapy such as brachytherapy or radiosurgery are used. The role of radioprotective agents is being explored to reduce the risk of radiation toxicity.

Chemotherapy has not been a primary treatment for malignant astrocytomas. Its benefit is thought to be limited by the blood–brain barrier: the glial foot processes and the endothelial cells prevent the passage of systemically administered hydrophilic chemotherapeutic agents. The most commonly used agents are the lipid-soluble nitrosoureas carmustine (BCNU) and lomustine (CCNU). Recently, the recognition that some subtypes of glial tumors are chemosensitive has increased enthusiasm for chemotherapy for primary brain tumors. The anaplastic astrocytoma, especially in younger patients, is considered to be chemosensitive. The preferred combination of therapeutic agents for this tumor is procarbazine, CCNU, and vincristine (the PCV regimen). Oligodendrogliomas and mixed oligoastrocytomas are also chemosensitive, and most experience has been with the PCV regimen. Unfortunately, survival benefit of chemotherapy for glioblastoma is limited, although clinical trials suggest that some patients receiving chemotherapy have an increased chance for long-term survival at 18 months. BCNU is the most widely used single agent for glioblastoma.

To circumvent the limitations of the blood–brain barrier, alternative methods of administering chemotherapy have been used for malignant astrocytomas. Intra-arterial chemotherapy utilizes a first-pass benefit to increase the concentration delivered to the area of perfusion, with diminished risk of systemic toxicity. Chemotherapeutic agents including BCNU and cisplatin have been administered by this route. Unfortunately, intra-arterial administration of chemotherapy appears to increase the risk of neurotoxicity. The procedure, involving repeated arterial catheterizations, is cumbersome. Tumors that involve multiple vascular territories require injections into multiple vessels.

Constant systemic infusional chemotherapy alters the pharmacokinetics of chemotherapy and may offer benefit over conventional chemotherapy. The combination of BCNU and cisplatin has been administered by constant systemic infusion. Intratumoral chemotherapy has been attempted in various ways over the past several years using various agents including bleomycin, methotrexate, and BCNU. The recent development and availability of a biodegradable drug delivery system containing BCNU has made the concept of intratumoral chemotherapy more practical (Fig. 20-1). This treatment modality has demonstrated modest benefit for the treatment of recurrent glioblastoma in patients eligible for reoperation. Investigations using this new drug delivery system with other agents, as well as in combination with other treatment modalities, are currently underway. Agents to modify the blood–brain barrier, such as mannitol, have been explored to enhance the effectiveness of chemotherapy. More recently, RMP7 has been under investigation to selectively modify the blood–brain barrier in the area of the tumor, thus allowing enhanced chemotherapy delivery just to that area. Unfortunately, the combination of autologous bone marrow transplantation and high-dose chemotherapy has not offered benefit for the treatment of malignant glioma.

Newer experimental agents to treat malignant glioma by inhibiting angiogenesis include thalidomide. Other agents inhibit the activity of tumor growth factors and their receptors. As we better understand the mechanism of tumorogenesis, we hope to find newer agents to specifically target and inhibit tumorogenesis. Chemotherapeutic agents such as paclitaxel have demonstrated activity against glioma. Given the limited prognosis and the predictable outcome for patients with high-grade glioma, it is important for the physician caring for these patients to be aware of the clinical protocols available and to make the appropriate referral for patients interested in investigational treatment. Ethical decisions involving the appropriateness of participation in experimental protocols for astrocytoma are very difficult when the survival rate using known treatment modalities is limited and the investigational treatments are yet unproven and potentially hazardous. In a national survey, less than 8% of patients with astrocytoma were enrolled in treatment protocols. As participation in investigational protocols by patients with other malignancies has resulted in improved treatment modalities, it is important to encourage participation.

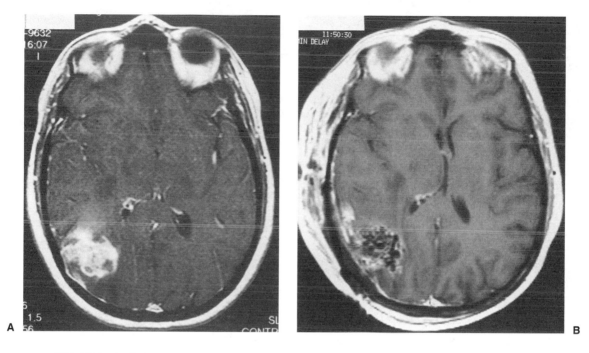

FIG. 20-1. A. Gadolinium MRI of a woman who presented with a seizure. The diagnosis was glioblastoma multiforme. **B.** Gadolinium MRI following resection of glioblastoma multiforme and intratumoral implantation of biodegradable chemotherapy disks containing carmustine (Gliadel).

Given the availability of radiosurgery and the frequency of its use for various CNS malignancies including astrocytoma, it is important to be aware of its potential complications. Radiosurgery has for the most part replaced brachytherapy or interstitial radiation therapy. Brachytherapy utilizes surgically implanted catheters loaded with radioactive seeds, usually iodine-125 or iridium-131, for local administration of irradiation with limited exposure to surrounding normal tissue. This treatment approach has been used in conjunction with external beam radiation therapy, and it has also been utilized for recurrences. A national brain tumor study group did demonstrate a benefit of brachytherapy in younger patients with small, well-circumscribed tumors in which catheters could be surgically implanted. However, the procedure has been shown to be quite cumbersome and associated with risks such as hemorrhage, infection, and radiation necrosis. Local recurrence, usually within 2 cm of the original tumor, is the pattern for the majority of patients receiving conventional treatment. In long-term survivors treated with brachytherapy, distant tumor recurrence, including leptomeningeal disease as well as systemic metastases, was seen with increased frequency. The development of radiation necrosis increases the need for dexamethasone and the possibility of reoperation.

Radiosurgery allows controlled delivery of localized radiation without the invasiveness of brachytherapy. It is currently being used both as initial therapy, usually in combination with conventional external beam radiation therapy, and at the time of recurrence. Radiation injury and radiation necrosis remain its main limitations (Fig. 20-2).

Various forms of immunotherapy have been used for the treatment of malignant glioma. Interferon-alpha and interferon-beta have been of limited use. The benefit of interleukin-2-activated lymphocytes (LAK cells) appears limited, possibly because of the concomitant use of dexamethasone necessary to control the tumor-associated edema.

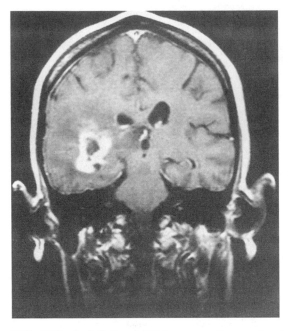

FIG. 20-2. Gadolinium MRI demonstrating contrast-enhancing radiation necrosis mimicking tumor recurrence. The patient had a history of glioblastoma multiforme and had been treated with combined conventional radiotherapy and radiosurgery.

NEUROLOGIC DETERIORATION AND TUMOR PROGRESSION

A decline in neurologic function usually marks the recurrence or progression of an astrocytoma. However, other medical and neurologic problems may mimic tumor progression, and the physician should be aware of the differential diagnoses for neurologic deterioration in patients with an astrocytoma. Complications from radiation therapy may mimic tumor progression or recurrence. In general, radiation therapy for an astrocytoma is initially well tolerated. However, an acute encephalopathy may develop, particularly if large radiation fractions are delivered to a large volume of brain in patients with increased intracranial pressure. The patients may complain of increased headaches, somnolence, lethargy, nausea, or worsening of focal neurologic symptoms. The symptoms of acute radiation toxicity are the result of disruption of the blood–brain barrier resulting in cerebral edema, and they usually improve with corticosteroid therapy. If the symptoms are not responsive to corticosteroid therapy, the radiation therapy may need to be temporarily postponed.

Subacute or "early delayed" complications from radiation therapy usually begin within 2 weeks of completing radiation therapy and may persist up to 4 months after completion of radiation therapy. This disorder is thought to be a reversible injury to the oligodendroglial cells resulting in demyelination, and it is responsive to corticosteroid therapy. During this phase, the neuroimaging study may demonstrate an increased mass effect and increased contrast enhancement, suggesting tumor progression. However, symptoms may be controlled with dexamethasone and the clinical situation may stabilize over time. This phase of radiation injury is often mistaken for tumor progression.

The late or "delayed" effect of radiation therapy for astrocytoma usually consists of a process known as radiation necrosis. This process cannot be distinguished from tumor recurrence by contrast-enhanced CT or MRI studies. Attempts have been made to differentiate between the two processes by various metabolic neuroimaging studies, such as positron emission tomography (PET) and single photon emission computed tomography (SPECT): radiation necrosis results in a hypometabolic abnormality, whereas recurrent tumor results in a hypermetabolic area. Often, both radiation necrosis and recurrent tumor are present simultaneously. If treatment options are available, a biopsy may be necessary. Reoperation with attempted resection and debulking may reduce chronic corticosteroid needs and improve neurologic symptoms. Reoperation for a recurrent astrocytoma is usually considered when additional treatment modalities are also available. Reoperation alone offers very limited benefit.

Late effects of radiation therapy also may result in a diffuse leukoencephalopathy, manifested by gait disturbance, urinary incontinence, and dementia. Unfortunately, the symptoms do not respond to shunting, although the ventricles appear large on CT scan. Central endocrinopathies, including central hypothyroidism and adrenal insufficiency, may also occur as a late complication of radiation therapy. An elevated prolactin level may be seen as the result of radiation injury to the hypothalamus.

The possibility of anticonvulsant toxicity should be excluded in a patient with progressive neurologic deficits. Chronic corticosteroid therapy may result in hyperglycemia. Hyperosmolar coma, the extreme of this condition, has been seen in these patients. This patient population is also at increased risk for systemic infections as a result of chronic corticosteroid therapy or chemotherapy. Intracranial infections (i.e., a brain abscess) may mimic recurrent tumor. Cerebrovascular accidents (CVAs) have been reported in patients with astrocytomas treated with radiotherapy or intra-arterial chemotherapy. A steroid myopathy resulting in proximal weakness may be mistaken for tumor progression. The patient with an astrocytoma has a particularly high risk for developing thrombophlebitis and pulmonary embolism. This risk, which appears to be the result of a generalized hypercoagulable state from the brain tumor, is added to the risks associated with a postoperative state or a nonambulatory patient with hemiparesis. This medical complication occurs with such a high frequency that any astrocytoma patient who complains of shortness of breath, atypical chest pain, leg pain, asymmetric peripheral edema, or atypical syncope should be evaluated. There is no consensus as to whether filter or umbrella placement in the inferior vena cava or anticoagulation is the preferred therapy. Clinical judgment is important, but there does not appear to be a significantly increased risk for intracranial hemorrhage using anticoagulation, and, therefore, an astrocytoma is not an absolute contraindication to anticoagulation.

Tumor progression or recurrence usually occurs locally within 2 cm of the original tumor margin. Tumor growth occurs via the white matter and therefore contralateral spread with deep midline tumors is not unusual. Multifocal gliomas are uncommon, occurring in 5% of patients at the time of presentation and 10% to 15% of patients at the time of tumor recurrence. Leptomeningeal or distant tumor spread is quite rare. Similarly, systemic metastases are extremely rare. Usually, the patient becomes progressively more dysfunctional with increasing somnolence that no longer responds to increasing dexamethasone doses. For the most part, pain is not a major complication of this type of malignancy.

PRIMARY CNS LYMPHOMA

Primary CNS lymphoma (PCNSL) is a non-Hodgkins lymphoma usually of B-cell origin that arises within the brain, spinal cord, or leptomeninges. This tumor may occur in otherwise healthy patients with normal immune systems, usually in older men, but it more often occurs in patients with immune compromise. It is seen with increasing frequency as a result of the growing population with human immunodeficiency virus (HIV). This tumor does not tend to metastasize systemically and is a separate entity from systemic lymphoma with CNS metastasis. Patients with inherited, acquired, or iatrogenically induced immune deficient states are at an increased risk for developing this tumor, particularly transplant patients and up to 10% of patients with acquired immune deficiency syndrome (AIDS). The clinical presentation may include headache, personality changes, seizures, and focal neurologic symptoms. Often the lesions are multifocal, frequently involving deep midline structures with contrast enhancement and minimal surrounding edema on neuroimaging studies. The diagnosis is usually established by biopsy, and surgical resection is usually not an option. The use of corticosteroid steroid therapy prior to biopsy may decrease the opportunity to obtain positive pathology and therefore should be avoided if possible.

The management of the immune-compromised patient may be somewhat different from that of the immunocompetent patient. The presentation may resemble CNS toxoplasmosis clinically. Therefore, it is common to treat a patient with known immune deficiency empirically for toxoplasmosis for a limited period, and to follow him clinically and radiographically. If the lesions improve, the assumption is that the patient has toxoplasmosis, whereas if the lesions progress or do not improve, then the possibility of CNS lymphoma increases and a biopsy may be performed. Occasionally, an immune-compromised patient may have simultaneous toxoplasmosis and CNS lymphoma, complicating the interpretation of the empiric trial. A lumbar puncture with cytologic examination may be helpful if the tumor is in the midline or if the leptomeninges are involved. Proper studies of the cerebrospinal fluid (CSF) may demonstrate a neoplastic monoclonal lymphocytosis as opposed to an inflammatory process. Intraocular involvement does occur and a slit lamp examination or vitreous biopsy may be helpful to establish the diagnosis. A systemic evaluation including a bone marrow biopsy may help to exclude the possibility of systemic lymphoma or other small-cell malignancies. Most often, a brain biopsy is indicated.

Once the diagnosis of PCNSL has been established, corticosteroid therapy may offer improvement of neurologic symptoms. For many years, radiation therapy has been the mainstay of treatment, but the prognosis was limited. The median survival of immunocompetent patients with primary CNS lymphoma is approximately 14 months, and it is much less in patients with immune deficiency. A recent approach using combined modalities with chemotherapy and radiation therapy has resulted in improved survival. Unfortunately, relapse remains common and late neurologic toxicity from combined therapy is a significant complication resulting in a progressive dementing leukoencephalopathy. Chemotherapy has generally not been used in patients with CNS lymphoma associated with immunodeficiency because of the overall poor prognosis and response rate. Future directions for treatment of primary CNS lymphoma include the use of various combinations of chemotherapy at the time of diagnosis, reserving radiation therapy for recurrence.

OLIGODENDROGLIOMA

The oligodendroglioma is a type of glial tumor derived from the oligodendrocyte, the myelin-producing cell within the CNS. Histologically, this tumor is identified by its characteristic "fried-egg" appearance and a positive stain for myelin basic protein. The tumor tends to be slow growing and therefore it is most often considered to be a low-grade tumor. However, varying degrees of anaplasia, and therefore aggressiveness, do occur. Most often, the tumor presents as a nonenhancing hypodense lesion on CT scan or abnormalities on T1 images on MRI scan. The tumor may be calcified. Enhancement may suggest a more aggressive tumor or the presence of a mixed oligoastrocytoma. Occasionally, the onset may be abrupt as the result of hemorrhage. The pluripotential glial cell may differentiate into either an astrocyte or an oligodendrocyte, which may explain the development of the mixed oligoastrocytoma.

Management of the oligodendroglioma depends on location, clinical presentation, and neuroimaging appearance. Surgical resection is generally attempted if possible. The oligodendroglioma has been identified as a chemosensitive tumor and therefore chemotherapy has played a major role in its treatment in recent years. The use of chemotherapy for low-grade oligodendroglioma is being studied. However, in anaplastic oligodendrogliomas, chemotherapy has been found to be beneficial. The chemotherapy most commonly used for this tumor has been the PCV regimen. Although radiation therapy has been shown to improve survival of patients with oligodendroglioma, the role of radiation therapy remains controversial, especially if total resection has been accomplished. However, if subtotal resection or biopsy has been performed, radiation therapy has some survival advantage. Survival benefits of treatment are difficult to assess because of the slow growing nature of this tumor.

EPENDYMOMA

The ependymoma is a glial tumor arising from the ependymal cells lining the ventricles and the CSF-filled spaces. This tumor usually occurs during childhood in the posterior fossa arising from the floor of the fourth ventricle, but it may present in the supratentorial cerebral hemispheres in the lining of the lateral ventricles or spinal cord. When the tumor occurs in the posterior fossa, it usually presents with symptoms of increased intracranial pressure, including headache, nausea, and vomiting, and it often causes obstructive hydrocephalus. The treatment of choice is surgical resection and the prognosis depends on the degree of resection. A 45% overall 5-year survival is reported in the literature, with an increased chance of long-term survival after complete resection. This tumor lines the CSF pathways and may seed the neuraxis, although the majority of tumor recurrence is local within the posterior fossa. Local radiation therapy is usually recommended for supratentorial and spinal lesions. Local or craniospinal radiation therapy may be appropriate for ependymomas of the posterior fossa.

CNS COMPLICATIONS OF SYSTEMIC CANCER

INTRACRANIAL METASTASES

Systemic cancer may spread to the CNS to involve the skull, dura, parenchyma, or leptomeninges. Specific tumors may metastasize in predictable patterns, and understanding these trends is important to correctly diagnose metastases and offer palliative therapy. Tumors of the breast, prostate, and lung; malignant melanoma; and cancers of the head and neck region have a propensity to metastasize to the skull. Symptoms are most common if the tumor involves the base of the skull, resulting in localized pain, headache, or cranial nerve dysfunction (Fig. 20-3). Special views on a CT or an MRI scan may be necessary to identify base-of-the-skull metastases. Standard screening studies may not image this region well, giving the false impression of a negative study, and thus the opportunity to offer effective palliative therapy may be missed. The nuclear bone scan is not a very sensitive study (despite the fact that the symptoms are the result of bony metastases) because of the overlapping nuclear isotope uptake by the venous sinuses in this region. Localized radiation often offers effective palliation of symptoms, especially pain.

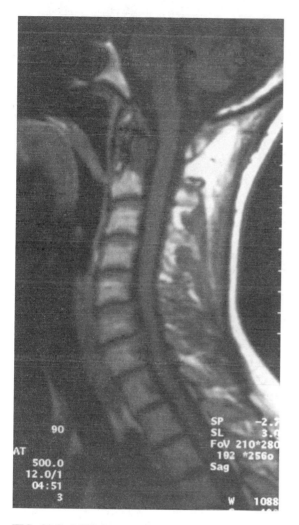

FIG. 20-3. MRI demonstrating metastatic cancer to the upper cervical spine in a man with lung cancer and severe, localized occipital pain. Metastasis to the base of the skull was clinically suspected from the location of the pain. However, interestingly, the pain was aggravated by neck movement.

Intraparenchymal brain metastases occur in nearly 25% of patients with systemic cancer. Patients with tumors of the breast and lung and malignant melanoma have a propensity to develop brain metastases. Less commonly, tumors of the gastrointestinal tract, kidney, or genitourinary system spread to the brain. The majority of tumors metastasize to the cerebral

hemispheres and less commonly to the brainstem and cerebellum in the posterior fossa. Metastases to the pituitary region, often from tumors of breast origin, have been described.

The risk of developing brain metastases from lung cancer varies with the pathology of the primary lung tumor. Small cell lung cancer has the highest risk (60%), adenocarcinoma has an intermediate risk (40%), and squamous cell carcinoma is the least likely to spread to the brain (20%). From 25% to 30% of patients present with neurologic symptoms and do not have a known primary cancer. Nearly half of these patients have a tumor of lung origin. Although brain metastases occur with high frequency in both lung and breast tumors, brain metastases often occur early in lung cancer (within months), whereas brain metastases are more likely to occur much later in breast cancer (i.e., in years). Although malignant melanoma is a relatively uncommon tumor, it has a very high propensity (80%) to spread to the CNS, often with multiple metastases.

Brain metastases originate from hematogenous spread, and therefore the majority of patients develop multiple lesions. Approximately 20% to 30% of patients have a single metastatic tumor. Treatment options are often determined by whether the lesion is single or multiple.

The signs and symptoms are determined by the size, number, and location of the tumors. Metastatic tumors of the cerebral hemispheres may cause progressive hemiparesis, language disturbance, confusion, seizures, sensory symptoms, visual field abnormalities, or personality changes. The development of depression in a cancer patient should raise the suspicion of brain metastases, in particular if he has never been previously prone to depression. Tumors in the cerebellum may result in dizziness, unsteadiness of gait, dysarthria, clumsiness of an extremity, or headaches from obstructive hydrocephalus. Cranial nerve dysfunction, motor and sensory signs, unsteadiness, and incoordination result from brainstem involvement. Hemorrhage into a metastasis may result in the abrupt onset of neurologic symptoms. Metastatic tumors with a tendency for hemorrhage include melanoma, renal cell carcinoma, choriocarcinoma, and various lung tumors.

The diagnosis of metastatic brain tumor is established by a neuroimaging study, either CT or MRI. A CT scan without contrast is the diagnostic study to assess for a hemorrhage. A contrast-enhanced CT scan may then demonstrate an enhancing tumor, usually with surrounding vasogenic edema. An MRI with gadolinium is the most sensitive test for detecting metastatic disease and is often performed to search for small, multiple tumors, especially when surgery is being considered to remove a presumably single brain metastasis.

When a patient presents with brain metastases without a known primary tumor, diagnostic studies are performed to identify the primary tumor, with special attention to imaging of the chest, remembering that approximately half of these patients will subsequently be found to have a primary lung cancer.

Corticosteroids, usually dexamethasone, are very effective in treating patients with symptoms that result from vasogenic edema. The appropriate dosing is determined by the number, size, and location of lesions, and by the severity of the symptoms. The most common initial dosage of dexamethasone is 4 mg four times daily. It is often used in conjunction with an H_2-receptor antagonist to reduce the risk of gastric complications from the corticosteroid therapy.

An anticonvulsant medication is indicated if the patient has experienced a seizure. The role of prophylactic use of an anticonvulsant is less clear, and many physicians prefer to avoid the risk of side effects from the medication in patients who have not experienced a seizure. Perhaps this approach is appropriate for patients with lesions in the deep white matter, cerebellum, or brainstem. It may be prudent to consider the use of a prophylactic anticonvulsant medication for lesions in potentially epileptogenic areas of the cerebral hemispheres such as near the motor cortex. Serum drug levels should be monitored appropriately.

Conventional treatment of brain metastases includes whole brain radiation therapy (3,000 cGy over 10 fractions). The whole brain is treated because of the high likelihood of multiple lesions and the chance of multiple microscopic foci of metastatic tumor from hematogenous dissemination. Advances in neuroimaging and neurosurgical techniques and the development of radiosurgery have increased the options for treatment of metastatic tumors. In general, surgery is reserved for removal of a single lesion in a surgically accessible area, for example a tumor in the posterior fossa causing hydrocephalus or a large tumor in the cerebral hemispheres (Fig. 20-4). Shunting is also considered for treatment of hydrocephalus if the cause of the hydrocephalus cannot be surgically excised. Stereotactic biopsy may be considered in patients presenting with neurologic symptoms without a known primary tumor or in patients in whom the specific tumor type cannot be established otherwise. Current recommendations regarding the role of whole brain radiation therapy are being reviewed now that radiosurgery is available. The current trend

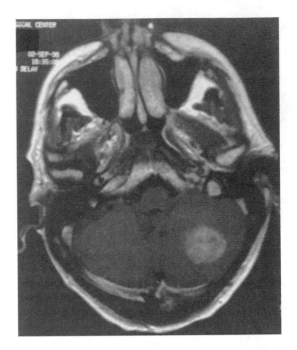

FIG. 20-4. Gadolinium MRI demonstrating contrast-enhancing single metastasis of the cerebellum in a patient with gastric carcinoma. His headaches, nausea, and unsteadiness improved after surgical resection.

is to use radiosurgery (1) to boost the effect of whole brain radiation therapy, or (2) to treat recurrences of metastatic tumors after whole brain radiation therapy. Some clinicians are using radiotherapy alone for the treatment of metastatic tumors. The maximal number of tumors that may be treated with radiosurgery is under investigation.

Untreated, the median survival for patients with brain metastases is 4 to 6 weeks. Appropriate therapy offers an improved quality of life and prolongation of survival. The overall median survival of patients treated for metastatic brain tumors is 6 months. Long-term survival is usually described in patients treated with surgery. The cause of death in patients with brain metastases is most often progression of systemic disease.

LEPTOMENINGEAL METASTASES

Systemic tumors may diffusely seed the leptomeninges, resulting in a condition known as neoplastic meningitis. Terms used in the literature to describe this condition (*carcinomatous meningitis, carcinomatosis of the meninges,* and *lymphomatous meningitis*) reflect the tumor of origin. The incidence of this serious complication is thought to be increasing as control of systemic disease improves. The CNS, including the leptomeninges, serves as a sanctuary site from systemic therapy as a result of the blood–brain barrier. Neoplastic meningitis may occur as the only CNS involvement or in combination with other sites of CNS involvement, such as intraparenchymal brain metastases. Most commonly, the solid tumors causing neoplastic meningitis include tumors of the breast and lung and malignant melanoma. Less commonly, tumors of the gastrointestinal tract, ovary, prostate, uterus, and bladder spread to the leptomeninges. Various types of lymphoma and leukemia have a tendency for leptomeningeal spread. The clinical presentation of neoplastic meningitis is variable and often subtle. Symptoms and signs reflect the diffuse involvement of the neuraxis at three levels: (1) the cerebral cortex, resulting in confusion, headache, and seizures, (2) cranial nerves, resulting in diplopia, facial numbness, hearing loss, visual loss, and tongue weakness, and (3) spinal and nerve roots, with a propensity for the lumbosacral spine region, resulting in low back pain, leg numbness and weakness, and sphincter dysfunction. Communicating hydrocephalus develops in 15% to 20% of patients with neoplastic meningitis. The diagnosis should be suspected in a cancer patient with neurologic symptoms and signs at various levels of the neuraxis. Often the findings on clinical examination are multiple and out of proportion to the symptoms described by the patient. The diagnosis of neoplastic meningitis is established by positive cytology of the CSF. The literature stresses the importance of repeated CSF examinations to establish the diagnosis. The CSF examination may also demonstrate elevation of opening pressure, mild pleocytosis with a lymphocytic predominance, a depressed glucose level, or protein elevation. Elevated biochemical markers may be used to diagnose the condition as well as to follow the response of treatment. Such markers include carcinoembryonic antigen (CEA), beta human chorionic gonadotropin (β-HCG), and alpha-fetoprotein (AFP). If a sufficient number of lymphocytes are present, specific immunohistochemical studies may help differentiate reactive inflammatory lymphocytes from neoplastic lymphocytes in lymphoma and leukemia patients.

Gadolinium MRI of the brain and spinal cord may demonstrate leptomeningeal enhancement, excluding the possibility of intracranial brain metastases that would contraindicate a lumbar puncture. Bulky disease that may be treated with localized radiation therapy may also be identified. In general, MRI with gadolinium is more sensitive than CT with contrast (Figs. 20-5, 20-6).

Treatment of neoplastic meningitis includes the use of intrathecal chemotherapy by lumbar puncture or through an Ommaya reservoir into the lateral ventricles. A limited number of chemotherapeutic agents are available for intrathecal use, including methotrexate, cytosine arabinoside, and thiotepa. Newer treatments, including liposome-encased chemotherapy and monoclonal antibodies, are being explored. Systemic chemotherapy is not thought to be effective. Radiotherapy is reserved for localized treatment of bulky disease. Patients with sphincter dysfunction may benefit from local radiotherapy to the conus medullaris and cauda equina. In patients with cranial nerve dysfunction, radiotherapy to the basal cisterns may be beneficial. Dexamethasone may improve symptoms. Untreated, the median survival of neoplastic meningitis is 6 weeks. The overall median survival with treatment is 4 to 6 months. A chance for longer survival in select patients has been described in patients with chemosensitive tumors such as breast cancer. Patients with neoplastic meningitis from malignant melanoma have a particularly poor prognosis. Often, a patient with neoplastic meningitis will have concomitant progression of systemic cancer.

SPINAL METASTASES

Spinal cord dysfunction from metastatic cancer may be the result of tumor metastasis to vertebral bodies, extension of a paravertebral mass, or intramedullary metastases from hematogenous spread to the spinal cord (5%). The most common cause of spinal cord compression is metastasis to the vertebral body from tumors with a tendency to spread to bone, such as multiple myeloma and tumors of breast, lung, or prostate origin. Pain is present in the majority of patients and the presence of back or neck pain in a patient with known cancer should raise the suspicion of a spinal metastasis and prompt appropriate investigation. Pain may be localized or radicular and often directs the clinician to the appropriate spinal level. The absence of pain in a patient with spinal cord dysfunction should suggest the possibility of another etiology for the patient's symptoms such as radiation myelopathy, intramedullary spinal cord metastases, or a paraneoplastic syndrome. The neurologic examination is very important to determine the level of spinal cord involvement. Symptoms may include motor and sensory abnormalities and sphincter dysfunction. The

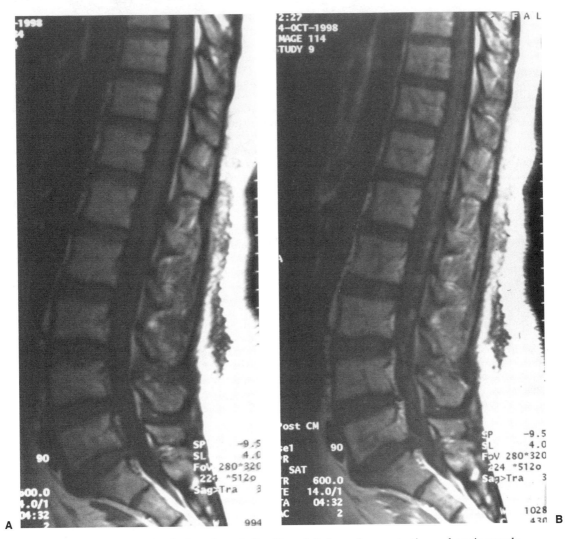

FIG. 20-5. MRI of spine before **A.** and after **B.** gadolinium, demonstrating enhancing nodular defects in the leptomeninges of a woman with metastatic breast cancer, who presented with paraparesis and urinary retention. CSF examination from Ommaya reservoir confirmed diagnosis of neoplastic meningitis.

neurologic examination may demonstrate hyperreflexia and dorsal column signs, with impairment of position sense and vibration. Spinothalamic dysfunction may result in abnormalities of pain and temperature sensitivities. A knowledge of the anatomy of the spinal cord is important in interpreting the neurologic examination.

Spinal cord compression from metastatic tumor represents one of the true neurologic emergencies in the cancer patient. The rate of progression is variable and failure to diagnose and treat spinal cord compression may result in irreversible neurologic injury, thus limiting the quality of life as well as potentially the survival of the cancer patient. In general,

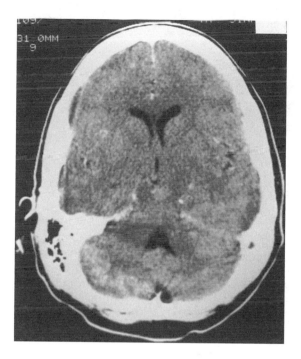

FIG. 20-6. Contrast-enhanced CT scan demonstrating multiple metastatic tumors in the woman (with metastatic breast cancer) seen in Figure 5. The patient required focal radiotherapy to the cauda equina, whole brain radiotherapy, and intrathecal chemotherapy.

the neurologic outcome is determined by the neurologic status at the time treatment is initiated. A patient who is ambulatory at the time of treatment has a good chance of remaining ambulatory, whereas it is unlikely that the nonambulatory patient will regain significant function. Sphincter involvement is considered to be a poor prognostic sign and often occurs later in spinal cord compression. Early involvement should alert the clinician to consider conus medullaris or cauda equina involvement.

Spinal MRI with gadolinium is the neuroimaging study of choice for evaluation of spinal cord dysfunction, since 15% to 30% of patients with spinal cord compression may have involvement at multiple levels. The entire length of the spine should be imaged for optimal planning of radiotherapy. A gadolinium MRI may also identify leptomeningeal involvement or intramedullary metastasis.

Corticosteroids, usually dexamethasone, are administered when the diagnosis of spinal cord compression is made. Initial doses range between 20 and 100 mg. The subsequent dosing is determined on symptoms, rate of progression, and extent of disease. Radiotherapy and surgery are the main therapeutic options. Radiotherapy is usually initiated urgently in a patient with known cancer. Surgery is appropriate for patients without a known cancer or in the setting of deterioration despite radiotherapy. Newer approaches to surgical decompression utilizing anterior and anterolateral approaches address the location of tumor involvement and may be preferred to the more traditional posterior surgical decompression. However, often the cancer patient in this situation has extensive systemic disease with a limited life expectancy, and surgery is not well tolerated.

NONMETASTATIC COMPLICATIONS

CEREBROVASCULAR COMPLICATIONS

Patients with cancer are at increased risk for a variety of cerebrovascular complications resulting either from the effects of malignancy or from treatment. The cerebrovascular complications may be either ischemic or hemorrhagic. Accelerated atheromatous disease resulting in thrombotic strokes may occur following radiation therapy to the head and neck region. Systemic cancer may cause a hypercoagulable state, resulting in arterial or venous sinus occlusion. Patients with mucin-producing adenocarcinomas, in particular, have been described to be at risk for the development of a hypercoagulable state and suffer subsequent cerebral infarction. Mucin deposits have been found in the venous walls at the sight of the infarct. Nonbacterial thrombotic endocarditis is a well-recognized complication of cancer and may result in cerebral embolism.

Bacterial endocarditis may occur as a complication of tumor therapy, because of neutropenia, and it may cause septic emboli resulting in stroke. Less commonly, a mycotic aneurysm may develop with the risk of subarachnoid hemorrhage.

Thrombocytopenia, either as a direct result of the malignancy (usually one of a hematologic origin) or a consequence of tumor therapy, may cause hemorrhagic complications including subdural hematoma, spinal epidural hematoma, or intracerebral hemorrhage. Lumbar puncture should be performed with a sufficient platelet count and appropriate coagulation parameters to avoid an iatrogenic spinal epidural hematoma with spinal cord compression. The cancer patient may be receiving warfarin for thrombotic complications related to the cancer-induced hypercoagulable state. In such a situation, the warfarin needs to be discontinued and the coagulation parameters corrected prior to performing a lumbar puncture.

A noncontrast CT scan is performed in patients in whom a hemorrhage is suspected. MRI is more sensitive than CT for identifying nonhemorrhagic cerebrovascular insults. A magnetic resonance angiogram (MRA) provides a noninvasive means to visualize the extracranial and intracranial circulation to evaluate a thrombotic stroke. The treatment depends on the type of cerebrovascular complication and the underlying cause.

METABOLIC AND NUTRITIONAL COMPLICATIONS

Metabolic abnormalities may develop as a direct result of systemic cancer or secondary to cancer treatment, and they affect both the peripheral and central nervous system. Metabolic derangements may cause a diffuse encephalopathy, resulting in generalized confusion, personality changes, alteration of alertness, seizures, and coma. The physical and neurologic examination may suggest a metabolic etiology by the presence of tremor, myoclonus, asterixis, and fluctuation of symptoms. The cancer patient is often on multiple medications, including narcotics for pain management. A thorough review of the medication list is essential in evaluating the cancer patient with neurologic symptoms. Although narcotics and pain medications are most commonly implicated to cause neurologic symptoms in the cancer patient, the clinician needs to be aware of the potential neurologic side effects of all medications the patient is receiving. The author has been impressed with the spectrum of neurologic symptoms caused by a drug such as metochlopramide including gait disturbance (initially thought to be spinal cord compression by a medical oncologist), tremor, rigidity resembling Parkinson's disease, physical and mental restlessness (akathisia), and confusion.

Corticosteroids are used for a variety of reasons in the cancer patient. Systemic and neurologic complications are common (Table 20-1). Anxiety, somnolence, and emotional lability, also common, may be managed either by altering the schedule (e.g., to avoid a late-night dose that causes insomnia), or by the administration of an antianxiety medication such

TABLE 20-1. Complications of Corticosteroids

Medical
Weight gain, striae
Diabetes mellitus
Skin fragility
Insomnia
Infection susceptibility
Candidiasis (oral thrush, esophagitis)
Neurologic
Anxiety, emotional lability
Psychosis, confusion
Proximal myopathy
Spinal lipomatosis (rare)

as a benzodiazepine. Chemotherapeutic agents can affect the peripheral and central nervous system in a variety of ways (Table 20-2). Toxicity depends on the age, specific agent, drug dosage, and associated therapies. It is imperative that the clinician caring for a cancer patient be aware of the neurotoxicity associated with each chemotherapeutic regimen.

Nutritional status, often poor in the patient with cancer, should be addressed if there are neurologic symptoms. Neurologic syndromes from deficiencies of thiamine, folate, and B_{12} are well recognized.

PARANEOPLASTIC SYNDROMES

Several distinct syndromes have been recognized in patients with systemic cancer that are not related directly to metastatic disease or treatment toxicity. These syndromes are considered to be remote effects of the cancer and are known as paraneoplastic syndromes. The paraneoplastic syndromes are of clinical significance for two reasons:

1. The neurologic symptoms may cause significant morbidity and therefore have a significant impact on the quality and survival of life of the cancer patient.
2. The neurologic symptoms may develop prior to the actual diagnosis of the systemic cancer; therefore, if the clinician is familiar with the various paraneoplastic syndromes, an earlier diagnosis of the systemic malignancy is potentially possible.

The disorders have been thought to be related to an autoimmune process, and various antineuronal specific antibodies have been identified (Table 20-3).

TABLE 20-2. Neurotoxicity of Chemotherapy

Cerebral hemispheres
  Acute encephalopathy
    Procarbazine
    Interferon
    Interleukin-1,2
    Ifosfamide
    Methotrexate (high-dose intravenous or intrathecal)
    Asparaginase
    Vincristine
  Chronic encephalopathy
    Methotrexate (high-dose intravenous or intrathecal)
    Fludarabine
  Leukoencephalopathy
    Methotrexate
    5-Fluorouracil + levamisole
    Carmustine (intra-arterial)
Cerebellum
  5-Fluorouracil
  Cytarabine
Visual system
  Tamoxifen (reversible retinopathy)
  Fludarabine (cortical blindness)
  Cisplatin (cortical blindness)
  Intra-arterial chemotherapy (optic neuropathy)
Myelopathy
  Methotrexate (intrathecal)
  Cytarabine (intrathecal)
  Thiotepa (intrathecal)
Peripheral nerves
  Vincristine
  Cisplatin
  Paclitaxel
  Suramin
  Etoposide

From Emergent and Urgent Neurology, 2nd Edition, 1999, p. 366.

QUESTIONS and DISCUSSION

1. A 50-year-old woman enters a walk-in clinic. She had had an unexplained episode of loss of consciousness while home alone. She was aware of being incontinent of urine and complained of a very sore tongue. You determine that she probably had a seizure. She does not have a history of seizures. As the physician, you:

A. Send her home and tell her to see her doctor if it happens again.
B. Start her on phenytoin and tell her to see her doctor if it happens again.
C. Order a CT scan of the brain and tell her to see her doctor.
D. Perform a complete neurologic examination, order appropriate tests for toxic and metabolic causes of a seizure, order a CT or MRI scan of the brain, and arrange for hospital admission or appropriate follow-up.

The answer is (D). An underlying cause for this seizure needs to be investigated. The onset of idiopathic epilepsy at this age is quite unusual. This patient should not be sent home if she is alone. She should not be allowed to drive. Hospitalization for observation and evaluation is preferred, although each situation should be individually reviewed.

2. The patient's MRI with gadolinium contrast demonstrates multiple ring-enhancing lesions in various parts of the cerebral hemispheres. She is neurologically intact. You then:

A. Start her on dexamethasone and an H_2-blocker.
B. Request an oncology consult.
C. Start her on an anticonvulsant medication.
D. All of the above

The answer is (D). If she has no evidence to suggest these lesions may be infectious, then metastatic tumor is the most likely diagnosis. Dexamethasone is very ef-

TABLE 20-3. Paraneoplastic Syndromes

SYNDROME	ASSOCIATED AUTOANTIBODIES	ASSOCIATED TUMORS
Cerebellar degeneration	Anti-yo (Anti-Purkinje cell)	Ovarian, breast
Encephalomyelitis	Anti-Hu	Lung
Opsoclonus-Myoclonus	Anti-Ri	Breast, bladder, lung
Subacute sensory neuropathy	Anti-Hu	Lung
Lambert–Eaton syndrome	Anti-VGCC (antisynaptotagmin)	Lung (small cell)

fective at reducing the vasogenic edema. In view of the abnormalities on the MRI and the fact that she has already experienced a seizure, prescribing an anticonvulsant medication is prudent.

3. An evaluation to establish a diagnosis and identify the primary site of tumor may include:

A. Chest x-ray and chest CT scan
B. Mammogram
C. Abdominal CT scan
D. Complete blood count, urinalysis, and liver function tests
E. Serum tumor markers
F. All of the above

The answer is (F). About half of patients presenting with metastatic brain tumors, without a known primary tumor, will subsequently be found to have a primary lung cancer. Unfortunately, although metastatic brain tumors most often present later in patients with breast cancer, synchronous presentation may occur in the most aggressive forms of breast cancer. Renal cell carcinoma, tumors of the gastrointestinal tract, and lymphoreticular neoplasms should also be considered. The various scans will also assist in establishing the extent of metastatic disease.

4. The chest CT scan is abnormal and a diagnosis of adenocarcinoma of the lung is confirmed histologically by bronchoscopy. The patient is treated with whole brain radiation therapy in 10 fractions. She returns to the clinic 1 month after therapy with headache, fatigue, and mental slowness. Your evaluation should include:

A. Carbamazepine level
B. Serum electrolytes, including sodium, potassium, and calcium
C. Serum glucose
D. All of the above

The answer is (D). Carbamazepine was chosen as the anticonvulsant medication because of the risk of dermatologic toxicity from the combination of phenytoin and whole brain radiotherapy. However, phenytoin is still the most commonly used anticonvulsant in this situation. Carbamazepine may cause the syndrome of inappropriate antidiuretic hormone (SIADH), as may the underlying lung cancer. Dexamethasone may cause significant hyperglycemia. The increasing symptoms may also be related to tapering the dexamethasone, so increasing the dose may treat the symptoms effectively.

5. The lung tumor was also treated with radiotherapy because it was thought to be blocking a bronchus. Four months later, the patient returns with urinary frequency and bilateral leg weakness. You then:

A. Assume it is a side effect from the chest radiotherapy.
B. Order a contrast MRI of the spine, using the neurologic exam to guide localization
C. Consider a lumbar puncture
D. Assume the patient has a steroid myopathy

The answer is (B) and (C). The major clinical concerns are epidural spinal cord compression from bony metastases and neoplastic meningitis. Epidural spinal cord compression most often causes pain. The MRI of the spine should be performed with gadolinium. Neoplastic meningitis may produce leptomeningeal enhancement. Lumbar puncture with cytologic examination should be considered to confirm the diagnosis of neoplastic meningitis. Steroid myopathy does not cause urinary frequency. Radiation-induced myelopathy is a rare diagnosis usually occurring later, and it should be considered only if the other direct metastatic complications have been excluded.

SUGGESTED READING

Bindal AK, Bindal RK, Hess KR et al: Surgery versus radiosurgery in the treatment of brain metastasis. J Neurosurg 84:748, 1996

Cairncross JG, MacDonald DR, Ramsay DA: Aggressive oligodendroglioma: A chemosensitive tumor. Neurosurgery 31:78, 1992

Chamberlain MC: Current concepts in leptomeningeal metastasis. Curr Opin Oncol 4:533, 1992

Cohen N, Strauss G, Lew R et al: Should prophylactic anticonvulsants be administered to patients with newly diagnosed cerebral metastases? A retrospective analysis. J Clin Oncol 6:1621, 1988

Friedman HS, Oakes WJ: New treatment options in the management of childhood brain tumors. Oncology 6:27, 1992

Graus FG, Rogers LR, Posner JB: Cerebrovascular complications in patients with cancer. Medicine 39:522, 1985

Heros DO: Neuro-oncology. In: Weiner WJ, Shulman LM (eds): Emergent and Urgent Neurology. New York, Lippincott Williams and Wilkins, 1999

Hochberg FH, Miller DC: Primary central nervous system lymphoma. J Neurosurg 68:835, 1988

Kori SH, Foley KM, Posner JB: Brachial plexus lesions in patients with cancer: 100 cases. Neurology 35:8, 1985

Moll JWB, Antoine JC, Brashear HR, et al.: Guidelines on the detection of paraneoplastic anti-neuronal-specific antibodies. Neurology 45:1937, 1995

Patchell RA, Tibbs PA, Walsh JW et al: Surgery versus radiosurgery in the treatment of brain mestastasis. J Neurosurg 84:748, 1996

Perrin RG, McBroom RJ: Metastatic tumors of the spine. In: Rengachary SS, Wilkins RH (eds): Principles of Neurology. St. Louis, Wolfe, 1994

Portenoy RK, Lipton RB, Foley KM: Back pain and the cancer patient: An algorithm for evaluation and management. Neurology 37:134, 1987

Posner JB: Neurologic Complications of Cancer. Philadelphia, FA Davis, 1995

Smalley SR, Laws ER, O'Fallon JR et al: Resection for solitary brain metastasis: Role of adjuvant radiation and prognostic variables in 229 patients. J Neurosurg 77:531, 1992

Thomas JE, Cascino TL, Earie JD: Differential diagnosis between radiation and tumor plexopathy of the pelvis. Neurology 35:1, 1985

Weissman DE: Glucocorticoid treatment for brain metastases and epidural spinal cord compression: A review. J Clin Oncol 6:543, 1988

Neurology for the Non-Neurologist, Fourth Edition,
edited by William J. Weiner and
Christopher G. Goetz. Lippincott
Williams & Wilkins, Philadelphia © 1999.

CHAPTER 21

Neurologic Evaluation of Low Back Pain

Russell H. Glantz

The purpose of this chapter is to distinguish non-neurologic from neurologic causes of back pain. The physician must frequently determine whether back pain from disease of the spine and its surrounding structures has involved the nervous system by spinal cord or spinal root compression. Neurologic involvement has specific prognostic and management implications.

The most common form of back pain is *spondylogenic*. This pain originates in the vertebral spinal column and associated soft-tissue structures. These soft tissues are most frequently incriminated in the causes of back pain and include diseases of the associated tendons, muscles, joints, and, most importantly, intervertebral discs.

Vascular back pain may result from abdominal aneurysms and is often a deep-seated, boring lumbar pain. In addition, vascular insufficiency of the superior gluteal artery may give rise to buttock pain of a claudicant nature. These symptoms may even radiate down the leg. The pain of vascular insufficiency is, however, not aggravated by other stresses on the lumbar spine, such as bending, twisting, or stooping.

Viscerogenic back pain may result from retroperitoneal tumors or diseases of the kidneys or pelvic viscera. Backache, however, is rarely the sole symptom of a visceral disease. Furthermore, this pain is neither aggravated by activity nor relieved by rest. Patients with severe visceral pain frequently writhe around to obtain relief.

Primary neurogenic pain is caused by a disease of the nervous system, which is reflected as back pain. Some causes are neurofibromas, ependymomas, astrocytomas, and other lesions within the dural contents but outside the spinal cord itself. These conditions are uncommon, however, and it is beyond the scope of this chapter to discuss the differential diagnosis of all primary neurogenic back pains. The emphasis is placed instead on accurate diagnosis of the more common causes of nerve root compression in the lumbar spine. A physician most frequently sees nerve root compression as a result of acute or chronic intervertebral disc degeneration.

ANATOMY AND PHYSIOLOGY

Each vertebra has three functional components: (1) the vertebral bodies, (2) the neural arches, and (3) the bony processes (spinous and transverse). The vertebral bodies are connected by the intervertebral discs, and the neural arches are joined by the zygapophyseal joints. The vertebral bodies are braced front and back by the anterior and posterior longitudinal ligaments (Fig. 21-1). The stability of the spine depends on two types of supporting structures: the ligamentous (passive) structures and the muscular (active) structures. Although the ligaments are strong, they alone cannot resist the enormous forces

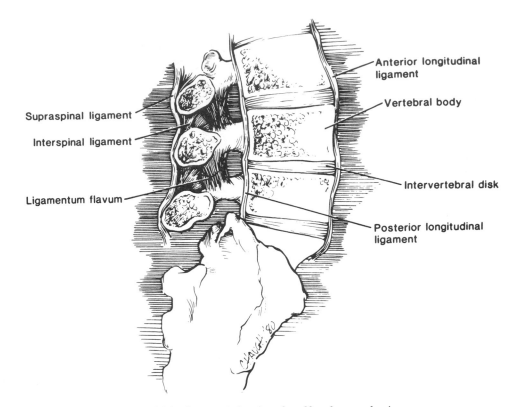

FIG. 21-1. Anatomic landmarks of lumbosacral spine.

on the spinal column. Most of the stability is dependent on the reflex contractions of the sacropinalis, abdominal, glutei, and hamstring muscles.

One of the most important anatomic features of the lumbar spine is the relationship that the neural elements bear to the bony skeleton and the intervertebral discs. The spinal cord ends at L1. From this point, all the lumbar, sacral, and coccygeal nerve roots run as distinct entities within the dural sac and exit through the lumbar, sacral, and coccygeal intervertebral foramina. The nerve roots course downward and outward. They cross the intervertebral disc and pass anterior to the superior articular facet, hugging the medial aspect of the pedicle before emerging into the intervertebral foramen. The nerve root, therefore, is vulnerable to compression by pathologic changes occurring at several points during its course down the spinal canal. The L4 root emerges between L4 and L5, in other words, *below* the vertebra that is numerically similar (Fig. 21-2). In the same way, the L5 root emerges between L5 and S1. However, in syndromes caused by

disc protrusion, an L4–L5 disc protrusion will usually compress the L5 root. This is because the more usual protrusion is posterolateral, and it catches the more medially placed downcoming root from a higher segment (Fig. 21-3). If a protrusion is far lateral, the L4 root is compressed in an L4–L5 syndrome; however, this situation is unusual. An L5–S1 protrusion generally implies an S1 root compressive syndrome. Similarly, an L3–L4 protrusion would give rise to an L4 root compressive syndrome, and an L2–L3 protrusion will cause an L3 root compressive syndrome.

The anatomy is different in the cervical region: The root emerges above the vertebra from which it takes its name. The C6 root emerges between C5 and C6; the C7 root emerges between C6 and C7; the C8 root emerges between C7 and T1 (see Fig. 21-2). The root, from this level downward, emerges below the vertebra from which it takes its name. *As a general rule,* for both cervical and lumbar compressive syndromes, the clinical lesion corresponds to the lower vertebral segment (C5–C6 = C6 syndrome, L5–S1 = S1 syndrome).

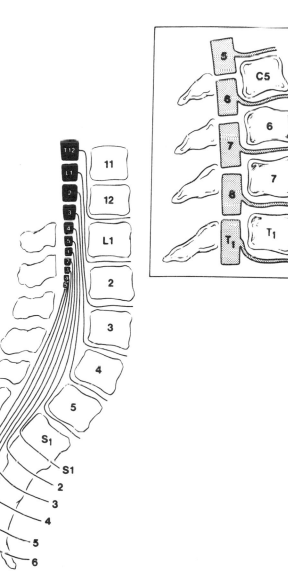

FIG. 21-2. Cervical *(upper right)* and lumbosacral *(lower left)* spine, showing the emergence of spinal roots.

DIAGNOSIS

Back pain of non-neurogenic or neurogenic origin may be (1) local, (2) referred, or (3) radicular (or root). Once a diagnosis is made in terms of these simple guidelines, the physician may focus on the differentiation between non-neurogenic causes (e.g., spondylogenic, viscerogenic, or vascular) and neurogenic causes.

Local pain is caused by any pathologic process that irritates sensory endings in the back. The fact that nerve endings are irritated does not necessarily mean that the cause is primarily neurogenic. The final expression of any pain, whatever the cause, has to be through nerve endings. Local pain may be due to the involvement of bone, muscle, ligaments, or periosteum. The pain is usually steady; it may be sharp or dull; and it is always felt in or near the affected part of the spine. The pain may change with a variation in

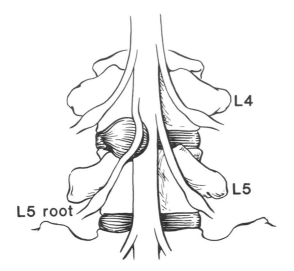

FIG. 21-3. Herniated disc at L4–L5 compressing the L5 rootlet.

position or activity. Firm tissue pressure in the region involved usually evokes tenderness and thus helps in localization. Most local pains fit generally into the spondylogenic category.

Referred pain may be projected from the spine into viscera and other structures lying within the area of the lumbar and upper sacral dermatomes. Referred pain may also be projected from the pelvic and abdominal viscera to the spine. Pain due to upper lumbar spine disease is usually referred to the anterior aspects of the thighs and legs. This pain may have to be distinguished from L3 radicular pain, which has a similar distribution. Pain from the lower lumbar spine is usually referred to the lower buttock; it is caused by an irritation of lower spinal nerves that activate the same pool of neurons that also serve the posterior thighs and calves. The referred pain often parallels in intensity the local pain in the back, thus maneuvers that alter local pain have a similar affect on referred pain. This is not the case with lancinating radicular pain, which may shoot suddenly and may be unassociated with a maneuver that causes aggravation of local pain. Furthermore, referred pain is rarely felt below the knees, whereas pain due to root irritation may spread into the calf or even the foot.

Radicular or root pain relates to an irritation or damage of neural structures by primary neurologic diseases or non-neurologic disease (e.g., discs) and hence must be specifically distinguished from local or referred pain. The misdiagnosis of local or referred pain as radicular pain often results in unnecessary investigations and unwarranted treatment. Root pain has some of the characteristics of referred pain but differs in its greater intensity, distal radiation, circumscription to the territory of a root, and, very importantly, the factors that induce it. Typically, any maneuver that raises the pressure of the spinal fluid (with secondary pressure on nerve roots) usually aggravates radicular pain. Hence, coughing, sneezing, and straining at stool characteristically evoke this sharp radiating pain.

Most root pain is the result of nerve root compression by a herniated intervertebral disc. True neurologic causes of the same syndrome include neurofibromas, ependymomas, and cysts, and these may give rise to similar symptoms and signs. Furthermore, the root entrapment may be bony in etiology, as in spinal stenosis, but here the problem is asymmetrical and bilateral.

The symptoms of nerve root compression may present in three ways: (1) backache only, (2) pain resulting from radiation only (sciatica), or (3) pain and backache together. The onset is frequently dramatic in the fully developed syndrome. There is a severe knife-like pain that is aggravated by any movement or Valsalva maneuver (e.g., sneezing or coughing). Most patients lie still in bed with legs flexed at the knees and hips. Some patients find a lateral decubitus position more comfortable. Not infrequently, patients will contort themselves into strange postures to alleviate their pain. A sitting position is frequently painful. Some patients with nerve root tumors, simulating radicular disc compression symptoms, find relief by walking around.

When examined, the patient's posture is characteristic. The lumbar spine is flattened and slightly flexed. The patient usually leans toward the side of his pain, and this action becomes more obvious when he is trying to bend forward. Symptoms may be improved by standing with the hip and knee slightly flexed and with the forced scoliosis to the sound side. This posturing diminishes any stretch on the sciatic nerve. Pain may be typically provoked by pressure over the involved vertebral spines and along the course of the sciatic nerve (sciatic notch, retrotrochanteric gutter, posterior surface of thigh, head of fibula). Pressure at one point may cause pain and tingling to radiate down the leg. It would be unusual not to find local vertebral spine pain when direct pressure is applied in a disc syndrome. Its lack, or the presence of symptoms with more lateral pressure, should cast some doubt on the diagnosis.

On further assessment of the degree of root involvement, it is important to test specifically for root tension. The two most useful tests are the straight-leg-raising and bowstring signs (Figs. 21-4, 21-5). The patient should be lying on a flat surface and the leg should be raised slowly. The knee must be fully extended. If the test is positive, pain will be produced in the back or the leg. Pain in the popliteal fossa produced by simple stretching of the legs does not signify a positive test. Two additional maneuvers add significance to straight-leg raising: (1) aggravation of pain by forced dorsiflexion of the ankle at the limit of straight-leg raising, and (2) relief of pain by knee flexion. Sciatic pain is almost always relieved by flexing the knee. The bowstring sign can be another important indication of root compression. The straight-leg-raising test is carried out to the point at which the patient experiences some discomfort. At this level, the knees are allowed to flex and the examiner allows the patient's foot to rest on his shoulder. The test demands sudden firm pressure applied to the popliteal nerve behind the knee. The reproduction of pain in the leg or in the back is irrefutable evidence of nerve root compression. As in the case of straight-leg raising, local popliteal fossa pain does not indicate a positive result. These maneuvers aim to diagnose radicular pain but do not distinguish the specific causes of such pain (e.g., disc or tumors).

Lesions of the fifth lumbar and first sacral roots are the most common. The former lesions usually give symptoms of pain in the hip, groin, posterior lateral thigh, lateral calf, and dorsum of the foot including the first to third toes. Paresthesias in this distribution may be of great diagnostic aid. There may be a weakness of dorsiflexion of the foot and great toe. The extensor hallucis (great toe extensor) is a powerful muscle and should not be overcome even in a slightly built or generally weakened patient. A weakness in this muscle is, therefore, very significant in the diagnosis of an L5 lesion. No reflex change will be present, the knee and ankle jerks being subserved by L2–L4 and S1, respectively.

Lesions of the first sacral root give rise to pain in the midgluteal region, the posterior thigh, the posterior calf to the heel, and the sole of the foot extending over to the dorsum and involving the fourth and fifth toes. Weakness, if present, involves the flexors of the foot and toes, the abductors of the toes, and the hamstring muscles. The ankle reflex is invariably decreased or lacking, and this finding forms an important diagnostic criterion in S1 root compression.

Symptoms of nerve root compression may be confined to back pain. In patients who have recurrent episodes, the presentations may be difficult on each

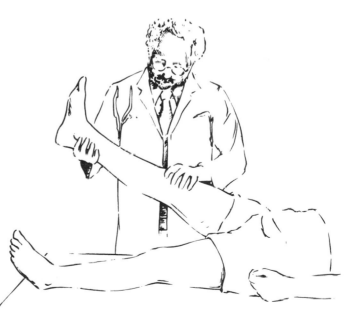

FIG. 21-4. Straight-leg-raising sign. Note that the examiner maintains the knee in the extended position.

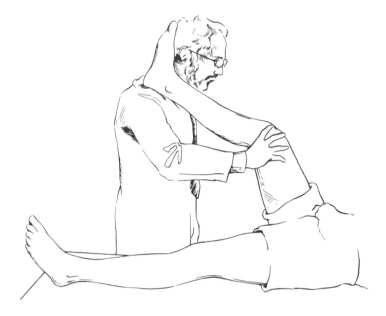

FIG. 21-5. The bowstring sign.

occasion. For example, the patient may initially present with the complete syndrome, and subsequently, with back pain only. The physician, therefore, must take an accurate history when trying to formulate the anatomy of any particular pain complex. Root entrapment due to disc protrusion has been mentioned. It is certainly the most common and frequently the most dramatic type of pain. Chronic lumbar spondylosis (which is more insidious than disc degeneration) and osseous overgrowth may also cause nerve entrapment. Pain due to these latter causes is usually chronic and has a local and referred component. Typical back and radicular pain are lacking. There may, however, be appropriate neurologic signs (e.g., loss of ankle reflex) indicating nerve root dysfunction.

SPECIAL DIAGNOSTIC INVESTIGATIONS

SPINAL RADIOGRAPHY

Spine x-ray films will not diagnose disc disease, but they are still useful in the initial workup of all acute and chronic low back pain syndromes. This noninvasive test may reveal a tumor deposit, marked osteophytosis, or even inherent bony anomalies such as lumbarization or sacralization.

MAGNETIC RESONANCE IMAGING, COMPUTED TOMOGRAPHY, AND MYELOGRAPHY

Magnetic resonance imaging (MRI) is the imaging technique of choice in the evaluation of low back disorders when the clinical situation or plain x-ray films suggest the need for further evaluation. MRI is particularly good at producing a detailed picture of soft tissues, and it is an excellent way to visualize the state of the intervertebral disc (Fig. 21-6). The computed tomography (CT) scan is also a powerful tool in the diagnosis of low back disease. Unlike MRI, which does not involve ionizing radiation, the CT scan involves significant radiographic exposure. However, the CT scan gives information not only about the state of the disc but also about bony structures (Figs. 21-7, 21-8).

Magnetic resonance imaging is useful for diagnosis not only of lumbar disc herniation, but also of spinal tumors, spinal trauma, and sometimes even failed low back surgery because the paramagnetic contrast medium gadolinium produces images that can distinguish between scar and disc. In cases of suspected spinal stenosis, MRI imaging is still an excellent tool, but CT may be preferred because of its ability to evaluate bony abnormality to a greater degree.

The role of myelography (Fig. 21-9) has changed since the advent of MRI and CT scanning. Even

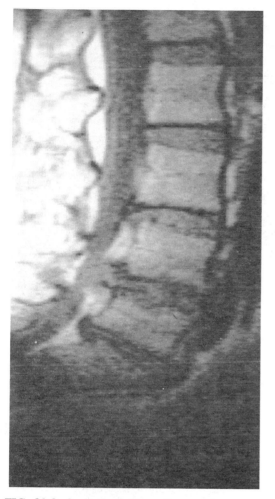

FIG. 21-6. Sagittal spinal cord magnetic resonance imaging showing evidence of extruded disc material between L4 and L5.

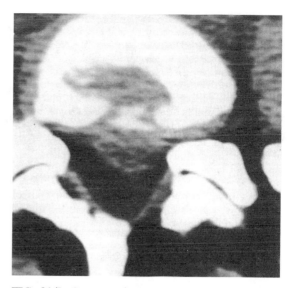

FIG. 21-7. Computed tomography scan of the lumbar spine showing prominent disc protrusion into the spinal canal.

though water-soluble dyes are now used in the performance of myelography, it is not a benign procedure: Complications occur in 10% to 20% of patients undergoing this examination, used to identify the cause of headache and, more rarely, seizures. Myelography is used today in situations where the MRI or CT scan give an equivocal result. When the myelogram is followed by a CT scan, smaller, previously missed lesions may be visualized.

ELECTROMYOGRAPHY

Electromyography (EMG) is the only test that may reveal functional impairment. The aim of this test is to localize the level of root or nerve involvement and also to help distinguish nerve damage from non-neurogenic disease, which may be the source of back pain. A normal muscle is silent at rest, but a denervated muscle gives rise to involuntary electrical discharges. These discharges take the form of fibrillation potentials or altered wave forms (positive waves). On voluntary contraction of a normal muscle, the motor unit potentials are biphasic or triphasic in form. With partial denervation, the quantity of motor units recorded is diminished and polyphasic potentials are seen (see Chapters 2 and 13).

The paraspinal muscles are supplied by the posterior primary rami of the emerging lumbosacral roots. No electrical activity is seen in the paraspinal muscles in a normal person who is completely relaxed. The physician may sample the high lumbar, mid lumbar, and low lumbar areas, thereby gaining a fairly accurate localization of proximal nerve damage. These findings can be corroborated with the results of needle studies on other muscles. For example, the gluteus medius and tibialis posterior muscles are almost purely innervated

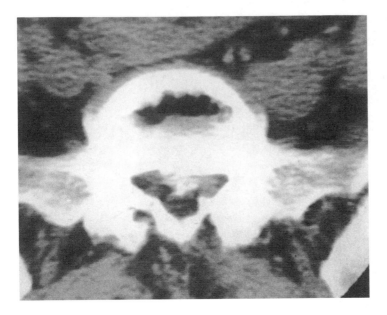

FIG. 21-8. Computed tomography evaluation of lumbar spine showing a markedly narrowed spinal canal as a result of protrusion of disc material as well as encroachment by bony hypertrophy and spurring. The vacuum disc phenomenon caused by disc degeneration is noted in the *upper half* of the picture.

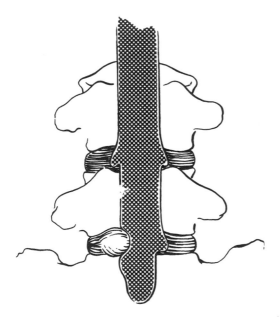

FIG. 21-9. Diagram depicting myelographic sign of indentation from extradural defect (*speckled area* represents dye column).

by L5. Conversely, the soleus muscle has almost a pure S1 innervation; therefore, finding denervation in the gluteus medius, tibialis posterior, and low lumbar paraspinals without soleus denervation is strong evidence for L5 denervation. Similar inferences can be made with S1, L3, L4, and so forth.

The H reflex is a subtle electrical test of S1 function. The physician stimulates the afferent limb of S1 in the popliteal fossa and measures the time it takes to travel up the dorsal root, through the reflex arc, and back down the lower limb, eventually producing a contraction of the gastrocnemius. This is equivalent to the ankle jerk, except that the stretching of the Achilles tendon is bypassed. The H reflex may elicit minor degrees of S1 root involvement before clear evidence of motor, reflex, and sensory dysfunction is clinically seen.

The EMG may also reveal root lesions at many levels, such as may be seen in lumbar spondylosis and stenosis with multilevel nerve root encroachment.

OTHER DIAGNOSTIC TECHNIQUES

Other techniques can be used in special cases when the previously mentioned procedures have not led to a satisfactory diagnosis. Discography combined with CT provides "disco-CT," which may demonstrate disruption of the disc and tracking of the dye toward the side of symptoms. Functional testing with somatosensory evoked responses has also been used in the evaluation of lower back pain. Although this type of testing has become fairly widely used for the diagnosis of spinal cord lesions, there is controversy as to whether these tests are more or less sensitive than EMG in diagnosing radiculopathies. When their results are clearly abnormal, these tests may be the only way of documenting a purely sensory radiculopathy; in those instances, they may be better than EMG. Overall, however, EMG is the preferred test to evaluate suspected radiculopathy.

TREATMENT

The treatment of low back pain varies widely according to the severity of the syndrome. The initial treatment, at least, of back pain from any cause is rest, whether the cause of pain is ligamentous, tendinous, muscular, or discal problems. However, when the neurologist examines a patient with nerve root compression that is probably caused by a disc protrusion, the question is always whether to use conservative or operative therapy. The decision depends on the history and physical examination. There are only three absolute indications for laminectomy: (1) marked muscular weakness pertaining to a nerve root or roots, (2) progressive neurologic deficit despite absolute bed rest, and (3) bladder or bowel dysfunction. The relative indications for operative intervention are (1) pain unrelieved by complete bed rest, and (2) recurrent episodes of severe pain and sciatica.

The hallmark of conservative management is complete bed rest. Traction is indicated only if severe pain persists despite 48 hours of bed rest and analgesia. If after 48 hours, the patient is comfortable, he may then carefully get up to use the toilet. In many instances, the bed rest can be carried out at the patient's home, where he is comfortable and in familiar surroundings. If, however, adequate home facilities are lacking, the patient should be admitted to the hospital. The patient should lie on a firm mattress if available. A bed board is unnecessary and, in some instances, may even increase the level of discomfort that the patient experiences. While in bed, the patient should be placed in a position such that the hips and knees are flexed to a moderate and comfortable degree. The amount of bed rest recommended varies, but most physicians require the patient to spend 1 to 2 weeks in bed, with 4 weeks being the maximum amount of time. Patients previously received 6 weeks of bed rest. However, today such a length of time spent in bed may be financially disastrous, especially since there is no guarantee of recovery.

The intelligent use of drug therapy is an important adjunct during the period of conservative therapy. Because diminution of inflammation around the degenerated disc is the primary aim of therapy, an anti-inflammatory drug should be used. There are many classes of nonsteroidal anti-inflammatory drugs currently available, and no one drug has been clearly shown to be better than another with respect to treatment of low back pain. During the weeks of therapy, the stomach should be coated with food or milk to prevent gastric irritation. Some patients who fail to respond to these drugs may obtain dramatic relief from a short course of systemic steroids.

If there is a prominent amount of paravertebral muscle spasm, which may be present especially in the acute phase, a muscle relaxant may be therapeutically effective. A drug such as cyclobenzaprine hydrochloride (Flexeril) may be tried.

Although the anti-inflammatory drugs also have an analgesic action, this latter effect might not be sufficient, and additional pure analgesia might be required, especially in patients with severe pain. Narcotics should be used only if the symptoms are extreme. The use of non-narcotic analgesia is preferable.

In the subacute phase of the disease, as the patient is recovering and his pain is disappearing, lumbar flexion exercises should be started. The overall aim of these exercises is to reduce the lumbar lordosis and strengthen the lumbosacral area of the spine. In practice, they should not be started sooner than about 3 weeks after the initiation of conservative therapy. The exercises should be started gently and should be discontinued immediately if a flare-up of symptoms appears.

If the response to conservative treatment is not adequate, and surgery is not contemplated at that time, lumbar epidural steroid injections are used. This has become a popular method of treatment and involves up to three injections given over a period of weeks.

QUESTIONS AND DISCUSSION

Answer *true* or *false* to each of the following statements.

1. The most common cause of low back pain is nerve root compression from disc protrusion.

The answer is *false*. The most common cause of low back pain is spondylogenic: This includes bone, muscle, tendon, and disc abnormalities. Thus, although disc abnormalities are frequent, secondary nerve root compression is less common. The neurologist, however, is frequently consulted about whether nerve compression exists or not.

2. The L1 nerve root emerges between L1 and L2.

The answer is *true*. The nerve root exists below the vertebra from which it takes its name in the thoracic, lumbar, and sacral regions. In the cervical region, the root emerges *above* the vertebra with which it is associated numerically. For example, the C2 root emerges between C1 and C2. However, disc lesions that compress roots clinically follow the lower vertebrae for both cervical and lumbar areas.

3. Tingling or numbness on the lateral aspect of the leg extending to the great toe signifies an S1 root lesion.

The answer is *false*. This sensory distribution strongly suggests an L5 lesion. Supportive evidence would be weakness of the great toe extensor. An S1 lesion usually causes numbness of the posterior calf and sole and also a diminution of the ankle jerk.

4. The H reflex is an electrically obtained equivalent of the ankle reflex.

The answer is *true*. The H reflex tests the same reflex as the ankle jerk. However, stimulation of the Achilles tendon is bypassed in this case. When ankle reflex diminution is equivocal, the prolongation of the electrical H reflex may be useful, especially in the diagnosis of S1 root lesions.

5. In a patient with clinical symptoms and signs of nerve root compression unresponsive to conservative therapy, MRI is the radiologic investigation of choice for further evaluation.

The answer is *true*. MRI is the preferred imaging technique and is best for evaluation of a protruded disc.

SUGGESTED READING

Adams RD, Victor M, Ropper A: Principles of Neurology, 6th Edition. New York, McGraw-Hill, 1997

Boden SD, Lee RR, Herzog RJ: Magnetic resonance imaging of the spine. In: Frymoyer JW (ed): The Adult Spine: Principles and Practice, 3rd ed. New York, Lippincott-Raven, 1997

Glantz RH, Haldeman S: Other diagnostic studies: Electrodiagnosis. In: Frymoyer JW (ed): The Adult Spine: Principles and Practice, 3rd Edition. New York, Lippincott-Raven, 1997

Zinreich S, Heithoff KB, Herzog RJ: Computed tomography of the spine. In: Frymoyer JW (ed): The Adult Spine: Principles and Practice, 3rd Edition. New York, Lippincott-Raven, 1997

Neurology for the Non-Neurologist, Fourth Edition,
edited by William J. Weiner and
Christopher G. Goetz. Lippincott
Williams & Wilkins, Philadelphia © 1999.

C H A P T E R 2 2

Sleep Disorders

Ružica Kovačević-Ristanović

Sleep is a subject that has fascinated physicians
and the public since antiquity. A search for a "sleep
center" in the brain has demonstrated the complexity of the sleep process, the multiplicity of structures
involved in sleep, and the reciprocal interactions
necessary for the initiation and maintenance of this
behavior.

The structures found to facilitate sleep are the
basal forebrain (i.e., the preoptic area of the hypothalamus), the area surrounding the solitary tract in
the medulla, the dorsal raphe nuclei, and the midline thalamus. It has been proposed that the sleep
promoting role of the anterior hypothalamus results
from its inhibitory action on the posterior hypothalamic awakening neurons (probably tuberoinfundi-
bular histaminergic neurons projecting widely to the
cortex). Structures found to facilitate waking are the
ascending reticular activating system of the pons, and
the midbrain and posterior hypothalamus. The functions of these structures appear to be modulated by
serotonin, catecholamines, acetylcholine, and other
neurotransmitters. Two antagonistic systems, aminergic and cholinergic, are suggested by Hobson and
McCarley to be involved in the control of alternating
sleep stages. The aminergic and cholinergic systems
are also involved in the process of cortical activation
of arousal. The discovery of the involvement of different neurotransmitters in different stages of sleep
has raised the possibility of more specific treatments
of sleep disorders. The important clinical, diagnostic,
and therapeutic features of some sleep disorders are

described in this chapter. Useful guidelines for diagnosis and therapy are also presented, although there
are few universally accepted treatments for common
sleep complaints.

SLEEP ARCHITECTURE

Since the workup of many patients with sleep disorders involves the use of a sleep laboratory, it is important to understand the tests available and the parameters measured. A portion of the sleep recording,
referred to as a polysomnogram (PSMG) of a normal
subject, is shown in Figure 22-1. Three basic parameters are needed to define the stage of sleep: an
electroencephalogram (EEG), an electrooculogram
(EOG), and an electromyogram (EMG). The normal
EEG of an alert, resting subject with closed eyes shows
an 8- to 12-Hz posterior activity known as alpha. Two
major sleep stages are distinguished: nonrapid eye
movement (NREM) and rapid eye movement (REM)
sleep. Electroencephalographically, NREM sleep is
composed of four stages: Stage 1 sleep is the stage of
NREM sleep that directly follows the awake state. An
EEG shows a low-voltage tracing of mixed frequencies
predominantly in the theta band with alpha activity
less than 50%, vertex sharp activity, and slow eye
movements. Stage 2 sleep is the stage of NREM sleep
that is characterized by the presence of sleep spindles
(12 to 14 Hz) and K-complexes against a relatively low-

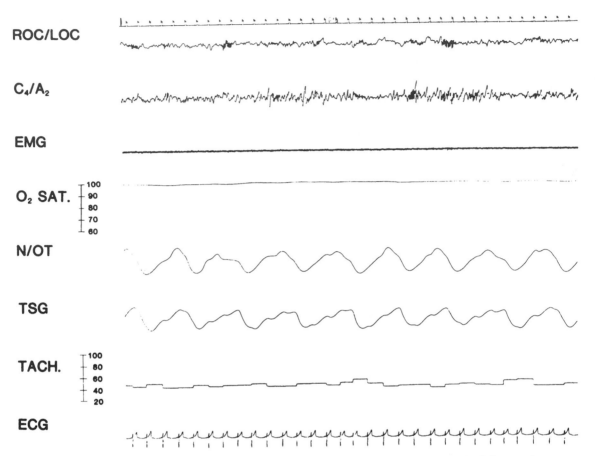

FIG. 22-1. A typical eight-channel polysomnogram recorded from a normal adult man in Stage 2 of NREM sleep. Electro-oculogram (ROC/LOC) recorded from right outer canthus referred to left outer canthus; electroencephalogram (EEG) (C_4/A_2) recorded from the right central lead referred to the right mastoid; electromyogram (EMG) recorded from the submental musculature; arterial oxygen saturation (O_2SAT) transduced by an ear oximeter; nasal and oral airflow (N/OT) recorded by a thermocouple mounted in a plastic respiratory mask; thoracic movement (TSG) recorded by a strain gauge; heart rate recorded by a cardio-tachometer; electrocardiogram (ECG) recorded from V_5 referred to the left mastoid.

voltage, mixed-frequency background. High-voltage delta waves may constitute up to 20% of Stage 2 sleep. In Stage 3 of NREM sleep, at least 20% but not more than 50% of the period consists of EEG waves less than 2 Hz; if more than 50% of the period contains such slow waves, the stage is Stage 4 NREM sleep. Both Stages 3 and 4 are often combined into a Stage Delta NREM sleep because of the lack of documented physiologic differences between the two

stages. This sleep usually appears only in the first third of the sleep period (Fig. 22-2).

Rapid-eye-movement sleep alternates with the NREM sleep at about 90-minute intervals in adults and 60-minute intervals in infants. The EEG pattern during REM sleep resembles Stage 1 sleep but is accompanied by rapid eye movements. In addition, EMG activity is low. There is a general activation of the autonomic system, with a higher average respi-

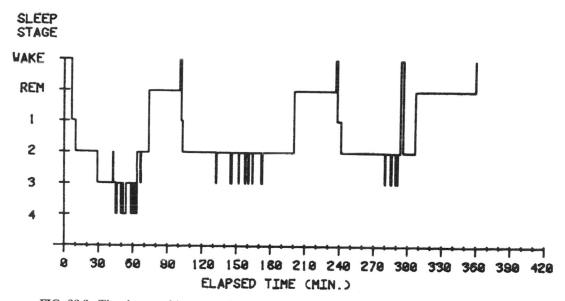

FIG. 22-2. The sleep architecture of a normal adult man. The progression of EEG stages of sleep demonstrates a concentration of Stages 3 and 4 within the first half of the sleep period. Episodes of REM sleep occur at approximately 90-min intervals, and the majority of REM appears within the latter half of the sleep period. Waking arousals are few.

ratory rate, heart rate, and blood pressure, and, more importantly, much more pronounced variability throughout the REM period. In about 80% of awakenings from REM sleep, people recall vivid dreams, compared to only 5% of awakenings from NREM sleep. However, in about 60% to 80% of awakenings from NREM sleep, people may recall thoughtlike fragments. Population studies have shown that the percentage of time spent in each stage varies with age and sex. Figures 22-1 and 22-2 represent a sleep PSMG and architecture plot from a normal adult.

NEUROCHEMICAL ASPECTS OF SLEEP

Understanding the neurochemistry of sleep is important for practical reasons. Perhaps better sleep-promoting and sleep-inhibiting compounds can be synthesized if the systems on which these drugs act are defined. Most current treatments for sleep disorders do not relate to the known neurochemical substrates for sleep. Even more important, the myr-

iad effects on sleep of currently used medications (both those used to alter sleep and those employed for an unrelated purpose) should be understood. Although serotonin was postulated to represent the transmitter governing NREM sleep, it appears that a complex interaction of serotonin, catecholamines, and acetylcholine is necessary for a modulation of the sleep–wake cycle. Noradrenergic, histaminergic, and serotonergic neurons, which are active during the waking state, are virtually silent during REM sleep, when most other neurons are highly active. It has been accepted that the activation of forebrain structures during REM sleep is generated and transferred rostrally by brainstem cholinergic nuclei, and that the shut-off of dorsal raphe serotonergic neurons is one of the major factors underlying the disinhibition of these cholinergic nuclei. In addition, long-acting hormones or peptides have been isolated in some species and have been considered to represent a "hypnogenic factor." The presence of vasoactive intestinal peptide in the suprachiasmatic nucleus was considered to imply its role in the control of circadian rhythmicity. The effects of these hormones and peptides on humans have not yet been defined.

SLEEP ABNORMALITIES

The new International Classification of Sleep Disorders divides the primary sleep disorders into (1) the *dyssomnias,* or disorders that produce a complaint of either insomnia or excessive daytime sleepiness, and (2) the *parasomnias,* or disorders that intrude or occur during sleep but do not produce a primary complaint of insomnia or excessive daytime sleepiness. The dyssomnias are further subdivided into *extrinsic, intrinsic,* and *circadian sleep disorders.* Thus, the causes of insomnia and hypersomnolence may be either within the body (intrinsic) or outside the body (extrinsic). These definitions of both types of primary sleep disorders differ from the medical–psychiatric definitions of sleep disorders. Future advances in understanding of the pathophysiology of sleep disorders will result in improved classification along the lines of pathology.

INSOMNIA

Insomnia is a perception of inadequate, disturbed, insufficient, or nonrestorative sleep despite an adequate opportunity to sleep, accompanied by daytime consequences of inadequate sleep. A recent Gallup phone survey found that 36% of Americans suffer from some type of sleep disorder. Occasional insomnia was reported by 27% of respondents, and chronic insomnia by 9%.

The intrinsic sleep disorders include disturbances such as psychophysiologic insomnia, sleep-state misperception, restless legs syndrome, and idiopathic insomnia, all of which produce the complaint of insomnia. Similarly, many extrinsic sleep disorders, such as inadequate sleep hygiene, environmental sleep disorder, altitude insomnia, adjustment sleep disorder, limit-setting sleep disorder, food allergy insomnia, hypnotic-dependent sleep disorder, and alcohol-dependent sleep disorder, are likely to be accompanied by insomnia. Among circadian rhythm sleep disorders, delayed sleep-phase syndrome is associated with a complaint of sleep-onset delay, while advanced sleep-phase syndrome is accompanied by a complaint of an early awakening. In general, the pattern of insomnia may be primarily (1) difficulty falling asleep (sleep-onset delay), (2) early morning arousal (premature awakening with inability to fall asleep again), or (3) sleep fragmentation (repeated awakenings).

Insomnias can be transient (lasting less than 3 to 4 weeks) or chronic (lasting longer than that). Multiple factors can trigger transient insomnia, including life stress, brief illness, rapid change of time zones, drug withdrawal, use of central nervous system (CNS) stimulants, and pain. Transient insomnia is experienced by everyone, and recovery is usually rapid.

Chronic insomnia may be lifelong. It is usually related to chronic psychophysiologic arousal, psychiatric disorders, use of drugs and alcohol, and other medical, toxic, and environmental conditions. However, it may also represent a primary sleep disorder in the form of sleep apnea syndrome, alveolar hypoventilation syndrome, sleep-related (nocturnal) periodic limb movements, and "restless legs."

SLEEP-ONSET DELAY

Sleep-onset delay is a common problem and probably accounts for most patients who present with a complaint of insomnia. It usually has psychogenic causes. Sleeplessness may develop from a continued association with stimulating practices and objects at bedtime. Such patients sleep better away from their bedrooms and usual routines. A conditioned internal factor may also develop in the form of apprehension about unsuccessful and excessive efforts to sleep. Conscious efforts to fall asleep result in CNS arousal. These patients consider themselves "light sleepers." They often have multiple somatic complaints such as back pains, headaches, and palpitations that lead to occasional abuse of alcohol, barbiturates, and minor tranquilizers. The sleep of such patients in the sleep laboratory is usually good, because the conditioning factors that are active at home are reduced in the laboratory. Multiple specific psychiatric illnesses associated with anxiety, such as personality disorders (e.g., anxiety and panic disorders, hypochondriasis, obsessive–compulsive disorders), and schizophrenia can also be associated with sleep-onset difficulty.

Drugs can also compromise the initiation of sleep. When obtaining a history, the physician should inquire specifically about possible precipitants of drug-induced insomnia. In addition to steroids and dopaminergic agents, xanthine derivatives (e.g., caffeine and theophylline) may cause sleep disruption. A frequently overlooked class of agents is the beta-adrenergic agonists, such as terbutaline and phenylethylamine derivatives (used as stimulants, appetite suppressants, and decongestants). If such medications are taken late in the day, and in increasing amounts because of the development of tolerance, they can easily cause sleep-onset delay, as well as sleep fragmentation and "lightening" of sleep. Such inadequate sleep provokes daytime symptoms such as sleepiness, which is responsible for a further increase of ingestion of the drug in order to promote alertness.

In addition to the psychological and drug causes of sleep-onset delay, patients who have a disturbed circadian rhythm may have the same sleep complaint. In delayed sleep-phase syndrome, patients naturally fall asleep at 2 or 3 AM, or later: They cannot fall asleep if they go to bed at conventional times. If they must get up for a job or school at 6 AM, they will be sleepy in the morning. However, they have no trouble going to sleep and getting full rest if they can go to bed late and sleep until mid day. A change in lifestyle and a course of chronotherapy at a sleep disorder center can correct this problem. Chronotherapy, an individually designed sleep schedule consisting of a gradual sleep-onset time delay until a desired time is reached, may also help patients with irregular sleep–wake patterns, who sleep for short and variable periods of time throughout the 24 hours. These people have difficulty falling asleep at conventional times because they have napped recently. Shift workers and those who travel frequently across time zones often experience sleep-onset delay (in addition to jet lag). Most patients affected by sleep-onset delay do not require drug treatment for therapy.

The treatment of chronic insomnia provides a significant challenge. The physician should first identify any underlying conditions, which may include psychiatric disorders such as depression, alcohol or substance abuse, chronic medical disorders, sleep apnea, aging, and alteration in the circadian rhythm. Treatment should then be based on concurrent problems, age, and hepatic and renal function. Pharmacologic treatment should be used judiciously and combined with nonpharmacologic treatments.

Counseling appears to play an important role in the therapy of sleep disorders. If the physician spends time talking with these patients, he may find that they are actually attempting to discuss problems that they find difficult to raise, such as impotence, marital discord, or alcoholism in a family member. The complaint may be resolved if attention is given to these problems, regardless of whether sleep behavior is actually altered.

Sleep hygiene includes setting a fixed hour for retiring each night, eliminating daytime naps, avoiding caffeine-containing beverages and anxiety-producing activities at night, and ensuring that the bedroom is quiet, dark, and comfortable. Because patients may not think of over-the-counter preparations as drugs, mentioning the need to avoid sympathomimetic substances may prove fruitful.

Only a few practical points concerning behavioral therapies need to be reviewed here. Techniques that attempt to increase relaxation, either through biofeedback or more conventional learning paradigms, may be valuable if they are aimed at a specific physiologic disturbance. For example, a patient whose PSMG indicates a large amount of muscle activity prior to falling asleep might benefit from EMG biofeedback. These techniques will generally require the facilities of a sleep laboratory. Attempts at operant and classic conditioning as aids in treating insomnia have also had some limited success. A widely accepted behavioral modification technique (stimulus control) is especially useful in correcting maladaptive association of arousal with bedtime routine. Other techniques aimed at reducing tension include progressive muscular relaxation and autogenic training.

Sleep restriction relies on restricting time spent in bed to the estimated sleep time the patient accumulates during the night, as documented by sleep logs, and then gradually increasing it until an optimal sleep time is achieved. This treatment is based on the observation that insomniacs spend too much time in bed in an attempt to obtain more sleep. Reduction of time spent in bed leads to a state of mild sleep deprivation, which is likely to result in faster sleep onset, improved sleep continuity, and deeper sleep.

Cognitive therapy focuses on maladaptive thoughts that produce an emotional arousal, such as unrealistic expectations about sleep requirements, negative consequences of insomnia, and misattributions of daytime difficulties to poor sleep.

Sleep-promoting medications can be used in the management of insomnia; however, their use must be considered carefully. These medications are most helpful when their use is self-limited, such as during acute hospitalization or as part of a more comprehensive program of sleep hygiene. In the latter case, they may allow the physician time to explore the roots of the sleep disturbance more thoroughly.

The choice of a sedative agent is dictated primarily by the duration of clinical sedation; ideally, the hypnosedative effect should cease by the time the patient arises. An effective hypnotic drug should decrease sleep latency and increase the total sleep time. The value of a hypnotic depends on the balance of its efficacy and side effects. The efficacy is defined by its ability to induce and maintain sleep, and it directly depends on the drug's dose, absorption, and duration of action. Thus, an efficacious hypnotic is rapidly absorbed and has duration of action consistent with the sleep period (usually around 8 hours). Ideally, such a hypnotic has no adverse effects. However, hypnotics with a duration of action that exceeds the sleep period usually lead to residual sedation during daytime. In contrast, use of short-acting hypnotics in doses higher than required is often associated with major adverse effects such as rebound insomnia and anterograde amnesia. Dependence is also an undesirable possibility with the use of hypnotics. This possibility can be minimized by the intermittent use of low doses, together with limited duration of drug intake and gradual withdrawal if treatment has been continuous for more than a month. The available drugs have a surprisingly heterogeneous set of effects on sleep architecture.

Although almost all agents employed as hypnosedatives will suppress REM sleep when given in sufficiently large quantities, two patterns of effects are seen at lower doses. Barbiturates, chloral hydrate, anticholinergics, tricyclics, and ethanol demonstrate REM suppression, whereas most benzodiazepines decrease Stages 3 and 4. They all appear to decrease sleep latency and reduce the number of spontaneous awakenings. Although the drugs that have the least effect on sleep architecture may offer a theoretical advantage in the therapy of insomnia, there is no clear demonstration that they induce "better" sleep.

Data on commonly used sleep-promoting medications and some miscellaneous agents are summarized in Table 22-1. Sleep latency is decreased, except where indicated. There is seldom a reason to use more than a single agent in the treatment of insomnia. A failure to obtain an adequate response on the first night does not imply a need to increase the

TABLE 22-1. Commonly Available Hypnosedative Drugs

MEDICATION	DOSAGE*	EFFECTS ON SLEEP ARCHITECTURE
Barbiturates		
Amobarbital	200 mg	Decreases REM; increases REM latency
Heptobarbital	400 mg	Decreases REM
Pentobarbital	100 mg	Decreases REM; increases REM latency
Phenobarbital	100 mg	Decreases REM
Secobarbital	100 mg	Decreases REM
Amobarbital and secobarbital (Tuinal)	—	Decreases REM
Ethanol	100 ml	Decreases REM, first half of night
	200 ml	Decreases REM, entire night
Benzodiazepines		
Chlordiazepoxide	50 mg	Decreases Stage 4
Diazepam	10 mg	Decreases Stage 4
Flurazepam	15 mg	Slight decrease REM and Stages 2 and 4
	30 mg	Slight decrease Stages 3 and 4
Lorazepam	2 mg	Decreases REM
Oxazepam	10 mg	Increases REM
Triazolam	0.1–1 mg	Decrease REM
Tricyclics		
Amitriptyline	50 mg	Increases Stage 4; decreases REM
Desipramine	50 mg	Increases Stage 4; decreases REM
Doxepin	25 mg	Increases Stage 4; decreases REM
Imipramine	50 mg	Increases Stage 4; decreases REM
Nortriptyline	25 mg	Increases Stage 4; decreases REM
Protriptyline	5 mg	Increases Stage 4; decreases REM
Miscellaneous		
Chloral hydrate	500–1500 mg	No significant effect
Diphenhydramine	50–100 mg	Decreases REM
Glutethimide	500–1000 mg	Decreases REM
Meprobamate	400–800 mg	No significant effect
Methaqualone	300 mg	No significant effect
Triclofos	1000 mg	No significant effect
Tryptophan (L- form)	1–10 g	Normal sleep architecture
	10 g	Decreases REM

* Dosages are suggestions for initial therapy only and will depend on usual factors influencing a patient's tolerance to medication.

dosage immediately; a trial of at least 2 or 3 nights is indicated. Sleep induction is related to the rate of absorption. Flurazepam is absorbed rapidly and temazepam is absorbed slowly. Sleep maintenance is related to dosage and half-life. The timing of the intake of the medications is, therefore, important. Hypnotics with longer half-lives (lasting more than 24 hours) show increased efficacy with two or three nights of administration, but they also show increased residual daytime effects. Some benzodiazepines, such as flurazepam (Dalmane), produce persistent long-acting metabolites and cause definite impairment in alertness, motor performance, and cognitive function in the morning.

When the initial therapy is unsuccessful, changing classes of medications may be useful. A barbiturate (with REM suppressant effect), for example, may be useful when a benzodiazepine fails. L-tryptophan was removed from the market because a potentially fatal condition, eosinophilia–myalgia syndrome, is presumably related to its use. Because of the intrinsic "tapering" effect of compounds with long half-lives, rebound and/or withdrawal phenomena appear to be unlikely; when they do occur, such effects are delayed in onset and are relatively mild. On the other hand, there is a much higher likelihood of rebound or withdrawal effect after abrupt discontinuation of short-half-life hypnotics, for which dose tapering is appropriate.

In the last decade, benzodiazepines have almost completely replaced barbiturates. Only five benzodiazepines are marketed for hypnotic purposes in the United States: triazolam, (Halcion), temazepam (Restoril), quazepam (Doral), flurazepam, and estazolam (Prosom). Various benzodiazepine anxiolytics [for example, diazepam (Valium), alprazolam (Xanax), lorazepam (Ativan), or oxazepam (Serax)] are also prescribed for insomnia associated with anxiety disorders. Unfortunately, there is limited evidence to support their efficacy for these disorders. The drug of choice for sleep-onset insomnia differs from that for sleep-maintenance insomnia (i.e., triazolam for the former, temazepam for the latter).

Onset of action after an oral dose depends on rapidity of absorption from the gastrointestinal tract. For instance, the capsule preparation of temazepam is very slowly absorbed, with peak concentration reached in an average of 2 to 3 hours after dosing. Duration of action of a single dose of a benzodiazepine hypnotic depends on its distribution (e.g., it may concentrate in sites such as adipose tissue, where it exerts no pharmacologic activity), and on elimination and clearance. With repeated administration at a fixed dosing rate, a drug will accumulate in plasma and brain until a steady state is reached. Time necessary to reach a steady-state condition depends only on the drug's elimination half-life. For a drug such as triazolam with a very short elimination half-life, accumulation will be complete within 1 day; that is, the mean plasma concentration will be no higher after multiple days of therapy than after the first day. At the other extreme is a drug such as flurazepam, with its principal active metabolite des-alkylflurazepam. This compound has a very long elimination half-life; 2 weeks or more of long-term treatment will be necessary for a steady state to be attained. The rate of drug disappearance following discontinuation after long-term treatment will mirror the rate of accumulation; that is, the longer the elimination half-life, the more time will be needed for the drug to disappear. A potential benefit of accumulating a benzodiazepine is that persistence of drug at the receptor sites throughout each 24-hour dosing interval increases the likelihood of a daytime anxyolitic effect, a potential benefit for patients with both anxiety and insomnia. For short half-life hypnotics such as triazolam, on the other hand, increased daytime anxiety has been reported in some studies, possibly attributable to wide fluctuations in plasma and receptor-site concentrations between doses. Pregnant women, alcoholics, and sleep apneics should *not* be given hypnotics, except in low doses and only in special circumstances. Preference for benzodiazepines over barbiturates is based on the former's lower tox-icity (less respiratory and cardiac depression) and less marked tolerance, rather than on its superior hypnotic effect. The prescribing of hypnotics to children is not recommended, except for rare use in the treatment of night terrors or severe somnambulism. Benzodiazepine metabolism varies and is largely age dependent. The elimination half-life of diazepam in healthy men may increase three- to fourfold from 20 years of age to 80 years of age. The elimination of hypnotics is decreased in elderly people who might have a low renal glomerular filtration rate, a reduced hepatic blood flow, and a decreased activity of hepatic drug-metabolizing enzymes. Benzodiazepine dosage should be halved in the elderly, and even then daytime functioning may be impaired significantly.

The choice of hypnosedatives for elderly patients with sleep-onset delay, especially when they are acutely hospitalized, is complicated by the risk of a paradoxical excitation at nighttime ("sun-downing"), which may be precipitated or exacerbated by medication. Although diphenhydramine has been useful in many of these patients, there is a risk of increasing their confusion because of its anticholinergic effect. These problems can be minimized by adjunctive measures, such as leaving a light on in the patient's room, and by frequently reorienting the patient to the unfamiliar surroundings. A family member may occasionally be required to stay with the patient.

Because of the intrinsic "tapering" effect of long-half-life compounds, rebound and withdrawal phenomena appear to be unlikely; when they do occur, such effects are delayed in onset and are relatively mild. On the other hand, there is a much higher likelihood of rebound or withdrawal effect after abrupt discontinuation of short-half-life hypnotics, so dose tapering is appropriate.

Estazolam, a relatively new benzodiazepine, remains effective as a hypnotic for at least 6 weeks of continuous administration at a dosage of 2 mg at bedtime, with no evidence of clinically significant tolerance. It improves sleep latency and total sleep time, reduces the number of nocturnal awakenings, and improves both depth of sleep and sleep quality in adults with chronic insomnia.

Zolpidem is another hypnotic, a benzodiazepine receptor ligand structurally unrelated to benzodiazepines (an omega 1-selective nonbenzodiazepine hypnotic). It has an elimination half-life of 3.5 to 5.1 hours (mean, 4 hours). In young adults, zolpidem leads to a marked increase in slow-wave sleep, with reduction of Stage 2 and no change in REM sleep. In the middle-aged, there is a reduction of awake time and increase of Stage 2 NREM sleep, without changes in REM sleep.

Zopiclone, a cyclopyrrolone compound, is another hypnotic that is chemically unrelated to benzodiazepines. Enhanced binding of gamma-aminobutyric acid (GABA) to the GABA-chloride ionophore complex occurs to a lesser extent with zopiclone than with benzodiazepines. Recently, a separate site of cyclopyrrolones on the benzodiazepine receptor complex has been identified. Zopiclone has a half-life of 5 hours and no long-acting metabolites. Its use is accompanied by an increase of NREM sleep without REM sleep reduction. Rebound phenomena have not been shown consistently. Zopiclone is not available in the United States.

Although many of these drugs, especially the benzodiazepines, have been marketed with emphasis on their short duration of action, many have long-acting active metabolites. This is often a problem in the patient who experiences a decrement in liver function. Sedative effects are additive and may convert what would have been a mild metabolic encephalopathy into a coma days after the initiation of treatment.

EARLY MORNING AWAKENING

Early morning awakening can be seen in numerous clinical settings, including depression, use of some drugs, and advanced sleep-phase syndrome. Endogenous depression is characterized by a typical premature awakening and an inability to fall asleep again, with variable sleep-onset disturbance depending on the individual's component of agitation. A key polysomnographic finding is shortened REM sleep latency, which is considered by some experts to be a biologic marker of depression, in addition to an increased intensity of REM sleep. Deep (delta) NREM sleep is also reduced; this is a relatively nonspecific feature. In contrast, bipolar depression is frequently associated with hypersomnia; however, this state is again accompanied by a shortened REM latency and reduced Stages 3 or 4 NREM sleep. The onset of sleep is delayed and sleep is short in mania and hypomania. Insomnia may precede all other symptoms of depression, and restoration of sleep may be the first sign of recovery.

In patients with early morning awakening, sedative therapy is usually accompanied by an unacceptable degree of morning sedation. Antidepressants appear to offer the best results and should be the initial form of therapy. Tricyclic antidepressants with sedative properties, such as amitriptyline (Elavil) and trimipramine (Surmontil), reduce sleep latency and improve sleep continuity. Trazodone, a nontricyclic, is also widely used for treatment of insomnia in depressed patients. Although an improvement in sleep often precedes an improvement in mood, changes of affect should determine the end point in therapy.

Drug-induced early morning awakening may occur with the use of some short-acting benzodiazepines, such as oxazepam or lorazepam. They are almost completely inactivated by a conjugation in the liver, and they have few residual morning aftereffects. Patients who drink alcoholic beverages prior to sleep may develop early morning awakening, apparently related to an increase in REM sleep ("REM rebound") after the alcohol is metabolized. An underlying psychiatric problem should be considered, as in any patient with an alcohol-related problem. Therapy involves a slow withdrawal of the causative agent.

Advanced-sleep-phase syndrome may mimic a pattern of early morning awakening typical of depression. It is seen most frequently in elderly people. There are no established treatments for this condition, although reverse chronotherapy or exposure to light in the evening accompanied by light deprivation in the morning may be helpful. Either treatment requires the skills of experts in sleep disorders centers.

SLEEP FRAGMENTATION

A major complaint of frequent awakenings at night often signals the presence of a primary sleep disorder, specifically sleep apnea or periodic limb movements. Multiple medical conditions can also interfere with sleep maintenance, whereas a psychiatric etiology is a less likely explanation.

In sleep apnea, sleep disruption is caused by cessation of breathing during apneic periods and subsequent frequent awakenings associated with occasional gasping for air or a choking sensation. In most cases, it is predominantly central sleep apnea occurring during sleep. Patients usually report daytime-"tiredness," but they do not take naps.

Periodic limb-movement disorder is a condition in which insomnia is associated with the occurrence during sleep of periodic episodes of repetitive and highly stereotypical leg jerks. These are consistently followed by a partial arousal. Patients are often unaware of the movements at night; rather, they report frequent nocturnal awakenings and unrefreshing sleep. A bed partner can usually provide accurate description of the movements. Insomnia can be also associated with the so-called restless-legs syndrome, when the patient has disagreeable deep sensations of creeping inside the calves whenever sitting or lying down, causing an almost irresistible urge to move the legs, and thus interfering with the sleep onset. Almost all patients with restless-legs syndrome also have sleep-related periodic limb movements. In some cases, restless legs and periodic limb movements are caused or exacerbated by identifiable medical problems (e.g., uremia or iron deficiency), dietary substances (e.g., caffeine), or medications (e.g., neuroleptics and tricyclic antidepressants)

Accepted and fairly successful treatments for restless and periodic limb movements include dopaminergic drugs, opioids, and some miscellaneous drugs. The dopaminergic agent carbidopa/levodopa (Sinemet) improves all of the features of both restless-legs syndrome and periodic-limb-movement disorder, including discomfort in the legs, involuntary movements during the waking state (dyskinesias while awake), periodic limb movements during sleep, and sleep fragmentation. Typical doses of carbidopa/levodopa are 25/100 to 100/400 mg, taken either in divided doses before bedtime, once only before bedtime, or occasionally during the night as well, if prolonged awakening in the middle of the night is a result of the recurrence of the restless legs. Side effects include gastrointestinal discomfort, nausea, and vomiting. The dopaminergic agonists bromocriptine (Parlodel) and pergolide (Permax) have been used successfully. Typ-

ical doses range from 5 to 15 mg for bromocriptine and from 0. 1 to 0.6 mg for pergolide, taken in divided doses before bedtime. Nasal stuffiness, gastrointestinal discomfort, and especially hypotension are adverse effects of concern. Numerous opioids have been used, such as codeine, propoxyphene (Darvon), oxycodone (Percodan), pentazocine (Talwin), levorphanol (Levo-Dromoran), and methadone. Their effectiveness has been tested formally by only a few studies. Open label trials using gabapentin (Neurontin) demonstrated subjective improvements in many patients with restless-legs syndrome. The most widely accepted and successful treatment of periodic limb movements is obtained by the use of clonazepam.

Medical conditions that sometimes lead to insomnia include alveolar hypoventilation, which in adults could be secondary to massive obesity, chronic obstructive pulmonary disease, myopathy, cordotomy, or lesions involving structures that control sleep and breathing. Primary alveolar hypoventilation is usually reported in infants and is associated with a further worsening of hypercapnia and hypoxemia in sleep. Gastro-esophageal reflux with regurgitation, heartburn and dyspepsia, nocturnal angina, sleep-related asthma, nightmares, and cluster headaches may all cause a serious insomnia due mainly to severe sleep fragmentation. Other medical and neurologic conditions can be associated with this form of insomnia, including CNS infections, head traumas, nocturnal epilepsy, fibrositis syndrome, cardiovascular disorders, pulmonary disease, any painful condition, toxic conditions, and endocrine diseases such as hyperthyroidism and Addison's disease. In these patients, treatment of the underlying disorder can be expected to alleviate the sleep disturbance and thus obviate the need for hypnotics. Hypercortisolism (especially iatrogenic) should be considered if sleep fragmentation is prominent. Parkinsonian patients receiving therapy with levodopa (or carbidopa/levodopa) are also subject to this complaint. Daytime napping is frequently reported. The response to hypnosedatives and tricyclics is unpredictable. Avoidance of dopaminergic drugs after supper is helpful for many patients. Another cause of sleep fragmentation is bruxism (teeth grinding).

SLEEP DISORDERS ASSOCIATED WITH HYPERSOMNOLENCE

Included in this category are intrinsic and extrinsic sleep disorders as well as parasomnias and disorders associated with medical/psychiatric disorders. The chief symptoms include an inappropriate and undesirable sleepiness during waking hours, decreased cognitive and motor performance, an excessive tendency to sleep, unavoidable napping, an increase in total sleep over 24 hours ("true" hypersomnia), and a difficulty in achieving full arousal on awakening. The term "hypersomnolence" in a strict sense, be reserved for patients who have a demonstrable tendency to fall asleep in the waking state when sedentary or who have sleep "attacks." There may also be diminished alertness in the waking state, described by the term *subwakefulness*. In all patients presenting with these symptoms, it is important to separate excessive daytime somnolence from less specific symptoms of fatigue, malaise, or depression.

The major causes of excessive daytime sleepiness are sleep apnea syndrome (43%), narcolepsy (25%), and insufficient sleep.

SLEEP APNEA

A potentially lethal condition, sleep apnea is an abnormal breathing pattern during sleep defined as a cessation of airflow at the level of the nostrils and the mouth, lasting for at least 10 seconds. The estimated prevalence of sleep apnea syndrome ranges from 2% to 4% of the adult population. It is the most frequent diagnosis in sleep disorder centers and the most frequent cause of daytime sleepiness. Apneas are subdivided by type:

1. Obstructive or upper airway apnea is secondary to a sleep-induced obstruction of the airway (Fig. 22-3).
2. Central or diaphragmatic apnea is secondary to decreased respiratory muscle activity.
3. Mixed apnea combines both phenomena: It usually starts as a central apnea (with no respiratory effort) and develops into an obstruction later. Either obstructive or central apnea predominates in each patient.

Obstructive sleep apnea seems to be caused by a concentric pharyngeal collapse during inspiration and not by an active musculature contraction. Contributing factors may include the following:

1. Abnormal anatomic relationships among the muscular or bony structures of the naso-, oro-, or hypopharynx (e.g., a short thick neck, macroglossia, a relatively small and *low-positioned* hyoid bone, or a narrow pharynx)
2. Inappropriate involuntary respiratory control of the pharyngeal and diaphragmatic muscle tone
3. Increased compliance of the pharyngeal walls, especially fatty or redundant pharyngeal and submucosal folds

4. The amount of inspiratory intraluminal negative pressure

Although many patients with obstructive sleep apnea are moderately overweight, morbid obesity is present only in a minority. These apneas are more prevalent with increasing age and worsen after alcohol or sedative drug intake.

Clinical symptoms usually include snoring, persistent daytime sleepiness, tiredness and fatigue, unrefreshing sleep attacks, deterioration of memory and judgment, early morning confusion, automatic behavior at times (i.e., amnestic attacks), serious morning headaches, personality changes, and a generally depressed outlook. Waking respiratory functions are usually within normal limits. Hypertension has been reported in 48% to 96% of patients with obstructive sleep apnea syndrome. Alveolar hypoventilation, associated with an elevated waking $PaCO_2$, occasionally accompanies obstructive sleep apnea. Increased $PaCO_2$ of 45 mm Hg or higher has been reported in 23% of obese patients with obstructive sleep apnea. Marked cyclic sinus arrhythmia appears during sleep and apnea. This rhythm pattern is characterized by progressive sinus bradycardia during apnea (heart rates of less than 30 beats/min are not uncommon) with an abrupt reversal and sinus acceleration at the onset of ventilation. Second-degree atrioventricular (AV) block, prolonged sinus pauses, limited runs of ventricular tachycardia, and paroxysmal atrial tachycardia episodes also occur. Furthermore, systemic and pulmonary artery pressures rise in association with obstructive apneas. About 22% to 30% of patients with systemic hypertension were found to suffer from obstructive sleep apnea. Although both conditions are also more frequent in men and obese people, the association of hypertension and obstructive sleep apnea seems to be independent of obesity. When episodes of apnea occur in rapid succession, pressures do not return to baseline but show a stepwise increase. Apneas are more prevalent with increasing age and worsen following alcohol or sedative drug intake.

Central sleep apnea is not a single disease entity but results from any one of a number of processes that produce instability of respiratory control. In contrast to patients with obstructive sleep apnea, these patients are older (i.e., their mean age is 63 as opposed to 46 years); they complain mainly of sleep fragmentation; they are not overweight; and they have less pronounced oxygen desaturation and a more moderate hemodynamic impact. There is no definite sex distribution.

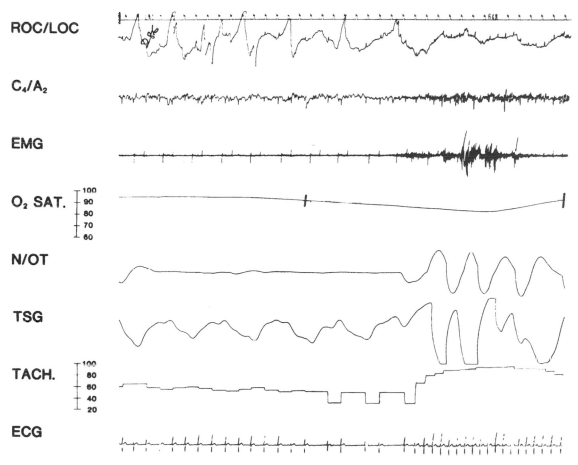

FIG. 22-3. Obstructive apnea. During the REM stage, airflow ceases for 21 sec while unsuccessful respiratory effort continues, indicating obstruction of the upper airway. Oxygen saturation falls to 81%. Immediately prior to the resumption of ventilation, the ECG demonstrates second-degree A-V block. When ventilation occurs, sinus rhythm appears in the EEG and tachycardia is evident in the ECG.

Upper airway patency does not need to be fully compromised for symptoms of daytime sleepiness to develop. The recently described upper airway resistance syndrome is accompanied by subjective and objective evidence of pathologic sleepiness. In some individuals, even a minor reduction of airway patency with sleep onset may lead to a modest increase in upper airway resistance and a slight drop of tidal volume without hypoxemia. In response to increased resistance, inspiratory muscles increase their effort to maintain normal tidal volume. This compensatory increase in respiratory effort usually triggers a brief alpha EEG arousal (3 to 14 seconds in duration), interrupting further development of obstruction before oxygen desaturation occurs. If the alpha EEG arousals are frequent, clinically significant daytime sleepiness may arise. Snoring is noted in most, but not all, of these individuals.

Both central and obstructive sleep apnea can be a complication of another medical or neurologic disorder, including brainstem infarction, lateral medullary syndrome, bulbar poliomyelitis, medullary neoplasms, syringomyelia and syringobulbia, olivopontocerebellar atrophy, Alzheimer's disease, encephalitides, Jakob–

Creutzfeldt disease, postencephalitic parkinsonism, cervical cordotomy, neuromuscular disorders affecting intercostal muscles and the diaphragm (such as myasthenia gravis), higher cervical spinal poliomyelitis, Guillain–Barré syndrome, limb–girdle dystrophies, and especially myotonic dystrophy. Hypoventilation and daytime drowsiness are prominent in all these disorders. Predominantly obstructive sleep apnea may result from enlarged tonsils (an especially important factor in the etiology of sleep apnea and snoring in children), myxedema, micrognathia and other facial and mandibular abnormalities, platybasia, neck infiltration secondary to Hodgkin's disease and lymphoma, acromegaly, and familial or acquired dysautonomia (usually mixed central and obstructive sleep apnea).

Of special interest is the development of postpolio syndrome years after the acute stage of poliomyelitis. It starts with fatigue, new muscular weakness, musculoskeletal pain, and dysphagia. During sleep, patients experience central and obstructive sleep apnea, which is worse during REM sleep because of the combined REM sleep–induced atonia and abnormal motor (phrenic) output caused by medullary dysfunction. Poliomyelitis can also cause atrophy of respiratory accessory muscles and thoracoabdominal muscles, leading to severe chest deformity such as kyphoscoliosis. Furthermore, impairment of cranial motor nerves (hypoglossal, facial, and trigeminal) may adversely affect tongue and other upper airway muscles. As a consequence, all types of apneas may occur. These patients are vulnerable to develop respiratory failure with acute respiratory infection and may require assisted ventilation in intensive care units until the infection is controlled.

The evaluation of patients suspected of having sleep apnea syndrome includes a history obtained not only from them but also (and most important) from their bed partner. A physical examination should concentrate on blood pressure, evidence of right heart failure, and abnormal skeletal and muscle configurations of the face and neck. The ear, nose, and throat examination is of primary importance. Chest radiographs and electrocardiograms are useful for evaluating pulmonary hypertension, determining the status of the right and left ventricles, and establishing possible coexistence of other cardiopulmonary disorders. A hemogram documents the presence of polycythemia. In selected patients, thyroid studies are necessary to rule out hypothyroidism. Pulmonary function studies may be necessary to investigate for primary hypoventilation during the waking state and responsiveness to CO_2 stimulation. These studies should be followed by an all-night polysomnographic (PSG) study, which is essential for an accurate diagnosis and an estimation of the severity of oxygen desaturation. The severity of sleep apnea, defined by the so-called apnea-hypopnea index (i.e., the number of episodes per hour of sleep), the degree of oxygen desaturation, and the presence of significant arrhythmias will be derived from sleep study and will guide future treatment (Fig. 22-4).

The treatment of sleep apnea syndromes depends on the associated abnormality, which must be defined before it can be treated. An important general treatment is weight loss, the only potentially curative measure for overweight apneics, provided the loss of weight is not only achieved but also maintained. Similarly, abstinence from alcohol and avoidance of hypnosedative drugs and beta blockers are advocated.

Pharmacologic approaches including acetazolamide, theophylline, naloxone, medroxyprogesterone, and clomipramine have not been studied systematically on large numbers of subjects. The only widely used drug is protriptyline, which may exert a beneficial effect in an occasional patient with obstructive sleep apnea. Its effect may be due to a reported direct action on the muscle tone of the upper airway. A recent crossover unblinded trial of protriptyline and fluoxetine suggests equal effectiveness of either drug, with about 30% to 50% of patients showing improved oxygenation during sleep.

A number of studies suggest that the administration of oxygen may be a useful method of treating central sleep apnea, although the mechanism by which it reduces central apneic events has not been established. It is hypothesized that the potential destabilizing influence of the hypoxic ventilatory response on respiratory control may in fact be counteracted by the administration of oxygen. However, in some cases, hypercapnia and the frequency of obstructive sleep apnea may increase.

The most widely used treatment of obstructive sleep apnea is nasal continuous positive airway pressure (CPAP), which acts by establishing a "pneumatic splint" to the upper airway. The key element of its effect is that it causes elevation of the pressure in the oropharynx, thus reversing the transmural pressure gradient across the oropharyngeal airway.

Nasal CPAP is the only treatment as effective as tracheostomy. The major reasons for CPAP failure are poor compliance for social or cosmetic reasons, and nasal obstruction. Some patients whose apneas are eliminated with CPAP continue to have nonapneic desaturations, especially during REM sleep. Usually, these patients are obese, with chronic obstructive pulmonary disease (COPD) in addition to sleep apnea. In such situations, supplemental oxygen may be ben-

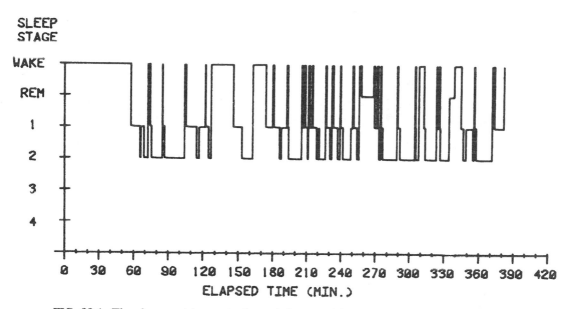

FIG. 22-4. The sleep architecture of an adult man with obstructive sleep apnea syndrome. Stages 3 and 4 are lacking; frequent arousals occur, which fragment the sleep cycle; REM sleep is much reduced as a proportion of the sleep period; and REM periodicity is abolished. The majority of the sleep period consists of NREM Stages 1 and 2.

eficial. The benefits derived from oxygen treatment should be polysomnographically verified.

Bilevel positive airway pressure (BiPAP) offers an effective alternative for patients who are uncomfortable while expiring against the high pressures delivered by CPAP. This device allows independent titration of expiratory and inspiratory airway pressure and has been very helpful in cases of comorbid obesity, intrinsic lung disease, and chest deformity, conditions associated with hypoventilation.

Sometimes, correction of nasal obstruction can result in significant reduction of sleep apneas. Adenoidectomy, tonsillectomy, and surgical correction of the maxillofacial anomalies will abolish apneas. Patients with serious mandibular deformities can undergo surgical procedures of maxillary, mandibular, and hyoid bone advancements, but a significant number of failures occur, primarily in patients with the most severe mandibular deficiencies.

Attempts to promote uvulopalatopharyngoplasty (UPPP) as an alternative surgical treatment of sleep apnea have not been successful. Multiple studies indicate at best a variable success rate, ranging from 33% to 70%. The success rate may improve somewhat, provided selection of patients is based on the determina-

tion of the level of obstruction prior to the surgery. More encouraging are results of UPPP in the treatment of snoring: A 75% to 100% sucess rate for the elimination of snoring has been reported, which is not unexpected because structures generating the sounds of snoring are surgically removed. This may be misinterpreted as a sign of apnea cure, but the apneas may persist despite the disappearance of snoring. Laser-assisted uvulopalatoplasty (LAUP), involving partial resection of the uvula and soft palate using a laser, is a simple surgical procedure that can be done on an outpatient basis in two to seven sessions without general anesthesia. It seems highly effective in eliminating habitual snoring, with success rates from 70% to 84%. The American Sleep Disorders Association, however, does not recommend this procedure for treatment of sleep apnea. Prosthetic devices focus on the nasopharyngeal inlet and position of the base of the tongue. The only two devices tested in a sleep lab for their effectiveness are a tongue-retaining device (TRD) and Snore-Guard (Hayes & Meade, Inc., Albuquerque, NM). TRD is most effective in patients demonstrating positional apnea who are not excessively obese. For some positional apneics, just being trained to sleep on their sides may be an effective cure.

NARCOLEPSY

Narcolepsy is a syndrome consisting of excessive daytime sleepiness and abnormal manifestations of REM sleep. The latter includes frequent sleep-onset REM periods, which may be subjectively appreciated as hypnagogic hallucinations, and dissociated REM sleep-inhibitory processes: cataplexy and sleep paralysis. The appearance of REM sleep within 10 minutes of sleep onset is considered evidence for narcolepsy. In narcolepsy, the patient falls asleep in the midst of activities, although most people will stay awake during animated conversation, walking, eating, or coitus.

The cardinal symptoms are excessive daytime sleepiness, sleep attacks, and cataplexy. Although sleep attacks are characteristic of this disease, excessive sleepiness is equally disturbing (i.e., a permanent, sometimes profound, impairment of vigilance or wakefulness between attacks). Sleep attacks usually last about 15 minutes. The patient awakens refreshed and there is a definite refractory period of 1 to 5 hours before the next attack. Cataplexy is a sudden decrease in, or abrupt loss of, muscle tone that is either generalized or limited to particular muscle groups. Cataplexy ranges from weakness in the muscles supporting the jaw, or a sense of weakness in the knees, to a complete muscular weakness causing the patient to slump to the floor, unable to move. Cataplectic attacks are characteristically initiated by laughter, surprise, outbursts of anger, or a feeling of exaltation. These attacks generally last for only a few seconds or as long as 30 minutes.

Auxiliary symptoms of narcolepsy include sleep paralysis, which occurs while the patient is falling asleep or waking from sleep. Consciousness is preserved and it is accompanied by an intense feeling of fear. Hypnagogic hallucinations also occur at the onset of sleep or on awakening, and they are usually frightening. Automatic behavior, sometimes reported as "blackouts," is a reflection of severe sleepiness. Nocturnal sleep is also disturbed with frequent awakenings, frequent sleep-onset REM periods, and vivid dreams.

A diagnosis of narcolepsy is based on the following:

1. A history of excessive daytime sleepiness, sleep attacks, cataplexy, and other auxiliary symptoms
2. Objective documentation of pathologic sleepiness by the Multiple Sleep Latency test (MSLT), showing a mean sleep latency of 5 minutes or less
3. Two or more sleep-onset REM periods during the naps

The onset of symptoms appears to involve a combination of environmental and genetic factors. More than 85% of all narcoleptics with definite cataplexy share a specific human leukocyte antigen (HLA) allele, HLA DQB1-0602 (most often in combination with HLA DR2), compared to 12% to 38% of the general population in various ethnic groups. DQB1-0602 may represent a genetic marker for the disorder, indicating the presence of the possible narcolepsy-susceptibility gene on chromosome 6. A negative test for DQB1-0602 does not rule out diagnosis of narcolepsy, because a rare narcoleptic patient with cataplexy may be DQB1-0602 negative. Genetic factors other than HLA are also likely to be involved. Only 8% to 10% of narcoleptics are aware of another member of the family with narcolepsy/cataplexy. The risk of a first-degree relative of a patient having narcolepsy with cataplexy is 1% to 2%. Usually, narcoleptic patients can be reassured that the illness will not develop in their relatives. However, a 1% to 2% risk is 10 to 40 times higher than the prevalence observed in the general population, suggesting the existence of genetic predisposing factors.

In rare patients, successful treatment involves only improved sleep hygiene, as previously described. Most patients, however, will need CNS stimulants, primarily dextroamphetamine (Dexedrine), methylphenidate (Ritalin), or pemoline (Cylert). Stimulants are likely to reduce but not eliminate excessive daytime sleepiness and performance deficits. Methamphetamine (Desoxyn) in doses higher than those recommended for treatment of obesity was found to normalize sleepiness and performance in eight subjects studied, but it is rarely used because of concerns about abuse and related adverse behaviors. Cataplectic attacks respond to imipramine (Tofranil), nortriptyline (Pamelor), and protriptyline (Vivactil). One of the most effective drugs for treatment of cataplexy is clomipramine (Anafranil), a potent serotonin-uptake inhibitor. Side effects such as impotence and xerostomia may limit its usefulness. Newer antidepressants with more exclusive inhibition of serotonin uptake [e.g., fluoxetine (Prozac), paroxetine (Paxil), and sertraline (Zoloft)] may also be useful in management of cataplexy, with fewer anticholinergic side effects. Mazindol (Sanorex or Mazanor), an anorectic imidazoline derivative with pharamacologic activity resembling the amphetamines, and selegiline (Eldepryl), a monoamine oxidase B–inhibitor that is converted to L-amphetamine and methamphetamine, improve daytime alertness and may have fewer side effects than amphetamines, but none has been shown to be more effective than amphetamines in treating narcolepsy. Modafinil (Provigil) is a new wake-promoting agent, pharmacologically distinct form currently available stimulants.

Unlike amphetamines and methylphenidate, modafinil does not appear to significantly alter the release of dopamine or norepinephrine. Although it does not stimulate release of norepinephrine directly, it does require an intact alpha-adrenergic system for its stimulant effect to occur. Modafinil has been evaluated in clinical trials in Europe and the United States. Recently published results of a double-blind, randomized, parallel-group, 18-center study of the effectiveness of modafinil in treatment of pathologic sleepiness in narcolepsy suggest that it is effective and safe. Patients refractory to other treatments may sometimes require the use of monoamine oxidase (MAO) inhibitors.

Improvements observed with the use of L-tyrosine, codeine, or propranolol have not been documented in controlled trials. When sleep fragmentation is a major complaint, judicious use of short-acting hypnotics once or twice per week may be helpful. The improvement of nocturnal sleep with gamma-hydroxybutyrate did not result in demonstrable improvement of diurnal symptoms. The use of amphetamines produces common adverse effects such as restlessness, agitation, tachycardia, dizziness, and sometimes psychotic episodes. Stimulants may all be associated with dependence.

Pharmacologic approaches are generally not entirely satisfactory, and many patients benefit from social support provided by groups such as the American Narcolepsy Association. Idiopathic CNS hypersomnolence is a condition resembling narcolepsy, but without sleep-onset REM periods, cataplexy, or auxiliary symptoms. Treatment with stimulants is usually less effective.

INSUFFICIENT SLEEP

Insufficient sleep is a frequent cause of daytime somnolence. The individual is voluntarily, but often unwittingly, chronically sleep deprived. Although this relationship may seem self-evident, most patients are unaware that their chronic sleep deprivation is responsible for their continuous excessive sleepiness. When these individuals obtain adequate sleep, their complaint of somnolence during the day disappears.

Various other medical and medicinal causes of excessive daytime somnolence deserve mention. Hypnosedatives, anticonvulsants, antihypertensives, antihistamines, and antidepressants are common causes. A withdrawal from stimulants may also give rise to severe sleepiness. Multiple medical and toxic conditions may be associated with drowsiness: hyperglycemia (prior to ketoacidosis or nonketotic coma), hypocortisolism, hypoglycemia, hypothyroidism, panhypopi-

tuitarism, hepatic encephalopathy, hypercalcemia, renal insufficiency, vitamin B_{12} deficiency, chronic subdural hematoma, encephalitis, intracranial neoplasm (primary or secondary), meningitis, or the aftereffects of trauma. Hypersomnolence is a misnomer in many of these conditions since more often a state of obtundation occurs. There are also two rare periodic disorders of excessive sleepiness: (1) Kleine–Levin syndrome, characterized by recurrent periods of extended sleep, megaphagia, sexual disinhibitions, and social withdrawal if awake, and (2) menstruation-associated hypersomnia, a period of sleepiness during a patient's menstrual period (without observed changes in behavior).

PARASOMNIAS

Parasomnias, which include a heterogeneous group of behavioral disturbances that occur only during sleep or are exacerbated by sleep, do not have a common pathophysiologic mechanism. They represent disorders of arousal, partial arousal, and sleep-stage transitions. Arousals from delta sleep are characterized by confusion, disorientation in time and space, and slow speech and mentation. These confusional arousals usually occur in children and may progress into sleepwalking (somnambulism) or sleep terror (pavor nocturnus, incubus). Typically, there is very little if any recall for the event the following morning, and minimal if any recall of dreamlike mentation. Most somnambulistic episodes last a few seconds to few minutes. A sleep terror is an arousal from NREM sleep accompanied by a piercing scream or cry and behavioral manifestations of intense anxiety indicating autonomic arousal. Autonomic manifestations include mydriasis, perspiration, piloerection, rapid breathing, and tachycardia. Morning amnesia for the episode is the rule.

There is often a concurrence of more than one of these disorders in the same child, and a hereditary predisposition to parasomnias has been noted. Somnambulism in children is not considered to be caused by psychological factors, although its persistence into adulthood represents a serious problem and may be associated with diverse forms of personality disturbance and psychopathology. Most children grow out of this condition between the ages of 7 and 14. It is important to protect patients against injury by, for example, installing safety rails at the head of stairways and placing locks on windows. In cases of frequent sleepwalking, diazepam may reduce the episodes, probably through the suppression of delta sleep. The usual dose is 5 to 10 mg at bedtime.

Sleep-related enuresis is involuntary micturition beginning usually during deep NREM sleep in an individual who has or should have voluntary waking control of the bladder. In contrast to this idiopathic nocturnal enuresis, symptomatic enuresis is due to urogenital or other diseases and is generally less benign. Idiopathic enuresis and somnambulism tend to disappear by late childhood or adolescence, probably representing a phenomenon of delayed maturation. At 5 years of age, 15% of boys and 10% of girls are enuretic. Recommended treatment includes tricyclic antidepressants [e.g., imipramine, 25–75 at bedtime (approximately 1.0–1.5 mg/kg/day)] and daytime bladder exercises aimed at increasing bladder capacity. Oxybutynin chloride (Ditropan) has been used with variable success. Intranasal desamino-D-arginine vasopressin (DDAVP, Desmopressin) at low doses has been shown to have a definite effect, especially in children over 9 years and adults. Conditioning with a buzzer and pad is the most successful treatment for enuresis, but success may depend on continued use of the buzzer.

A nightmare is an arousal from REM sleep with the recall of a disturbing dream, accompanied by anxiety and much less prominent autonomic arousal. The awakened patient is instantly oriented and alert. Vocalization, fear, and motor activity are less intense than in sleep terrors. Nightmares are more likely to occur in the second half of the night, when more prolonged REM episodes are likely to occur. Withdrawal from alcohol, amphetamines, or hypnotics may lead to REM sleep rebound and cause nightmares.

Rapid-eye-movement sleep behavior disorder (RBD) is a parasomnia characterized by vigorous motor activity, instead of atonia, in response to dream content, often resulting in an injury. Manifestations of acting out dreams include laughing, talking, chanting, singing, yelling, swearing, gesturing, reaching, grabbing, arm flailing, punching, kicking, sitting up, jumping out of bed, crawling, and running movements. One third of people with RBD have a demonstrable underlying neurologic disorder. Most of the cases are, however, idiopathic and tend to occur in the elderly. Transient RBD has been seen in association with acute drug intoxications and withdrawal states. Clonazepam is the drug of choice for treatment of RBD.

Parasomnias also include a cluster headache and the related (but more chronic) condition of paroxysmal hemicrania. Cluster headaches occur in REM sleep and may be related to an increased cerebral blood flow during REM sleep. About 45% of patients with seizure disorders have seizures mainly during sleep. Generalized seizures are markedly activated by NREM sleep; specifically, generalized tonic–clonic seizures are most common during Stages 1 and 2 NREM sleep. Focal seizures may occur during NREM and REM sleep. Prolonged EEG monitoring may be necessary in some difficult cases when a diagnosis of epileptic (as opposed to nonepileptic) episodic behavior is needed. Sleep-related eating disorders may occur in association with obstructive sleep apnea, somnambulism, daytime eating disorders, medication abuse, or in isolation. They are characterized by almost nightly eating, and weight gain that patients attribute to the nocturnal eating. Most patients are only partially conscious during the eating episode. Two thirds of patients with this condition are women who are generally concerned over the weight gain. Daytime binge eating or obsessive–compulsive disorder is absent. Treatments include clonazepam (Klonopin), carbidopa/levodopa (Sinemet), and fluoxetine (Prozac).

Other parasomnias that may occur in childhood as well as in adulthood include bruxism, head banging (jactatio capitis nocturna), abnormal swallowing, and painful penile erections. Whether these conditions require a polysomnographic evaluation and treatment depends entirely on the persistence of the symptoms and the degree of the patient's disability. Bruxism affects up to 15% of children. This condition may contribute to periodontal disease and temporomandibular joint dysfunction.

USE OF SLEEP LABORATORIES AND EVALUATION OF NON-SLEEP-RELATED COMPLAINTS

The examination of nocturnal penile tumescence during sleep represents a useful tool for the evaluation of impotence. Sleep-related erections are inconsistent with organic impotence: Impotence is more likely to be psychogenic in nature if sleep-related erections are normal. Attention should be paid to a careful drug history, because many drugs have the potential to cause an impairment of erectile mechanisms.

QUESTIONS AND DISCUSSION

1. A 23-year-old man presents with a chief complaint of "narcolepsy." His history indicates the presence of sleep attacks, cataplexy, sleep paralysis, and hypnagogic hallucinations for the last 4 years. He states he has never been treated for the disorder and

recognized his problem from reading about narcolepsy in a magazine. The neurologic examination is normal. The physical examination reveals a nervous man with a heart rate of 102 beats/minute but otherwise normal vital signs. The remainder of the physical examination is normal. A routine complete blood count (CBC), SMA-25, electrocardiogram (ECG), and chest x-ray film are normal. A thyroid battery is within normal limits. Management at this point would consist of:

A. Prescription of D-amphetamine, 5 mg three times daily
B. Administration of D-amphetamine in combination with a tricyclic antidepressant
C. Routine all-night PSMG
D. Urine screening for amphetamine metabolites
E. Scheduling for a series of daytime naps in the sleep laboratory

The answer is (D). The usual practice is to screen the urine for amphetamine metabolites before doing a more involved study. It is usually a bad sign to have a patient who knows the classic symptoms of narcolepsy and maintains he has never been diagnosed or treated. In most cases of narcolepsy, excessive daytime sleepiness and sleep attacks are initial symptoms of the disease, whereas associated symptoms develop later. A patient with all components of the syndrome early in the course of the disorder is subject to suspicion. Once urine samples are known to be "clean," all-night polysomnography and nap studies are useful to establish the diagnosis. If a patient is suspected of covert stimulant use, a prolonged period of abstinence should be documented before assuming that an REM-onset sleep episode is narcolepsy (since the same pattern may appear as part of stimulant withdrawal). Empirical therapy with stimulants is a practice that should be avoided.

2. A 36-year-old schoolteacher is referred for an evaluation of excessive somnolence. The patient states that he feels extremely drowsy unless he is actively involved in a novel behavior. The problem has been present for at least 3 years but seems to be getting worse. He has fallen asleep at the wheel of his car twice in the last 6 months. He denies a significant history of alcohol ingestion and is not taking medications. The physical examination reveals a large (1.6-m, 82-kg) individual with normal vital signs. The physical and neurologic examinations are normal. After leaving the room to answer a call, you return to find the patient sleeping. A routine blood count reveals a hemoglobin

(Hb) of 17 g/dl, with normal indices and white blood cell count. Biochemical screening is normal. A routine ECG is normal. Thyroid hormone levels and cortisol determinations are unremarkable. A reasonable differential diagnosis at this point would include:

A. Sedative drug abuse
B. Narcolepsy
C. Sleep apnea
D. Depression
E. Idiopathic hypersomnia

Which of the following studies might be of value in evaluating these possibilities?

A. EEG
B. Computed tomography (CT) of the head
C. Magnetic Resonance Imaging (MRI) of the brain
D. All-night polysomnographic (PSG) study, with respiratory and cardiac monitoring
E. Urine drug screen
F. Diagnostic psychiatric interview
G. A series of daytime naps in the sleep laboratory
H. An empirical trial of D-amphetamine without additional testing

This is a fairly typical history—it lacks the important details that would help clarify the diagnostic possibilities: history of snoring, cataplectic episodes or episodes of sleep paralysis, episodic amnesia, morning headache, or a family history of a similar problem. Any of the possibilities could be entertained from this history. The patient's weight and sex make sleep apnea statistically more likely, but sedative drug abuse is too frequently a cause of this symptom to overlook it as a possibility. Our usual approach is to screen for sedatives, then to proceed with an all-night PSG, with respiratory and cardiac monitoring. If the results are negative, daytime naps are studied the following day to exclude narcolepsy. The studies in answers (A), (B), and (C) are rarely of any value in evaluating these patients. In this particular case, an all-night PSG documented the presence of a severe obstructive sleep apnea with associated cardiac arrhythmias. The elevated red blood cell count appeared to be a secondary complication of nocturnal apnea.

3. A 71-year-old man is receiving carbidopa/levodopa for Parkinson's disease. After 2 years of therapy, he complains of severe insomnia and daytime somnolence. By history he awakens at 2 AM each night and cannot return to sleep before 4 AM. He falls asleep at 11

PM with no difficulty. Each day he finds it necessary to take one or two 1-hour naps. His wife complains that he often awakens the household during the night with loud screams. The patient is not aware of this behavior and denies any abnormal dreams. This history reflects:

A. Probable dementia in association with Parkinson's disease
B. Psychotic depression
C. A side effect of chronic dopaminergic therapy
D. An unrelated sleep disorder

Management would include:

A. Administration of a hypnosedative before retiring
B. Antidepressant therapy
C. All-night sleep study
D. Discontinuation of antiparkinsonian medications
E. Restriction of antiparkinsonian medications, avoiding administration in the evening

The answer to the first part is (C). Although there is some debate on the relationship of dementia to sleep disruption in this patient group, symptoms usually clear when dopaminergic therapy is stopped. In most cases, continued therapy is necessary, and in these patients, avoiding drug administration after 6 PM often improves the insomnia and daytime napping. Nightmares in patients receiving levodopa appear to arise out of Stage 2 sleep, and patients are frequently amnestic for the episodes. Furthermore, REM sleep behavior disorder may have developed. Hypnosedatives and antidepressants are unpredictable in their response in these patients and frequently exacerbate the complaint. In most cases, answer (E) seems to be the most appropriate management.

4. You are consulted by a 23-year-old man who described episodes of "amnesia." On several occasions, he has found himself at various locations with no recollection of having traveled to them. He recollects being at another location hours before; his memory for previous events is good, and he denies any other symptoms preceding the attack. Observers have seen him during an episode, and he appeared distracted but carried on social conversations appropriately and on one occasion drove a car without incident. He appears relatively stable, and attacks occur in situations that seem devoid of any emotional importance. The patient does not drink. The neurologic examination is normal. A sleep-deprived EEG without sedation is read as normal, although it is noted that drowsiness is followed quickly by the onset of low-voltage fast activity. Biochemical studies including a 6-hour glucose tolerance test are all normal. An MRI of the brain is normal. Empirical therapy with phenytoin (100 mg three times daily) leads to worsening of the symptoms. Your differential diagnosis at this point should include:

A. A pseudoseizure
B. Narcolepsy–cataplexy syndrome
C. Somnambulism
D. Recurrent transient global amnesia
E. Sleep apnea syndrome
F. Complex partial seizure
G. Amnestic migraine

The appropriate answers are (B) and (E). The episodes described are typical of "automatic behavior" syndrome. This behavioral abnormality is associated with the appearance of "microsleep" episodes which electroencephalographically are Stage 1 sleep. Sleep apnea and narcolepsy are associated with this disorder. Although the diagnosis of complex partial seizures is difficult to rule out on the basis of a normal EEG, the adverse response to empirical anticonvulsants is more typical of an "automatic behavior" syndrome. Transient global amnesia presents a similar clinical picture but is an entity restricted to late middle life; frequent recurrences are unusual in this syndrome. Somnambulism is a similar phenomenon but is more frequent in childhood and arises from a period of normal sleep; it is usually a Stage 4 sleep event. Psychiatric disorders are frequently present in adults with somnambulistic disorders.

Amnestic migraine may produce recurrent amnestic episodes but usually does so in the presence of more typical migrainous episodes. There is some question of whether this is a *sui generis* disorder or represents the coexistence of two phenomena in a single individual.

Pseudoseizures are rarely characterized by global amnesia and are usually situationally related.

Appropriate management in this case would include an all-night PSMG followed by the Multiple Sleep Latency test the next day as well as a routine 16-channel EEG. A careful history-taking directed specifically toward cataplexy, daytime napping, nocturnal apnea, and snoring would help in a differentiation of the underlying condition. Treatment with amphetamine is usually not entirely successful. Hypnosedatives, anticonvulsants, and diazepam usually cause worsening of the symptoms. In patients with sleep apnea of any cause, proper medical or surgical management has been reported to alleviate this symptom complex.

SUGGESTED READING

Bootzin RR, Perlis ML: Nonpharmacologic treatment of insomnia. J Clin Psychiatry 53 (6) (Suppl):37, 1992

Cartwright RD, Ristanovic R, Diaz F et al: A comparative study of treatments for positional sleep apnea. Sleep 14:546, 1991

Dement WC: Rational basis for the use of sleeping pills. Int Pharmacopsychiatry 17 (Suppl 2):3, 1982

Diagnostic Classification Steering Committee: International Classification of Sleep Disorders: Diagnostic and Coding Manual. Rochester, MN, American Sleep Disorders Association, 1990

Engelman HM, Martin SE, Deary IJ et al: Effect of CPAP therapy on daytime function in patients with mild sleep apnoealhypopnoea syndrome. Thorax 52:114, 1997

Findley L, Unverzagt M, Guchu R et al: Vigilance and automobile accidents in patients with sleep apnea or narcolepsy. Chest 108:619, 1995

Fletcher EC: The relationship between systemic hypertension and obstructive sleep apnea: Facts and theory. Am J Med 98:128, 1995

Fletcher EC, Munafo DA: Role of nocturnal oxygen therapy in obstructive sleep apnea. Chest 98:1497, 1990

Fry JM (ed): Current issues in the diagnosis and management of narcolepsy. Neurology 50 (2) (Suppl 1):S1, 1998

Gottlieb GL: Sleep disorders and their management: Special considerations in the elderly. Am J Med 88 (Suppl 3A):29S, 1990

Guilleminault C: Narcolepsy 1985. Sleep 9 (Vol 1, Pt 2):285, 1986

Guilleminault C, Stoohs R, Quera-Salva M-A: Sleep-related obstructive and nonobstructive apneas and neurologic disorders. Neurology 42 (Suppl 6):53, 1992

Hanly PJ: Mechanisms and management of central sleep apnea. Lung 170:1, 1992

Hla KM, Young TB, Bidwell T et al: Sleep apnea and hypertension: A population-based study. Ann Intern Med 120:382, 1994

Hobson JA: Sleep: Order and disorder. Behav Biol Med 1:1, 1983

Hoffstein V: Is snoring dangerous to your health? Controversies in sleep medicine. Sleep 19 (6):506, 1996

Hudgel DW: Mechanisms of obstructive sleep apnea. Chest 101:541, 1992

Hudgel DW: Pharmacologic treatment of obstructive sleep apnea: Review. J Lab Clin Med 126:13, 1995

Hudgel DW: Treatment of obstructive sleep apnea: A review. Chest 109:1346, 1996

Kales A (ed): The Pharmacology of Sleep. New York, Springer-Verlag, 1995

Kovacevic-Ristanovic R, Dyonzak J: Sleep disorders associated with respiratory dysfunction. In: Goetz CG, Tanner CM, Aminoff MJ (eds): Handbook of Clinical Neurology, Vol. 19 (63): Systemic Diseases, Part I. Elesevier Science, pp. 449—475, 1993

Mahowald MW, Schenk CH: REM sleep behavior disorder. In: Kryger MH, Roth T, Dement WC (eds): Principles and Practice of Sleep Medicine, pp 389—401. Philadelphia, WB Saunders, 1989

McCarley RW: Sleep neurophysiology: basic mechanisms underlying control of wakefulness and sleep. In Chokroverty S (ed), Sleep Disorders Medicine, Second Edition. Butterworth/Heinemann, 1999, pp. 21—50.

Mignot E: Behavioral genetics '97: Genetics of narcolepsy and other sleep disorders. Am J Hum Genet 60:1289, 1997

Millman RP, Rosenberg CL, Kramer NR: Oral appliances in the treatment of snoring and sleep apnea. Clin Chest Med 19 (1):69, 1998

Montplaisir J, Boucher S, Poirier G et al: Clinical, polysomnographic, and genetic characteristics of restless legs syndrome: A study of 133 patients diagnosed with new standard criteria. Movement Disord 12 (1):61, 1997

Morin CM: Insomnia, Psychological Assessment and Management. New York, Guilford Press, 1993

Mortimore IL, Marshall I, Wraith PK et al: Neck and total body fat deposition in nonobese and obese patients with sleep apnea compared with that in control subjects. Am J Respir Crit Care Med 157:280, 1998

Parkes JD: Sleep and Its Disorders. Philadelphia, WB Saunders, 1985

Pierce MW, Shu VS: Efficacy of estazolam: The United States clinical experience. Am J Med 88 (Suppl 3A):6S, 1990

Powell NB, Riley RW, Robinson A: Surgical management of obstructive sleep apnea syndrome. Clin Chest Med 19 (1):77, 1998

Roth T, Roerhs TA, Stepanski EJ et al: Hypnotics and behavior. Am J Med 88 (Suppl 3A):43S, 1990

Sherin JE, Shiromani PJ, McCarley RW et al: Activation of ventrolateral preoptic neurons during sleep. Science 271:216, 1996

Strohl KP, Redline S: State of art, recognition of obstructive sleep apnea. Am J Respir Crit Care Med 154:270, 1996

Strollo PJ Jr, Sanders MH, Atwood CW: Positive therapy pressures. Clin Chest Med 19 (1):55, 1998

Thase M: Depression, sleep and antidepressants. J Clin Psychiatry 59 (Suppl 4):55, 1998

US Modafinil in Narcolepsy Multicenter Study Group: Randomized trial of modafinil for the treatment of pathological somnolence in narcolepsy. Ann Neurol 43 (1):88, 1998

Walters AS, and the International Restless Legs Syndrome Study Group: Toward a better definition of the restless legs syndrome. Movement Disord 10 (5):634, 1995

Weiss WJ, Remsburg S, Grapestad E et al: Hemodynamic consequences of obstructive sleep apnea: State of the art review. Sleep 19 (5):388, 1996

Williams RL, Karacan I: Sleep Disorders: Diagnosis and Treatment. New York, John Wiley, 1978

Winkelman JW: Clinical and polysomnographic features of sleep-related eating disorder. J Clin Psychiatry 59:14, 1998

Young T, Palta M, Dempsey J et al: The occurrence of sleep-disordered breathing among middle-aged adults. N Engl J Med 328 (17):1230, 1993

Neurology for the Non-Neurologist, Fourth Edition, edited by William J. Weiner and Christopher G. Goetz. Lippincott Williams & Wilkins, Philadelphia © 1999.

C H A P T E R   2 3

Eye Signs in Neurologic Diagnosis

James A. Goodwin

This chapter is intended as a survey of visual signs and symptoms that are of use for localization and etiologic diagnosis in neurologic disease. The organization of the chapter reflects both anatomic and functional classifications, and in all cases the close relation between anatomic and physiologic details and a practical clinical diagnosis is drawn. This chapter includes a discussion of the afferent or sensory visual system, the pupillomotor, and the oculomotor systems. The localizing value of examining the visual systems for lesions of the cerebral hemispheres, brainstem, spinal cord, and peripheral anatomic pathways is emphasized.

AFFERENT (SENSORY) VISUAL SYSTEM: SENSORY OR MOTOR?

It seems so simple to refer to one part of the visual system as afferent, and another as efferent or oculomotor, but the two parts must function together to such an extent that the separation is artificial, although useful in a practical sense.

Man is a foveate animal, which means that retinal morphology and function are not uniform throughout: They are specialized for high-resolution vision in a small central area called the fovea, or pit. The special architecture of the retina at the fovea and the immediate surrounding region, the macula lutea (so-called because of its concentration of yellow pigment), underlies its capacity to resolve fine detail in the visual scene.

The general structure of the retina is such that groups of photoreceptors are connected by bipolar cells to a ganglion cell that provides input to the central nervous system (CNS) by way of its axon. This basic arrangement is complicated by a host of horizontal interactions mediated by other cells in the retina.

A roughly circular array of photoreceptors that send input to a ganglion cell is referred to as the *receptive field* of that ganglion cell. Light captured by one of the photoreceptors within a receptive field can signal to the ganglion cell only that a visual event has occurred within its receptive field, not where in the field the photon has been captured. In areas of the retina where receptive fields are large and many hundreds of photoreceptors are connected to a single ganglion cell, the capacity for fine spatial resolution is poor. At the fovea, where there are only a few photoreceptors in the receptive field of a ganglion cell, the spatial resolution is very fine.

For example, consider two points of light near the foveal representation of the visual field (called the fixation area). These are likely to activate two photoreceptors that are connected to different ganglion cells, thus signaling the presence of two separate lights. The same two points of light at a peripheral position in the visual field would likely activate two photoreceptors connected to the same ganglion cell. The only information provided to the CNS is that light is on somewhere within that receptive field. Because there are two spots of light, the encoded brightness is greater than if only one spot were present, but information on the spatial distribution of the spots is lost.

For us to see an object clearly, the image of the object must be positioned on the fovea (an act that involves the oculomotor system interacting intimately with the afferent visual system). The afferent system must perceive that a potentially interesting object exists in the peripheral visual field and must then provide coordinates for the motor system to turn the eye so the image of that object is on the fovea. There are stages in this process that are neither clearly visual (afferent) nor motor (efferent), but are in between. Our concepts of sensory and motor are inadequate in this gray zone between taking information in and putting it out in the form of executive or motor commands. This activity possibly takes place somewhere in the higher-order visual centers of the occipitoparietal convexity. Bilateral lesions in this region produce a clinical syndrome in which there is an unraveling of the afferent and the efferent command structure. Balint called it *optic ataxia,* and the syndrome now bears his name. Patients who have *Balint's syndrome* have special difficulty in directing their gaze in an orderly manner to scan or *palpate* an extended visual scene. The world for them is a fragmentary and disordered array of images, none organically articulated in a meaningful way. This perceptual difficulty can be shown to accompany a disorder of motor scanning behavior. The patient acts as though the coordinates by which to direct his gaze have been scrambled. As an example, these patients lose the highly learned and orderly *scan path* used by normal viewers to investigate a human face, using many fixations on areas of high information such as the eyes, nose, mouth, and brows. Instead, these patients shift their line of gaze aimlessly, often fixing on low-information areas such as an ear or a bit of hair. They fail to conceive of the object as a human face in the course of this random scanning. It can be shown that the basic afferent function, including visual acuity and visual field, are normal when tested in the usual way. Although large scenes are improperly synthesized, small objects that can be encompassed in a single fixation are recognized correctly. These patients should be tested with pictures of objects that can be shown in both small and large versions to demonstrate this special difficulty of spatial synthesis with preserved visual acuity and visual field. Visual field testing may be particularly difficult in these patients because of their inability to simultaneously perceive two points in the field. When they are aware of the central fixation point, they fail to respond to the peripheral target; however, when they lose the fixation point, they can see the peripheral target with near-normal sensitivity. This facet of the disease has been called *simultanagnosia* or *amorphosynthesis.*

These brief introductory remarks on the shady limits of the sensory and motor visual systems serve to promote a sense of mystery about vision. This is certainly appropriate at these limits and at every stage of visual processing. Even the retina is poorly understood in all its physiologic aspects. The neural signal that is conducted to the lateral geniculate body is highly processed even at this early stage. We are only beginning to learn the complexity of visual disorders that originate from retinal disease.

The more usual disorders of the afferent visual system and the standard office methods for testing them will now be examined. The following discussion is aimed at the practicalities of office or bedside testing without further discussion of the controversies that might be involved. The information can be considered "safe" in that it has been in common clinical usage for a long time and has proved its reliability for localizing and etiologic diagnosis.

TESTING VISUAL ACUITY

Visual acuity as tested with *Snellen's optotypes* is probably the best-known and most widely used visual examination. It is important to realize, however, that some conditions are poorly characterized by visual acuity testing. These conditions are diseases in which the early manifestations involve loss of the peripheral visual field. Glaucoma and papilledema are notable examples. Even total hemifield defects do not degrade the visual acuity unless they are bilateral, thus all the hemianopic disorders from lesions behind the optic chiasm cannot be adequately characterized by acuity testing.

In neuro-ophthalmology, reduction of central visual acuity is an important sign of optic nerve disease. The fact that visual acuity is also degraded by several other conditions unrelated to nerve function is unfortunate for diagnostic purposes. Optical blur from improper refraction is a common one, but clouding of the ocular media by corneal opacity, by cataract, or by blood or other debris in the vitreous is also a consideration. In addition, visual acuity is reduced by *amblyopia ex anopsia,* which is the practically permanent visual defect that accompanies childhood strabismus or early life anisometropia (unequal refractive error in the two eyes). The differential diagnosis of poor visual acuity also includes retinal disorders that affect the macula (another broad category of diseases).

All the clinical features of a case are important to establish a diagnosis of optic nerve disease as the cause of reduced visual acuity. Once the diagnosis is established, visual acuity is the most useful and the most universally used test for following the course of optic nerve disease. Visual field examination is also required in this regard and must be used as a complement to acuity determination in the follow-up of optic neuropathies.

The ophthalmologist usually measures acuity in an *examination lane,* a long testing room in which letters of calibrated size are projected on a screen that the patient views. The original letters were made to be viewed at a distance of 20 feet, but the economics of office building construction have led to modifications. The commercially available projection devices can be made to project the letters small enough to make a valid test at viewing distances as short as 10 feet, and mirrors can be used to test a patient in even more cramped conditions.

An optical supply company representative should be consulted for instructions on how to set up a regular eye lane in an office. Non-ophthalmologists will probably not wish to purchase an expensive projection system for occasional use; however, inexpensive wall-mounted reading charts are available for use at various reading distances from 10 to 20 feet. Adequate lighting must be provided, and standard ceiling fluorescent lights are usually sufficient.

THE NEAR CARD

Most non-ophthalmologists, including neurologists, internists, and family physicians, test visual acuity on a *near card,* which is intended for viewing at 14 inches (a comfortable reading distance). The distance from eye to card should be measured if the near card is the only acuity measurement used. Once the examiner gets used to the distance, he can usually judge it without measuring.

Some other features need attention to make the near card approximately equivalent to a formal testing lane. The light must be sufficient and should be provided either by good fluorescent lights from the ceiling or by a bright lamp that can be positioned to illuminate the card without shining into the patient's eyes. This is not difficult to provide in the office, but I have found that hospital beds are seldom well lighted. It is best to carry a bright handlight that provides illumination even for bedside testing. The best handlights are the *Finoff heads,* which are angled bulb carriers that

attach to the battery handle of the ophthalmoscope. Penlights seldom stay bright, and most have uneven zones of illumination. The handlight is especially useful for testing near-card acuity, because the beam can be positioned to indicate which set of letters you want the patient to read. The handlight should not be held too close, however, because the diminished contrast of the spotlighted letter makes it difficult to see. It is best to create an elliptical zone that illuminates one entire line of letters by shining the handlight onto the card from one side. Oblique illumination also eliminates glare from the surface of the card.

Proper refraction is mandatory regardless of the method used to test visual acuity. Reduced acuity from needing glasses is of no neurologic interest and creates a great deal of confusion on hospital charts. A brief discussion of lenses and refraction follows. A basic understanding of these optical principles is useful for anyone planning to do visual acuity testing or a field examination, even though the non-ophthalmologist will not actually be doing refraction.

LENSES AND REFRACTION

Light travels in a straight line through a homogeneous refractive medium such as air, glass, transparent plastic, or water. When light encounters an interface between refractive media of different density, its path is bent. A sheet of plate glass with flat parallel surfaces does not, however, alter the path of entering light. Light rays are bent as they enter the glass from air, but they are bent back to an equal degree as they go from the glass into air on the other side (Fig. 23-1A). Flat (plano) glass does not, therefore, alter the *vergence* of light.

A glass wedge bends light rays toward the base (Fig. 23-1B, C), but parallel entering rays remain parallel on exit. These pyramids are useful optical devices called *prisms* that are often used to measure eye deviation by shifting images to meet the line of sight of a deviated eye. Wide-based prisms bend light more than narrow-based ones (Fig. 23-1B, C), and quantitative units called *prism diopters* can be used to measure this degree of deviation. The patient views a small light while the examiner introduces prisms of increasing power in front of one eye. The patient specifies the amount of eye deviation by telling the examiner when the false image from the deviating eye overlies the centered (foveated) image from the other eye (the power of the prism needed to do this provides the measure of deviation).

Lenses are defined as refractive objects that *change the vergence of light:* Light rays that enter parallel will be

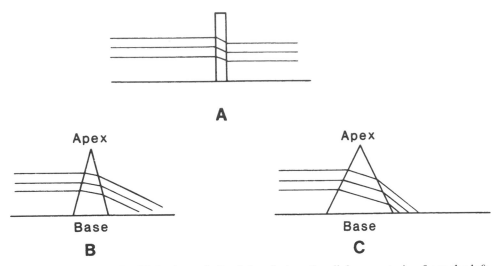

FIG. 23-1. A. The path of light through flat (plano) glass. Parallel rays entering from the left, exit parallel to the right and the *vergence* of light is not changed. **B.** A *prism* bends light toward its base (*down* in the figure). Parallel rays remain parallel, and the vergence of light is not changed. **C.** A "stronger" prism has a broader base and a less acute angle at the apex. It bends light more drastically than the "weaker" prism in B.

nonparallel when they emerge at the other side. A *convex* lens causes *convergence* of light rays and is called a *positive* or *plus* (+) lens; an upright image is created at the focal plane behind the lens, or on the side opposite the object, and is called a *real* image (Fig. 23-2A). A *concave* lens produces a *divergence* of light rays and is called a *negative* or *minus* (−) lens; the object is imaged inverted at the focal plane in front of the lens, or on the same side as the object, and is termed a *virtual* image (Fig. 23-2B). Figures 23-A and B illustrate parallel rays of light from an infinitely distant *point* source of light rather than rays emanating from an object with dimensions. They do not illustrate the upright or inverted quality of images. *Cylindrical* lenses act as lenses in one plane and as plano or flat nonlenses in a plane orthogonal to the first plane (Fig. 23-2C). A *plus* (+) *cylinder* converges light rays in its plane of power and a *minus* (−) *cylinder* diverges rays in this plane. A person whose natural optical system— the cornea, aqueous humor, crystalline lens, and vitreous humor—creates a focused image of an infinitely distant point on the fovea is *emmetropic* (Fig. 23-3A).

Ametropia refers to a significant deviation from emmetropia. A nearsighted person, or *myope*, brings the image of a distant point to focus in front of the retina (Fig. 23-3B) and needs a concave or diverging

lens to move the focal point of an infinitely distant point *back* to the retina (Fig. 23-3D). A *hyperope*, or far-sighted person, creates a focused image of an infinitely distant point behind the retina (Fig. 23-3C) and needs a convex or *converging* lens to move the focal plane forward to the surface of the retina (Fig. 23-3E). The natural optical system of a person with *astigmatism* has varying power in different planes and requires a *cylindrical* lens to correct the aberration (not illustrated in Fig. 23-3).

Once a person has achieved the focus of distant objects, either naturally or through spectacles or contact lenses, he must alter the power of the crystalline lens of the eye to maintain focus for objects nearer than infinity. Specifically, the *plus* (+) power of the eye's crystalline lens must be increased to focus on objects near the eye. Contracting the ciliary muscle, which increases the convexity of the lens, does this. This process is called *accommodation*. The power of accommodation is lost progressively with age: when a person reaches his mid forties, he needs an additional plus lens to correct for this normal condition, which is called *presbyopia*. Emmetropes (normal focus for distant objects), as they become presbyopes, usually require reading glasses that they take off for distant viewing (the images of distant objects are blurred to

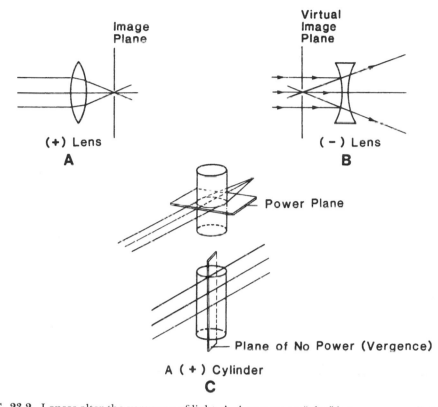

FIG. 23-2. Lenses alter the vergence of light. **A.** A convex or "plus" lens converges light rays to a focal point in the *image plane* on the side opposite the light source, which is the *object plane*. **B.** A concave or "minus" lens causes *divergence* of light rays. A "virtual" image is formed on the same side of the lens as the source of light rays in the object plane. **C.** Light rays converge through a "plus" or convex cylinder in the *power plane* (*upper figure*) and remain parallel as they pass through the cylinder in a plane orthogonal to the power plane (*lower figure*).

the emmetrope wearing his reading glasses). Those individuals who must constantly look from near to far in the course of daily activities require *half eyes* (i.e., those narrow glasses that ride low on the nose) or bifocals with no correction in the upper segment. Moderately nearsighted (minus distance refraction) presbyopes may simply take off their distance glasses to read at 14 inches—this is what nearsighted means. Highly nearsighted people have their natural focus at distances shorter than 14 inches. Although they can see clearly at such a distance, they usually find it too close for comfortable reading. These people may have bifocals in which the lower segment is still *minus,* but less minus than the upper segment. The relative plus

power needed for near vision is added arithmetically to the distance refraction.

This information will help the non-ophthalmologist to make sure that the patient is optimally corrected for an assessment of visual acuity, either in a distance lane or on the near card. The presbyopic patient should always use reading glasses or the bifocal segment when testing is done on the near card. The poor acuity that results from uncorrected presbyopia is not interesting in a neurologic assessment and creates great confusion when it is noted in the patient's chart without regard to the state of refraction. Visual acuity tested at a distance of 10 to 20 feet will require the distance correction for an ametrope. The patient should be asked to

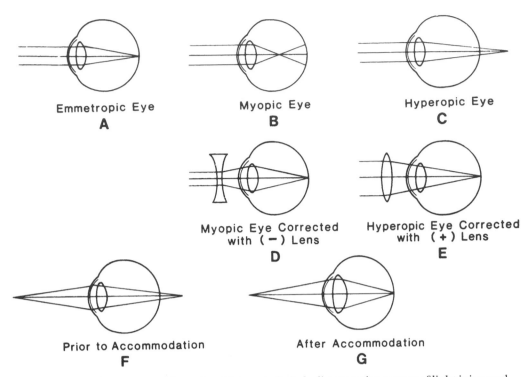

Emmetropic Eye
A

Myopic Eye
B

Hyperopic Eye
C

Myopic Eye Corrected
with (−) Lens
D

Hyperopic Eye Corrected
with (+) Lens
E

Prior to Accommodation
F

After Accommodation
G

FIG. 23-3. A. An emmetropic eye in which an infinitely distant point source of light is imaged on the retina by the natural refractive media of the eye (cornea, aqueous, lens, vitreous). **B.** A myopic eye in which an infinitely distant point source of light is imaged in front of the retina. **C.** A hyperopic eye in which an infinitely distant point source of light is imaged behind the retina. **D.** A myopic eye corrected with a minus lens. The lens superimposes divergence on the overconverged light rays and moves the focal plane back to the retina. **E.** A hyperopic eye corrected with a plus lens. The lens superimposes convergence on the overdivergent light rays and moves the focal plane forward to the retina. **F.** A point source of light near the eye produces divergent rays entering an emmetropic eye as in A. Without the act of accommodation, the refractive power of the eye is unchanged and the rays are brought to a focal plane behind the retina. In **G.**, the crystalline lens has become more convex or has increased its plus power by virtue of ciliary muscle contraction. The near source of divergent rays is now imaged on the retina because of the added convergent power that results from the act of *accommodation*.

put on his distance correction or, if he has bifocals, to be sure that he is looking through the top part. The lower segment of the bifocal generally contains the *near add,* which refers to the additional plus power for reading distance.

PINHOLE

Those not wishing to trust themselves with the vagaries and complexities of optics can depend on

the *pinhole.* The pinhole, known since the earliest days of the camera obscura, was the earliest focusing device. The hole is small enough to admit only the central rays from the object, eliminating the divergent rays that would not reach focus in the image plane. This has the disadvantage of admitting only a fraction of the light and thus creating a dim image. Most significant refractive errors can be bypassed, however, by having the patient read through a pinhole placed in front of the eye, approximately where a spectacle lens would sit. The hole should measure about 2 mm in diameter and can be punched in a card with a pin, or purchased as a manufactured item made of plastic with numerous holes in an array. This arrangement makes it easier for the patient to find the chart through one of the holes.

TECHNIQUE OF TESTING AND RECORDING VISUAL ACUITY

Most of the technique issues have been covered. Near-card acuity is done at 14 inches for most printed cards, but the card should be checked for this information. As mentioned, the light should be good, and a *standardized* lighting condition in the office is preferable if the near card is to be the only method of testing. The best refraction for a near card must be used. This usually means reading glasses or the bottom segment of bifocals for the presbyope.

Ophthalmologists have a convention in which they record near-card acuity using *Jaeger*, which is a printer's notation system (e.g., J_1 print is equivalent to 20/25). The near cards usually show both Jaeger and Snellen fractions. Notation should be made of the reading distance chosen, so that the test conditions can be reproduced, and of the optical conditions used (e.g., "patient's bifocal segment" if the exact refractive correction is not known, or "with pinhole" if that is how the test was performed).

The Snellen fraction is not really an arithmetic fraction, although it is sometimes expressed as a decimal equivalent. For instance, 20/40 can be written as 0.5, and 20/20 would be 1.0. An acuity of 20/40 means that the patient reads at 20 feet (the numerator) that which a normal person could read at a viewing distance of 40 feet (the denominator). The definition of 20/20 as normal visual acuity was determined by doing population studies; however, this definition is too liberal. The 20/20 figures are calibrated so that at the retina, the image of each letter measures (subtends) 5 minutes of arc and the width of each stroke is 1 minute of arc. Since the retina is on the back surface of a sphere, angular measure (degrees, minutes, and seconds of arc) is more convenient than linear or tangent measure (e.g., millimeters of height or width).

OPTIC NERVE DISEASE AND VISUAL ACUITY

It was mentioned earlier that hemianopia does not degrade visual acuity. Any disorder that is constrained to affect only one half of the visual field will leave the patient with 20/15 vision on the eye chart as long as there is no coexisting condition that diminishes visual acuity. A more inclusive corollary is that if any half of the fovea is functionally intact, then the resolving power of the fovea is not disturbed. This extends the rule to *altitudinal* visual field defects, in which either the upper or lower half of the visual field is selectively affected. Let us examine the anatomic underpinnings of this axiom and of the contrary rule that optic nerve diseases commonly affect visual acuity.

The functional midline in the retina is an imaginary vertical line drawn through the center of the fovea (the *vertical hemianopic midline*). Ganglion cells to either side of this line send axons through the optic nerve in an intermingled array without any systematic segregation of axons that arise from nasal or temporal ganglion cells. It is not until the axons reach the chiasm that there is a systematic separation of nasal fibers that cross the chiasm and temporal fibers that go through the chiasm uncrossed. Because of this, optic nerve diseases most often affect afferent units on both sides of midline and thereby degrade visual acuity. Measuring visual acuity is an important aspect of assessing either the response to treatment or the natural course of an optic nerve disease.

VISUAL FIELDS

Analysis of visual fields provides another key to localizing a diagnosis in the CNS. The principles in the following paragraphs deserve emphasis because they pertain to field defects that accompany lesions at all locations. Some particulars that relate to lesions at specific locations will then be outlined.

GENERAL FEATURES

MONOCULAR VERSUS BINOCULAR DEFECTS

Field defects limited to one eye suggest a lesion anterior to the optic chiasm, whereas binocular defects, when caused by a single lesion, localize to the visual pathways at or behind the optic chiasm.

Of course, bilateral multiple lesions anterior to the chiasm can give binocular field defects; however, for this discussion we are concerned primarily with signs of localizing value for single lesions.

LOCATION IN THE VISUAL FIELD

The location of defects in the visual field provides at least broad information regarding the responsible lesion. Central scotomas are associated with a wide variety of optic nerve lesions but are especially char-

acteristic of optic neuritis, compressive optic neuropathy, and toxic-metabolic optic neuropathy. Nasal
quadrant defects are associated commonly with glaucoma, a degenerative condition of the optic nerve
head in which ganglion cell axons at the upper and
lower poles of the nerve head are preferentially lost.
Temporal defects, usually binocular, are characteristic of chiasmal compression. Homonymous hemianopic defects, which are on the same side in both
eyes, characterize lesions anywhere from the optic
tract to the calcarine cortex.

These broad principles relating lesion location
with shape and locus of visual field can be used for
analysis of confrontation fields. Confrontation field
data usually lack precision as to the shape and density
of the defect, but one can generally determine which
quadrants are involved and whether a central or
paracentral defect is present. The technique of con-
frontational visual field testing will be presented after
a description of field defects.

SHAPE OF THE VISUAL FIELD DEFECT

The shape of the defect corresponds to the morphology of the fiber bundles in the afferent pathways.
This morphology is unique for each part of the CNS,
and the details for each part are discussed in the
particular sections on each locus. The shape of the
defect is thus one of the most important features of
the visual field.

DENSITY OF THE FIELD DEFECT

The density or severity of light sensitivity loss in the
field defect gives some indication of the etiology. This
is not as fine a distinction as some of the other features;
however, vascular lesions, especially infarctions, generally produce dense or severe defects. Tumors, in particular the slowly growing ones, tend, on the other
hand, to produce field defects of lesser severity, because the tissue is more likely to be affected in a graded
manner.

CONGRUITY OF THE VISUAL FIELD DEFECT

For a single lesion behind the chiasm, congruity refers
to the degree to which both the density and extent of
the defects are similar in the two eyes. This has practical meaning only for subtotal homonymous field
defects. Total hemianopia is often associated with complete tract lesions as well as with complete calcarine
infarctions; total hemianopia, therefore, has no localizing value apart from placing the lesion behind the
chiasm.

To understand congruity, it is necessary to imagine
the overlapping fields of the two eyes, a condition
effected by the binocular fusion of the foveal repre-
sentations of the two eyes (Fig. 23-4). Within the
binocular field, every point in visual space is regis-
tered by a particular ganglion cell in each eye (an
example is point AB in Fig. 23-4).

Lesions of the optic tract characteristically produce
incongruous field defects; a monocular *hemianopia* is
one extreme case. In the optic tract, the ganglion cell
axons serving receptive fields for the homologous
points in visual space are not necessarily adjacent to
one another. Hence, a disease process may affect the
axon from one eye serving a particular point in binocular visual space without affecting the axon for the
homologous point in visual space from the other eye.
Axons A and B are shown separate from one another
in the left optic tract in the midportion of Figure 23-4.

The calcarine cortex, area 17 of Brodmann, is organized so that the axons from homologous points in
space (here the axons are those of lateral geniculate
cells) project to the same column of cortical cells. A
cortical disease will, therefore, affect the visual fields
of the two eyes in exactly the same way, producing
congruous defects.

Lesions in the geniculocalcarine pathways produce
an intermediate degree of congruity, thus this feature
is much less reliable in determining the anteroposterior position of lesions than is the case with tract and
cortex lesions. The geniculocalcarine projections A
and B are shown in Figure 23-4 as being separate
anteriorly, near the geniculate body. They converge
progressively as they near their point of entry into the
calcarine cortex.

SLOPE OF THE VISUAL FIELD DEFECT

The slope of a visual field defect refers to the amount
of lateral increase in the defect's size with a reduction of stimulus visibility. A steeply sloping region
changes little in horizontal dimension with a major
reduction in stimulus visibility. A gently sloping area
of defect becomes much larger with reduced visibility. A gentle slope thus denotes a region of transition
between a severe dysfunction and a milder dysfunction in the visual pathways. The marginal area of
field, which is sensitive enough to see the more visible target but which is reduced in sensitivity and
unable to see the less visible target, is what constitutes
the sloping region.

Gentle slope denotes change. Vascular lesions that are
healing and tumors that are advancing will have a
dense core of total dysfunction surrounded by an area

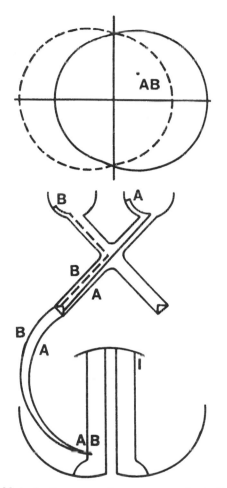

FIG. 23-4. A diagrammatic representation of the binocular visual fields and the afferent fibers serving a point in binocular visual space, point *AB* in the upper figure. A hypothetical photoreceptor, *A* in the right eye and *B* in the left eye, connects with the central nervous system by way of a ganglion cell axon from each eye, also labeled *A* and *B*, respectively. The ganglion cell axon from the right eye crosses in the chiasm (point *AB* is in the temporal field of that eye), while that from the left passes through to the ipsilateral optic tract (point *AB* is in the nasal field of that eye). Each ganglion cell axon synapses in the left lateral geniculate body and second-order neuron axons continue in the geniculocalcarine radiations to the occipital cortex, area 17 in the bottom figure (see text for further explanation).

of relative dysfunction, probably related to tissue compression and edema. This gradual transition to normal function in afferent pathways brings about the gentle slope to the visual field defect. Old vascular lesions in which the dense core of infarcted tissue remains, but in which the surrounding pathways have returned to normal sensitivity, are characterized by a *steeply sloped* transition from defective to normal field. The defect in Figure 23-5A is gently sloping in the right lower quadrant, typical of a fresh infarct or hemorrhage with surrounding edema. The defect in Figure 23-5B is steeply sloping in the same region, as would be expected of an old infarct in which the necrotic zone leaves a field defect of absolute density, but in which the transition to normal function is abrupt. The slope is readable only in subtotal *hemianopia* in which there is some sparing of either upper or lower sectors. The slope should also be analyzed only along the margin of the defect, where there is the opportunity of transition to normal across a gradient (i.e., adjacent to the spared sector). There is almost always an abrupt transition at the vertical hemianopic midline, because here the lesion has produced maximal effects in the involved half field and has no opportunity of causing *any* defect in the other half field because the other half is served by the opposite cerebral hemisphere. The transition at the vertical midline is *always* steep, and here no information is provided on the temporal course of the lesion.

TOPICAL FEATURES OF THE VISUAL FIELDS

RETINA AND OPTIC NERVE

Figure 23-6 indicates the arrangement of ganglion cell axons in the retina and optic nerve. Bundles of axons coming into the optic nerve from all sides follow a converging course from ganglion cells widely distributed in the retina. On the nasal side of the optic disc (left side in the figure), the bundles have a straight trajectory in the form of a wedge whose apex is at the optic nerve head. Accordingly, interruption of a nasal retinal bundle gives rise to a wedge-shaped visual field defect with the apex at the *physiologic blind spot*. This normal blind spot in the visual field corresponds to the optic nerve head, where there are no photoreceptors. The papillomacular bundle (region 1 in Fig. 23-6) occupies most of the temporal side of the optic nerve head. Because of this, ganglion cells in the periphery of the retina on the temporal side of the fovea must send their axons in an arcuate course (regions 2 in the figure) around the papillomacular bundle to gain access to the optic nerve at the upper and lower poles.

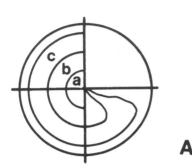
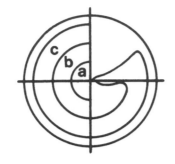

A

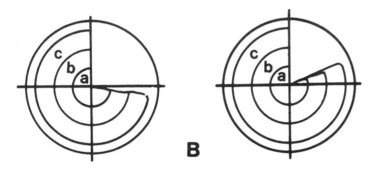

B

FIG. 23-5. **A.** A *gently sloped* right homonymous upper quadrant defect. The extent of field defect for isopters *a* and *b* is greater than for *c* in the right lower quadrant. **B.** A *steeply sloped* defect. The extent of all isopters is the same. The defects in *A* and *B* are also *incongruous.*

Embryologically, the fovea began at the margin of the retina. With development, invagination carried the fovea toward its adult position near the optic nerve with final fusion of the upper and lower halves of the retinal margin that formed the invagination. The embryonic discontinuity between the upper and lower halves in the temporal retina is reflected in the adult distribution of retinal ganglion cell axons. The term *temporal raphe* is used to denote the imaginary line separating the upper and lower halves of the temporal retina.

All the ganglion cells immediately above the raphe must send their axons into the upper pole of the disc via the upper arcuate region, while all the ganglion cells below the raphe are constrained to send their axons into the lower pole via the inferior arcuate region.

This forced discontinuity provides for arcuate visual field defects with an abrupt transition to normal at the *nasal horizontal midline* (the famous *nasal step*). It is typical of glaucoma to produce these arcu-

ate defects with nasal steps; they were described long ago by Bjerrum and are still referred to by his name.

The location and shape of visual field defects are potent indicators of the site of an optic nerve lesion but also give some indication of etiology. Ischemia of either the retina or the optic nerve tends to produce upper- or lower-half field defects that "respect" or have a sharp border along the horizontal midline of the visual field. These are called *altitudinal* field defects and can be thought of as extended arcuate bundle defects in which the temporal quadrant is affected as well as the nasal quadrant. Since there is no *retinal raphe* serving the temporal quadrant, the reason for the sharp border at the horizontal midline must be sought in the patterns of vascular supply.

The reason for altitudinal-type field defects is intuitive for the case of inner retinal infarction, since the retina is supplied by an upper and a lower primary branch of the central retinal artery and selective branch occlusion may occur [*branch retinal artery occlusion* (BRAO)]. The altitudinal quality of visual field

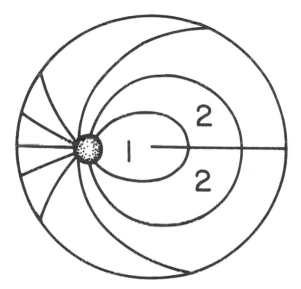

FIG. 23-6. The arrangement of retinal ganglion cell axons in a left eye fundus. Region 1 is the *papillomacular bundle* serving foveal function. Region 2 is the *arcuate bundle* or *Bjerrum region*, where ganglion cell axons from the temporal retinal periphery arch over the massive papillomacular bundle.

defects in ischemia of the optic nerve [*acute anterior ischemic optic neuropathy* (AION)] is more difficult to understand, however, since the anterior optic nerve is supplied by an array of arterioles that stem from an anastomotic vascular circle just behind the globe (the *circle of Zinn and Haller*). This arterial circle is in turn supplied by a variable number (two to five) of *short posterior ciliary arteries* that supply the nerve head and the adjacent vascular choroid layer of the eyeball. It has been suggested that sector infarction of the optic nerve head occurs when there is critically low perfusion in the ciliary distribution and a watershed zone between adjacent posterior ciliary artery choroidal vascular territories cuts across the optic nerve head. The orientation of these watershed zones does not always conform to an upper- or lower-half distribution, and this seems to leave the stereotyped altitudinal character of the resulting visual field defects unexplained.

Another common optic neuropathy is *optic neuritis* of the demyelinating type, which is strongly associated with multiple sclerosis. We used to teach that the most common type of visual field defect in optic neuritis is the central scotoma, a roughly circular area of

low visual sensitivity centered on the fixation point. The scotoma may be large enough to engulf the physiologic blind spot, and then it is called a *centro-cecal* scotoma. The recently concluded *Optic Neuritis Treatment Trial* (ONTT), in which 448 patients with optic neuritis were randomly assigned to different treatment groups, provided a unique opportunity to study the visual field and other clinical characteristics of the disease. Among affected eyes at onset, 48.2% had diffuse field loss, but among those with focal defects (the remaining 51.8%), the most common pattern was *altitudinal* in 15%. The investigators concluded that the morphology of field loss is an unreliable criterion for differentiating optic neuritis from ischemic optic neuropathy. Differentiating features include pain exacerbated by eye movement, subacute evolution, and visual field abnormalities in the fellow eye, all of which are frequent in patients with optic neuritis. Features suggestive of AION include more acute onset, lack of pain, and upper- or lower-half swelling of the optic disc with flame hemorrhages.

OPTIC CHIASM

Axons from ganglion cells on either side of the retinal hemianopic midline, which run a mingled course in the optic nerve, separate at the optic chiasm (Fig. 23-7A). This divergence of pathways is the anatomic feature that creates the *hemianopic midline* and determines the existence of field defects that *respect* the midline (i.e., the lateral half-field defects that denote lesions at and behind the optic chiasm).

Fibers from the inferior retina (i.e., the upper temporal visual field) loop forward in the opposite optic nerve as they cross the midline. A lesion at the posterior end of one optic nerve will first encounter these inferonasal fibers of the other eye at the chiasm junction, which creates a distinctive combination of field defects in the two eyes (Fig. 23-7B1). The field defect ipsilateral to the lesion is any of those typical for optic nerve disease (a central scotoma or other nerve fiber bundle defect). In the opposite eye there will be a midline respecting upper temporal defect, or "pie in the sky" defect according to J. Lawton Smith. This is the *anterior junctional syndrome* of the chiasm.

Some fibers from the nasal retina, especially papillomacular bundle fibers, loop backward in the ipsilateral optic tract before crossing. Thus, a lesion at the junction of the posterior chiasm and optic tract will produce a characteristic *posterior junctional syndrome* of the chiasm (Fig. 23-7B3). The basic defect is a homonymous *hemianopia* contralateral to the lesion. *Homonymous* means that the hemifield defect is on the same side in both eyes. A left tract lesion, for instance,

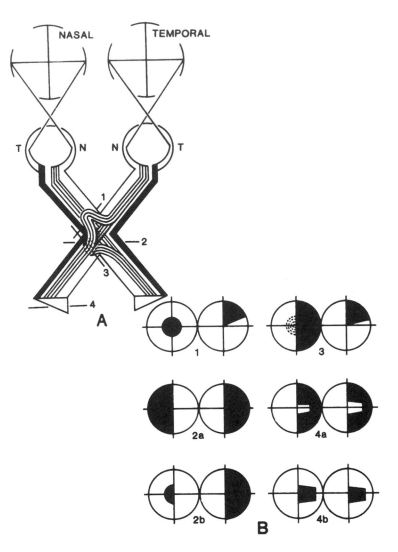

FIG. 23-7. The optic chiasm region. **A.** The arrangement of crossing and noncrossing fibers. Inferior nasal fibers from the right eye loop forward into the left optic nerve before continuing back in the left optic tract. Papillomacular bundle fibers from the left eye loop backward into the ipsilateral optic tract before decussating into the right optic tract. Lesions at levels 1, 2, and 3 produce characteristic field defects that are illustrated in **B.** *B1* is the anterior chiasm junctional syndrome; *B2a* is a typical midchiasm bitemporal field defect; *B2b* is a variation with a scotomatous temporal field defect in the left eye and a peripheral temporal defect in the right; *B3* is a posterior chiasm–tract junctional syndrome; *B4a* is an anterior choroidal artery–geniculate infarct.

gives rise to a right-sided field defect in either eye (the defect is in the nasal half field of the left eye and is also in the temporal half field of the right eye). As the tract lesion spreads anteriorly and encounters the posterior chiasm, the first chiasmal fibers affected are those from the ipsilateral nasal retina that loop back into the tract before crossing. These fibers serve central vision because the papillomacular bundle crosses in the posterior chiasm. Thus, in the ipsilateral eye there is the nasal *hemifield* defect that is part of the homonymous pair, plus some loss of *central temporal field* secondary to

the involvement of the posterior looping nasal retinal fibers. The field defect thus involves both sides of the foveal field in the ipsilateral eye and reduces the visual acuity, whereas the purely hemianopic defect in the temporal field of the opposite eye leaves acuity normal, in accord with the axioms previously described.

The typical central chiasmal defects will now be considered. Most symptomatic lesions of the chiasm are tumors, and most of these encounter the chiasm from below. *Chiasmal compression is most often accompanied by bitemporal visual field defects.* The crossing fibers are apparently least able to tolerate mass effects, probably because they are *tethered* across the middle, whereas the uncrossed fibers are free to splay out over the mass. Whatever the mechanism, nine times out of ten, compression of the chiasm will first cause midline-respecting temporal field defects in both eyes. This can involve any combination of central (scotomatous) defects and peripheral defects in the two eyes. The most common variations for chiasmal field defects are demonstrated in Figure 23-7B2a,b.

LATERAL GENICULATE BODY

Two highly characteristic field defects caused by vascular lesions of the lateral geniculate body are shown in Figure 23-7B. Frisén has provided elaborate detail on the dual vascular supply of the geniculate by the *anterior choroidal* and the *lateral (posterior) choroidal* arteries. Anterior choroidal artery occlusion can be associated with upper and lower quadrant homonymous defects that spare a rectangular area along the horizontal midline (Fig. 23-7B4a). Lateral choroidal artery occlusion has been associated with a rectangular homonymous scotoma along the horizontal midline (Fig. 23-7B4b)—the exact complement of the other geniculate syndrome.

GENICULOCALCARINE RADIATIONS

Figure 23-8 illustrates how the axonal outflow from the lateral geniculate radiates within the deep white matter of the cerebral hemispheres. These radiations form a thin band just external to the lateral ventricle. They take the form of a ribbon that is broad in the vertical plane but very thin in the horizontal plane (Fig. 23-8A,B). Thus, lesions must extend deep into the white matter to encounter the geniculocalcarine radiations.

Parietal lobe lesions encounter the upper radiations on the way to the upper bank of the calcarine cortex (area 1 in Fig. 23-8B) and cause inferior quadrantic homonymous visual field defects. Temporal lobe lesions interfere with the anterior looping fibers that are destined for the lower bank of the calcarine cortex (area 3 in Fig. 23-8B) and produce upper quadrantic homonymous field defects. The anterior temporal contingent of fibers in the geniculocalcarine radiations is called *Meyer's loop* after Adolph Meyer who described them.

CALCARINE CORTEX

A semifinal way station in the afferent system is the primary visual cortex, area 17 of Brodmann on the mesial surface of the occipital lobe. The localization of lesions can be very precise here, because of the sometimes-restricted nature of the lesions. Small infarcts from branch occlusions of the calcarine artery may produce exceedingly localized, but always congruous, homonymous field defects.

There are two basic axes of localization: from anterior to posterior in the calcarine cortex, and from lip to depth of the calcarine fissure (Figs. 23-8, 23-9). The anteroposterior dimension translates to an axis from center (fixation point) to periphery in the visual fields (see Fig. 23-8C). The fixation area is represented at the posterior end of the calcarine cortex, a portion of which wraps around onto the convexity of the occipital pole. The periphery of the visual field is represented at the anterior end of the calcarine fissure, near the splenium of the corpus callosum.

Sparing of the visual field, either at the center or at the far periphery, is a useful sign that localizes a homonymous *hemianopia* to the occipital cortex.

Central Sparing, or Sparing of Fixation

Many cases of *hemianopia* result from infarction of calcarine cortex with occlusion or stenosis of the posterior cerebral artery. The occipital pole receives a collateral blood supply from the middle cerebral artery and may be spared when the flow in the posterior cerebral artery reaches a critical status, and infarction occurs in the more anterior portions of the calcarine cortex.

Testing for this spared circle around fixation can best be done at the tangent screen, or even on a wall, as long as a vertical line through the fixation point can be drawn or imagined. The problem with eliciting fixation sparing is the fact that patients often shift their gaze a few degrees to either side of fixation, and the examiner cannot always see these little eye movements. Of course, the whole hemianopic midline will shift with the angle of gaze, and the patient may then seem capable of perceiving test objects a little way into his hemianopic field.

The examiner should use two vertically aligned test spots to avoid mistaking these ocular refixations for *central sparing*. Most instances of "central sparing" from occipital lobe lesions involve an area no larger than 5 to 15 degrees in diameter, so the examiner should present the two stimulus spots vertically aligned, bringing one inward along the horizontal midline and the other one 20 degrees above or below the central one. The patient is asked to call out "one" or "two" when he first sees any test spot, depending on how many spots he sees. Under these test conditions, if the patient says "two," there has

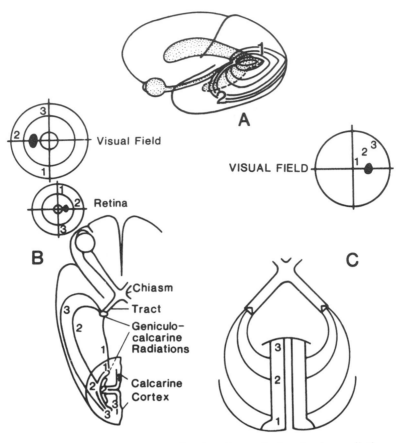

FIG. 23-8. A. Lateral view of the brain showing the geniculocalcarine radiations emanating from a focal point deep to the lateral ventricle (the location of the lateral geniculate body) and fanning out to occupy the parietal and temporal lobes on the way to the calcarine cortex. The anterior looping contingent in the temporal lobe is called *Meyer's loop.* **B.** Diagram of the geniculocalcarine radiations in a mixed horizontal and coronal section of the brain (*lower figure*) together with a diagram of the left eye retina (*middle figure*) and corresponding left eye visual field (*upper figure*). The numbers correlate lesion locations in the lower figure with affected retinal and visual fields in the middle and upper figures, respectively. **C.** A horizontal section through the calcarine cortex is depicted in the lower figure, with successive zones from the left occipital pole to the anterior end of the left calcarine cortex numbered 1 through 3. Corresponding zones in the right visual field are shown in the *upper figure.* The fixation area is represented at the occipital pole, and the periphery of the visual field is represented at the anterior end of the calcarine cortex (see text and Fig. 23-9 for further details).

been a shift of the whole hemianopic midline; if the patient says "one," then the central target has fallen into a circular area of real central sparing whereas the other (above or below) is still in a hemianopic field.

Sparing of the Unpaired Temporal Crescent

The nasal field (with a maximal extent of 60°) is smaller than the temporal field (with a maximal extent of 75° to 80°) in both eyes. Therefore, with

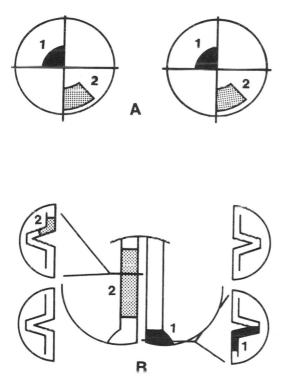

FIG. 23-9. Two practice field defects are depicted in **A.** The corresponding localization in the calcarine cortex is shown in **B.** both in the horizontal plane (*central figure*) and in the coronal plane (*lateral figures*).

binocular fusion, there is a large area of binocular field, beyond which is a crescent of 20° or so in which the temporal field of one eye has no corresponding nasal field of the other—this is the *unpaired temporal crescent*. Posterior cerebral lesions, basically those in the occipital lobe, may spare the anterior fibers of the geniculocalcarine radiations and the anterior calcarine cortex, leaving some preserved peripheral field in an otherwise dense and complete homonymous hemianopia. If the extent of preserved periphery is all beyond 60° of eccentricity, there will be no corresponding nasal field spared in one eye, and the spared crescent of field will exist only in the eye with the temporal field on the side of the hemianopia.

Imagine a right occipital lesion and a dense left homonymous hemianopia. There is some sparing of the unpaired crescent. This means that the left eye, which has its temporal field on the left (the side of

the hemianopia), will perceive objects in the far periphery, but the right eye (with nasal field toward the hemianopic side) will have no peripheral sparing.

This sparing of the unpaired crescent is an important sign of occipital localization in hemianopia. It can be detected most consistently with confrontation techniques. I have seen several patients with *total* homonymous hemianopia by perimetry who can perceive hand motion in the far temporal periphery of the one eye but not in the nasal periphery of the other. When testing for this, the patient should cover one eye at a time and the examiner should extend his arm beside and just behind the patient's head on the side of the patient's hemianopia. The examiner should bring his hand forward, wave it up and down, or wiggle his fingers. This motion can be a more potent stimulus for the far visual periphery than light.

The other important dimension for occipital localization is a series of sectors extending from the *lip* of the calcarine fissure, which faces the opposite occipital cortex across the inter-hemispheric fissure, to the *depth* of the calcarine fissure. The corresponding visual field dimension is a series of pie-shaped sectors extending from an apex at fixation to a broader base at the periphery. The sector abutting the *vertical hemianopic midline* corresponds to the lip of the calcarine cortex, and the sector abutting the *horizontal midline* corresponds to the depth of the calcarine cortex. Intermediate field and tissue sectors lie between these limits. The upper bank (lip to depth) serves the inferior homonymous field quadrant, and the lower bank (lip to depth) serves the superior quadrant. Thus, we have a dimension that extends all the way around one half of the visual field from the upper vertical midline through the horizontal midline to the lower vertical midline in a series of pie-shaped sectors. The more sectors the pie is divided into, the more pieces there are, and the finer the localization. At the cortex, this dimension flows from the inferior lip of one (right or left) calcarine cortex by way of the depth of the calcarine fissure to the upper lip.

Once the location of the pie-shaped sector has been established, localization within the sector should be established along the dimension from fixation to periphery, which is from occipital pole to anterior calcarine cortex.

An exercise in calcarine cortex localization is shown in Figure 23-9. Two small field defects, one in the left upper quadrant, the other in the right lower, are depicted. A horizontal section through the calcarine cortex is flanked on either side by coronal sections in Figure 23-9B. Consider first lesion 1. It extends to fixation, but not far into the periphery; thus, in the horizontal section, it is represented at the pole with little anterior extension. It occupies a series of pie-shaped sectors all the way from the vertical midline to the horizontal midline. In the coronal section to the right, the lesion extends all the way from the inferior lip to the depth of the calcarine cortex. The lesion must be in the inferior bank because the field defect is in the upper quadrant.

The reader should try to map the lesion that would accompany field defect 2 in Figure 23-9A before reading on or looking at the answer in Figure 23-9B. Set up the cortical diagrams as in Figure 23-9B and draw in the lesion.

The field defect caused by lesion 2 does not extend to fixation or to the periphery; hence, the lesion is in the middle of the calcarine cortex in the horizontal section, extending neither to the pole nor to the anterior end. The field defect occupies pie-shaped sectors abutting the inferior vertical midline but not extending all the way to the horizontal midline. The lesion, therefore, is in the upper bank of the left calcarine cortex; it involves the lip but does not extend all the way to the depth of the calcarine fissure.

It is fun to draw these diagrams and take them to the radiologist as you read the computed tomography (CT) scan or the magnetic resonance imaging (MRI) results. Small cortical lesions can often be identified that were radiographically questionable without the ironclad visual field correlation.

CONFRONTATION VISUAL FIELD EXAMINATION

Many patients must be tested with confrontation techniques because their overall condition and lack of mobility preclude formal testing. Bedside methods are most practical for physicians other than ophthalmologists.

Confrontation test results must be used in a special way, however, because they do not have the specificity or the quantitative detail of well-done perimetry. Nonetheless, confrontation results can indicate the proper direction for a further workup and may thereby save a great deal of time and expense.

This method is called *confrontation* because the examiner faces the patient and presents targets while he watches the patient's eyes. Eye movement during examination is a problem, as with all visual field testing, and the examiner must be able to monitor fixation. It is best always to start with the right eye, because it will be easier to remember the sequence of findings and to relate them to the correct side when recording the results.

Ask the patient to cover his left eye with the palm of his left hand, and be sure that the fingers are all the way up onto the forehead so that no peeking is possible between them. To peek is human. The examiner faces the patient and closes his right eye so his open left eye is directly in front of the patient's right eye (being tested). The patient is asked to fix his gaze on the examiner's open eye. In this configuration, the examiner can watch for small eye movements and monitor fixation. Also, the patient's and examiner's hemianopic midlines are aligned, so the examiner can determine if a visual field defect "respects" that midline. The setup is reversed to test the patient's left eye.

The presentation of targets follows. The best initial test is *finger counting*. Although form resolution is the key function of the fovea, motion detection is performed with great sensitivity by the peripheral visual system. A waving motion of the hand or a wiggling of the fingers is, therefore, the grossest stimulus one can present to the periphery. This means that peripheral field function must be almost gone before there is failure to detect motion. Motion, then, is too gross a stimulus to be sensitive, and thus it is not the ideal screening test. Form discrimination, on the other hand, is poorly done in the peripheral parts of the visual field. Thus, finger counting, which requires spatial analysis of a stationary form, is a sensitive test for peripheral dysfunction—it will be abnormal with only minor reduction of field function.

Fingers should be presented *en face* to the patient. Obviously, the patient must be able to see all the fingers to make it a valid test, and if you orient your hand so that all the fingers are lined up one behind the other from the patient's perspective, he will be unable to count them.

The test can be done quickly. All that is necessary is to present enough combinations of fingers to be sure the patient is not succeeding by guesswork. Combinations should include all fingers, one, two, or none—it is difficult to present three fingers because of the way the tendons in our hands are arranged. Present the combination once in each of the four quadrants and then go around again in a random sequence of quadrants. Two presentations for each quadrant should be sufficient. If errors are made, then more presentations may be required to be sure whether an apparent defect is real.

Some quantitation of confrontation fields is possible, although it will never match formal quantitative perimetry. If the fingers are counted correctly in all quadrants, there may still be a field defect. First, some defects are scotomas occupying only the central 10° to 20° field. Finger counting will often miss these defects. Second, the degree of peripheral defect may be so minor that fingers are still adequately counted.

Color perception is an extremely sensitive, though subjective, measure of visual field dysfunction. It is common for patients to report that colors are less vivid in defective field areas—they seldom mention this, but they will agree to it when specifically asked. Present a fairly large bright red object in the four quadrants and ask the patient if there is any difference in the redness of the object in any field. *Desaturation* is the term applied to a subjective loss of color intensity in the defective field. Patients may report that the reds are shifted to a darker amber color, or bleached toward a lighter, pinkish, or yellowish color; however, in either case, the stimulus is perceived as *less red*. Try to avoid the term *brightness,* because it is a separate parameter of visual function and should be inquired about separately.

If color saturation is lost in a quadrant, the boundaries should be explored by moving the test red object and by asking the patient to indicate quickly if it becomes *redder*. The most important area to screen is the vertical midline. To do this, two red spots, one on either side of the midline, may be presented either above or below the examiner's eye (i.e., the fixation point), and the patient should be invited to compare the redness of the two spots. This may bring out a difference across the midline that the patient was unable to describe by viewing the spot sequentially in different quadrants. The examiner should then present one red spot as a stationary target in the normal quadrant and he should move the other spot horizontally from the defective field. The patient is told to indicate immediately when the two spots become equal in redness, and the examiner determines if this transition corresponds to the vertical hemianopic midline. The examiner easily senses the location of the midline: It is an imaginary vertical line through the examiner's line of sight to the patient's eye.

If the patient has trouble counting fingers in a defective field, then other stimuli can be presented to determine the relative density of the defect. Moving fingers or a waving hand is a grosser stimulus than stationary fingers. If motion is not detected, a bright light may be moved within the defect and its margins plotted to light.

Thus, we can develop a hierarchy of stimuli by which to grade the density of a visual field defect. From most intense to least, this hierarchy of stimuli is ordered as follows:

1. Moving light
2. Moving hand or fingers
3. Finger counting
4. Subjective judgment of color saturation

Using the hierarchy, one can even derive information on the relative slope of the defect. Consider a patient who is unable to perceive light or hand motion in the upper right field, who is able to see movement, but who is unable to count fingers in the lower right field. This finding would indicate a *hemianopia* that is denser in the upper than in the lower quadrant; in other words, there is a sloping defect with a transition from an upper to a lower field.

PUPILLARY SYSTEM

The eye has many structures and functions that are analogous to those of a camera, and the eye shares some common optical requirements with the latter. Among them is the capacity to limit the amount of light entering the optical system; this is a function of the adjustable camera diaphragm. The iris of the eye is essentially an opaque diaphragm with an adjustable central opening (i.e., the pupil). Diameter adjustments are accomplished by coordinated action of the concentrically arranged sphincter muscle together with a set of radially oriented dilator fibers. The sphincter is a 1-mm-wide band of smooth muscle surrounding the pupillary margin. The radial fibers, also smooth muscle, originate at the iris root near the limbus of the cornea, and insert within the collagenous substance of the iris near the pupil and the sphincter muscle. Although the sphincter is innervated by the parasympathetic nervous system and the dilators are innervated by the sympathetic system, the two muscle groups function together as an organized unit; that is, when the sphincter is activated, the dilators are concomitantly inhibited at the CNS level. There is always a resting tonus in both systems—they are in a state of mutual opposition when the pupil is at rest. Of the two groups, however, the sphincter is stronger and tends to dominate the equilibrium determining pupil size at average levels of illumination. This is in accordance with the common observation that anticholinergic sphincter inhibitors, such as tropicamide (Mydriacyl), are much stronger pupil dilators than are sympathomimetics such as phenylephrine.

EXAMINATION OF THE PUPILS

PUPIL SHAPE

Under normal circumstances, the entire sphincter/dilator network functions in a coordinated manner and the pupil margin remains round as diameter changes occur. There are pathologic states, however, in which an altered function in the CNS brings about unequal contraction and dilatation of the pupil in various sectors. Wilson called this condition *corectopia pupillae* or *ectopic pupil*. This condition might involve either unequal segmental sphincter contraction or independent activation of a small sector of the dilator fibers. Irregular pupils are, however, more commonly the result of direct iris muscle damage, as in trauma or infection in the eye.

PUPIL SIZE AND REACTIVITY

The diameter of the pupil at any particular time reflects the coordinated activity of the sphincter and the dilator systems. As already mentioned, the former is the stronger of the two but can be overcome in the presence of a massive increase in dilator tone caused by activation of the sympathetic system. The adequate sensory stimulus for activating the sphincter is light falling on the retina, whereas "psychosensory" inputs cause dilator activation by way of the sympathetic nervous system. Pupil size tends to be small in infants, with progressive enlargement through early childhood, and eventual return to a smaller diameter in the elderly.

In a fixed ambient light, the pupils constrict as the subject becomes drowsy, and they dilate with arousal or startle. Fear and anxiety are thus commonly associated with larger-than-average pupils for a particular light level. Dilator system activation resulting from anxiety can even inhibit the pupil's contraction in response to light. When testing pupil function, it is common to obtain only a small response to the first series of light stimuli. The amplitude of contraction usually increases as the patient becomes less fearful and more relaxed with the situation. One should never conclude that the pupils are nonreactive or sluggish until several stimuli have been delivered and the patient has been put *at ease,* if possible. This anxiety-related fixity of the pupil seldom lasts more than 20 or 30 seconds under usual conditions.

Pharmacologic agents can cause prominent effects on the size of the pupil. This subject is too vast for review, but some examples are worthy of mention. Glutethimide (Doriden) is a sedative/hypnotic drug that is sometimes the causative agent in drug overdose cases. In toxic doses, it characteristically causes widely dilated pupils that do not react to light or near effort. Opiates generally cause small pupils, as do sedative drugs. Therefore, in coma resulting from an overdose with opiates, barbiturates, and other sedative/hypnotic drugs (except glutethimide), pupils that are widely dilated should raise suspicion of anoxic damage to the CNS secondary to ventilatory suppression. The effects of atropinic substances introduced directly into the eye are discussed later. Systematically administered sympathomimetics can cause widely dilated pupils, but this is seldom observed clinically. Such a finding has occasionally been described among patients taking levodopa for treatment of Parkinson's disease. Pupillary dilatation occurs with the systemic administration of amphetamines, most commonly in the setting of drug abuse. The size of pupils in all of these situations, however, may reflect the psychic state of the patient due to factors other than the presence of pharmacologically active substances in the system. Furthermore, the examiner must have considerable experience to know the range of expected pupil sizes among normal persons in the usually varying sorts of illumination in which patients are examined. The light intensity in the examination area is uncontrolled in most cases; thus judgments about pupil size are often unreliable. Fortunately, in most cases, anisocoria or asymmetry of pupil diameter is more important for a diagnosis than is absolute pupil size.

TECHNIQUE OF PUPIL EXAMINATION

Every physician should take time to define a certain reproducible type of lighting in which he will always perform his pupil examination. As his experience increases, he will better be able to assess whether a patient's pupils are abnormally large or small. The ideal area is one that can be both brightly and dimly illuminated in a standard way. Bright light causes relative activation of the sphincter system and can enhance anisocoria resulting from parasympathetic (i.e., third cranial nerve) system lesions. Similarly, dim light shifts the balance of tone to the sympathetically innervated dilator systems and may serve to uncover anisocoria caused by Horner's (oculosympathetic) syndrome. The pupils in Horner's syndrome may even be equal in bright light.

Thus, the degree of anisocoria, or the *difference* between diameters of the pupils in defined dim and bright light, is important in pupil diagnosis. Approximately 15% of normal individuals have anisocoria of up to 1 mm without any lesion in either the sympathetic or parasympathetic systems. The difference in size remains the same in bright and dim lighting, which serves to distinguish this *physiologic anisocoria* from pathologic states. Irene Loewenfeld calls this "simple central or see-saw anisocoria" and notes that the degree of difference may vary or the smaller pupil may even reverse sides over the course of minutes, days, or weeks.

The light reaction is usually observed with the patient in a dim room. Contraction of the sphincter is evoked by shining a bright light into each eye for 0.5 to 2 seconds at a time. The most commonly used light source is a penlight, but any bright light that can be directed into one eye at a time will do. Penlights tend to become dim rapidly and also to flicker because of cheap on/off switches. The Finoff head is an angled carrier that attaches a halogen bulb to the battery handle of the ophthalmoscope. It provides a bright, steady light source that is ideal for testing the pupil. It is a small accessory that is easy to carry in the examining bag along with the ophthalmoscope and otoscope.

Light delivered to one eye causes equal contraction of both pupils. The *direct* light response refers to pupil constriction in the eye stimulated, and the *consensual* response is that which occurs when the eye opposite the observed pupil is illuminated.

The contraction of the pupils to near stimulation should be approximately as brisk and extensive as that to light. This contraction is best elicited by having the patient attempt to focus on his own thumb held about 2 or 3 cm from his nose. The resulting proprioceptive cues, together with common narcissistic tendencies, make this a more compelling target for *near effort* than any external object, even the examiner's finger. Simple *awareness of near* is said to be an effective stimulus for activation of the neurally linked *near triad*. This triad consists of (1) pupillary constriction, (2) (crystalline) lens accommodation (increase of plus lens power to focus at close range), and (3) convergence of the optic axes (to maintain binocular fusion on a near object). There is often pupil constriction even if the patient does not make any convergent eye movements or accommodative changes in the lens of the eye.

FORMAT FOR REPORTING THE PUPIL EXAMINATION

The notation "pupils equal, round, regular, and reactive to light and accommodation (PERRLA)" is best avoided except under battlefield conditions, when the main distinction to be drawn is between the living and the dead. Many cases do not demand an intense, systematic examination of the pupil, so abbreviated formats are sometimes warranted. A good brief form is presented in Table 23-1. The *near reaction* is not included in the brief examination, as it is generally unimportant if the light response is normal. The important *light/near dissociated* pupils, which will be discussed later, involve a failure of the light reaction with preservation of the near response (never the reverse). When the pupil is the central issue for a clinical case, extended notation can used, as shown in Table 23-2.

TABLE 23-1. Brief Form for Pupil Examination

PUPIL	SIZE IN DIM LIGHT (MM)	LIGHT REACTION	RELATIVE AFFERENT PUPILLARY DEFECT
Right	5	Brisk	None
Left	5	Brisk	None

OVERVIEW OF CENTRAL PUPILLARY PATHWAYS

The importance of the pupil in neurologic diagnosis rests on the fact that structures determining pupil size and motility occupy extensive portions of the CNS in addition to the circuitous pathways of the peripheral ocular sympathetic innervation in the head and neck. Lesions in widely separated portions of the body will thus lead to specific disorders of pupil function.

The cerebral hemispheres probably contribute to pupil tone, although (for practical purposes) the hemispheres do not have localizing pupillary significance, because lesions and irritative states at this level do not produce any reliable changes in the pupils. It is useful to envision the pupillary motor systems as reflex arcs analogous to those in the spinal cord. Each system (parasympathetic and sympathetic) has an afferent side and a motor side to its reflex arc, which is similar to the organization at the segmental level. The optimal afferent stimuli, however, are different in the two systems. This is discussed later in more detail, but stated briefly, the parasympathetic system operates the pupillary reaction to light falling on the retinas, whereas the dilator system functions in response to *psychosensory* inputs.

The afferent arc of the parasympathetic reflex is mediated by way of inputs from the retina to the midbrain, where connections exist with the Edinger-Westphal subnucleus of the third cranial nerve nucleus. The motor side is mediated by way of axons of the Edinger-Westphal nucleus passing in the third cranial nerve to the ciliary ganglion, where synapses with the postganglionic fibers are found. These postganglionic fibers form neuromuscular junctions with the pupillary sphincter muscle.

Within the sympathetic system, the afferent arcs come from ascending sensory pathways, with collateral branches to the brainstem and diencephalic reticular formation. Inputs from the cerebral hemisphere are not anatomically well defined, but they probably feed into the descending reticular system, perhaps at the hypothalamic level along with other

TABLE 23-2. Complete Form for Pupil Examination

PUPIL	SIZE IN DIM LIGHT (MM)	SIZE IN BRIGHT LIGHT (MM)	LIGHT RX (D/C)	NEAR RX	RELATIVE AFFERENT PUPILLARY DEFECT
Right	5	3	3+/3+	3+	None
Left	5	3	3+/3+	3+	0.6 log[a]

D = direct; C = consensual.

[a] Quantitation of relative afferent pupillary defect (RAPD) using neutral density (gray) filters over the better-seeing eye.

limbic–diencephalic interfaces. The efferent side is mediated by way of descending polysynaptic pathways within the brainstem and spinal cord, which then make contact with preganglionic neurons, the cell bodies of which are in the intermediolateral cell column of the spinal cord. The preganglionic and postganglionic fibers for the sympathetic system follow a complex pathway through the head and neck to reach the iris dilator fibers.

This brief overview will serve to emphasize that there is tremendous diversity of sensory inputs to the pupil systems. These afferent pathways, together with pupillomotor efferent pathways, occupy an extensive and functionally critical portion of the nervous system.

PARASYMPATHETIC PUPIL SYSTEM (LIGHT REFLEX)

The parasympathetic system provides a mechanism for reflex adjustment of pupil size in response to the amount of light entering the eye. This serves to maintain the image quality by limiting excessive quantities of light, and it also increases the depth of focus by reducing spherical aberration of the eye's optics. The same optical phenomena occur in a camera when the aperture (f-stop) of the diaphragm is reduced.

Figure 23-10 is a diagrammatic representation of the afferent and efferent sides of the reflex pupillary pathway for light. Changes of luminous intensity in the environment normally enter the system through both eyes simultaneously. However, for purposes of clarity, we have chosen to illustrate the more usual mode of clinical testing, in which a light is introduced selectively into one eye. In this diagram, the flashlight is directed at the right eye, and the photoreceptors of the right retina are activated. Through several intermediate neurons in the retina, excitation is conveyed to the retinal ganglion cells, the axons of which constitute the optic nerves. An important aspect of this system is the fact that when light is introduced into one eye, both pupils constrict to an equal degree. The extent of pupillary constriction was once considered to

be greater on the side of the light stimulus, but pupillographic studies have disproved this contention. The anatomic substrate for a bilateral symmetrical pupil constriction with monocular stimulation will become clear on inspection of this diagram. When the right eye is stimulated (Fig. 23-10), the optic nerve carries impulses to the optic chiasm, where the fibers originating nasal to the macula (serving temporal fields) cross into the opposite optic tract, and the fibers originating temporal to the macula (nasal fields) pass undecussated in the ipsilateral optic tract. At some point anterior to the termination of these fibers in the lateral geniculate nuclei (LGN), a collateral pathway leads to the pretectal region of the midbrain just ventral to the collicular plate. Neurons in this pretectal nuclear (PTN) region are depicted in Figure 23-10 by triangle symbols (*open arrows*, PTN). Right eye stimulation produces bilateral activation of pretectal nuclei because of the hemidecussation at the chiasm. Some of the pretectal neurons send axons across the midline to the opposite Edinger-Westphal nucleus, whereas others send fibers to the ipsilateral nucleus (Fig. 23-10) Thus, there are crossing fibers at two levels in the afferent system to explain the observed symmetrical pupillary contraction when light stimulates one eye.

The efferent arm of the light reflex is generally considered to begin with cell bodies in the Edinger-Westphal nucleus, a subunit of the third cranial nerve (oculomotor) nuclear group. The third cranial nerve innervates quite a number of extraocular muscles as well as the pupils, and the architecture of its nucleus is complex (Fig. 23-11). For the moment, we will consider only the pupillomotor fibers that exit from the midbrain within the third cranial nerve, bound for the orbit. The upper left-hand inset of Figure 23-11 shows the location of pupillary fibers within the nerve—they are depicted as the black band at the periphery of the nerve trunk. This is important in the diagnosis of third cranial nerve lesions, because the peripheral pupillomotor fibers are vulnerable to the effects of external compression by aneurysms (Fig. 23-11).

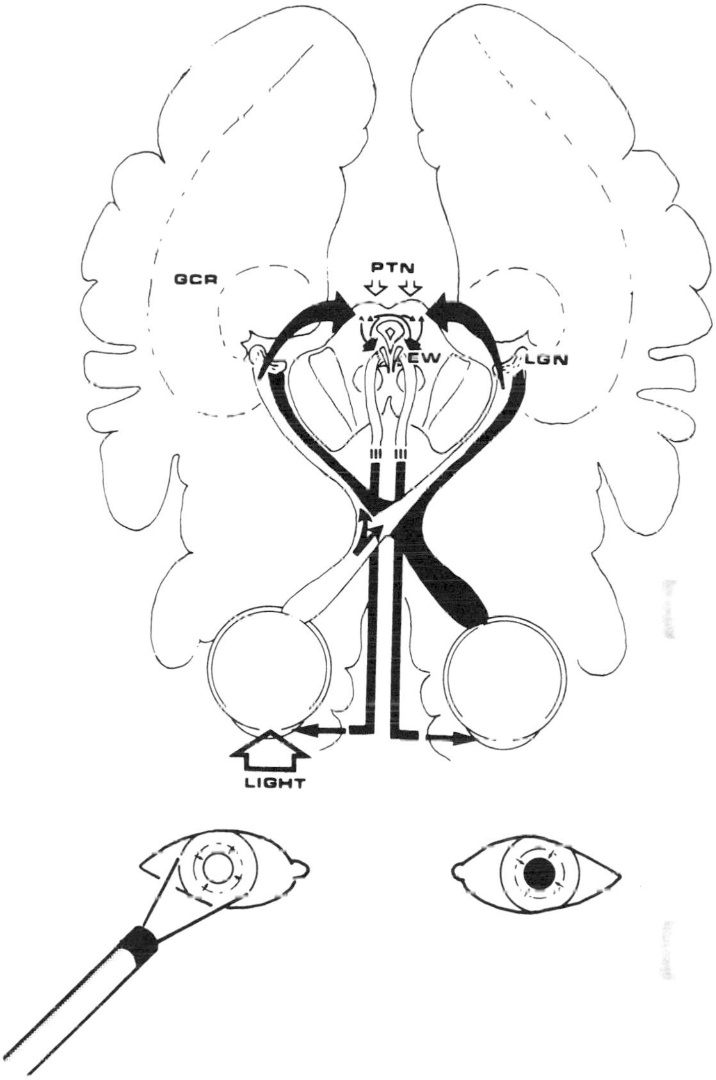

FIG. 23-10. Pathways for the parasympathetic light reflex. The upper portion of the figure illustrates afferent pathways from the retina of the right eye to both sides of the midbrain by way of the hemidecussation at the chiasm. Afferent fibers of retinal ganglion cells leave the optic tracts anterior to the lateral geniculate bodies and innervate pretectal nuclei (PTN, *open arrows*). *Closed triangles* just below the superior colliculi in the midbrain section indicate neurons of the *pretectal nuclei*. Pathways from either PTN innervate the Edinger–Westphal (EW) nuclei bilaterally, constituting a second hemidecussation in the afferent side of the reflex arc. The outflow pathways from the Edinger–Westphal nuclei are in the third cranial nerves to the ciliary ganglion, where a synapse occurs with postganglionic neurons (not shown) that innervate the iris sphincter muscle. The *inset* below illustrates that both pupils constrict to an equal degree when light is applied to one eye as a consequence of the twin hemidecussations in the afferent pathways.

Within the orbit, the parasympathetic fibers synapse with postganglionic cell bodies in the ciliary ganglion. The postganglionic fibers enter the anterior segments of the eyes as the *long posterior ciliary* nerves and form neuromuscular junctions with the pupillary sphincter muscle. The synaptic neurotransmitter at the ciliary ganglion level and at the neuromuscular junction is acetylcholine. The transmitter at the pretectal level and at the Edinger-Westphal nucleus is unknown. Pharmacologic manipulation of the cholinergic neuro-muscular junction at the eye is important in the diagnosis of pupil sphincter paralysis.

CLINICAL DISORDERS OF THE PARASYMPATHETIC PUPILLARY SYSTEM

Relative Afferent Pupillary Defect (Marcus Gunn)

A neural signal that varies with the amount of light entering the eyes is conveyed by retinal ganglion cell axons to the pretectal nuclei, where it is translated into

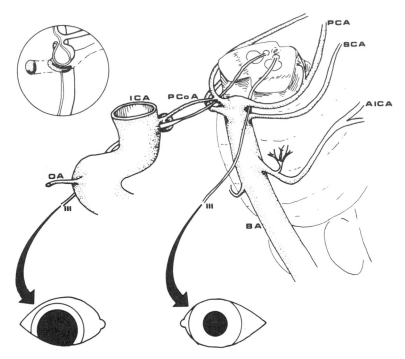

FIG. 23-11. The third cranial nerve is depicted in relation to an aneurysm of the right posterior communicating artery (PCoA). The main body of the figure illustrates the anatomic relationship of the right third cranial nerve to the posterior cerebral artery (PCA) and the superior cerebellar artery (SCA) as the nerve exits from the brainstem and crosses the subarachnoid space. It also illustrates the close relationship between the nerve and the internal carotid artery (ICA) at its junction with the PCoA more anteriorly. The figure shows that an aneurysm of the PCoA at its origin from the ICA is in an ideal position to compress the third nerve. The *upper left-hand inset* shows the relationship of an aneurysm to the passing third nerve. Note that the pupillary parasympathetic fibers, indicated by a *solid black band,* are peripherally placed and especially vulnerable to sudden enlargement of the aneurysm or to breach of the nerve surface by localized hemorrhage. The *lower inset* indicates a typical aneurysm-type right third nerve palsy. The right eye is abducted and depressed with maximum pupillary dilatation. BA = basilar artery; OA = ophthalmic artery; AICA = anterior inferior cerebellar artery.

a motor command for the appropriate pupil size. The signal is relayed by way of the third cranial nerve to the iris sphincters of both eyes. The system functions as if there were a fixed relationship between the amount of light entering the two eyes and the neural code for the resultant pupil size. Anything that reduces the amount of light entering will cause the pupils to attain a larger diameter, all other stimuli remaining equal. This can be demonstrated by covering one eye of a subject and then noting that the uncovered pupil dilates slightly.

Both pupils are dilating, but the pupil under cover cannot, of course, be seen. This type of observation led Marcus Gunn to describe the *relative afferent pupillary defect* (RAPD), which is now routinely tested by the *swinging flashlight* technique. Marcus Gunn's original observation, made in 1904, was that when an eye has an optic nerve lesion, covering it causes relatively little dilatation of the pupil, because almost all the light-induced signal comes to the midbrain from the opposite eye. As the cover is switched to the normal eye, however, the pupils dilate strikingly, because all the light information now comes from the eye with the defective afferent function. This *variance* of pupil size with alternating occlusion (when one eye is providing most of the brightness signal) is the basis of the swinging flashlight test.

Rather than alternately covering each eye in bright ambient light as Marcus Gunn did, the RAPD is now tested by illuminating each eye separately with a focal light source. Both pupils dilate as the light is swung to the defective eye, and both pupils constrict as it is swung to the normal eye. The test is best done in the dark, and only the eye illuminated by the flashlight can be seen at any one time. The unseen fellow eye, however, is undergoing the same pupillary constriction and dilatation that can be observed in the illuminated eye. The swinging flashlight technique provides a sensitive means of comparing afferent function in the two eyes. If one eye is totally blind, and the other has normal visual acuity and fields, the difference in magnitude of the direct light reflex between eyes will be evident without the swinging flashlight technique. The test becomes useful when the difference in direct light reflex between the eyes is less, in which case observation of the extent and velocity of pupil constriction may seem the same when either eye is stimulated alone. Nonetheless, a clear difference is usually apparent when the eyes are stimulated alternately in rapid succession.

Under the best circumstances, an afferent pupillary defect is easy to detect, even when small. However, certain variances of pupil function among normal individuals sometimes makes interpretation of the swinging flashlight test difficult. The presence of a Marcus Gunn pupil, or RAPD, indicates a lesion in the afferent pupillary reflex arc between the eye and the midbrain, although the type of lesion is not directly specified by the test.

One should not conclude, however, that the RAPD has no specificity as to the cause of visual loss in the defective eye. Cataracts and other opacities in the ocular media do not produce a significant RAPD even with major visual loss. This is probably true because such opacities *diffuse* light within the eye and degrade the visual image but do not significantly reduce the total quantity of light that reaches the retina until the cataract becomes brown (brunescent) in its late stages. Dark or brown cataracts can induce a mild RAPD. Visual loss resulting from opacities in the media of the eye is not generally a major diagnostic problem, since these are easily seen on ophthalmoscopic examination.

There is greater difficulty in distinguishing among macular lesions, optic nerve lesions, and childhood amblyopia. In any of these cases, the fundus appearance may not give a clue as to which is causing the visual loss. Although macular lesions usually cause an observable change in the optic fundus, the findings may be subtle and may even require adjunctive examinations, such as fluorescein angiography, to demonstrate them.

The usefulness of the afferent pupillary defect in this type of situation lies in the relationship between the degree of afferent defect and the degree of visual dysfunction. In the presence of minimal functional impairment (nearly normal visual acuity and fields), a prominent afferent pupil defect signifies a high probability that the lesion is in the optic nerve. A macular lesion must produce a more extensive visual acuity loss than an optic nerve lesion to result in an equivalent RAPD. If the visual acuity is severely impaired from a macular lesion, there may be a fairly prominent RAPD, so the test is specific for optic nerve lesions mainly when visual impairment is minor. Amblyopia (strabismic or anisometropic) may be associated with a mild to moderate RAPD, but oddly enough the degree of RAPD does not correlate well with the level of visual acuity reduction.

The afferent pupil defect is decisive in evaluating monocular functional visual loss, which can result from either hysteria or malingering. Most commonly, the differential diagnosis falls between functional visual loss and retrobulbar (behind the globe) optic neuropathy, because the fundus is normal in both cases.

If a patient has visual acuity worse than 20/40 in one eye with normal visual acuity and visual field in the other eye without RAPD, it is reasonably safe to conclude that the problem is functional. A problem exists if a person has reduced acuity in one symptomatic eye and an asymptomatic peripheral visual field defect in the other eye. The peripheral field loss may be sufficient to balance the central visual loss in the symptomatic eye, in which case there will be no RAPD. The swinging flashlight technique is a comparative test that uses the fellow eye as an internal control. The phenomenon that has been called Marcus Gunn pupil should, therefore, be referred to as the *relative* afferent pupillary defect.

It is important to keep in mind that the absence of an RAPD in a patient with symptomatic reduction of visual acuity in one eye is a useful sign of hysteria or malingering only if one has detailed information on the visual function in the fellow eye.

Occasionally, there is confusion between the Marcus Gunn pupil and *hippus,* which is random, often rhythmic pupillary oscillation that can be observed in many normal individuals during steady illumination of the eyes. The term *hippus* is usually reserved for those pupils that oscillate with fairly large amplitude; almost every pupil has small sinusoidal oscillations of size with steady illumination. High-amplitude oscillation is a curiosity, but not a disease—there are no currently accepted disease associations with the phenomenon. It often complicates the interpretation of the swinging flashlight test, however, because there can be an interaction between the rhythm of flashlight alternation and that of the spontaneous pupil fluctuation. The examiner sometimes swings the light between the eyes in such a way that a false afferent defect is produced on one side, or a real afferent defect is masked by the interaction of stimulus alternation and natural oscillation. To avoid this problem, the examiner should probably swing at *different rhythms* during a single examination, including at least one trial of very slow alternation, changing eyes every 3 to 5 seconds. During the steady illumination of each eye, the examiner can observe whether there is significant hippus; if there is, the results should be interpreted carefully. An apparent afferent defect that is not seen with most alternation rates may be spurious.

A person can see his own pupil oscillate by his sense of the brightness of the stimulus light, which brightens as the pupil widens and dims as the pupil contracts. When you shine a light in your own eye, the pupil first constricts and then dilates slightly. This is normal *early release* and does not in itself indicate an afferent defect; many normal pupils behave in this manner, although others assume a new smaller size with illumination and do not redilate. This early contraction and slight redilatation should be equal in amplitude between eyes to qualify as a normal variant. If there is significant early release, the swinging flashlight test should be done at slow alternation rates to let the new steady-state pupil size be expressed before changing eyes.

A pupil that dilates right away when it is illuminated, without any early constriction, strongly indicates a Marcus Gunn pupil. However, an afferent defect may be manifest only in that there is less early constriction in one eye than in the other during the swinging flashlight test. It is not necessary for all early constriction to be abolished in mild degrees of unilateral optic neuropathy. The asymmetry of pupil behavior is the important feature to look for.

Preganglionic Ocular Parasympathetic (Third Cranial Nerve) Lesions

The diagnosis of third cranial nerve lesions based on an abnormal eye position with weakness of the extra-ocular muscles is discussed in a later section. Here, we will concern ourselves with the involvement or sparing of the *pupil* in oculomotor nerve lesions, because a good deal of clinically important information revolves around this issue. Since the large studies of lesions involving third, fourth, and sixth cranial nerves were published from the Mayo Clinic in the 1950s, 1960s and 1990s, the importance of the pupil in etiologic diagnosis of third cranial nerve lesions has been recognized. In these studies, and in subsequent clinical investigations, it has become well established that paralysis of the pupillary sphincter is the rule in third cranial nerve lesions resulting from aneurysms (see Fig. 23-11). On the other hand, older patients (generally older than 65) who develop third cranial nerve palsies on the basis of presumed microvascular occlusive disease within the nerve itself seldom have major pupillary involvement. Many patients in this latter category have risk factors for accelerated atherosclerosis, including diabetes mellitus or hypertension, but the lack of these factors should not rule out the diagnosis. These "medical" lesions tend to improve and most often make a nearly full recovery within 3 to 6 months.

Although there are only a few pathologic studies of third cranial nerve ischemia, consistent morphologic changes have been observed. The lesion is dominated by demyelination in the acute stages, and the lesion shrinks with fibrosis in the late "recovery" stages. In both the acute and chronic phases there is relatively little, if any, disruption of axons as they pass through the lesion. This correlates well with the usual clinical outcome in which complete or nearly complete recovery of function occurs over several weeks or months.

Since axons are not disrupted, there is no opportunity for the development of *aberrant* or *misdirected regeneration* of fibers in the late stage of recovery. This contrasts with the outcome when the third cranial nerve is damaged by hemorrhage from aneurysms in which there is often loss of axonal continuity. A fairly high incidence of *aberrant regeneration* tends to be seen in the late stages of recovery from aneurysmal third nerve palsy. The most commonly observed clinical manifestation of this is inappropriate contraction of the levator palpebrae muscle linked with activation of either the medial rectus or inferior rectus muscle on attempted adduction or depression of the eye. This causes the striking appearance of lid elevation as the affected eye moves inward (adduction) or downward (depression). These phenomena are caused by a misdirection of axons that had been destined originally for one of the extraocular muscles but which on regrowth attain the wrong channel in the peripheral portion of the nerve and end up at the wrong muscle.

Both the *medical* third cranial nerve palsies and *surgical* cases caused by aneurysms tend to present acutely with considerable pain in the eye and orbit at the onset. There is a tendency to accept painful third cranial nerve palsy caused by aneurysms without much need for explanation. The cause of pain in microvascular occlusive lesions, however, is not readily apparent. On close examination, the cause of pain in the presence of aneurysms is not entirely explained. Although there is often evidence for enlargement of an aneurysm prior to the occurrence of small hemorrhages into the nerve, this is by no means always the case. Whether or not the aneurysm has enlarged, it is always possible that a direct irritation of pain-carrying afferent pathways from the artery wall at the site of the aneurysm is responsible for the pain. The important point is that pain is characteristic both of aneurysmal third cranial nerve lesions *and* of those secondary to ischemia within the nerve substance. The criterion of pain should not, therefore, be used to differentiate between medical and surgical causes.

The importance of making a differential diagnosis prior to angiography is that patients with an intraneural lesion caused by small vessel disease are at high risk for angiographic procedures, and the angiogram does not lead to any beneficial therapy. It is, therefore, optimal to avoid angiography in these patients. Fortunately, sparing of the pupil is sufficiently reliable evidence of a *medical* cause that most of these patients can be managed without angiography.

Although this seems simple and clear-cut in abstract discussion, the evaluation of individual cases presents ambiguities. Since all biologic phenomena tend to fall along continua rather than in all-or-none fashion, it is not surprising that this occurs in relation to pupillary involvement with third cranial nerve lesions. The safest formulation is that in aneurysm-induced third cranial nerve palsies, the pupil is strongly involved, whereas in microvascular lesions, the pupil is *relatively* spared. This means that the degree of pupillary involvement in relation to the degree of extraocular muscle involvement is the critical factor. There is little difficulty in diagnosis when a person presents with a total involvement of all extraocular muscles, including complete ptosis, while the pupil is only slightly larger than that of the other eye and remains reactive to light. This would be the profile of a clear-cut *medical* third cranial nerve palsy. Unfortunately, some patients present with *partial involvement of the extraocular muscles*, and then, even though the pupils are normal, or nearly so, it is difficult to exclude an aneurysm. Newer methods, such

as intravenous (IV) or intra-arterial digital subtraction angiography, rapid sequence CT with bolus IV contrast injection, magnetic resonance angiography (MRA) (i.e., a type of angiogram), or duplex scanning methods, all have the capacity to visualize larger aneurysms. There is presently, however, no definitive test to exclude smaller aneurysms except standard angiography, and some patients with nonaneurysmal third cranial nerve palsies have to be studied using this invasive technique when the characteristics of the cranial nerve involvement are not definitive.

Pupillary involvement in slowly progressive third cranial nerve compressive lesions such as meningioma, pituitary adenoma, and nasopharyngeal carcinoma is much less predictable. The onset and course of the third cranial nerve dysfunction may be the most valuable clue to the presence of one of these other compressive lesions. The onset is generally much less explosive than that resulting from aneurysms or microvascular infarction. Furthermore, the lesions caused by aneurysm or infarction are usually complete within hours or days, whereas the level of pupillary and extraocular muscle dysfunction caused by tumor compression tends to be slowly progressive over weeks or months.

It would seem practical to undertake a small-scale workup on each patient in whom the diagnosis of microvascular infarction of the third cranial nerve is considered. CT or MR of the sella turcica, cavernous sinus, ethmoid sinus, and sphenoid sinus regions, may follow laboratory screening, especially for diabetes, depending on the degree to which alternate diagnoses are suspected. If the patient is hypertensive and diabetic and in the mid- to late sixties, it may be appropriate to stop testing after the blood studies. If the patient is without risk factors for accelerated atherosclerosis, or is under the age of 55 or even 60, it is wise to proceed to MRI or CT scan with special attention to the parasellar and posterior orbital areas. Angiography remains the definitive test for an aneurysm.

Herniation Syndromes

Supratentorial masses large enough to cause herniation of the medial temporal lobe over the tentorium cerebelli bring pressure to bear against the midbrain and third cranial nerve, which results in pupillary dilatation. Once the stage of third cranial nerve dysfunction has commenced in the course of the transtentorial herniation syndrome, there is often only a matter of minutes or hours until irreversible brain damage occurs, and this is clearly a medical emergency. As with more distal third cranial nerve lesions—caused by aneurysms, infarcts, and tumors—the pupillary involvement is on the *motor* side of the reflex arc. Although it is axiomatic that a lesion on the afferent side of the reflex arc does not cause anisocoria, lesions on the motor side of the arc do so routinely. It is also the rule that a lesion in the efferent pupillary pathway will result in a sluggish pupillary response to either direct or consensual light stimulation on the involved side. It is thus always possible to distinguish an afferent pupillary lesion from one at or distal to the Edinger-Westphal nucleus in the third cranial nerve complex. In the latter instance, the neural message from the midbrain is not conducted on one side only—that is, on the side of the eye being stimulated with light. In other words, both the direct and the consensual light response is diminished on the side of a third cranial nerve lesion.

Depending on the location of the supratentorial mass lesion causing herniation, one can distinguish *central* and *lateral herniation syndromes.*

Central herniation, caused by lesions near the midline, commonly in the parasagittal regions, tends to present with symmetrical pupillary paralysis in both eyes. In these cases, the entire substance of the diencephalon and midbrain are shifted downward, with a tendency for bilateral dysfunction from the onset. It is not uncommon for both pupils to be small and sluggishly reactive in the early stage of central herniation. The *lateral herniation syndrome* occurs in conjunction with laterally placed supratentorial masses, commonly in the temporal lobe. The third cranial nerve findings tend to be unilateral until the final stages of global midbrain dysfunction.

In both central and lateral herniation syndromes, there is sufficient disruption of function in the ascending reticular activating system that the patient is usually obtunded by the time that pupillary signs emerge. The end stage of both central and lateral herniation is bilateral pupillary paralysis, which is accompanied by large nonreactive pupils, probably caused by severe ischemia, often with hemorrhages (Duret) in the midbrain and pons. At this stage, it is usually not possible to determine whether the antecedent herniation was of the central or the lateral type.

It is worthy of repeated emphasis that the patients who are in the midst of cerebral herniation syndrome do not present to the office or hospital complaining of pupillary dilatation, or of anything else for that matter. They are usually severely obtunded by the time the pupillary phenomena have begun. Gradual somnolence and outright stupor evolve during the earlier *diencephalic* phase of herniation, when the level of functional compromise is at the thalamus, above the midbrain level.

POSTGANGLIONIC PARASYMPATHETIC LESION (ADIE'S SYNDROME, TONIC PUPIL, AND VARIATIONS)

Confusion often occurs when an ostensibly healthy, alert patient presents to the emergency room complaining of a dilated pupil, which is not a rarity. This clinical presentation must, therefore, be dealt with effectively in the emergency department, and a firm differential diagnosis of the *monosymptomatic dilated pupil* is important for all emergency room physicians to keep in mind. Tonic pupil with or without Adie's syndrome and pharmacologically blocked pupil sphincter (atropine-like substances) are the two most common disorders to present in this way.

Adie's Pupil

In 1932, Adie published findings concerning a group of generally healthy young women who presented with a unilaterally dilated pupil. He found that the affected pupil had a peculiar *tonic* light reaction: it responded slowly to light stimulation and had a more brisk, although still pathologically slow, response to near-vision effort. The pupil seemed totally fixed or unresponsive to light in the usual examination setting—a dim environment with a bright light flashed into either eye briefly (Fig. 23-12). When the patient was observed in a bright environment for several minutes, the "tonic" pupil would gradually decrease in diameter. When the environment was dimmed again, the normal pupil would dilate briskly and the "tonic" pupil would remain small for several minutes, although it would redilate slowly, given enough time.

The absolute diameter of the affected pupil, therefore, depends on the *immediate past light experience* of the individual: the tonic pupil may be, at a particular time, smaller or larger than the normal pupil, depending on the ambient illumination and the immediate past illumination. It is important to keep this in mind, because the tonic pupil is usually described in textbooks as being pathologically large. The average diameter of a tonic pupil generally decreases as months and years go by. These pupils tend not to recover their normal function once the tonic state has begun. An old tonic pupil is often small and does not dilate in dim light over any period of time.

Adie observed that there was a high incidence of areflexia in his group of patients. Many had lost all of their deep tendon reflexes, although others retained some reflexes in a patchy manner. The etiology of this syndrome has never been elucidated; it remains an *idiopathic dysautonomic state.*

The presence of normal deep tendon reflexes does not rule out the diagnosis, because a significant per-

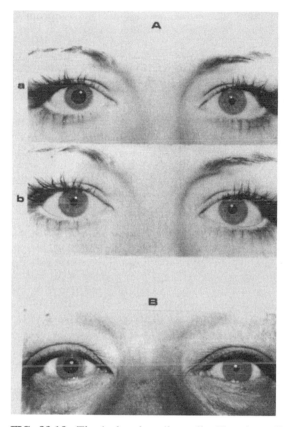

FIG. 23-12. The isolated, unilaterally dilated pupil. **A.** Adie's syndrome: (*a*) The right pupil is widely dilated and unreactive to light. There is no ptosis or extraocular muscle weakness. (*b*) The right pupil is constricted to a greater extent than the left after instillation of "weak" ⅛% pilocarpine in either eye. **B.** Atropinized pupil. The right pupil was widely dilated and fixed to light. It failed to constrict on instillation of "strong" 4% pilocarpine.

centage of patients have normal reflexes, at least when the syndrome first presents, and the features of the pupil syndrome do not distinguish between those with reflex loss and those without. Any of the limb reflexes may be diminished, and asymmetrical loss is found in nearly half the patients. The reflexes generally become less active as time passes, although in some patients they become a little more brisk (Thompson et al., 1979).

Aside from simply noticing the large pupil in the mirror, occasionally symptoms lead the patient to be indirectly aware of the problem. The pupil normally limits the amount of light entering the eye by reacting to variations in ambient illumination. When too much light enters the eye, it creates the sensation of *glare*. Furthermore, the large pupil alters the optics of the eye toward a state in which there is a *shallower depth of focus* and an increased *spheric aberration*. This tends to cause a sensation of blurred vision in both bright and dim environments. The accommodative mechanism is also affected in Adie's syndrome: The change in diopteric power (convexity) of the lens to *accommodate* for near vision takes many seconds to occur, and then the focus remains for many seconds after the patient has shifted his gaze from a near to a distant object. Vision from the affected eye will, therefore, be blurred for the first few seconds of any near-vision effort and will remain blurred for several seconds as the patient subsequently attempts to use his eyes for distant viewing. The tonic accommodation with a sustained effort at near vision occasionally causes a *ciliary spasm*, which is manifested as pain in the eye, usually in the vicinity of the brow and inner canthus during close work.

The patient with an Adie's pupil is completely alert without any of the CNS signs that accompany transtentorial herniation. Nonetheless, many such patients are subjected to needless cerebral angiography, often as an emergency procedure.

The *tonic pupil* is caused by a postganglionic parasympathetic lesion. Some authors believe that this is a viral infection of the ciliary ganglion; however, no definitive data exist as to the cause of the lesion. The lesion is in the postganglionic parasympathetic system, because there is *denervation supersensitivity* to weak cholinergic substances. This seems to follow the same principles as denervation supersensitivity in skeletal muscle that has lost its direct innervation. Normally, the muscle can be activated only through its motor end plate; however, 4 or 5 weeks after an acute loss of direct nerve supply, the functional muscle end plate begins to expand until nearly the entire sarcolemmal membrane becomes responsive to circulating or experimentally applied acetylcholine. This procedure forms the basis of a definitive test for Adie's pupil. Since acetylcholine is unavailable as a pharmaceutical solution, the physician can choose another direct-acting cholinergic such as *methacholine chloride* (Mecholyl) or *pilocarpine* for the test. The physician must select a solution that is too weak to cause a normally innervated sphincter muscle to contract. For these purposes, we have selected 1/16% pilocarpine, because we found that it does not cause a significant contraction of a normally innervated sphincter muscle, unlike 1/8% pilocarpine, which can cause more than 1 mm miosis in some normal persons (unpublished study). Pilley and Thompson recommended 1/8% pilocarpine, but Cohen and Zakov found 1/16% to be ideal, as have we. Methacholine had been advocated earlier for testing denervation supersensitivity of the iris sphincter, but this drug is no longer readily available and it has actually been shown to be less sensitive than 1/8% pilocarpine in demonstrating iris denervation supersensitivity.

The normal pupil serves as an internal control in this test. One drop of 1/16% pilocarpine is placed in either eye, and a second drop is applied 10 minutes later. The pupil size is measured approximately 30 to 60 minutes from the first application. In most cases, the Adie's pupil will become smaller than the fellow pupil under the influence of this weak solution of pilocarpine, thus demonstrating the presence of denervation supersensitivity. This is categorically different from the failure of a contraction to weak pilocarpine that characterizes the dilated pupil of an intracranial third cranial nerve lesion, in which case the postganglionic innervation is intact. Preganglionic lesions of the intracranial third nerve result in a dilated pupil, but there is not significant denervation supersensitivity and the pupil does not constrict in the presence of 1/16% pilocarpine. Ponsford and coworkers found that among 10 patients with aneurysms causing third cranial nerve palsy, 2.5% methacholine caused pupillary constriction equal to that in 14 patients with Adie's syndrome. These authors had no explanation for this finding, and others have not had similar experience, so it is still generally accepted that significantly greater miosis on the side of a dilated pupil is strongly indicative of a postganglionic (orbital) lesion.

It should be mentioned that the weakest solution of pilocarpine available commercially is 1/4%, so the interested physician will have to arrange for having it dilated fourfold to 1/16%, possibly by a local pharmacist.

One can, therefore, distinguish the Adie's pupil from the dilated pupil caused by aneurysms, transtentorial herniation, and intracranial mass lesions that directly compress the third cranial nerve. The dilated pupils caused by all of these central lesions, together with all normal (nondilated) pupils, will remain the same size after the instillation of a weak pilocarpine solution. There is seldom great difficulty in distinguishing Adie's syndrome from compressive lesions of the third cranial nerve even without pharmaco-

logic tests. The intracranial lesions that compromise functions in the third cranial nerve generally cause clinical findings related to the extraocular muscles in addition to the pupil. Some cases of intracranial aneurysms that cause isolated pupillary involvement have been documented. In these rare instances, the extraocular and lid muscles become involved shortly after the pupil, and there are often subtle lid and ocular motility findings even when the pupil seems to be involved in isolation. My experience has not included any aneurysms that caused enough denervation sensitivity of the pupil to cause a clearly positive weak cholinergic test. The reader should be aware that the differential value of weak cholinergic testing is being scrutinized.

Up to this point, we have been discussing the diagnosis of the unilateral denervated pupil in which the normal fellow pupil is used as an internal control. Bilateral denervation may be encountered in patients with autonomic neuropathies such as occur in diabetes mellitus. Both pupils are affected in these cases, and thus one pupil cannot serve as a control for the other. In testing for bilateral denervation, the pilocarpine solution must be weak enough that it will not cause *any* constriction of normal pupils. For this type of test, 1/16% pilocarpine is recommended. If there is any contraction of either pupil, denervation can probably be diagnosed without reference to the other pupil.

Atropinized Pupil

The second major category of patients who present to the emergency room with an isolated large pupil is that of postsynaptic sphincter blockade by atropinic substances. The old term *belladonna* (alkaloid), indicating atropine and its congeners, derives from the use of these agents by women (donna) who wanted to enhance their beauty (bella). It was once considered attractive for one's eyes to appear as bottomless pools, and this was accomplished by dilating the pupils. This seldom adequately accounts for the situation today. Two groups of people end up with atropinics in one eye—those who do so accidentally and those who put the drug in the eye willfully. The first category includes those people whose work involves the use of atropine, such as nurses and other paramedical personnel, and those who manipulate plants. Many plants have naturally occurring atropinics in the sap and on the surfaces of stems, leaves, and roots. The willful application of atropine to one eye is less easy to understand. In many cases, such a person will present to the emergency room with a large pupil and a history of either blurred vision or headaches, as though there were some secondary gain attached to the frequent sequel of cerebral angiography. It stretches the imagination to assume that all these patients are aware of the relationship between pupil size and cerebral herniation syndromes. Some of the patients, though, are medical personnel who are aware of the relationship and its medical implications. It must be concluded that certain individuals are motivated to seek invasive diagnostic procedures, and the physician must be prepared to rule out CNS causes of the dilated pupil in these cases. This is easily done by the instillation of a strong solution (4% to 6%) of pilocarpine in each eye. A potent cholinergic activator of the iris sphincter that will produce a pinpoint pupil in normal eyes, 6% pilocarpine will also constrict all pathologically denervated pupils including the postganglionic parasympathetic lesions of Adie's syndrome and the preganglionic third cranial nerve lesions. The only condition that will cause a failure of the pupil to constrict with 6% pilocarpine is a postsynaptic receptor blockade at the sphincter muscle—atropinization. If the pupil is large because of iris trauma or infection, with muscle atrophy or synechiae causing an adhesion to the lens capsule, there will also be a failure of constriction; however, this situation should not present a diagnostic problem because the anterior segment appears abnormal. It may require slit lamp biomicroscopy of the anterior segment to observe iris damage or lens capsule adhesions, and an ophthalmologic consultation should be obtained if this is considered a possibility.

The use of strong pilocarpine, therefore, unequivocally segregates those with a large pupil caused by lesions or pharmacologic blockade at the iris sphincter from normal persons and from those with large pupils caused by intracranial lesions of all types. There are few diagnostic procedures in medicine for which such a claim can be made!

It is theoretically possible for an aneurysm or other mass to compress the third cranial nerve in such a way as to cause isolated paralysis of the pupil. The pupillary fibers are superficial in the subarachnoid portion of the nerve and might be selectively disrupted by any lesion that compresses the nerve. Such a presentation is rare, and only a few cases have been documented. In most of these cases, the extraocular muscles and levator palpebrae are affected within days of isolated pupillary involvement. I have found that subtle, often fluctuating lid and oculomotor signs are present in patients who are said to have isolated pupil dilatation caused by aneurysms. A carefully repeated examina-

tion often gives evidence that leads to the proper diagnosis of these cases. Any patient with a dilated pupil that contracts to strong pilocarpine must, therefore, be observed carefully, because there may be a serious intracranial cause such as an aneurysm.

OCULAR SYMPATHETIC SYSTEM

The sympathetic system produces a dilator tone in opposition to the iris sphincter. The dilator system functions by way of a reflex arc just as the sphincter system does; however, the afferent arm is much less circumscribed than that of the light reflex, which probably accounts for the fact that the sympathetic system is often not thought of as a reflex circuit.

Afferent stimulation along pain and temperature pathways from the spinal cord generally causes pupil dilatation that is abrupt in onset and lasts on the order of 20 to 60 seconds. More sustained dilatation often attends mental states involving fear, anxiety, or surprise. Since the sympathetic afferent pathways are anatomically ill defined, especially at rostral levels of the CNS, the subsequent discussion will focus on efferent sympathetic pathways.

Anatomic studies have shown sympathetic fiber degeneration in the upper brainstem after experimental lesions in the hypothalamus. These degeneration studies document widely dispersed fiber tracts in the upper midbrain and diencephalon but no reliably demonstrated pathways in the pons and medulla. The descending system is most likely, therefore, a polysynaptic one, even though in clinical usage it is referred to as the *central neuron* in the chain leading to the iris dilator.

Clinical studies have documented that dorsolateral lesions throughout the brainstem often produce ocular sympathetic dysfunction ipsilaterally, whereas medial and ventral lesions do not. This is the basis for the widely accepted view that the polysynaptic descending system is dorsolaterally disposed in the brainstem. This pathway continues into the spinal cord to the C8 through T2 segmental levels, where the "central" fibers synapse with cells in the intermediolateral gray horns; this zone between C8 and T2 is commonly known as the *ciliospinal center of Budge and Waller*. The central pathways through the cervical spinal cord are located superficially (near the pia) in the lateral columns. The preganglionic cells from the ciliospinal center send axons to the *paravertebral sympathetic ganglion chain* by way of the C8–T2 ventral roots. These preganglionic fibers travel upward in the sympathetic chain through the *stellate* (combined upper thoracic and lower cervical ganglion) and the *middle cervical* ganglion. They synapse with postganglionic cells in the *superior cervical ganglion,* which is usually found high in the neck, often under the angle of the mandible. This means that the common lesions that cause ocular sympathetic palsy (Horner's syndrome) interfere with preganglionic fibers as they course through the upper thorax. Virtually all the lesions producing postganglionic sympathetic dysfunction are intracranial and intraorbital in location, since the superior cervical ganglion is so near the base of the skull.

The postganglionic axons at first travel in the adventitia of the carotid artery. Those supplying vascular and sweat gland structures in the lower face travel with external carotid branches, whereas the ocular sympathetics and those serving vasomotor and sudomotor function for the forehead go with the internal carotid into the middle cranial fossa. A contingent of ocular sympathetic fibers takes a "side path" through the otic ganglion in the middle ear. This apparently explains the occasional occurrence of Horner's syndrome with middle ear infections. The main ocular sympathetic pathway, however, follows the carotid artery through its *siphon* region and then joins the *first division (ophthalmic)* of the *trigeminal nerve,* which carries it into the orbit. A sympathetic contingent passes through the parasympathetic ciliary ganglion, constituting the so-called sympathetic root of the ganglion, but no sympathetic synapses occur there. In the orbit, the ocular sympathetics innervate the iris dilator muscles together with small smooth muscles in the lids, which contribute to upper lid elevation and lower lid depression. Defective contraction of these sympathetically innervated *Mueller's muscles* causes a low-grade ptosis or a descent of the upper lid. Less well recognized, however, is the fact that the weakness of Mueller's muscle in the lower lid causes the latter to elevate. Upper lid ptosis and elevation of the lower lid together cause a narrowing of the *palpebral fissure.* This contributes to an illusion that the involved eye is displaced backward in the orbit, the so-called apparent enophthalmos that has been described with Horner's syndrome. It used to be stated that the enophthalmos was real in Horner's syndrome; however, only frogs have a sympathetically innervated muscle that normally holds the eye forward in the orbit, the weakness of which allows the eye to move backward. Thus, the enophthalmos in Horner's syndrome is truly *apparent*—an illusion caused by the narrowed palpebral fissure.

Sympathetic fibers serving the skin of the forehead just above the brow travel with the nasociliary branch of the first or ophthalmic division of the trigeminal nerve. With postganglionic sympathetic lesions, a triangular patch of altered vasomotor tone and decreased sweating may present just above the brow extending to the midline.

CLINICAL DISORDERS OF THE OCULAR SYMPATHETICS

The defective function of the sympathetically innervated Mueller's muscle in the upper lid results in the minor degree of ptosis that occurs typically in Horner's syndrome. The position of the upper and lower lids and thereby the width of the palpebral fissure is determined by the relative tone in the orbicularis muscle, which closes the lids, compared with the tone of the levator palpebrae plus Mueller's muscles, which open the eyes. The levator palpebrae, a striated muscle innervated by the third cranial nerve, provides most of the upper lid's elevation, whereas Mueller's muscle produces some upper lid elevation and lower lid depression. Thus, the levator and Mueller's muscle work together and in opposition to the orbicularis muscle, which encircles the palpebral fissure. When assessing lid position, one must be careful of illusions crated by asymmetrical skin folds, by altered position of the eye in the orbit (extraocular muscle palsies and strabismus), and even by anisocoria. The observer's eye uses all of these landmarks for assessing where the lid margin is expected to fall and whether its position is the same in the two eyes. Eyelid position and the relation of lid margins to landmarks such as skin folds is often asymmetrical for various non-neurologic reasons. It is useful, therefore, to measure the distance between a central corneal light reflex and the upper and lower lids, respectively, and also to compare these for symmetry between eyes. This reflex, produced when a point source of light such as a penlight or handlight is directed toward the eyes from a position in front of the patient, does not move appreciably with a variation in eye position as long as it still falls on the cornea. By convention, the distance from the light reflex to the upper lid margin has been called the margin-reflex-distance-1 (MRD1) and the distance from the reflex to the lower lid margin, margin-reflex-distance-2 (MRD2). A useful and succinct way to note this measurement in the chart is shown in Table 23-3.

A pitfall that occurs not uncommonly is the false diagnosis of a facial or seventh cranial nerve palsy caused by apparent widening of one palpebral fissure (orbicularis oculi weakness) when the fissure is really narrowed on the other side from an ocular sympa-

TABLE 23-3. Width of Palpebral Fissures

	RIGHT EYE	LEFT EYE
MRD1	4	4
MRD2	5	5

MRD1 = margin-reflex-distance-1 (the distance from the light reflex to the upper lid margin); MRD2 = margin-reflex-distance-2 (the distance from the light reflex to the lower lid margin).

thetic lesion. This error is more likely to occur if the normal range of facial asymmetry produces an apparent flattening of the nasolabial fold on the side of the wider palpebral fissure and if the pupillary miosis is minimal or lacking in the ocular sympathetic palsy. Pharmacologic pupil testing can be a useful arbiter in this setting.

ETIOLOGIC DIAGNOSIS IN HORNER'S SYNDROME

The most common ocular sympathetic palsies are those caused by an interruption of preganglionic fibers in relation to lesions of the lung apex and the neck. The bulk of these lesions are malignant tumors, often primary in the lung or metastases to cervical nodes, that can complicate a wide variety of carcinomas, lymphomas, and leukemias.

Some of these cases of preganglionic Horner's syndrome will be secondary to trauma and will usually include penetrating neck wounds and root involvement in spinal injuries. These cases should be obvious from the history and physical findings. Inflammation, caused by suppurative infections and granulomatous diseases such as sarcoidosis or tuberculosis in cervical lymph nodes, is an occasional nonmalignant cause for preganglionic ocular sympathetic palsy.

Central nervous system lesions (e.g., of the hypothalamus, brainstem, or upper cervical cord) are an uncommon cause of Horner's syndrome. They are almost always recognizable by the associated cranial nerve, cerebellar, and sensorimotor long-tract findings. A classic example is *Wallenberg's lateral medullary syndrome,* which is usually caused by an occlusion of one vertebral artery with an infarction in the distribution of the *posterior inferior cerebellar artery.* The attendant dorsolateral medullary lesion produces a syndrome that includes ocular sympathetic palsy, along with facial numbness ipsilateral to the lesion, loss of pain and temperature sensation in the contralateral extremities, vertigo, dysphagia, and dysarthria. This typical central lesion is distinct from the usually isolated, frequently asymptomatic Horner's syndrome that accompanies preganglionic peripheral lesions.

Postganglionic ocular sympathetic palsy is commonly associated with pain in the ipsilateral orbit and eye. In the early part of this century, a Norwegian ophthalmologist named Raeder reported this combination of pain, miosis, and ptosis as a *"paratrigeminal"* *syndrome* with a localizing value for mass lesions in the middle cranial fossa. All four of his patients had, in addition to ocular sympathetic palsy, findings referable to the third through sixth ipsilateral cranial nerves, either singly or in combination. During the past two decades, there has been an increasing awareness of patients with painful ocular sympathetic palsy without demonstrable middle fossa mass lesions. These patients often have histories of episodic retrobulbar and orbital pain that in many cases is typical of *cluster* or *histamine headache.* The ocular sympathetic lesion comes about during a cluster of headaches and sometimes resolves spontaneously after the cluster has ended, although it sometimes remains as a permanent sequel. This benign condition, which is considered a migraine variant, has acquired the name *Raeder's paratrigeminal syndrome, type II.* To qualify for this benign diagnosis, the patient must have no objective neurologic deficit of the third through sixth cranial nerves; the presence of cranial nerve findings strongly favors the presence of a middle fossa lesion. It has been speculated that in type II Raeder's syndrome, the postganglionic ocular sympathetic fibers are affected by edema in the wall of the carotid artery. Vascular wall changes, probably including edema, are presumed to occur during severe migrainous episodes. The exact sequence of events leading to the ocular sympathetic palsy in this setting is, however, unknown.

Figure 23-13 presents the ocular findings in a man 46 years of age who had frequent episodes of steady intense pain in the left orbit. Each headache lasted 45 to 60 minutes and occurred daily, often at predictable times. These findings had been present for 2 weeks prior to the examination. He had had similar bouts of frequent headaches in previous years. These headaches lasted 1 to 3 weeks at a time. During this symptomatic period, however, a physician had noted left ptosis and miosis of which the patient was unaware. The neurologic examination was otherwise completely normal. This was a typical case of type II Raeder's syndrome with a presumed migrainous etiology. The pupillary pharmacologic aspects of this diagnosis will be discussed later.

PHARMACOLOGIC WORKUP OF OCULAR SYMPATHETIC LESIONS

The objectives of pharmacologic testing in the sympathetic system are twofold. In some cases, the objec-

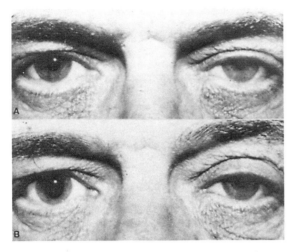

FIG. 23-13. Left ocular sympathetic lesion with ipsilateral orbital headache of migraine type (Raeder's syndrome type II). **A.** The asymmetrical position of the upper lid margin with respect to the overlying skin fold is the most prominent feature of this man's ptosis. The relation of the lid margin to the iris and globe is relatively symmetrical between eyes. **B.** The left pupil failed to dilate on instillation of 1% para-OH-amphetamine, indicating a postganglionic ocular sympathetic lesion.

tive is to document the presence or absence of an ocular sympathetic lesion without regard to further localization. A typical example would be a case of isolated anisocoria or isolated ptosis in which the evidence is insufficient for the reliable diagnosis of a sympathetic lesion. The second objective of pharmacologic diagnosis is to identify the level of involvement (pre- or postganglionic) in a case in which there is reasonable certainty that an ocular sympathetic lesion exists.

There is great practical value in segregating patients with Horner's syndrome into those with preganglionic and those with postganglionic lesions. The group with preganglionic lesions has a high incidence of malignant disease requiring extensive investigation, whereas the group with postganglionic involvement has primarily benign causes (usually a vascular headache).

The physiologic basis of clinically useful pharmacologic tests is noradrenergic transmission at the iris dilator neuromuscular junction, where the sympathetic postganglionic axon terminals contact the muscle cells. The drugs of greatest clinical usefulness are the

indirect-acting sympathomimetics: cocaine and para-*p*-hydroxyamphetamine (Paredrine). The schemes for clinical usage have been worked out primarily by Thompson and coworkers (1971). Transmission in the sympathetic system at the superior cervical ganglion is cholinergic, but there are no clinically useful diagnostic tests for evaluating the function at this level.

At the postganglionic axon terminal, norepinephrine (NE) is maintained in storage vesicles by metabolically active processes. The bound vesicular NE is in equilibrium with a pool of unbound NE in the vesicle and in the cytoplasm of the nerve terminal. A small portion of the vesicular pool is released as each nerve action potential arrives along the postganglionic cell axon. The released NE interacts with specific receptors on the dilator muscle membrane, causing a contraction. As in other adrenergic systems, the effect of the released transmitter is terminated by a metabolically active reuptake from the neuromuscular junction into the postganglionic nerve terminals. Cocaine exerts its primary effect by blocking reuptake at this stage. This potentiates pupil dilator tone due to ongoing tonic neural activity and neurotransmitter release in the ocular sympathetic efferents. Failure of this potentiation in the presence of ocular sympathetic lesions at all levels is useful evidence for Horner's syndrome. The reason that cocaine fails to dilate pupils with central and preganglionic sympathetic dysfunction is related presumably to the fact that the tonic release of NE at the postganglionic terminal is reduced, even with these proximal lesions, so that the blockage of NE reuptake has little effect compared to the normal other eye. A positive cocaine test is defined as relative failure of the pupil to dilate on the side of the lesion with dilatation of the fellow pupil, which is used as an internal control. Cocaine is a weak dilator, thus if neither pupil enlarges, the test must be considered indeterminate and should be ignored.

Para-OH-amphetamine not only blocks reuptake of naturally released NE but promotes the release of any stored NE from the postganglionic axon terminals into the neuromuscular junctions at the iris dilator muscles. This means that regardless of the level of ongoing neural activity in the system, if the postganglionic cell and its terminals at the dilator muscles are intact, para-OH-amphetamine will release the stored NE and then will block its reuptake, both of which actions bring about pupillary dilatation. Para-OH-amphetamine, unlike cocaine, will thus dilate the pupil in the presence of both central and preganglionic Horner's syndrome. Only a pupil with the loss of postganglionic sympathetic fibers and the stored NE at their terminals will fail to dilate in response to para-OH-amphetamine. This is the basis of the localizing value of the para-OH-amphetamine test (see Fig. 23-13). It is used primarily to differentiate postganglionic lesions (pupil will not dilate) from preganglionic lesions (pupil will dilate), because central lesions are usually not a problem for localizing diagnosis on account of the associated neurologic findings. Of course, one must be sure that an ocular sympathetic lesion exists before using para-OH-amphetamine because this test will "miss" the central and preganglionic lesions by short-circuiting the neural chain and causing release of the NE stored at the postganglionic terminal, even though the level of spontaneous release was diminished because of the more proximal lesion. Para-OH-amphetamine should, therefore, be reserved for the localization of an ocular sympathetic lesion and not for the identification of the lesion. An exception may be a case in which only a postganglionic deficit is suspected, as for instance in a patient with orbital pain plus ptosis and miosis. A note of caution is in order at this point. Some patients have pain in the orbit ipsilateral to preganglionic ocular sympathetic lesions caused by trauma in the neck. The pathogenesis of this condition is obscure, but it often responds favorably to propranolol (Inderal) with relief of pain. The important point for this discussion is that one should not conclude a priori that the sympathetic lesion is postganglionic because of concomitant orbital pain or frontotemporal headaches. If the para-OH-amphetamine test is negative, a cocaine test should be done on another day.

The para-OH-amphetamine and cocaine tests should be done prior to any manipulations that might disrupt the corneal epithelium, because any breach of corneal integrity can lead to unequal drug absorption in the two eyes and false-positive or false-negative test results. Thus, corneal reflex testing, ocular pressure measurements (tonometers usually operate through pressure on the cornea), and use of any other topical ophthalmic agents should be done on a separate day, or at least after the completion of sympathetic testing. The usual protocol is installation of one drop of either a 10% solution of cocaine or of a 1% solution of para-OH-amphetamine in each eye, with a second dose 5 to 10 minutes later. The pupil size in standard dim illumination is measured before the first drop and 60 minutes after this dose. An increase in the amount of anisocoria is a positive test result. In other words, selective failure of the involved pupil to dilate *as much as* the normal eye after an adequate interval is the criterion for a positive test.

DETERMINING THE AGE OF THE LESION

Since malignant disease is such a prominent feature of recently acquired preganglionic ocular sympathetic lesions, it can be helpful to document that a newly observed Horner's syndrome is actually of long standing, so that an extensive workup for carcinoma can be avoided. The history is usually not helpful, since most patients are unaware of the lesion. The best way to prove that the lesion is not new is to inspect old photographs, which might reveal the ptosis and perhaps even anisocoria.

If the iris of the eye with Horner's syndrome is blue and the other is brown, one can establish that the lesion was probably present at birth, or at least during the first year of life. A sympathetic lesion, if present early in life, prevents the development of ipsilateral iris chromatophores in a person who is genetically destined to have brown eyes. This condition is known as heterochromia iridis. The color asymmetry will not be manifest if both eyes are blue.

ARGYLL ROBERTSON PUPIL

A good deal of confusing literature has accumulated concerning the pupillary manifestations of CNS syphilis, most notably that pertaining to the so-called Argyll Robertson pupillary phenomenon. The original report by Argyll Robertson appeared in 1896 under the title Four Cases of Spinal Myosis: With Remarks on the Action of Light on the Pupil. The thrust of the report centered on the association between spinal cord disease and the peculiar observation of very small pupils that failed to constrict to light but were still capable of response on near viewing effort. Argyll Robertson noted that although most of the patients had ophthalmoscopic evidence of mild optic atrophy, their vision was not significantly impaired. That is, of course, crucial because a person who is blind from optic nerve disease will have pupils that do not respond to light, but that constrict normally to near effort. In this setting, a dissociation between the light and near responses would have no specificity in itself. The differential diagnosis would simply be that of the optic neuropathy. Argyll Robertson was puzzled by the miosis that he felt must have been caused by involvement of the ciliospinal nerves by the spinal disease. When this classic observation was first made, there was neither serologic nor other method by which the spinal disease could be ascribed to neurosyphilis. In fact, syphilis was not mentioned in the discussion, and only one of the four patients was noted to have previously had syphilis.

In subsequent years, the link between "locomotor ataxia," now called tabes dorsalis, and syphilis came to be well recognized, and Argyll Robertson's sign attained common usage as a powerful diagnostic sign of neurosyphilis. It was noted to be present in 60% to 84% of tabetics and in up to 50% of patients with dementia paralytica or general paresis of the insane.

Much controversy has occurred concerning whether the miosis should be considered essential to the definition of the Argyll Robertson pupil. The problem arose with the observation that diseases other than syphilis can be associated with pupils that are fixed to light, but that constrict on near effort in patients with normal vision. This has been reported in a wide variety of disorders, including difficult-to-understand entities such as alcoholism, myotonic dystrophy, and diabetes mellitus. The phenomenon seems easier to accept as specific for the disorder when linked with midbrain lesions such as infarcts, hemorrhages, tumors, and encephalitis lethargica, all of which can produce destructive lesions in parts of the brainstem and spinal cord that are known to participate in pupil function. Most of these nonsyphilitic light-near dissociated pupils "or" Argyll Robertson-like pupils are not miotic, being of average size or larger, and this serves to distinguish the syphilitic from the nonsyphilitic cases. It would certainly be a wonderful universe if a differential diagnosis could be so simple and reliable! Irene Loewenfeld has shown by an exhaustive review of the literature and by extensive personal observations that the absolute size of the pupil does not definitely discriminate between syphilitic and nonsyphilitic Argyll Robertson pupils. Lawton Smith has shown that moderately large light-near dissociated pupils occur in many tabetics and paretics, so one cannot rule out syphilis in this setting if a workup fails to reveal an alternative cause. Fortunately, the situation is rendered somewhat academic by the availability of reliable and sensitive serologic markers for past syphilitic infection [e.g., fluorescent treponemal antibody absorption (FTA-ABS) and others], tests that usually remain positive for the life of the patient.

The anatomic pathology leading to the Argyll Robertson pupillary phenomenon must still be considered problematic. It is difficult to imagine a single locus in the nervous system at which the afferents from the retina to the pupillomotor centers (midbrain tectum and Edinger-Westphal nucleus) would be involved together with fibers or centers that oppose the mydriatic tone of the sympathetic system. Kerr (1968) reviewed pathologic studies indicating that syphilis tends to produce a superficial demyelination, or subpial encephalopathy, throughout the neuraxis. He postulated that, in neurosyphilis, subpial demyelination of the superficial pretectal area would affect the light reaction, whereas lesions of the lateral columns just under the pia at the cervical level could produce miosis by interfering with the descending central sympathetic pathways, the combined lesions resulting in the full Argyll Robertson syndrome.

In summary, the Argyll Robertson pupil sign is manifest as a variable miosis, but more crucially by fixity of the pupil to light stimulation with preserved ability to constrict on near-viewing effort (with convergence and accommodation) in a patient with normal or near-normal vision. This is most commonly bilateral but may be unilateral when first observed, often becoming bilateral as months or years pass. The phenomenon is frequently associated with neurosyphilis, particularly tabes dorsalis and general paresis, but may occur with all sorts of destructive lesions, suitably situated. Observation of the Argyll Robertson pupil in a patient should first prompt a serologic investigation and an appropriate history to establish or preclude past syphilitic infection. If such infection can be ruled out, a workup for structural lesions, in particular at the midbrain or diencephalic area, should be undertaken.

OCULAR MOTILITY IN NEUROLOGIC DIAGNOSIS

The importance of eye movements for daily visual activity is perhaps intuitively obvious. Humans are foveate: Our sharp or high-resolution vision resides in a small area (2° to 3°) of visual field surrounding the fixation point, which is the point in external space at which one is looking. The object of regard is then projected on the fovea centralis of the retina, where high-resolution vision is served. Perception of motion is acute outside the central visual field; however, the resolution of fine spatial details declines rapidly toward the periphery of the visual field. To adequately perceive an extended visual scene (as in daily viewing), therefore, one must "palpate" the environment by moving the fovea from point to point while compiling and storing a central image or engram of the scene. Accordingly, the eye movement system has developed in close association with the sensory or afferent visual system. This is reflected in the anatomy of the oculomotor system, particularly at the cerebral hemisphere level, where major intra- and interhemispheric connections link the so-called frontal eye fields (area 8 of Brodmann, just anterior to the primary motor strip) with temporal lobe and parieto-occipital visual centers. This is of practical significance, because lesions in the cerebral hemispheres often produce a diagnostically useful alteration of ocular motility.

SUPRANUCLEAR ORGANIZATION OF EYE MOVEMENT

The supranuclear organization of eye movement is discussed first because it is rich in diagnostically useful signs. Later sections will cover the final common pathway for the accomplishment of eye movement—third, fourth, and sixth cranial nerves, including their nuclei in the brainstem and their connections with the individual extraocular muscles. Finally, the characteristics of third, fourth, and sixth cranial nerve lesions and of primary disorders of the eye muscles will be discussed.

FUNCTIONAL ORGANIZATION

Images of objects in the visual environment must be brought onto the retinal fovea where a clear neural representation can be generated. This process of foveation is the central issue for the various supranuclear eye movement control systems. In general terms, one must be able to move the eye so as to bring the image of an object onto the fovea and then keep it there despite both object movement in space and head movement—these are unavoidable conditions of daily viewing. The control networks that serve these functions are the saccade system, the pursuit system, and the vestibulo-ocular system, each with a specific anatomic arrangement in the cerebral hemispheres, brainstem, and cerebellum.

All of the supranuclear systems are concerned with conjugate eye movements, meaning that the visual axes of the two eyes remain parallel during the movement. Dysconjugate eye movements indicate a disorder at or below (peripheral to) the third, fourth, and sixth cranial nerve nuclei, or the pathways joining these nuclei.

Saccade System

The saccade system generates high-velocity ballistic movements, or saccades, by which we foveate the elements of a stationary but large or extended visual scene. An adult scans a scene in a highly organized way, extracting data from the highest information areas but directing relatively few saccades to non-specific or uninformative areas in the display. This efficient palpatory behavior is highly learned: It develops progressively during infancy. The efficiency of ocular scanning is often degraded in the presence of cerebral lesions, particularly those associated with dementia, but this type of eye movement alteration is not accessible to bedside examination. It requires elaborate equipment to record exactly where on a visual scene the eyes are fixed at any particular time. This type of ocular motor behavior has organizational elements that encompass the highest levels of whole brain function. We will focus, however, on the motor aspects alone, because they can be observed directly at the bedside.

Lesions in the frontal lobes most commonly interrupt saccade function selectively. The system is represented also at the brainstem level where "burst" cells deliver high levels of innervation to oculomotor neurons and produce the high-velocity eye movements characteristic of saccades. The cerebellum also participates in the saccade system: Lesions here are associated with abnormal saccade characteristics such as low velocity or altered metrics (both overshoot and undershoot).

The parameters by which we can measure saccadic eye movement performance include latency, velocity, and metrics or accuracy.

The average normal human takes about 200 msec to generate a refixation eye movement or saccade to a new target presented in his visual periphery. The time required for each saccade varies widely, but most saccades occur between 180 and 250 msec. This latent interval includes time for the visual stimulus in the peripheral field to travel along afferent pathways to the cerebral cortex, where the spatial coordinates of the object to be foveated are turned into motor commands or vectors that have both direction and amplitude specifications. This computation of vectors and passage of the efferent commands to the brainstem require additional time. It has also been postulated that the system works by way of intermittent data samples rather than a continuous intake of afferent data. Thus, if a novel visual stimulus occurs just after a sample is taken, it will have to wait for the next sampling interval, which may be 40 to 50 msec later, before entry into the system. This would explain much of the latency variability observed for the generation of individual saccades. The real story is much more complex, however, and there is considerable controversy as to whether saccade vectors are calculated in an intermittent or continuous sampling way. It is also unclear at present whether saccade motor commands can be modified as the eyes are in motion during a saccade. Under ordinary circumstances, saccades behave as a ballistic movement—as with a thrown ball, the saccade trajectory is not modifiable after the movement begins. Under special test circumstances, however, some individuals are capable of modifying the saccade trajectory in mid flight. These special features of some saccades in normal patients have not yet been adequately explained by existing models of brainstem circuitry.

Saccades have characteristic peak velocities that bear a direct relationship to the size of the eye movement in normal persons. Larger saccades are faster than smaller ones, but it is impossible to perceive these subtle velocity variations by direct observation of the eyes in flight. Fortunately for diagnosis, pathology in the saccade system often slows refixational eye movements sufficiently that the movements are easily perceived to be slow on direct inspection. The best way to observe this is by asking the patient to redirect his gaze to stationary points right and left of primary gaze. A major reduction in saccade velocity generally indicates cerebellar or brainstem disorders, although minor slowing that usually requires electronic eye movement measurement to document can accompany cerebral hemisphere pathology, particularly if it involves the frontal lobes.

Another aspect of saccade abnormality is dysmetria, in which there is altered excursion amplitude—eyes either fall short of their goal (hypometric saccades) or overshoot the target (hypermetric saccades). When saccades are hypometric, the eyes achieve the target by a series of small saccades (usually three or more). This gives the movement a "jerky" or ratchet-like quality that is easily observed. It is useful to count the number of saccades necessary for the eyes to achieve a target 25° or 30° to either side of center (primary gaze). Normal persons often require two and occasionally three saccades, but a patient who consistently uses three or more saccades to make a 30° refixation can be considered abnormal. It is easier to be sure that saccade hypometria is significant if the number of saccades used for refixation to one side of primary gaze differs markedly from the number required to make an equal distance excursion to the other side.

Overshoot or hypermetric saccades are also easily observed. The eyes overshoot and attain the target by way of a series of decreasing amplitude reversals, each of which overshoots to a smaller degree than the preceding one. Each corrective saccade is separated from the last by the normal obligatory intersaccadic interval of approximately 200 msec. This gives the movement a discontinuous quality as opposed to a smooth to-and-fro, or pendular, appearance. In the acute stages of vascular lesions—infarctions or hemorrhages—of one frontal lobe, the eyes are usually deviated tonically to the side of the lesion because of the suddenly unopposed tonic influence of the normal hemisphere. It can be deduced from this that the normal tonus of a particular hemisphere, and perhaps of the frontal eye field specifically, brings about contralateral eye movements. This contraversive functional orientation is also observed in the disordered saccadic behavior that accompanies chronic frontal lobe lesions. In these cases, after the tonic eye deviation of the acute stage wears off and the patient is able to deviate the eyes fully in both directions, there remains a subtle disorder in which saccades directed away from the side of the lesion are hypometric. As an example, a patient with right frontal lobe infarction will have trouble looking volitionally to the left. During the first 4 or 5 days after the acute event, his eyes may be strongly deviated to the right, sometimes along with a forceful head and even torso deviation in the same direction. He will gradually be able to direct his gaze further to the left, and finally, full deviation will be possible. He may also require an abnormally long latency before initiating leftward eye movements during the acute stages. This directional latency effect must be distinguished from bidirectional increased latency, which may represent an altered mental function rather than a specific disorder of the saccade system. In the chronic stages of this right hemisphere vascular lesion, leftward refixations may continue to evoke numerous hypometric saccades, while normometric single saccades are generated for rightward refixations.

This contraversive organization is peculiar to the saccade system, because the pursuit system operates in an ipsiversive mode, controlling eye movements toward the hemisphere that is active. This fact of opposing functional orientation in the saccade and pursuit systems at the cerebral hemisphere level greatly enhances the diagnostic usefulness of eye signs related to these subsystems.

Pursuit System

The task of the pursuit system is the maintenance of a target on the fovea with motion of the target in space. If the viewer's head remains stationary, the tracking of a moving target is achieved by matching the angular velocity of the eyes turning in the orbits to the angular velocity of the target moving across visual space.

The visual system is oriented about the retinas, which are on the spherical back surfaces of the eyes, and angular measurements in degrees or minutes of arc are more convenient than the tangent measure, which would have to include the distance traveled in the frontal plane and the distance of that plane from the viewer in order to define the appropriate pursuit eye movement. The pursuit movement would also be awkward to specify in tangent measure because it involves rotation about a vertical axis rather than translational movement in a flat plane.

The normal behavior of the pursuit system can be specified as the gain (G), and $G = I/O$, where I is the input or target velocity in visual space (deg/sec) and O is the output, in this case pursuit eye velocity (deg/sec). Normal tracking involves a gain of 1.0 such that the eyes stay on the target as it moves.

The most frequently observed abnormality of pursuit is subnormal gain, in which the eyes fall progressively behind the target. The examiner cannot perceive the velocity of a patient's pursuit movements by inspection. Fortunately, the visual system will not tolerate the error that develops as the eyes fall behind the target, and an easily observed saccade is generated as soon as the eye is sufficiently far behind to generate a position error signal. Thus, low-gain pursuit is interrupted by a series of catch-up saccades aimed at refoveating the target. These inserted saccades occur rhythmically, since it requires about the same amount of time to generate the necessary position error throughout the course of the pursuit movement. Normal pursuit is smooth with no inserted saccades. Low-gain pursuit is indicated to the observer by the presence of rhythmic saccades rather than the slowness of the pursuit movement itself.

This pursuit abnormality, which is best referred to as low-gain pursuit with catch-up saccades, has engendered various descriptive names including saccadic pursuit, and even cogwheel pursuit in patients with Parkinson's disease. This movement should not, however, be linked to the pathophysiology of parkinsonian cogwheeling. The saccadic pursuit of parkinsonism is the manifestation of low gain in the pursuit system with a relatively normal saccade function so that forward saccades achieve refoveation during defective tracking. This does not differ from low-gain pursuit in other pathologic conditions.

The pursuit system is highly susceptible to degraded function, and bidirectional low-gain pursuit may be a nonspecific abnormality in various clinical settings in which the finding has no localizing value. Fatigue and the effects of many drugs bring about bidirectional symmetrical low-gain pursuit. Bidirectional low-gain pursuit is common in the elderly and has little prognostic or localizing value.

Unidirectional low-gain pursuit, however, is highly specific for a lesion of the horizontal gaze pathway on one side. The pursuit function in the cerebral hemisphere is ipsiversive, and a unidirectional defective pursuit suggests a lesion of the parieto-occipital convexity on the side toward which pursuit gain is low. For instance, a right-sided posterior hemisphere lesion will cause low-gain pursuit with catch-up saccades rightward, but it will leave leftward pursuit unaffected.

Large hemisphere lesions may involve both saccade and pursuit functions, in which case there will be hypometric saccades in one direction (opposite the lesion) and low-gain pursuit in the other (toward the lesion). Low-gain pursuit can also be observed as part of the supranuclear conjugate gaze disorder that accompanies lesions of the rostral pons and midbrain, usually in conjunction with altered saccade parameters, but here the saccades and pursuit are defective in the same direction.

A fundamental distinction must therefore be made between cerebral hemisphere and brainstem conjugate gaze syndromes. At the cerebral level, the direction of the saccade abnormality (contraversive) is opposite to the direction of the pursuit abnormality (ipsiversive), whereas at the brainstem level both are ipsilateral to the lesion side. Clinical evidence tells us that the saccade control pathways cross somewhere caudal to the diencephalon but rostral to the pons, whereas the pursuit pathways either do not cross at all, or they cross and recross such that their functional direction is ipsilateral to the disordered hemisphere. I have published a case in which a small hematoma at the posterior thalamus resulted in contraversive hypometric saccades and ipsiversive low gain pursuit with catch-up saccades. This indicates that the hemisphere bidirectionality is preserved as far caudal and as deep as the thalamus. This may indicate that the pursuit and saccade pathways both operate by way of the ipsilateral frontal eye field outflow through the thalamus. Alternatively, the pursuit system may have pathways in the corona radiata separate from the saccade system outflow, but these may funnel through the same region in the thalamus as the frontal system. Clinical evidence does not as yet discriminate between these two possibilities. The fact that some frontal lesions are associated with an ipsidirectional pursuit defect in conjunction with a contraversive saccade disorder supports the idea of a pursuit system outflow by way of a common frontothalamic brainstem pathway. The repeated observation of frontal lesions with isolated contralateral saccade disruption and normal pursuit weigh against a common pathway. Further clinical observations are required to specify more precisely how this might operate.

Saccade versus Pursuit Testing

Proper testing means the separate elicitation of saccade and pursuit-type eye movements. The examiner should stand about 1 meter in front of the patient. Visually guided saccades are tested by asking the patient first to look at the examiner's nose and then to look at an object about 30° to either side of the midline. Appropriately placed objects will be provided if the examiner holds his arms semiextended (elbows about 90° flexed) with hands slightly in front of his own facial plane. The patient should keep his head stationary in a straight-ahead position during this type of testing to avoid introducing vestibulo-ocular components. He is asked to refixate his gaze from the examiner's nose to one of his hands, then back to his nose, and finally to his other hand and back again. It is often useful to wiggle the fingers of the hand you want the patient to look at as an added stimulus for a visually guided saccade.

The clinical setting sometimes suggests the need to test for saccades without visual targets. This has to do with the ability to imagine coordinates for the saccade system, which can be selectively defective in some cases of higher cortical function abnormality with diffuse or widespread lateralized hemisphere lesions. In this case, simply ask the patient to "look left" or "look right" without providing any target.

A selective examination for pursuit system defects involves providing a slowly moving target for the patient to view. One can infer that pursuit function is pathologic if the normally smooth following or pursuit eye movement is interrupted by a series of "jerky"-appearing saccades. The target should not be moved too rapidly, since the pursuit system in normal persons falls behind when target velocities reach 40° to 50°/second, producing saccadic pursuit at faster target speeds. A target excursion that carries the patient's eyes from extreme right to extreme left gaze should take about 5 seconds.

Vestibulo-ocular System

The vestibulo-ocular system maintains the fixation of objects in visual space in the presence of head movement. The afferent arm of this reflex is initiated by acceleration receptors in the inner ear. A mathematical integration is performed on the acceleration data by virtue of the mechanics of the semicircular canal and cupula, and information on head rotational velocity in space is supplied to the vestibular nuclei by way of the eighth cranial nerve. The information is relayed from there to the brainstem gaze centers, where slow eye movements with velocity equal to and

direction opposite head rotation are generated. For instance, if the head rotates rightward at 10°/second, the vestibulo-ocular reflex produces a leftward eye movement at 10°/second, and the image of a viewed stationary object remains fixed on the fovea. The operation of this system, like that of the pursuit system, is conveniently expressed as "gain," that is, eye movement velocity divided by head rotation velocity in degrees per second. Naturally, a gain of 1.0 is needed to maintain foveation with head rotation. It turns out, however, that the vestibulo-ocular reflex does not supply the entire eye movement drive, since in total darkness the gain of this system falls to about 0.6 in normal persons. This means that the vestibulo-ocular reflex normally works together with the pursuit system, which optimizes function, since the vestibulo-ocular reflex has no retinal feedback by which to monitor its performance and keep its output accurate. Any inappropriate velocity drive from this "open loop" vestibulo-ocular system is adjusted by the "closed-loop" pursuit system, which receives direct retinal afferent feedback for fine control of the foveal position on the visual environment.

The key symptom of pathologic underactivity in the vestibulo-ocular reflex is oscillopsia, which is an illusory sense of movement in the visual environment as the head moves. This is a direct consequence of foveal image motion engendered specifically by head movement. The illusion ceases when the head is immobile. Vertigo, another common symptom of vestibular disorders, is often present when the head is still, although head movement usually aggravates it. Vertigo is a rotational illusion that is often accompanied by rhythmic oscillopsia as a consequence of nystagmus, in which case the rhythm is probably imposed by the regular fast phases of the nystagmus.

Nystagmus is defined as a repetitive bidirectional or multidirectional ocular oscillation in which the slow-phase movement is the pathologic one. When caused by vestibular disease, the nystagmus is created by tonic imbalance or bias in the vestibular subsystems on either side of midline, including the central connections and the peripheral labyrinthine apparatus. Tonic vestibular system imbalance passes a tonic directional bias to the brainstem gaze centers, which causes the eyes to drift toward the side with reduced activity. The tonic influence of each side is contraversive and a lesion creates underactivity of the ipsilateral system, with relative overactivity of the opposite system. The unopposed contraversive tone of the system opposite the lesion imposes eye drift toward the lesion side. This drift is checked by rhythmically occurring saccades in the opposite direction. The ensemble effect is rhythmic jerk-type nystagmus with slow-phase movements toward the side with the lesion and fast phases away from the lesion. This nystagmus is rhythmic because the slow-phase drift is at a constant velocity, determined by the degree of bias or imbalance between the two lateral vestibular subsystems, and the corrective saccades occur whenever a certain fixed amount of retinal position error between the object of regard and fovea occurs.

Vestibular disorders are discussed in Chapter 14. The discussion here is meant to provide the basis for understanding the more important ocular motility aspects of vestibular function.

BRAINSTEM ORGANIZATION OF EYE MOVEMENT CONTROL: THE FINAL COMMON PATHWAY

Zones within the tegmental reticular formation in the brainstem serve to combine the various eye movement commands and to present an integrated set of final motor commands to the oculomotor nuclei. The pontine paramedian reticular formation (PPRF) refers to the zone surrounding the seventh nerve nucleus on either side of midline in the pontine tegmentum. This area is specialized for integration of horizontal eye movement commands. The rostral interstitial nucleus of the medial longitudinal fasciculus (riMLF), the interstitial nucleus of Cajal (iC), the nucleus of Darkschewitsch (nD), the nucleus of the posterior commissure (nPC), and the adjacent portions of the mesencephalic reticular formation probably perform similar integration of commands for vertical eye movement and pass the final innervation pattern to the nuclei of the third and fourth cranial nerves.

Commands for saccades and pursuit come down to the brainstem by way of the supranuclear eye movement pathways outlined previously. In addition, the vestibular nuclei in the medulla and the flocculi and noduli of the cerebellum provide vestibular inputs to both the horizontal eye movement system in the PPRF and to the vertical eye movement zones of the mesencephalic reticular formation, primarily the riMLF and iC.

VERTICAL GAZE

The organization of the vertical eye movement system is complex and is not completely understood. The riMLF appears to contain primarily burst neurons that generate vertical saccades, whereas cells of the iC, nD, nPC, and MRF carry the fully assembled burst–tonic firing pattern needed to perform saccades, and pursuit and vestibulo-ocular movements, and to hold the eyes in eccentric positions of gaze. There is evidence that the iC provides vertical gaze–holding signals, while the nucleus prepositus hypoglossi (NPH) and medial vestibular nucleus (MVN) provide this function for horizontal eye movements. Nuclei at the pontine and medullary levels are important in the control of vertical eye movements. Bilateral lesions of the medial longitudinal fasciculus (MLF), which carries complex ascending influences from vestibular nuclei, NPH, and PPRF gaze centers to the iC, nD, and nPC, abolish vertical pursuit and vestibulo-ocular reflex movements but spare saccades. Thus, the riMLF apparently has functional connections with the cerebral hemispheres independent of supranuclear pathways that operate by way of the PPRF. Although vertical saccades are spared with bilateral lesions of the ascending pathways, the eye position signal is abolished and gaze paretic nystagmus occurs with up-and-down gaze effort.

For all practical purposes, there are no clinical disorders in which vertical gaze palsy is caused by cerebral hemisphere disease. Brainstem structures classically thought to mediate vertical gaze are situated in the midbrain tectum and pretectal areas. In this region, lesions commonly cause upward and downward gaze palsies along with certain other classic features, the constellation of which constitute the midbrain pretectal syndrome, also referred to as the periaqueductal gray matter syndrome, or Parinaud's syndrome. It is sometimes referred to as the syndrome of Koerber and Salus, who documented similar findings in a patient with a mass lesion in the sylvian aqueduct itself, whereas Parinaud described the findings related to pinealomas compressing the midbrain pretectum from the outside. The same clinical constellation results from infarction and hemorrhage involving these same anatomic structures as intrinsic lesions. The syndrome to be described is, therefore, of localizing value but does not provide evidence for a specific etiology in a particular case. For this, the tempo of evolution and the regression of signs and symptoms, along with other clinical details, are needed.

Aside from vertical gaze palsy, the common features of midbrain pretectal lesions include pupillary paralysis with unequal pupils that are sometimes large and sometimes small, loss of pupil reaction to light with preserved miosis on near viewing (light-near dissociation), convergence–retraction nystagmus, and variable degrees of ptosis or pathologic lid retraction. Rhythmic backward movement of the globes into the orbits in a nystagmus-like cycle characterizes retractory nystagmus. In conjunction with globe retraction, there may be convergence movements of the two eyes with respect to one another.

This constitutes the classic convergence–retraction nystagmus of midbrain pretectal lesions.

HORIZONTAL GAZE

Efferents from the PPRF on one side connect with large motor cells in the ipsilateral sixth nerve nucleus for abduction of the ipsilateral eye, and with small cells in the same nucleus. Axons from the small cells of the abducens nucleus ascend in the MLF and connect with cells in the opposite medial rectus subnucleus of the third nerve for adduction of the contralateral eye. Thus, a contraversive (opposite direction) saccade command from one hemisphere descends to the opposite-side PPRF, then to the abducens nucleus for both abduction of the eye ipsilateral to the active PPRF and adduction of the opposite eye. This produces conjugate gaze contralateral to the hemisphere issuing the command, ipsilateral to the activated PPRF.

Figure 23-14 illustrates schematically the brainstem and hemisphere pathways that participate in conjugate leftward gaze. Beginning at the right cerebral hemisphere, we can follow the path through the deep cerebral white matter and diencephalon to the midbrain, where a proposed crossing occurs just caudal to the third cranial nerve nucleus. This route continues to the PPRF on the left side of the brainstem, probably in the basis pontis. A synapse occurs here with PPRF neurons, which, in turn, make a relay to the ipsilateral sixth cranial nerve nucleus. Activation of the sixth nerve (abducens) nucleus causes abduction of the left eye. It is clear that conjugate leftward gaze will require coordinated adduction of the right eye, thus the next step is a requisite connection between the small cell population of the left abducens nucleus and the right third cranial nerve nucleus, specifically the medial rectus subnucleus. This connection is served by a paired bundle of fibers that run throughout the brainstem dorsally and just on either side of midline: the MLF. This is the basic connectivity that underlies conjugate horizontal gaze. Of course, there are a great many other contributory connections to and from the other nuclei having to do with the control of saccade, pursuit, and vestibular and gaze-holding functions.

These multidirectional systems are admittedly difficult to follow; however, it will make more sense if you trace the steps carefully from level to level and you work out the directions for yourself.

MEDIAL LONGITUDINAL FASCICULUS AND "INTERNUCLEAR OPHTHALMOPLEGIA"

To this point, our discussion has concerned only disorders that bring about conjugate disorders of gaze;

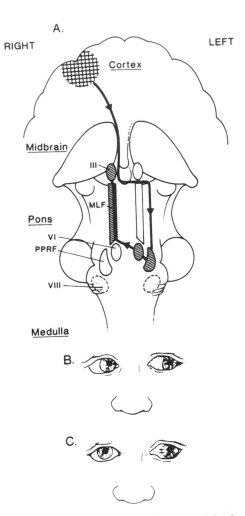

FIG. 23-14. A. Semischematic diagram of the brainstem pathways and centers that serve horizontal conjugate gaze. Multisynaptic pathways from the right frontal cortex decussate in the midbrain and form synapses in the left pontine paramedian reticular formation (PPRF), which relays innervation to two cell populations within the sixth cranial nerve nucleus. The large cells in the nucleus send axons to the lateral rectus muscle to abduct the left eye. The small cell population gives rise to a pathway that decussates and ascends in the contralateral medial longitudinal fasciculus (MLF) and makes synaptic contact with cells of the medial rectus subnucleus of the third cranial nerve complex. This pathway gives rise to coordinated adduction of the right eye to complete the act of con-

that is, if one eye fails to deviate leftward, the other eye also fails in the same direction and to an equal degree. Thus, the eyes in all these lesions remain "straight" with parallel visual axes when viewing objects at a distance. For simplicity, we will ignore the case of near-object viewing with convergence of the visual axes, because it is irrelevant for most neurologic diagnoses. After the supranuclear organizational systems supply input to the PPRF for horizontal eye deviation, the neural information must be conveyed to the ipsilateral sixth cranial nerve (lateral rectus nucleus for abduction) and the contralateral third cranial nerve (medial rectus subnucleus for adduction). The MLF provides the pathway that connects these two nuclei, and lesions of this pathway cause a clinical condition known as internuclear ophthalmoplegia (INO).

Lesions affecting the MLF cause failure of the adducting eye to move, whereas the abducting eye deviates laterally to its full extent. This striking pattern of dysconjugate eye movement is called internuclear ophthalmoplegia because the lesion in effect disconnects the sixth and the third cranial nerve nuclei by causing a failure of neural conduction in the internuclear pathway, the MLF.

In addition to failure of the eye on the side of the MLF lesion to adduct, there is usually "dissociated" monocular nystagmus of the abducting other eye in cases of INO. This peculiar monocular nystagmus can be either transitory (one or two beats) or sustained. The clinical importance of diagnosing the MLF syndrome is its exquisite localizing value for lesions deep in the substance of the brainstem tegmentum. This general area in the brainstem contains the ascending reticular activating system, which is necessary for alert consciousness, along with several adjacent cranial nerve nuclei and various ascending and descending sensory and cerebellar pathways. Therefore, the isolated occurrence of an MLF syndrome in an alert individual without other brainstem signs or symptoms suggests the presence of a discrete lesion. For practical purposes, in the adult this is caused by either a small demyelinating plaque of multiple sclerosis or by a tiny infarction due to small vessel disease. This type of tiny infarct is called a lacune and occurs

mainly in hypertensive patients older than 60 years. An MLF syndrome or INO is occasionally encountered as a result of trauma, and in children it can be the first sign of a brainstem glioma (astrocytoma).

Differentiating between multiple sclerosis and lacunar infarction can be a problem, because in either, the lesions tend to evolve acutely or subacutely and then resolve slowly over a period of days or weeks. Some generalizations can be helpful, however. The patient with an MLF lesion caused by multiple sclerosis will most often be under 40 years of age, whereas the patients at risk for lacunae are generally over 60 years. It has been said that a bilateral MLF lesion favors multiple sclerosis, because there is nothing to limit a plaque at the anatomic midline, whereas vascular lesions are often limited to one side by the vascular territory of a basilar artery paramedian-penetrating branch.

The clinical appearance of internuclear ophthalmoplegia can be mimicked in most details by myasthenia gravis, which can present with failure of adduction in one eye with dissociated nystagmus of the other eye. It is theoretically interesting that the dissociated, unilateral nystagmus of internuclear ophthalmoplegia is also present in myasthenia, which is, of course, a peripheral disorder. The mechanisms that cause the dissociated nystagmus in MLF lesions are not understood. The practical offshoot is that any patient presenting purely with findings of an MLF lesion, either unilateral or bilateral, without other brainstem signs or symptoms should have an edrophonium chloride (Tensilon) test as part of the workup. If the disorder of eye motility is caused by myasthenia, it will clear dramatically during the time the edrophonium chloride is in effect.

EYE MOVEMENT DISORDERS WITH NUCLEAR AND INFRANUCLEAR LESIONS

Lesions of the oculomotor (third), trochlear (fourth), and abducens (sixth) nerve nuclei and their outflow pathways produce dysconjugate eye movements. The pattern of the movement disorder is highly characteristic of the involved cranial nerve and serves to localize the problem. The medial recti cause adduction of the eye, whereas the lateral recti cause abduction or outward rotation of the eye. The anatomy and physiology of the vertically acting muscles are more complicated.

Elevation and *depression* are the terms applied to upward and downward rotations of the eyes about a horizontal axis. The term *torsion* has been applied to rotation of the globe about an anteroposterior axis.

---

jugate leftward gaze as illustrated in **B.** A lesion in the MLF causes internuclear ophthalmoplegia, which is characterized by a failure of adduction of the ipsilateral eye during attempted conjugate gaze as illustrated in **C.** The abducting eye often manifests dissociated or monocular nystagmus.

Intorsion refers to the rotation of the 12:00 meridian of the iris inward, toward the nose, and *extorsion* refers to the rotation of this reference point outward toward the ear. The names *incyclodeviation* and *excyclodeviation* have also been applied to torsional movements.

The superior and inferior recti function, respectively, as elevators and depressors of the globe when the eye is in abduction. The inferior and superior obliques serve, respectively, as elevators and depressors when the eye is in adduction. The torsional component for each of these muscles comes into play when the optical axis is not in alignment with the axis of pull for the particular muscle (Table 23-4).

THIRD CRANIAL NERVE PALSIES

The third cranial nerve innervates the medial rectus, superior rectus, and inferior oblique muscles, along with the pupil sphincter and the levator palpebrae, which elevates the upper eyelid. The third nerve originates in a rostrocaudally elongated group of subnuclei clustered in the midbrain just rostral to the level of the fourth cranial nerve nucleus. The architecture of this nuclear group has been the subject of intensive study over the years. The most widely accepted anatomic scheme is that of Warwick, which is represented in a stylized view in Figure 23-15. Warwick conceived of the subnuclei as columns of cells in elongated arrangement along the rostrocaudal dimension. Axons from the more dorsally situated subnuclei pass through the middle and inferior columns of cells on their way to the point of exit from the ventral aspect of the midbrain near the cerebral peduncles. The nuclei for the inferior rectus, inferior oblique, and medial rectus muscles send axons only to the ipsilateral third cranial nerve. The subnucleus for the levator palpebrae (caudal central nucleus) is a midline structure and sends axons to both nerves. The superior rectus subnucleus sends axons only to the contralateral third nerve trunk. These anatomic details lead to clinical rules by which one can determine whether a lesion is in the third nerve trunk or at the level of the nucleus. Figure 23-15 is set up to illustrate

the effects of a right third nerve nuclear lesion. The *filled triangles* and *solid lines* indicate uninterrupted neurons from the left subnuclei. The *open triangles* and *dotted lines* represent neurons that are affected by the lesion in the right third nerve nucleus. Lesioned neurons include those with cell body damage in the affected nucleus, and others with damage primarily to the axons as they pass through the lesioned nucleus. Note that with destruction limited to the right side of the nucleus, there is complete disruption of outflow to the right third cranial nerve. In addition, fibers coming from the left superior rectus and levator palpebrae subnuclei are shown as *solid lines* changing to *dotted lines*, indicating axonal disruption as they pass through the right-sided lesion. This is a necessary consequence of the fact that fibers flow through the other nuclear subgroups and are almost always involved in clinical lesions such as infarction or hemorrhage limited to one side. This mixture of crossed and uncrossed axonal involvement leads to the rule that nuclear lesions on one side cause partial bilateral ptosis and failure of elevation of both eyes. The contralateral ptosis is usually incomplete because there are some intact fibers to the levator contralateral to the nuclear lesion supplied by noncrossing neurons in the normal side of the caudal central nucleus.

Nuclear lesions are caused primarily by small infarctions secondary to occlusion of the medial penetrating vessels from the basilar artery. On rare occasions, small hemorrhages in this area may cause nuclear third cranial nerve palsies. More ventral lesions in the brainstem substance may cause a disruption of the fibers emerging from the third cranial nerve nuclei along with contralateral hemiplegia caused by the involvement of the cerebral peduncle (Weber's syndrome). The characteristics of these fascicular third nerve lesions are the same as those of any distal lesion, affecting only the axons of one nerve.

An important third nerve lesion is caused by aneurysms of the posterior communicating artery that involve the nerve trunk as it passes near this vessel at its junction with the supraclinoid portion of the internal carotid artery near the cavernous sinus. Figure 23-11 illustrates semidiagrammatically the anatomy of the third nerve course in relation to the posterior cerebral artery, the superior cerebellar artery, and the posterior communicating artery. This figure illustrates an aneurysm of the posterior communicating artery at its origin from the internal carotid. The inset shows an aneurysm in cross section, and its relationship to the adjacent third cranial nerve. The pupillary fibers from the Edinger–Westphal subnucleus are

TABLE 23-4. Muscle Action by Position

	POSITION	
MUSCLE	*ADDUCTION*	*ABDUCTION*
Superior rectus	Intorsion	Elevation
Inferior rectus	Extorsion	Depression
Inferior oblique	Elevation	Extorsion
Superior oblique	Depression	Intorsion

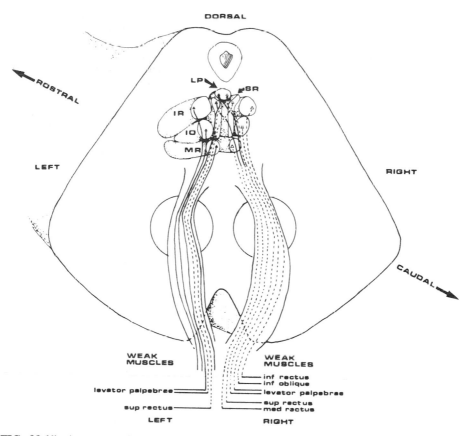

FIG. 23-15. A cross section through the midbrain showing the third cranial nerve nuclear complex. The subnuclei extend in rostrocaudally oriented columns as depicted in this three-dimensional representation modeled on Warwick's schemata. The letters superimposed on each nuclear group indicate the muscle innervated as follows: LP = levator palpebrae; SR = superior rectus; IR = inferior rectus; IO = inferior oblique; MR = medial rectus. A right nuclear third nerve lesion is illustrated. *Open triangles* and *dotted lines* indicate lesioned neurons and their axons. *Filled triangles* and *solid lines* denote normal neurons and their axons. All of the outflow to the right third nerve is lesioned. Crossed outflow from the right SR and LP subnuclei gives rise to paresis of contralateral eye elevation and ptosis. The left ptosis is partial since there is still ipsilateral (uncrossed) outflow from left LP subnucleus to the left LP. The crossed pathway from left LP subnucleus to right LP is affected at the axonal level as the fibers course through the damaged right third nerve complex (*transition of solid lines to dotted*), thus right ptosis is complete. The contralateral elevator palsy and ptosis thus distinguish nuclear nerve palsy from fascicular palsy in which the findings are limited to the ipsilateral eye.

shown as a black band at the periphery of the nerve. The fact that aneurysms commonly produce dilatation of the pupil on the side of the third nerve lesion was discussed previously. Figure 23-11 shows that the right eye is slightly abducted and depressed on account of a

weakness of the medial rectus, superior rectus, and inferior oblique muscles, with unopposed tone in the lateral rectus and superior oblique muscles.

The third nerve is often involved in lesions of the cavernous sinuses, commonly in conjunction with the other cranial nerves that pass in this structure, namely the fourth (trochlear), the sixth (abducens), and the first two divisions of the fifth (trigeminal). The most commonly encountered lesions in this area are inflammatory diseases of unknown etiology, aneurysms of the subclinoid internal carotid artery, and tumors. Granulomatous or primarily lymphocytic inflammation in the cavernous sinus and superior orbital fissure is known as the Tolosa–Hunt syndrome. It is manifest primarily by painful ophthalmoplegia from combined involvement of third, fourth, and sixth cranial nerves, and it nearly always improves with steroid treatment. This relatively benign inflammatory disease must be distinguished, however, from other infiltrating lesions such as lymphomas and carcinomas, which may also respond transiently to steroid administration. Meningiomas of the medial sphenoid ridge and pituitary tumors expanding laterally from the sella can also involve the cranial nerves within the cavernous sinuses. Mucocele of the sphenoid and ethmoid sinuses can, on rare occasions, also present in this way.

The subject of "medical" third cranial nerve palsy, referring to a microvascular occlusion with infarction in the nerve trunk, has already been discussed in the pupil section. Since the infarction is often limited to the center of the nerve, and the pupillary fibers occupy the periphery, the rule for diagnosis of this type of lesion is sparing of the pupil relative to the degree of palsy in the extraocular muscles.

FOURTH CRANIAL NERVE PALSIES

The trochlear nerve innervates the superior oblique muscle. Lesions affecting this cranial nerve produce a failure of the eye to depress in adduction with consequent vertical diplopia. With a right fourth cranial nerve palsy, the vertical diplopia would typically increase in gaze to the left (adduction of the right eye) and in downward gaze (into the field of action of the superior oblique). Since the superior oblique contributes to intorsional tone in primary gaze, the image from the involved eye is tilted. An astute patient with a right fourth nerve palsy may tell you, for instance, that the false image of a horizontal edge is not only below the image from the left eye but is also tilted with respect to the latter. Some patients develop a habitual head tilt, presumably to compensate for this torsional imbalance. A person with a right fourth cranial nerve palsy would tend to tilt his head to the left to bring the extorted eye back to the vertical position. The sound left eye can then increase its intorsional tone to make the two eyes parallel in the plane of rotation around the optic axis (anteroposterior axis). Since some intor-

sional tone can be contributed by the superior rectus, this muscle may be called into play to overcome the intorsional weakness caused by the fourth cranial nerve palsy. If, for instance, the examiner tilts the head of a person with right fourth nerve palsy to the right, even more intorsion than normal is required. The superior rectus is recruited in an effort to maximize intorsional power. This causes further inappropriate elevation of the right eye, because the primary effect of superior rectus contraction is an elevation of the eye.

This is the basis for the Bielschowski test for a fourth nerve palsy. The patient is directed to gaze straight ahead, and the head is then tilted to the right and to the left, making sure that there is no vertical or horizontal deviation away from primary gaze. If the degree of elevation of the eye on the side of the cranial nerve palsy increases as the head is tilted toward the side of the palsied muscle, the test is positive.

The fourth cranial nerve is unique in that it exits from the brainstem dorsally and crosses on the other side before encircling the brainstem on the way to the cavernous sinus. This renders it particularly susceptible to trauma in which forces are brought to bear on the dorsal midbrain. This usually occurs in the setting of severe head trauma in which the brainstem is forced downward and is angulated backward by a sudden shift of supratentorial structures. The dorsal midbrain and both fourth nerves are impacted in the crotch of the tentorium cerebelli, and both nerves tend to be contused together. Because of bilateral injury to the ascending reticular formation, the patient is usually unconscious for a protracted period of time after the injury, following which he complains of vertical double vision. On examination, one finds relative elevation of the right eye in left gaze and relative elevation of the left eye in right gaze. This reversal of vertical deviation indicates bilateral fourth cranial nerve palsies.

Unilateral fourth nerve palsy sometimes follows minor head trauma. There is reason to believe that many of these represent "decompensation" of long-standing or congenital fourth nerve palsies that were never previously symptomatic. Exactly how this comes about is unclear, but it is important to ask these patients to bring in childhood photographs to search for head tilt that would indicate a congenital condition.

Fourth cranial nerve palsies can occur secondary to intraneuronal microvascular ischemic disease as seen in elderly patients, often associated with diabetes and long-standing hypertension. These are presumably similar to the type of third and sixth cranial nerve palsies that one encounters in this same group of patients. The diplopia tends to improve over several weeks or months following the onset. Tumors in the region of the midbrain tectum can also occasionally present with fourth cranial nerve palsies.

SIXTH CRANIAL NERVE PALSIES

The abducens nucleus is medial and dorsal in the brainstem at the pontomedullary junction. Its axons course almost directly ventral and exit from the pons near the midline. The large cells of the abducens nucleus innervate the lateral rectus muscle, while a small cell population innervates the contralateral medial rectus subnucleus of the oculomotor complex (third cranial nerve) by way of the MLF.

The abducens nucleus is activated by input from the ipsilateral PPRF leading to coordinated abduction of the ipsilateral (to the active PPRF) eye, and adduction of the contralateral eye; this yoked deviation of both eyes is horizontal conjugate gaze.

Figure 23-16 illustrates a patient with weakness of the right lateral rectus caused by a sixth cranial nerve palsy. Note that in primary gaze the eyes are slightly crossed or convergent (esodeviated). This is caused by the unopposed tone of the medial rectus that is acting without the normal tonic innervation of the weak lateral rectus muscle. In left gaze, the eyes are parallel, but in right gaze there is a clear-cut failure of right eye abduction. In this case it is the right eye that is deviating inward in primary gaze, and it is the right lateral rectus muscle that is weak. Be aware, however, that in primary gaze the right eye might be used for fixation of the target, with deviation of the left eye, even with a weak right lateral rectus muscle. Which eye the patient chooses for fixation is a matter of habit that may not be disrupted by muscle paresis, even if the weakness is profound. There is also a strong tendency to fixate with the eye that has better vision.

The degree of esodeviation in primary gaze may be different depending on which eye is fixing. Primary deviation refers to the angle that results from fixation with the "good" eye. Secondary deviation results from fixation with the paretic eye and it is larger than primary deviation. In primary gaze, the bad eye is "struggling" to abduct even to the midposition against the tone of the medial rectus, and a great deal of rightward innervation is required by the right eye. According to Hering's law of equal innervation, the yoked medial rectus of the opposite (left) eye will also get this large amount of innervation and will adduct a great deal, creating a large-angle esotropia. When the nonparetic left eye is fixing, a standard quantity of rightward innervation is required, and a lesser deviation results from the failure of the right eye to abduct completely.

This difference between primary and secondary deviation is a good clue to the presence of muscle paretic deviation, as opposed to deviation caused by squint or childhood strabismus in which the deviation remains the same whichever eye is fixing. Fixation with one or the other eye can be forced by occluding the fellow eye and then quickly uncovering it to observe the degree of deviation of the covered eye before fixation is shifted.

As with the third and fourth cranial nerves, sixth cranial nerve palsies can occur on the basis of microvascular lesions in hypertensive and diabetic patients, in which case the abduction deficit tends to improve over a 3- to 6-month period. In addition, the sixth cranial nerve is susceptible to all of the local lesions that one could imagine in the pons, including hemorrhage, infarction, demyelination, and neoplasia (e.g., pontine glioma in childhood; metastatic tumor and reticulum cell sarcoma in adults). The sixth nerve may also be involved in inflammatory and infiltrating lesions of the cavernous sinuses, as already mentioned, or of the leptomeninges (e.g., carcinomatous meningitis, and chronic or acute infectious meningitis). In addition to these standard lesions, the sixth cranial nerve is susceptible to stretching and distortion in a way that the other cranial nerves are not. This phenomenon results in the so-called false-localizing sixth

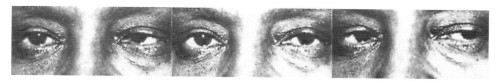

FIG. 23-16. Right lateral rectus palsy. In primary gaze (*center*), the eyes are slightly inturned with respect to one another (esodeviated). In right gaze (*left figure*) the angle of esodeviation increases as the right eye fails to abduct fully. In left gaze (*right figure*) the visual axes are parallel.

cranial nerve palsy in which the failure of abduction in one eye or both accompanies lesions that are remote from the sixth cranial nerve or its muscle, the lateral rectus. This occurs most commonly with raised intracranial pressure. Sixth nerve palsy has also been documented occasionally as a transient phenomenon following lumbar puncture. The pathophysiology in these cases is unclear, although presumably a transient shift of the brainstem secondary to cerebrospinal fluid pressure gradients is sufficient to cause the problem. The susceptibility of the sixth nerve to small brainstem displacement may be based on the fact that it is fixed on one end at its emergence from the pons, and at the other end at its entry point into the cavernous sinus—Dorello's canal in the petrous bone tip. The sixth nerve is between the proverbial rock and a hard spot.

WEAKNESS OF INDIVIDUAL EXTRAOCULAR MUSCLES

In the preceding sections, we have referred to a weakness of the muscles innervated by the third, fourth, and sixth cranial nerves and to lesions of these cranial nerves as though they were synonymous. This type of thinking should be avoided when one first encounters a patient with a weakness of one or several of these muscles. Disorders of muscle may mimic a lesion in any of these cranial nerves. Myasthenia gravis and thyroid eye disease are frequent offenders because they have a tendency to affect one or several extraocular muscles of one eye, or an asymmetrical array of muscles in both eyes. The level of the lesion may be difficult to determine when the nerve in question innervates only one muscle. In the case of the third cranial nerve, however, it should be easy to distinguish peripheral muscle disorders from those caused by an involvement of the cranial nerve. It is generally held that a lesion in the nerve trunk or at the nuclear level will involve, to some degree, all of the muscles within the distribution of the third cranial nerve. Isolated weakness of a superior rectus, or an inferior oblique, or a medial rectus muscle should engender suspicion that the disorder is peripheral, in the muscle or the terminal orbital branches of the third nerve, rather than in the more proximal intraorbital or intracranial portion of the nerve. Although an MLF lesion commonly causes isolated medial rectus weakness, the involvement of an inferior oblique or a superior rectus in isolation should immediately lead one to suspect that the disorder is in the orbit involving branches of the third cranial nerve or the muscles themselves. Myasthenia gravis and thyroid eye disease are the most likely etiologies. Myasthenia gravis can mimic INO (an MLF lesion) in all its aspects, including the dissociated

monocular nystagmus of the abducting eye. An edrophonium chloride test is therefore warranted in cases in which there are no brainstem signs or symptoms other than the ocular motility disorder of INO. Masses and infiltrating diseases within the orbit may affect one or the other of the muscles in the third cranial nerve group, but in these cases orbital signs (e.g., proptosis, lid edema, and conjunctival chemosis) should be evident.

QUESTIONS AND DISCUSSION

1. A 58-year-old man presents with a history of pain in the left orbit. He denies diplopia. The pain is described as intense and "boring" in quality without throbbing. He has no previous neurologic or ophthalmologic history. You have been monitoring him for 5 years for fairly well controlled adult-onset diabetes mellitus treated with diet restriction alone.

There is a complete left ptosis and the left eye is externally rotated (exodeviated) and depressed (deviated downward, hypodeviated). The pupil is 8 mm and fixed to light (direct stimulation). The patient is able to elevate and depress the eye through only about 10% of the expected range. There is no adduction past midline, but the left eye abducts fully. Your differential diagnosis includes:

A. Myasthenia gravis
B. Thyroid eye disease
C. Third cranial nerve (oculomotor nerve) palsy secondary to diabetes mellitus
D. Third cranial nerve palsy secondary to a tumor in the left cavernous sinus
E. Third cranial nerve palsy due to an intracranial "berry aneurysm"

You would order the following:

A. Carotid angiography
B. Skull series
C. Tomograms of the sella turcica region
D. Nothing

As it happens, the patient leaves town because of a family crisis and is away for the next 3 months. When he returns, he is able to open the left lid almost completely, although ptosis is still easily observed. Elevation and depression of the globe are more complete, and he can now adduct the left eye through about 70% of normal range. On adduction and attempted depression (downward rotation), however, there is a peculiar "staring" appearance to the left eye in that the lid elevates farther than its resting position with eyes straight ahead. You now conclude:

A. The danger is over.
B. Despite no change in diabetic management, the lesion has begun to improve, thus no further intervention is warranted.
C. There is an "aberrant regeneration" of fibers.
D. Because there has not been a complete recovery, an aneurysm should be ruled out.

Starting with the first office visit, you can make an educated guess as to the cause of the patient's clinical picture. The problem is not myasthenia gravis because the pupil is involved (internal ophthalmoplegia) as well as the extraocular muscles (external ophthalmoplegia). Thyroid eye disease must be considered in a patient with external ophthalmoplegia; however, ptosis and pupillary involvement in this condition is rare, if it occurs at all. The combination of ptosis; dilated pupil; weakness of medial, superior, and inferior recti; and weakness of inferior oblique reliably establishes the diagnosis of third cranial nerve (oculomotor nerve) palsy. It is left to decide what is the most likely cause. The differential diagnosis should include (C), (D), and (E) in the first question.

The primary physician is commonly required to make the basic and important decision as to whether a particular patient's third cranial nerve palsy is "medical" or "surgical." Medical third cranial nerve palsies are common in the age group past 55 years, and they are generally thought to represent ischemic lesions in the substance of the cranial nerve caused by insufficiency of vasa nervora. The scant available pathologic material relating to "medical" third cranial nerve palsies shows that healed lesions are characterized by fibrosis and acute lesions by demyelination. Axons are not disrupted to any appreciable degree in early or late lesions, which accounts for the recovery of function within a few months, and which underlies the fact that aberrant regeneration does not occur late in the course. The ischemic lesion is also restricted to the center of the nerve trunk, which is the anatomic basis for another characteristic feature of "medical" third cranial nerve palsies—the pupil is relatively spared. Anatomic studies have shown that the pupillary (sphincter) fibers run in the periphery of the nerve, which is spared from the more centrally distributed ischemia.

These ischemic lesions are commonly associated with long-standing hypertension or diabetes mellitus but can occur without these systemic risk factors for atherosclerosis, in which case the cranial nerve palsy is, by default, called idiopathic, although they are probably based on arteriosclerosis in patients over 60 years of age. These palsies generally clear within 3 to 6 months, and persistence of the deficit beyond this time calls for a further diagnostic workup.

Surgical third cranial nerve palsies are most commonly caused by berry aneurysms, particularly those that originate from the junction of the posterior communicating artery and the internal carotid artery. Observations at surgery or autopsy suggest that small bleeds from the aneurysm break into the parenchyma of the nerve, causing disruption of axons as well as local demyelination. This characteristically causes pupillary dilatation with little or no light reaction, because the superficially placed pupillary fibers are disrupted. This pupillary finding is the most reliable differential diagnostic feature to separate medical (ischemic) from surgical (aneurysms) third cranial nerve palsies, at least early in the course of the disease. Sparing of the pupil is most reliable as an indicator of "medical" third nerve palsy when the external ophthalmoplegia is complete. With partial external ophthalmoplegia, one must strongly consider angiography to make the distinction, even with relative sparing of the pupil. This is certainly true if the patient is under 60 years of age.

The disruption of axons caused by aneurysmal leakage into the nerve sets the stage for the misdirection of regenerating axons during the recovery phase. As an example of this, fibers destined originally for the medial or inferior rectus are sometimes misdirected to the levator palpebrae. Consequently, when the patient attempts to look down or to adduct the eye, the lid elevates.

Tumors compressing the third cranial nerve also cause pupillary involvement, but less frequently than do aneurysms.

This patient, therefore, has compelling evidence in favor of an aneurysm as the cause of his cranial nerve palsy, even though he is diabetic. One should be highly suspicious of this finding at the first office visit, because the pupil was large and fixed to light. After enough time has elapsed for the regeneration of axons and misdirection (aberrant regeneration) to occur, the finding of lid elevation on adduction and downward rotation of the eye further supports the diagnosis of an aneurysm or a tumor as opposed to an ischemic cause.

The best answers for the second question would, therefore, be (A) and (C). One would be justified in ordering carotid angiography in this case. If this study is negative for aneurysm, it may become necessary to order tomograms of the sella region in search of a meningioma or other tumor in the cavernous sinus or superior orbital fissure area. The angiogram or a routine CT scan is likely to reveal such a lesion, but may not if the lesion is an *en plaque* meningioma, in which case bony erosion or hyperostosis may require thin-section CT with bone windows to be visualized.

The answer to the third question is clearly (C), Response (D) is correct, but for the wrong reason.

2. An 18-year-old girl, brought in by her mother, complained that she had transiently gone blind in her right eye. The episode occurred in school and lasted 20 minutes. She noted that the right half of a large word on the blackboard seemed to be missing and that "everything seemed to be shimmering and wavy." She is in good general health, and the physical as well as neurologic examinations are normal. Useful questions you could ask include:

A. Where were you the night before this happened?
B. Did you cover the right or left eye to see if the vision changed?
C. Did you develop a headache during or after these visual symptoms?
D. Do you get sick headaches or sinus headaches?

Which of the following tests would be most appropriate for a workup of this patient?

A. Cerebral angiography
B. Pneumoencephalography
C. Carotid duplex examination
D. CT scan with enhancement, or MRI
E. Visual-field examination
F. Reassurance and a follow-up visit in 1 month or sooner should symptoms recur

Choices (B), (C), and (D) are potentially rewarding in the first part of this question. Patients, even those with reasonable intelligence, often fail to make a simple test of whether a visual defect exists in one or both eyes. People conceptualize vision as a unitary experience and are unaware of binocularity in daily life. As part of this unity of experience, many patients are unwilling to comprehend the concept of a homonymous field defect and doggedly stick to the contention that they lost vision in the right eye when, in fact, they experienced a right homonymous hemianopsia. Careful consideration of this patient's history indicates an inability to see the right half of a word written on the blackboard. This finding was experienced with both eyes open and must, therefore, represent a homonymous binocular loss of vision even though the patient's natural reaction was to ascribe the symptom to a loss of vision in the right eye.

It would be comforting in this case to elicit a history of left temporal throbbing headache, because this would almost undeniably label this patient's symptom complex as a classic migraine. It is important to realize, however, that many migraine patients have typical migrainous aura without a subsequent headache. A previous history of severe throbbing headaches with nausea, vomiting, diaphoresis, diarrhea, and vertigo would also identify the individual as one who is prone to common migraine. Such persons may occasionally have classic episodes (i.e., with aura) interspersed among common migraine attacks without aura. Patients with common migraine will often deny that they have migraine, because they ascribe their recurring, often unilateral frontal throbbing headaches to "sinus infections."

Choices (C), (D), and (E) would certainly be practical and justifiable noninvasive procedures for the second part of this question. Aside from migraine, which this patient almost certainly has, one should consider the less likely diagnosis of occipital arteriovenous malformation with small volume bleeding or transient steal syndrome and ischemia of the visual cortex, giving rise to the evanescent visual symptoms. Contrast-enhanced CT scan and MRI (D) should identify the vast majority of such lesions.

My personal choice when confronted with this patient, however, would be to give reassurance that the syndrome is common and would not be expected to produce any serious complications. Teenagers are often easily frightened by diagnostic procedures and may actually develop a functional overlay when confronted with the apparent seriousness of their condition engendered by a flurry of complex and dramatic examinations. The statistical chances of missing a significant structural lesion are small. Return visits are advisable, however, to ensure against missing progressive symptoms and to provide confidence on the part of the patient and family that they are not being abandoned. In treating patients who suffer from headaches, this sense of ongoing commitment is more important than the type of medicine prescribed.

3. A 38-year-old man presents with a 2-week history of frequent severe headaches in the right orbital area. The pain is steady, "boring" in character, and severe, but it lasts only 40 to 60 minutes. It tends to occur two to three times daily and can be anticipated regularly at 10 pm usually just after he retires. On examination, there is right ptosis and miosis but no other physical or neurologic findings. Workup should include:

A. Carotid angiography
B. CT scan including sphenoid and ethmoid paranasal sinuses

C. Instillation of 1% para-OH-amphetamine in either eye
D. Instillation of 4% cocaine in either eye

The most reliable indicator of a postganglionic lesion is failure of the pupil to dilate on instillation of 1% para-OH-amphetamine, which, like cocaine, blocks the reuptake of norepinephrine into the presynaptic sympathetic nerve terminals in the iris. In addition, however, it causes the release of any existing presynaptic norepinephrine stores. This means that, regardless of a lesion in the oculosympathetic preganglionic or central pathways, para-OH-amphetamine will release stores of norepinephrine and cause pupillary dilatation. Failure of dilatation, therefore, establishes the presence of a postganglionic oculosympathetic neuron lesion in which the normal stores of transmitter are pathologically absent.

Raeder described patients with painful oculosympathetic palsy and space-occupying lesions of the middle cranial fossa. All his patients also had findings referable to one or more of the third through sixth cranial nerves, and he put forth this combination as diagnostic of middle fossa masses. This original, or type I, form of Raeder's syndrome has now been separated from a benign, probably migrainous form, referred to as type II.

The original description of Raeder's syndrome type II included seven patients with painful oculosympathetic palsy. They all had unilateral brief steady headaches that conformed to the pattern of cluster or histamine headache, but they also had an ipsilateral oculosympathetic syndrome. None had findings of third, fourth, or sixth cranial nerve dysfunction. Lawton–Smith's concept that these patients with Raeder's type II have a form of migraine with secondary sympathetic involvement has come to be widely accepted. The patients are generally middle-aged, and men predominate. There must be no associated cranial nerve palsy, and the headache history should be typical of the cluster pattern. The oculosympathetic lesion should also be documented as postganglionic using the para-OH-amphetamine test. The theory is that the sympathetic lesion is caused by edema in the adventitia of the carotid siphon as a consequence of frequent and severe vascular headaches.

The diagnosis of Raeder's syndrome type II relieves the physician of the obligation to consider the patient to be a cancer suspect.

4. A 62-year-old man presents for a routine examination. He has no head or neck symptoms, but an examination reveals 1 to 2 mm of left ptosis. In the examining room, however, the pupils are noted to be equal in size at 3 mm. The patient denies awareness of the lid droop and denies head or neck trauma. A reasonable workup would include:

A. Chest roentgenogram
B. Sputum cytology with acid-fast bacilli (AFB) smear and culture
C. Examination of the pupils in a dim room
D. Instillation of 1% pilocarpine in either eye
E. Instillation of 4% cocaine in either eye
F. Instillation of 1% para-OH-amphetamine in either eye
G. Nothing
H. A request for old full-face photographs
I. Observation of iris color

The most serious concern on first observing a patient with Horner's syndrome is the possibility of cancer, which is one of the most common causes of an acquired ocular sympathetic lesion in the adult. Apical carcinoma of the lung (Pancoast's syndrome) is a common type that causes Horner's syndrome, but any neoplasm infiltrating cervical lymph nodes can present this way. Most often the patient is unaware of a change in his facial appearance, because the degree of ptosis is small and the onset is insidious without visual or other symptoms. The most practical approach is to determine (1) whether ptosis is actually due to oculosympathetic dysfunction, and (2) the age of the lesion.

Grimson and Thompson (1975) reviewed pharmacologic testing in Horner's syndrome with a logical approach to diagnosis. They found that the use of a weak direct-acting sympathomimetic (1:1000 epinephrine) was unreliable in clinical diagnosis. Four percent cocaine blocks the reuptake of norepinephrine into presynaptic terminals at the iris and causes pupillary dilatation in the normal eye. In the presence of Horner's syndrome, the release of norepinephrine is reduced and a reuptake block fails to dilate the pupil as much as it does in the fellow eye, which is used as a control. The cocaine test is useful to identify an oculosympathetic lesion in patients with ptosis and minimal or no anisocoria.

A simple preliminary approach is to observe the eyes for anisocoria in as dim an environment as possible consistent with adequate visualization of the pupils. In bright light, the iris (parasympathetic) sphincter dominates pupil size and can overcome minor asymmetry of tone in the radially oriented, sympathetically innervated dilator muscles. The sphincter relaxes in a dim light, and anisocoria, resulting from weakness of the pupil dilator muscles on the side of the oculosympathetic lesion, may become apparent.

If the ptosis has been present for several years, carcinoma can almost certainly be ruled out as the cause. An examination of old photographs will often settle the issue without an expensive workup, by demonstrating the ptosis to be long standing and unchanged over the years. Furthermore, an oculosympathetic lesion arising before birth, and perhaps in the first 1 to 2 years of life at the latest, will cause failure of iris chromatophores to develop. If the patient has one brown iris contralateral to the ptosis and a blue iris ipsilateral, the Horner's syndrome can be identified as ancient.

If the lesion cannot be documented as old and stable, a workup for carcinoma of the lung or carcinoma metastatic to cervical nodes could be undertaken. This presumes that there is no history of stroke, or of head or neck trauma, to explain the lesion. If the first round of tests is negative, it is important to follow the patient closely for emergence of signs or symptoms of underlying carcinoma. Frequent chest roentgenograms or CT scans with attention to apical regions are usually necessary. MRI will probably be the preferred method for examining the upper chest and neck.

SUGGESTED READING

Asbury AK, Aldridge H, Hershberg R et al: Oculomotor palsy in diabetes mellitus: A clinicopathologic study. Brain 93:555, 1970

Boniuk M, Schlesinger NS: Raeder's paratrigeminal syndrome. Am J Ophthalmol 54:1074, 1962

Borchert MS: Principles and techniques of the examination of ocular motility and alignment. In: Miller NR, Newman NJ (eds): Walsh and Hoyt's Clinical Neuro-Opthalmology, 5th Edition, Vol 1. Baltimore, Williams & Wilkins, 1998

Giles CL, Henderson JW: Horner's syndrome: An analysis of 216 cases. Am J Ophthalmol 46:289, 1958

Goldstein JE, Cogan DG: Diabetic ophthalmoplegia with special reference to the pupil. Arch Ophthalmol 64:592, 1960

Grimson BS, Thompson HS: Drug Testing in Horner's Syndrome, Vol 8, pp 265–207. St. Louis, CV Mosby, 1975

Hayreh SS: In vivo choroidal circulation and its watershed zones. Eye 4:273, 1990

Hayreh SS: The ophthalmic artery: III. Branches. Br J Ophthalmol 46:212, 1962

Keltner JL, Johnson CA, Spurr JO et al: Baseline visual field profile of optic neuritis: The experience of the Optic Neuritis Treatment Trial. Arch Ophthalmol 111:231, 1993

Kerr WL: The pupil: Functional anatomy and clinical correlation. In: Smith JL (ed): Neuro-Opthalmology, Vol 4, pp 49–80. Hollendale, FL, Huffman, 1968

Leigh JR, Zec DS: The Neurology of Eye Movement, 2nd Edition. Philadelphia, FA Davis, 1991

Leigh RJ, Averbach-Heller L: Nystagmus and related ocular motility disorders. In: Miller NR, Newman NJ (eds): Walsh and Hoyt's Clinical Neuro-Opthalmology, 5th Edition, Vol 1. Baltimore, Williams & Wilkins, 1998

Rucker CW: The causes of paralysis of the third, fourth and sixth cranial nerves. Am J Ophthalmol 61:1294, 1966

Rucker CW: Paralysis of the third, fourth, and sixth cranial nerves. Am J Ophthalmol 46:787, 1958

Sharpe JA: Neural control of ocular motor systems. In: Miller NR, Newman NJ (eds): Walsh and Hoyt's Clinical Neuro-Ophthalmology, 5th Edition, Vol 1. Baltimore, Williams & Wilkins, 1998

Smith CH: Nuclear and infranuclear ocular motility disorders. In: Miller NR, Newman NJ (eds): Walsh and Hoyt's Clinical Neuro-Ophthalmology, 5th Edition, Vol 1. Baltimore, Williams & Wilkins, 1998

Smith JL: Raeder's paratrigeminal syndrome. Am J Ophthalmol 46:194, 1958

Thompson HS, Bourgon P, Van Allen MW: The tendon reflexes in Adie's syndrome. In: Thompson HS (ed): Topics in Neuro-Opthalmology, pp 104–113. Baltimore, Williams & Wilkins, 1979

Thompson HS, Mensher JM: Adrenergic mydriasis of Horner's syndrome: Hydroxyamphetamine test for diagnosis of postganglionic defects. Am J Ophthalmol 72:472, 1971

Weber RB, Daroff RB, Mackey EA: Pathology of oculomotor nerve palsy in diabetics. Neurology 20:835, 1970

Neurology for the Non-Neurologist, Fourth Edition,
edited by William J. Weiner and
Christopher G. Goetz. Lippincott
Williams & Wilkins, Philadelphia © 1999.

CHAPTER 24

Central Nervous System Infections

Larry E. Davis

Central nervous system (CNS) infections can be caused by viruses, bacteria, fungi, and parasites, but bacteria and viruses are the most common. Infectious agents enter the body by way of the gastrointestinal tract or the respiratory tract, or following skin inoculation (e.g., animal or insect bite). The organism sets up the initial site of replication in the gastrointestinal tract, respiratory tract, or subcutaneous/muscle/vascular tissue. The majority of organisms then reach the CNS by way of the bloodstream, but occasional organisms reach the brain by way of peripheral nerves or by direct entry through adjacent bone from infected mastoid or air sinuses.

In spite of the many infections we develop during our lifetimes, few organisms ever reach the brain. Important protective systems include the reticuloendothelial system (which efficiently removes bacteria and viruses from blood), cellular and humoral immune responses (which destroy organisms from the blood and primary site of infection), and the blood–brain barrier [which prevents entry of organisms into the brain or cerebrospinal fluid (CSF)]. Organisms that do enter the brain or CSF from blood generally do so by infecting endothelial cells of the cerebral blood vessels (many encephalitis viruses), by penetrating the blood–CSF barrier in the meninges or choroid plexus (many bacteria), or by occluding small cerebral blood vessels with infected emboli from the heart or lung (brain abscess organisms). The brain and the CSF have less immune protection than the rest of the body: Normal CSF has about 1/200th the amount of antibody as blood and it has few white blood cells, and the brain lacks a lymphatic system. Thus, after invasion has occurred, individuals who develop a brain or meningeal infection often die without antimicrobial intervention.

Inflammation of the meninges or brain is the hallmark of CNS infection. Inflammatory cells (neutrophils and mononuclear cells) are seen in the meninges, in the perivascular spaces, or around an abscess. Lymphocytes in the inflammation show specific immune activity against the infectious agent.

The signs and symptoms of a CNS infection depend on the site of the infection, not on the organism, which primarily determines the time course and severity of the infection. In general, the time course for a viral infection to develop CNS signs is hours to 1 day; for aerobic bacteria, it is hours to a few days; for anaerobic bacteria, *Mycobacterium tuberculosis,* and fungi, it is days to weeks; and for parasites and *Treponema pallidum* (syphilis), it is weeks to years. Follow these steps to diagnose and treat CNS infections:

- Determine the site of infection
- Determine the class of organism (e.g., bacteria, virus)
- Begin initial treatment
- Determine specific organism and antimicrobial sensitivities, and modify treatment if necessary
- Watch for and treat complications

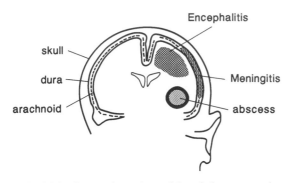

FIG. 24-1. Coronal section of head demonstrating locations of three major central nervous system infections.

There are three major sites where infections occur in the nervous system: diffusely in the meninges (meningitis), diffusely in the brain (encephalitis), and locally in the brain (abscess) (Fig. 24-1). Although patients may develop infections at other sites, such as epidural and subdural spaces, this chapter will focus on the most common infections.

MENINGITIS

CLINICAL FEATURES

A variety of viruses, bacteria, fungi, parasites, chemicals, and neoplasms may cause inflammation of the meninges. These patients all have common clinical findings:

- *Early features:* Prodromal illness, fever, headache, stiff neck, relative preservation of mental status, no focal neurologic signs, no papilledema
- *Later features:* Seizures, stupor and coma, cranial nerve palsies, deafness, focal neurologic signs

Clinical findings that suggest meningitis rather than encephalitis include stiff neck, relative preservation of mental status, lack of focal neurologic signs, and no papilledema. The time course of the meningitis may give clues as to its etiology. Viral meningitis is hyperacute, and patients develop acute symptoms and signs over a few hours. Patients with bacterial meningitis develop an acute illness over hours to 1 day. Patients with fungal meningitis or tuberculous meningitis develop symptoms over days to 2 weeks.

LABORATORY FINDINGS

In blood, the white blood cell count is usually elevated, as is the erythrocyte sedimentation rate. The CSF exam is the key to the diagnosis of meningitis, ascertainment of the class of infecting agent, establishment of the etiologic agent, and determination of antimicrobial sensitivities (Fig. 24-2). Viral, bacterial, tuberculous, and fungal infections of the meninges have different CSF profiles (Table 24-1). CSF culture determines the etiology of the infection as well as antimicrobial sensitivities. In general, cultures for bacteria take 1 to 3 days; for *M. tuberculosis* and fungi, 1 to 6 weeks; and for viruses, days to 3 weeks. Rapid diagnosis of bacteria can be made by Gram stain of CSF sediment and by testing CSF for common bacterial antigens. The Gram stain will detect bacteria in CSF sediment in over three fourths of patients with acute bacterial meningitis and often gives clues for initial antibiotic treatment. Latex agglutination antigen tests are commercially available to detect *Hemophilus influenzae, Streptococcus pneumoniae, Neisseria meningitidis,* and group A beta-hemolytic streptococci. Antigen tests have about the same sensitivity as the Gram stain. In the near future, polymerase chain reaction (PCR) tests should be available in clinical diagnostic laboratories to detect nucleic acid from common viruses and bacteria present in CSF. The PCR tests should have a sensitivity equal to or superior to culturing the infectious agent and can be performed within a few hours. This test, like a bacterial antigen test, will likely be available only for common bacteria and viruses that cause meningitis and will not yield antimicrobial sensitivities. Thus, the best diagnostic test is still to culture the CSF and blood for an infectious agent and use the isolate to determine antimicrobial sensitivities.

VIRAL MENINGITIS

Enteroviruses (echoviruses and Coxsackie viruses) are the most common cause of viral meningitis. Less common causes include herpes simplex virus type 2, mumps virus, and human immunodeficiency virus. Typically in viral meningitis, the CSF contains a pleocytosis with predominately lymphocytes, mildly elevated protein, normal glucose, and negative Gram stain of sediment. Viruses often can be isolated from CSF early in the meningitis. Treatment of viral meningitis is usually symptomatic and may include analgesics for the headache and antiemetics for nausea and vomiting. Hospitalization is often not required, but the patient should be observed at home by a responsible individual. The prognosis of viral menin-

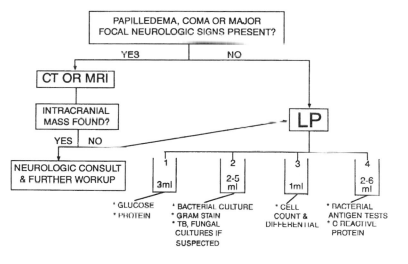

FIG. 24-2. Flow diagram for lumbar puncture and cerebrospinal fluid tests in suspected bacterial meningitis. With permission from Davis LE: Acute bacterial meningitis. In: Weiner WJ (ed): Emergent and Urgent Neurology, p. 139. Philadelphia, JB Lippincott, 1992.

gitis is excellent, and most patients fully recover within 1 to 2 weeks.

ACUTE BACTERIAL MENINGITIS

Aerobic bacteria, both gram-positive and gram-negative, cause meningitis mainly in young children, in the elderly, and in the immunosuppressed. *H. influenzae, S. pneumoniae,* and *N. meningitidis* are the most common offending bacteria. Unlike viral meningitis, patients with bacterial meningitis will progress to death if not treated with antibiotics. Therefore, prompt diagnosis and treatment are essential. If bacterial meningitis is suspected, the lumbar puncture becomes an emergency procedure (see Fig. 24-2). In general, it is not necessary to perform a computed tomography

(CT) or magnetic resonance imaging (MRI) scan before the lumbar puncture unless the patient is comatose, has focal neurologic signs, or has papilledema. The presence of these signs suggests the possibility of a space-occupying lesion and increased intracranial pressure. If there is to be a significant delay before the neuroimaging can be obtained, broad-spectrum antibiotics may be given before the lumbar puncture. One should always obtain a blood culture, as it is positive in about 60% of patients with bacterial meningitis.

Typically, the lumbar CSF has a high normal or elevated opening pressure and contains a pleocytosis with a neutrophil predominance, depressed glucose, elevated protein, and bacteria seen on the Gram stain of the sediment.

TABLE 24-1. Spinal Fluid Profiles in CNS Infections

	OPENING PRESSURE	WHITE BLOOD CELLS	PROTEIN	GLUCOSE	BACTERIAL OR FUNGAL CULTURE
Epidural abscess	N or sl ↑	0–20 (lymphs)	N or sl ↑	N	Negative
Subdural empyema	↑	10–1,000 (polys)	sl ↑	N	Negative
Viral meningitis	N or sl ↑	20–1,000 (lymphs)	sl ↑	N	Negative
Bacterial meningitis	↑	50–10,000 (polys)	↑	Low	Positive
Fungal or tuberculous meningitis	↑	50–10,000 polys & lymphs	↑	Low	Positive
Meningovascular syphilis	N or sl ↑	10–1,000 lymphs	↑	N	Negative
Brain abscess	↑	0–10 lymphs & polys	N	N	Negative
Viral encephalitis	sl ↑	10–200 lymphs	N or sl ↑	N	Negative

N = normal; sl ↑ = slight increase; ↑ = increased.

MANAGEMENT AND PROGNOSIS

The key to treatment of acute bacterial meningitis is the prompt administration of appropriate antibiotics. *General principles involved in the use of antibiotics include the following: (1) The antibiotic should be given early in the clinical course; (2) The bacteria must be sensitive to the antibiotic; (3) The antibiotic must cross the blood–brain barrier and achieve sufficient CSF concentrations to kill the bacteria; and (4) A bacteriocidal antibiotic is preferable to a bacteriostatic antibiotic.* Once the diagnosis of bacterial meningitis is made, one should begin treatment with a broad-spectrum antibiotic, which can be later modified when antibiotic sensitivities become available. The choice of an antibiotic for initial treatment depends on several factors: age of the patient, immune status of the patient, predisposing medical conditions, results of the CSF Gram stain, results of the CSF bacterial antigen tests, knowledge of the types of drug-resistant bacteria in the community, and the patient's drug allergies to antibiotics. Table 24-2 gives common initial antibiotic regimens for newborns, children, and adults.

Since many of the neurologic sequelae stem from the meningeal inflammation causing damage to brain or cranial nerves, there is a search for adjunctive therapies that will minimize the meningeal inflammation. At present, corticosteroids have been shown to have some benefit in children, particularly in reducing the incidence of hearing loss. Dexamethasone (0.15 mg/kg intravenously every 6 hours for 4 days) is often recommended in children. The dexamethasone should be given promptly, but only when the illness is highly suggestive of bacterial meningitis in an immunocompetent patient. No studies have proven efficacy in adults.

In general, the CSF becomes sterile 1 to 2 days after antibiotic treatment. The fever usually disappears within a few days but may persist for up to 2 weeks. CSF abnormalities such as pleocytosis, elevated protein, and depressed glucose may persist for several weeks. Dead bacteria may be seen on Gram stain of CSF for several days.

Even if the patient is promptly treated with appropriate antibiotics, serious complications may still develop. Seizures develop in about one third of patients. The seizures usually occur early in the meningitis and seldom recur after the hospitalization. Causes of seizures in meningitis include cerebral cortex irritation from bacterial toxins or meningeal inflammation, CNS vasculitis, brain infarction, high fever, and hyponatremia from the syndrome of inappropriate antidiuretic hormone release (SIADH) coupled with excess fluid administration. Treatment of the seizures is usually with phenytoin. At discharge, the anticonvulsant can be discontinued. Focal neurologic signs, which develop in up to 25% of patients, include cranial nerve palsies, especially cranial nerves VIII (deafness) and VI and III (diplopia). Brain damage resulting in hemiparesis, ataxia, aphasia, or visual loss may also occur. CT or MR of the head is often helpful in the evaluation of these complications and may demonstrate cerebral or cerebellar infarction, brain necrosis, subdural hygromas, or mild ventricular dilatation. Hydrocephalus, subdural empyema, and brain abscess occur but are uncommon.

Mortality from bacterial meningitis ranges from 5% to 25%, depending on the infecting bacteria, the age group, and the predisposing illness. In surviving children, 15% have language disorders or delayed language development, 10% mental retardation, 10% hearing loss, 5% visual impairment, 5% weakness

TABLE 24-2. Initial Antibiotic Therapy While Awaiting Identification of Infecting Organism

SETTING	THERAPY
Preterm and Newborn	Vancomycin (15 mg/kg IV every 6 hr); monitor renal function plus ceftazidime (50–100 mg/kg IV every 8 hr)
Under 3 mo	Ceftriaxone (50–100 mg/kg IV every 12 hr) plus ampicillin (100 mg/kg IV every 8 hr)
3 months to 18 yr	Ceftriaxone (50–100 mg/kg IV every 12 hr) plus Vancomycin (10 mg/kg IV every 6 hr)
18 years to 50 yr	Ceftriaxone (2 g IV every 12 hr) plus Vancomycin (1 g IV every 12 hr)
Over 50 yr	Ceftriaxone (2 g IV every 12 hr) plus ampicillin (2 g IV every 4 hr)
Immunocompromised adults	Ampicillin (2 g IV every 6 hr) plus ceftazidime (2 g IV every 8 hr)
Penetrating head trauma or ventricular shunt in adults	Vancomycin (2 g IV every 12 hr) plus ceftazidime (2 g IV every 8 hr); monitor renal function

Modified from Davis LE: Acute bacterial meningitis. In: Weiner WJ (ed): Emergent and Urgent Neurology, 2nd Edition. Philadelphia, Lippincott Williams & Wilkins , 1999, p. 114

or spasticity, and 3% seizures. Adults have a similar pattern of complications but less deafness.

Some bacterial meningitis requires chemoprophylaxis of immediate family members and close contacts because of their increased risk of developing meningitis. In *N. meningitidis* meningitis, treatment of all close contracts is indicated. Rifampin (600 mg for adults or 10 mg/kg for children, twice daily orally for 2 days) or ciprofloxacin (single oral dose of 500 mg for adults) may be given. If the patient has *H. influenzae*, type B meningitis, chemoprophylaxis is indicated for children less than 4 years of age who have been in close contact with the patient and not previously vaccinated with the *H. influenzae* vaccine. Rifampin (10 mg/kg twice daily orally for 4 days) is usually recommended. All close contacts should be observed carefully for the next week.

Many cases of bacterial meningitis can be prevented by immunizing infants with the *H. influenzae* vaccine and by immunizing high-risk populations with the meningococcal and pneumococcal vaccines.

SPIROCHETE MENINGITIS

Bacterial meningitis from spirochetes is a chronic infection with a time course over months to years. In Lyme disease (*Borrelia burgdorferi*) and neurosyphilis (*T. pallidum*), a chronic meningitis can cause headaches, cranial nerve palsies (especially cranial nerve VII), and occasionally brain infarctions from thrombosis of cortical blood vessels (meningovascular syphilis). Years later, the spirochetes invade the brain to cause a low-grade encephalitis (general paresis or CNS Lyme disease). The CSF contains a lymphocytic pleocytosis, elevated protein, and usually a normal glucose level. Spirochetes are seldom isolated from CSF, and the diagnosis is made by serologic tests [CSF-VDRL (Venereal Disease Research Laboratories) or Lyme antibody titers]. Workup for subacute meningitis is given in Table 24-3. Treatment is with high-dose penicillin or ceftriaxone for several weeks.

TUBERCULOUS AND FUNGAL MENINGITIS

Patients with tuberculous or fungal meningitides usually develop a subacute meningitis with the onset of CNS signs developing over days to weeks. These infections occur most often in individuals who are malnourished, debilitated, or immunosuppressed. Although initial entry is usually by way of the lungs, less than 50% will have an active pulmonary infec-

TABLE 24-3. Evaluation of Subacute Meningitis

Skin tests: Intermediate purified protein derivative tuberculin test (PPD) and anergy skin tests

Serum antibody serologic tests: Brucella, syphilis, toxoplasmosis, coccidioides, Lyme disease, and human immunodeficiency virus

CSF studies: Opening pressure, cells, glucose, protein, IgG, Gram stain, acid-fast stain, India ink, cytology, VDRL, coccidioides, and Lyme disease antibody tests and cryptococcal antigen test

Cultures for bacteria, brucella, tuberculosis, and fungi: CSF cultures repeated ×3, blood, urine, sputum or gastric aspirate, bone marrow biopsy, lesion biopsy

Computed tomography or magnetic resonance imaging

Chest x-ray

tion at the time of the meningitis. Culture of the CSF is the key to establishing the etiology. Since tuberculous or fungal organisms may be in low concentrations in the CSF, one should culture 5 to 10 ml of CSF on several occasions. Treatment of tuberculous meningitis usually requires administration of three drugs (rifampin, isoniazid, and pyrazinamide) for 2 months, followed by rifampin and isoniazid for another 7 months. Most patients with fungal meningitis are treated with intravenous and/or intrathecal amphotericin B for weeks to months. In patients with cryptococcal meningitis, flucytosine is often added to the amphotericin B. Fluconazole has been shown to be nearly as efficacious as amphotericin B in the treatment of cryptococcal and coccidioidal meningitis. Fluconazole has the advantage that it can be given orally and has less renal and hematopoietic toxicity. If patients with acquired immunodeficiency syndrome (AIDS), or who are otherwise immunosuppressed, have fungal meningitis in remission, continued use of fluconazole in lower dosage may prevent recurrence of the fungal meningitis. Neurologic sequelae are similar to those seen in acute bacterial meningitis. Mortality rates range from 20% to 50%, depending on the organism and predisposing factors.

ENCEPHALITIS

The majority of infectious agents that cause encephalitis (diffuse brain infection) are viruses that reach the brain by a hematogenous route. Once the virus reaches the brain parenchyma, a widely disseminated infection of neurons and glia ensues. Neuronal necrosis and lysis of glial cells result in secondary cerebral edema. The inflammatory response includes perivascular cuffing with inflammatory cells and infiltration of lymphocytes and macrophages into the adjacent brain parenchyma. The invading immune response often terminates the infection, but the patient may be left with permanent neurologic sequelae.

CLINICAL FEATURES

Acute encephalitis is a febrile illness characterized by the abrupt onset of headache and mental obtundation. Other common features include seizures, which may be generalized or focal, hyper-reflexia, spasticity, and the Babinski sign. Occasional patients develop hemiparesis, aphasia, ataxia, limb tremors, and cortical blindness. Patients often have a prodromal illness, which varies with the infectious agent and can include parotitis (mumps virus), or fever, malaise, and myalgias (togavirus). Encephalitis differs from meningitis primarily because patients with encephalitis develop prominent mental changes and a minimal or absent stiff neck.

LABORATORY FINDINGS

The electroencephalogram (EEG) is always abnormal and usually shows diffuse bilateral slowing with occasional seizure activity. A lumbar puncture in a patient with early encephalitis will have an opening pressure that is normal or slightly elevated. The CSF contains five to several hundred white blood cells per cubic millimeter (predominantly lymphocytes). CSF glucose is normal, while CSF protein is mildly elevated. Bacterial and viral cultures are usually sterile. Early in the course of encephalitis, the CT scan may be normal while the MRI scan shows areas of cerebral vascular permeability with parenchymal areas of increased signal on T2-weighted images. Later, both scans may demonstrate areas of necrosis or hemorrhage.

ETIOLOGIES OF ENCEPHALITIS

Viruses cause more than 90% of cases. Worldwide, togaviruses (arboviruses) are the most common cause. Since togaviruses require a vector (mosquito or tick), togavirus encephalitis often occurs in clusters or epidemics. In the United States, herpes simplex encephalitis is slightly more common than togavirus encephalitis. Herpes simplex virus is a latent infection in most individuals, following a primary stomatitis infection in childhood. Years later, the latent virus reactivates to cause an encephalitis that occurs sporadically year round. The remainder are usually caused by the spirochete bacteria (*T. pallidum, B. burgdorferi*), parasites (toxoplasmosis or falciparum malaria), or viruses (cytomegalovirus, varicella-zoster, adenovirus).

The diagnosis of viral encephalitis is usually made by serologic tests. Since most togaviruses produce a systemic viral infection before producing the encephalitis, immunoglobulin M antibodies to the virus are often present early in the encephalitis. The IgM-antibody-capture enzyme linked immunosorbent assay (MacELISA) can be used to detect togavirus antibodies during the first few days of the encephalitis. Acute and convalescent serum titers can be determined for many viruses and a fourfold increase in antibody titer is usually diagnostic. Unfortunately, serologic tests have not been useful in establishing the diagnosis of herpes simplex encephalitis. Previously, a brain biopsy was the only certain method of establishing this diagnosis. The diagnosis now can be made by detection of herpes simplex DNA in CSF by PCR. While herpes simplex virus is almost never cultured from CSF, enough viral DNA leaks into the CSF from the brain infection to be detected by PCR. The CSF PCR test is most sensitive when used in the first few days of the encephalitis.

MANAGEMENT AND PROGNOSIS

Treatment of encephalitis varies with the infectious agent. For most viruses, with the exception of herpes viruses, no antiviral treatment is available. All patients require excellent symptomatic care to minimize complications. If seizures develop, anticonvulsants are indicated. If increased intracranial pressure develops from vascular engorgement and cerebral edema, treatment includes hyperventilation or the administration of mannitol. Use of corticosteroids is controversial. In patients with herpes simplex encephalitis, treatment with acyclovir significantly improves outcome. Acyclovir should be administered as early as possible in the clinical course for maximal benefit. Current recommendations are to give 30 mg/kg/day of acyclovir that is divided into three doses per day for at least 10 days. The drug should be intravenously delivered slowly over 1 hour to prevent renal toxicity. Drug complications include transient renal failure, thrombophlebitis, and elevations of serum liver enzymes. Ganciclovir is antiviral for cytomegalovirus, and famciclovir is effective against varicella-zoster virus.

Prognosis of encephalitis depends on the infectious agent. Patients with mumps meningoencephalitis and Venezuelan equine encephalitis have an excellent prognosis. Patients with western equine, St. Louis, and California encephalitis usually have a good prognosis (2% to 10% mortality). Occasional patients may be left with dementia, seizures, or focal neurologic deficits. Patients with eastern equine, Japanese B, and Murray Valley encephalitis have mortality rates from 20% to 40%. Patients with herpes simplex encephalitis who are treated with acyclovir have a 20% mortality rate, and 55% are left with some neurologic sequelae. Rabies encephalitis is fatal.

BRAIN ABSCESS

While viruses tend to cause diffuse brain infections, most bacteria, fungi, and parasites cause localized brain disease. Brain abscesses (focal infections of the brain) may arise by direct extension from other foci of infection within the cranial cavity (mastoiditis and sinusitis), from infections following skull fracture or craniotomy, or as metastases carried by the blood from infections elsewhere in the body. The infection usually begins as a localized encephalitis with focal softening, necrosis, and inflammation. As the process continues, fibroblasts proliferate at the edges, forming a capsule wall with a variable amount of cerebral edema surrounding the lesion. If the etiology is bacterial or fungal, the space-occupying lesion slowly expands. Untreated, the expanding brain mass is lethal. However, parasites, such as in neurocysticercosis, develop a cyst that usually stops growing after it reaches about 10 to 15 mm in size.

CLINICAL FEATURES

Symptoms from localized brain infections typically are subacute in onset. Early symptoms include headaches, lethargy, intermittent fever, and focal or generalized seizures. Focal neurologic signs may develop depending on the site of lesion. Thus, lesions in the frontal cortex may produce hemiparesis, while lesions in the occipital cortex cause homonymous visual defects. As the mass expands, increased intracranial pressure becomes more pronounced, producing psychomotor slowing, lethargy,

and increasing confusion. Papilledema and horizontal diplopia from a sixth-nerve palsy may be seen. Focal neurologic signs become more prominent. Eventually, brain herniation and death occur as a result of the expanding mass.

LABORATORY FINDINGS

Computed tomographic and MRI scans are extremely helpful in diagnosing brain abscesses. The CT scan usually demonstrates a lesion with a low-density necrotic center, a well-developed contrast-enhancing capsule, and surrounding cerebral edema (Fig. 24-3). A similar picture is seen on MRI scan. Administration of gadolinium will cause the capsule wall to enhance. The EEG is often abnormal, with localized slowing (delta waves). A lumbar puncture is seldom helpful in establishing the diagnosis and may be contraindicated

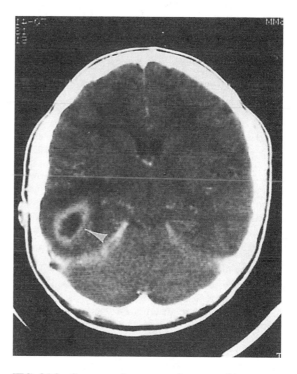

FIG. 24-3. Computed tomography scan with contrast demonstrating a brain abscess in the posterior temporal lobe. Arrow shows the enhancing capsule with necrotic center. There is some low-density surrounding edema.

since it increases the risk of brain herniation if the intracranial pressure is markedly elevated.

ETIOLOGY

Anaerobic bacteria are found in over half of brain abscesses. Anaerobic streptococci and *Bacteroides fragilis* are common organisms. Occasionally, multiple bacteria are found in abscesses. Brain abscesses following head trauma or neurosurgery may contain *Staphylococcus aureus*. *Nocardia asteroides* may cause a fungal brain abscess.

MANAGEMENT AND PROGNOSIS

Treatment of brain abscesses usually entails appropriate antibiotic therapy and surgical drainage. Broad-spectrum antibiotic treatment is usually given as soon as the clinical diagnosis is made. The antibiotics should be selected for effectiveness against all likely pathogens as well as for their ability to penetrate brain abscesses and surrounding brain parenchyma. Broad-spectrum antibiotic coverage should be given to cover both common anaerobic (especially *Streptococcus intermedius* and *B. fragilis*) and aerobic bacteria. Common combinations include the use of cefotaxime or high-dose penicillin G plus metronidazole or chloramphenicol. If staphylococci are suspected or isolated, nafcillin should be given. Once bacteria are isolated, therapy should be directed by their antibiotic sensitivities. Antibiotics should be administered intravenously, and treatment is normally continued for 6 to 8 weeks. Because the most immediate threat from brain abscesses is the mass effect, surgical aspiration of pus often diminishes the increased intracranial pressure. The simplest method of aspirating the pus is to use a CT-guided stereotactic technique. Pus should be Gram stained and cultured for anaerobic and aerobic bacteria, fungi, and tuberculous organisms. If the brain abscesses are multiple or deep, they may be treated only with broad-spectrum antimicrobial agents. However, careful clinical observation and repeated CT scans are needed to determine whether the abscess continues to expand. If expansion occurs despite antibiotics, neurosurgical intervention is required, as rupture of the brain abscess into the ventricles or brain herniation is usually fatal.

Mannitol or corticosteroids may be necessary initially to control cerebral edema, but corticosteroids should be used cautiously and tapered rapidly as they may interfere with capsule formation and host defenses against the organism.

Mortality from brain abscesses ranges from 30% to 65%, with the lower rates being for patients who receive combined therapy with antibiotics and surgery. About 50% of survivors have neurologic sequelae, including seizures and focal neurologic deficits.

PRION DISEASES

Creutzfeldt–Jakob disease (the most common form, with an incidence of 1/1,000,000/year), Gerstmann–Straüssler syndrome, fatal familial insomnia, and kuru are classified as prion diseases. Prions are infectious agents that break all the rules for conventional infectious agents. First, no nucleic agent has been identified in the infectious particle, which appears to be a protein that is made normally by brain and other cells and is somehow modified to become infectious. Second, patients with the illness do not present with typical signs of an infection. They lack fever and elevated white blood cell counts, and they have a normal-appearing CSF. No immune response is made by the host to the infectious particle. Third, the infectious particle is not killed by formalin, ethanol, or boiling, but it can be destroyed by autoclaving. Fourth, most patients present with a subacute to chronic progressive dementia that is fatal over the course of 6 months to 2 years. The prion infectious agent is present in CSF, the brain, the pituitary, and peripheral nerves that innervate cornea and dura. The infectious agent does not appear to be present in saliva, urine, sweat, and stool, so isolation of the patient is not necessary. Blood should be considered infectious, but no documented human cases have occurred from blood transfusions. Transmission of a prion infectious disease may occur through transplantation of infected human cornea, dura, pituitary, or surgical instruments, or it may be inherited, as in the Gerstmann–Straüssler syndrome and fatal familial insomnia. Most cases of Creutzfeldt–Jakob disease appear to be sporadic without a known source of transmission. Diagnosis may be difficult as there is no simple diagnostic test. Creutzfeldt–Jakob disease should be suspected in an adult with rapidly progressive dementia, myoclonic jerks, and normal CSF. An EEG may show characteristic abnormalities. Neuroimaging may show progressive brain atrophy without brain enhancement. The brain shows a characteristic spongiform encephalopathy without inflammation. Work is underway to develop a specific CSF diagnostic test. Currently, there is no available treatment to stop disease progression. Patients suspected of having this disease should not donate blood or autopsy organs.

QUESTIONS AND DISCUSSION

1. Western equine encephalitis:

A. Occurs sporadically all year
B. Is contagious to others for about 1 year
C. Begins with severe headache and a stiff neck
D. Produces widespread death of glia and neurons
E. Is best treated with acyclovir

The answer is (D). Western equine encephalitis virus is an arbovirus that is transmitted to man from the bite of infected mosquitoes during the summer and early fall. While meningitis begins with a headache and stiff neck, encephalitis usually begins with marked changes in mental status. The virus infects both glia and neurons, producing widespread cell death. Western equine encephalitis virus is not present in urine, saliva, or stool. Therefore, the patient is not contagious and does not need isolation. Acyclovir works as an antiviral drug only against viruses of the herpes family such as herpes simplex. Thus, current treatment is symptomatic and the prevention of severe increased intracranial pressure.

2. In a brain abscess, the best way to establish the etiology is to:

A. Isolate bacteria from CSF
B. Detect specific bacterial antigen in CSF
C. Identify bacteria in CSF by Gram stain
D. Isolate bacteria from abscess pus
E. Isolate bacteria from blood or urine

The answer is (D). In a brain abscess, the bacteria are surrounded by a capsule and confined to the pus. Therefore, the CSF does not contain any bacteria or bacterial products. In a few patients, the blood may contain the bacteria if the organism reached the brain from a bacteremia. Thus, patients with a brain abscess from an acute bacterial endocarditis may have a *S. aureus* bacteremia. The only certain method of isolating the bacteria causing the abscess is to culture the pus. This can be done by stereotactic aspiration of the pus or from a craniotomy and direct surgical aspiration or drainage. The pus should be cultured for anaerobic and aerobic bacteria, fungi, and *M. tuberculosis*.

3. In a right anterior frontal lobe brain abscess, the main signs and symptoms that the patient develops are caused by:

A. Increased intracranial pressure
B. Inflammation of adjacent meninges
C. Disruption of thalamofrontal tracts
D. Destruction of frontal eye fields
E. Compression of the anterior corpus callosum

The answer is (A). Brain abscess produces signs and symptoms by two major mechanisms. If the abscess is located in a critical area of the brain, such as the motor cortex, localized signs develop. The second mechanism is through mass effect. As the abscess expands in size, the mass effect increases intracranial pressure. Increased intracranial pressure causes headache, lethargy, and psychomotor slowing. Eventually, the increased pressure causes brain herniation and death.

4. Treatment of tuberculous meningitis requires multiple drugs. The combination that is often given is isoniazid plus:

A. Streptomycin and para-aminosalicylic acid (PAS)
B. Chloramphenicol and PAS
C. Rifampin and PAS
D. Rifampin and pyrazinamide (PZA)
E. Ethionamide and ethambutol

The answer is (D). Rifampin, isoniazid, and pyrazinamide cross the blood–brain barrier well and are effective against *M. tuberculosis*. PAS poorly crosses the blood–brain barrier, and chloramphenicol has weak activity against *M. tuberculosis*. Ethionamide and ethambutol are second-line drugs against *M. tuberculosis*. The Centers for Disease Control recommends that rifampin, isoniazid, and PZA be given for 2 months, and then rifampin and isoniazid continued for another 7 months. Streptomycin is active against *M. tuberculosis* and crosses the blood–brain barrier. It is often added if isoniazid or rifampin drug resistance is suspected. Streptomycin is potentially toxic and can cause cochlear and vestibular hair cell damage, resulting in hearing loss or imbalance.

5. Enterovirus meningitis:

A. Is transmitted by a mosquito bite
B. Can be treated with acyclovir
C. Follows a prodrome of cramps and diarrhea
D. Causes cranial nerve palsies in 10% of patients
E. Is the most common cause of aseptic meningitis

The answer is (E). In the United States, enterovirus causes about 75% of cases of viral meningitis and the majority of aseptic meningitis cases. The virus is transmitted to the gastrointestinal tract from infected water.

Most patients develop an asymptomatic gastrointestinal infection. In occasional patients, a viremia occurs that spreads virus to the meninges. No antiviral drugs are available for treatment, but the clinical course is benign, with over 99% of patients making a complete recovery.

SUGGESTED READING

Anderson NE, Willoughby EW: Chronic meningitis without predisposing illness: A review of 83 cases. Q J Med 63:283, 1987

Davis LE: Acute bacterial meningitis. In: Weiner WJ (ed): Emergent and Urgent Neurology, 2nd Edition. Philadelphia, Lippincott Williams & Wilkins, 1999, pp. 101–126

Davis LE, Reed WP: Infections of the central nervous system. In: Rosenberg R (ed): Comprehensive Neurology, 2nd Edition, pp. 281–353. New York, Wiley-Liss 1998

Davis LE: Aseptic and viral meningitis. In: Long SS, Pickering LK, Prober CG (eds): Principles and Practice of Pediatric Infectious Diseases, pp. 328–336. New York, Churchill Livingstone, 1997

DeArmond SJ, Prusiner SB: Etiology and pathogenesis of prion diseases: Review. Am J Pathol 146:785, 1995

Heilpern KL, Lorger B: Focal intracranial infections. Infect Dis Clin North Am 10:879, 1996

Johnson RT: Acute encephalitis. Clin Infect Dis 23:219, 1996

Leonard JM, DesPrez RM: Tuberculous meningitis. Infect Dis Clin North Am 4:769, 1990

Quaglarello V, Scheld WM. Treatment of bacterial meningitis. N Engl J Med 336: 708, 1997

Skoldenberg B: Herpes simplex encephalitis. Scand J Infect Dis 100(suppl):8, 1996

Neurology for the Non Neurologist, Fourth Edition, edited by William J. Weiner and Christopher G. Goetz. Lippincott Williams & Wilkins, Philadelphia © 1999.

C H A P T E R   2 5

Neurologic Emergencies

Lisa M. Shulman
José G. Romano

Neurologic emergencies are frequently encountered in the practice of medicine and, if unrecognized, they may rapidly progress to a permanent neurologic disability or death. The topics included in this chapter represent the more common and treatable conditions with which all health-care professionals should be familiar.

CENTRAL NERVOUS SYSTEM

ACUTE ISCHEMIC STROKE

With the development of new and effective treatments, stroke is increasingly becoming a treatable neurologic emergency. An ischemic stroke is defined as a sudden-onset event caused by insufficient blood supply to brain tissue. With over 500,000 strokes a year, about 3 million stroke survivors at any time, and 150,000 annual deaths, stroke constitutes the third most frequent cause of death and main cause of disability in the United States, as about 50% of survivors are unable to return to their previous activities. This ominous picture is offset by optimism regarding acute stroke treatment, particularly for ischemic strokes, which account for 85% of all cerebrovascular events, the rest being hemorrhagic.

Brain tissue requires approximately 50 cubic centimeters (cc) of blood flow per 100 grams (g) of tissue per minute (min) to meet its metabolic demands, but areas with flow greater than 20 cc/100 g/min are able to function. Tissue with less than 10 cc/100 g/min develops irreversible damage and dies; it represents the "core" of the stroke. However, brain tissue with blood flow between 10 and 20 cc/100 g/min is salvageable, albeit not functional, if reperfused within a certain amount of time; this area is the ischemic penumbra. Even without further drops in regional blood flow, irreversible changes in the penumbra will ensue within about 6 hours, mainly as a result of excitotoxic insults arising from the core of the stroke. This damage is mediated by various neurotransmitters, mainly glutamate, that through a number of cell membrane interactions result in increasing intracellular calcium levels leading to cell death.

The treatment of acute ischemic stroke is directed at saving the penumbra, which early on may represent up to 90% of the tissue at risk. The three main tenets of intervention include opening the occluded vessel, increasing collateral flow to the ischemic penumbra, and blocking excitotoxicity.

OPENING THE OCCLUDED VESSEL

Until recently, the use of thrombolytics in cerebral ischemia carried a prohibitive risk of cerebral hemorrhage. However, with U.S. Food and Drug Administration approval of recombinant tissue plasminogen activator (rt-PA) for intravenous (IV) thrombolytic therapy in acute ischemic stroke, its administration in appropriate patients is rapidly becoming standard of care, as one third of those treated have minimal or no deficits after treatment. The dose used is lower than the usual cardiac dose, 0.9 mg/kg, not to exceed 90 mg total dose, 10% given as a bolus and the rest over 1 hour. With a 6% incidence of hemorrhagic complications, it remains a potentially dangerous drug, and certain precautions should be observed to avoid a higher complication rate. Establishing the precise onset of symptoms is extremely important as rt-PA is approved for use within 3 hours of stroke onset. Administration after this period results in a significantly elevated rate of symptomatic cerebral hemorrhage. This results from postocclusive endothelial damage with leaking of blood after revascularization. Patients who wake up with neurologic deficits must be assumed to have had onset of symptoms at bedtime or the last time they were observed to be normal. A noncontrast brain computed tomography (CT) needs to be done urgently, as the presence of cerebral hemorrhage, which cannot be reliably excluded on clinical grounds alone, precludes the use of thrombolytic medications. Patients presenting within 3 hours of onset of symptoms may have a normal brain CT, or one with early ischemic changes, such as loss of distinction between gray and white matter, effacement of the insular ribbon, or loss of basal ganglia definition. A dense middle cerebral artery represents thrombus within this vessel. Further evidence of ischemia, particularly a well-established hypodensity, carries an increased risk of thrombolysis-induced hemorrhagic conversion, and should raise the possibility of a longer interval since initiation of ischemia. As diffusion–perfusion magnetic resonance imaging (MRI) and other techniques to quantify blood flow, such as xenon-CT, become more widely available, clinicians will be better equipped to estimate the relative benefits and risks of thrombolysis. Patients with large areas of penumbra tissue would benefit most, while those with large tissue volume with blood flow under 10 cc/100 g/min would not benefit and may be at increased risk for hemorrhage. Quantification of neurologic deficits is helpful in estimating the risk of administering thrombolytics and in assessing response to treatment; the National Institutes of Health Stroke Scale (NIHSS) is the most widely used. An NIHSS grade greater than 20 (a higher grade indicates more deficits) is associated with more intracerebral hemorrhagic complications after therapy, but it does not represent an absolute contraindication, as these patients have a bad prognosis if left untreated. Conversely, minimal deficits, such as isolated sensory symptoms, or an NIHSS less than 4, does not warrant the risk of thrombolytic therapy. A careful history should be taken for factors that may preclude thrombolytic use, such as recent surgery, cerebral aneurysms, cranial vascular malformations or tumors, or a potential source of systemic bleeding (i.e., active gastric ulcer). Laboratory screening tests for coagulopathic conditions or significant thrombocytopenia should be obtained. Intra-arterial administration of thrombolytic agents may prove to be a safer and more effective way of opening occluded cerebral vessels, and it may provide a longer window of opportunity for intervention than intravenous application.

INCREASING COLLATERAL FLOW TO THE ISCHEMIC PENUMBRA

The most important single measure to reach this goal is to avoid hypotension. As the hypertensive response after acute cerebral ischemia may be a normal compensatory response, it is not advisable to treat systolic blood pressure (SBP) under 220 mm Hg in the first 24 hours after onset of the event. If thrombolytics are employed, then the SBP should be kept under 180 mm Hg, and the diastolic BP under 110. If elevated BP needs to be reduced, beta-blockers are preferred. Labetalol (which also has alpha-blocking effects) may be used in 10 mg IV pushes or as a continuous infusion. Vasodilators, particularly nifedipine, should be avoided as they can produce a precipitous drop in BP resulting in reduction of cerebral blood flow to the ischemic penumbra. In the presence of overt cardiac failure, coronary ischemia, or aortic dissection, BP needs to be reduced more energetically. Patients with low BP may require intravenous fluids, colloids, and occasionally vasopressors to ensure adequate perfusion to the ischemic penumbra.

BLOCKING EXCITOTOXIC INFLUENCES

The use of neuroprotective agents to block the excitotoxic influence of core neurons on the penumbra is still experimental, although a multitude of compounds are actively being investigated; it is likely that one or more of these drugs will be available for general use in the near future. If a safe agent is developed, it may be administered in the prehospital setting by paramedics. Nevertheless, there are two very effective interventions with clear neuroprotective effects that should currently be employed: The first is avoidance of hyperglycemia, as it worsens ischemic injury. The second is treatment of hyperthermia: Even small increases of temperature adversely affect the reversibility of ischemic penumbra damage. Fever should be aggressively treated with antipyretics and even cold blankets if needed. Hypothermia has been shown to have beneficial effects on stroke outcome in animal studies; human studies are currently underway.

When the use of thrombolytic agents is not warranted, consideration should be given to antithrombotic or anticoagulant therapy. Anticoagulants are often empirically used in suspected embolic strokes for prevention of stroke recurrence or progression, but not for acute treatment of the ischemic insult. As embolic strokes may develop hemorrhagic conversion of the ischemic tissue upon spontaneous lysis of the thrombus, it is not recommended to anticoagulate large strokes, particularly those that involve more than a third of the distribution of a large cerebral artery. Most clinicians would anticoagulate small embolic strokes in the presence of atrial fibrillation, ventricular thrombus, or progression of stroke symptoms, particularly in the setting of a posterior circulation event. When IV heparin is used, infusion without a bolus to a partial thromboplastin time (PTT) of 1.5 to 1.8 times control is suggested. A recent large trial [the International Stroke Trial (IST)] suggested that while heparin does reduce early stroke recurrence, its benefits are annulled by an increase in hemorrhagic complications. Similarly, a recent trial of heparinoids [Trial of ORG-10172 in Acute Stroke Treatment (TOAST)] has been disappointing. Two large trials [IST and the Chinese Acute Stroke Trial (CAST)] have demonstrated that aspirin administration in the acute setting confers a small but statistically significant benefit. It should be noted that both antithrombotic and anticoagulant agents are contraindicated for 24 hours after thrombolysis.

As the therapeutic window for intervention is short, all medical centers should have a specific plan of action to deal effectively with the acute stroke patient. Stroke teams have been effective in fulfilling this purpose. To have patients arrive in a timely fashion to the hospital, the Brain Attack concept (following the model of Heart Attack) should be aggressively publicized to the community. Ideally, once acute therapy has been initiated, stroke victims should be admitted to a specialized unit familiar with the care of these patients, where prompt evaluation of the causative mechanism for the ischemic stroke is performed. Only with this knowledge can rational long-term therapy be instituted to prevent recurrent events.

ACUTE INTRACEREBRAL HEMORRHAGE

Intracerebral hemorrhage (ICH) represents only 10% of all strokes but accounts for 50% of all stroke-related mortality, most of it (43%) in the first 30 days. Almost 90% of survivors have some degree of disability. African-Americans and Asians have a higher incidence of ICH than Caucasians; heavy alcohol consumption and low cholesterol levels (under 160 mg/dl) appear to increase risk for ICH (the latter particularly in Asians). Over half of all ICH is attributable to hypertension; other common causes are listed in Table 25-1. The vascular anomaly associated with hypertension and believed to be responsible for the vascular rupture in ICH is lipohyalinosis of small penetrating arteries. This is the same process that results in lacunar infarcts, so it is not surprising that both affect similar brain regions: basal ganglia, thalamus, pons, and dentate nucleus of the cerebellum. Although the pseudoaneurysms of Charcot and Bouchard are often found in areas of hypertensive ICH, their causative role is controversial. Progressive enlargement of the hematoma in hypertensive ICH over the first 3 hours is well documented by serial CT scanning. One theory states that the pressure of the hematoma on adjacent small vessels results in their engorgement and rupture, thus initiating a cascade phenomenon.

The clinical presentation of ICH depends on two factors: the location of the hemorrhage and the resultant increased intracranial pressure. Headache, nausea, vomiting, and progressive deterioration in consciousness indicate the latter. Basal ganglia and thalamic lacunae most commonly present with dense contralateral hemiplegia and hemisensory loss. Large hemorrhages may also result in visual field defects, dysphasia, and gaze deviation toward the affected hemisphere. Rupture into the ventricles can produce obstruction of cerebrospinal fluid circulation and hydrocephalus. Lobar hemorrhages (occurring in one of the cerebral lobes, more peripheral than the deep nuclei) commonly have associated contralateral hemiparesis, gaze preference if in the frontal lobe, dysphasia if in the dominant hemisphere, and neglect in the nondominant hemisphere. Seizures are frequent as blood has

TABLE 25-1. Causes of Intracerebral Hemorrhage

Hypertension
Trauma
Tumors
Vascular malformations
Arteriovenous malformation
Cavernous angioma
Venous angioma
Saccular aneurysm
Hemorrhagic transformation of ischemic stroke
Amyloid angiopathy
Sympathomimetic agents
Coagulopathic conditions, including use of anticoagulants or thrombolytics

irritant effects on the cerebral cortex. Cerebellar hemorrhages are especially hazardous as they may result in obstructive hydrocephalus and compress vital brainstem structures (respiratory and cardiovascular centers). Small pontine hemorrhages affect cranial nerve function, commonly causing horizontal diplopia and facial weakness with contralateral hemiplegia; larger hemorrhages in this location are often fatal.

The best instrument to evaluate the presence and location of ICH is the CT, in which blood is radiodense or "white." MRI is less sensitive than CT in detecting blood in the acute period, but later it may be useful in defining the precise location and dating the age of the hemorrhage. The need for further evaluation is dictated in part by the CT findings. A hematoma in the typical hypertensive ICH location in a patient with known history or clinical findings of chronic hypertension (fundoscopic changes, left ventricular hypertrophy) may not warrant further investigations. Lobar hemorrhages may also result from hypertension, but they should alert the clinician to alternate diagnoses. Amyloid angiopathy is caused by deposition of amyloid protein in the media of small vessels, thus weakening them and leading to their rupture. It usually affects the elderly in a sporadic fashion and less commonly occurs in a familial pattern. A progressive dementing process ensues after repeated hemorrhages. Strict blood pressure control and the use of antiepileptics may prevent new episodes of bleeding.

Significant vasogenic edema surrounding the hemorrhage, bleeding in atypical sites such as the corpus callosum, or multiple lesions suggest a neoplastic etiology and should trigger a contrast imaging study. Contrast enhancement, often in a ringlike pattern, strongly raises suspicion for tumor, but the tumor may be obscured by the hematoma. In these cases, a contrast-enhanced MRI, 2 to 4 weeks later, may unmask the tumor. Brain metastases that commonly hemorrhage include melanoma, renal cell carcinoma, choriocarcinoma, and bronchogenic carcinoma. Of the primary brain tumors, glioblastoma multiforme is the one most frequently associated with hemorrhagic conversion. Pituitary adenomas are benign tumors that may develop hemorrhagic infarction or pituitary apoplexy, although this condition may occur in nontumorous glands. Pituitary apoplexy presents with an acute headache and meningismus, which can be confused with aneurysmal rupture. Superior extension with pressure on the optic chiasm leads to visual disturbances, and lateral expansion with pressure on the cavernous sinus may produce diplopia and facial numbness. It may even compromise carotid flow in its cavernous segment, resulting in contralateral hemi-

paresis. The anterior pituitary is usually involved, with deficiencies in prolactin, corticotropin, thyrotropin, growth hormones, and gonadotropins. Intravenous corticosteroid administration is vital; visual field monitoring and careful hormonal determination and replacement should be pursued. Early surgical evacuation is warranted in some cases.

Embolic infarcts may develop secondary hemorrhagic conversion once the thrombus is lysed and blood rushes into a vascular bed with damaged endothelium. CT often reveals punctate areas of hyperdensity in a hypodense area of ischemic infarct, but occasionally there may be a frank hematoma. The previous clinical and radiologic findings should guide the clinician into making the diagnosis of hemorrhagic conversion of an ischemic stroke. Patients treated with thrombolytics or anticoagulants are at an increased risk for this complication. When subarachnoid blood is present in addition to ICH, saccular aneurysmal rupture should be considered. Conventional catheter angiography remains the diagnostic gold standard in this condition, but new techniques such as CT angiography are playing an increasing role in the emergency room evaluation of acute subarachnoid hemorrhage.

The presence of engorged vessels near the ICH suggests a vascular malformation. Arteriovenous malformations should be studied angiographically to define their vascular characteristics and guide therapy, which may be achieved endovascularly (with coils and glue-like substances) or surgically. Cavernous angiomas and venous angiomas are best visualized by MRI and may be missed by conventional angiography. In general, they have a lower risk of rebleeding than arteriovenous malformations.

When the patient arrives in the emergency room, the first objective is to stabilize his vital signs and his general medical condition. Particular attention should be given to airway protection, and patients with a significantly diminished state of alertness should be prophylactically intubated even in the absence of respiratory failure. Adequate blood pressure control is then instituted. In the presence of increased intracranial pressure, optimal cerebral perfusion pressure (CPP) depends on systemic BP. In chronic hypertensives, the autoregulatory curve between mean arterial blood pressure and CPP is usually shifted to the right. For these reasons, to maintain an adequate CPP, it is vital not to lower systemic BP excessively; some authors recommend not lowering SBP under 180 mm Hg. Vasodilator agents such as nitroprusside, hydralazine, and nifedipine may increase ICP and should be avoided if possible; IV beta-blocking agents are ideal. Prophylactic antiepileptic medication is administered to patients with lobar or large deep ICH, as seizures increase ICP and cerebral metabolic demand. All patients with ICH need intensive care monitoring.

As to surgical intervention in the management of ICH, there is no doubt that ventriculostomy can be life-saving in acute hydrocephalus. Cerebellar hemorrhages smaller than 3 cc without fourth ventricular compression can be closely observed; larger hematomas with brainstem or ventricular system compression should be urgently evacuated. Evacuation of surgically accessible supratentorial hematomas remains controversial. In general, surgery is indicated only when medical therapy fails to control rising ICP, as studies have not demonstrated improved outcome from surgery versus medical management in the absence of life-threatening increased ICP. However, there are suggestions that early evacuation within 3 hours of onset may be beneficial, and a randomized controlled study is being planned to test this hypothesis. New techniques such as stereotactic or endoscopic aspiration with local instillation of fibrinolytics are promising. Lobar hematomas that are felt to be caused by amyloid angiopathy should not be approached surgically, if possible.

In general, the prognosis for survival is poor when the ICH has a volume greater than 60 cc or when there is depressed state of consciousness on arrival to medical attention. Survivors need to be enrolled in rehabilitation programs as soon as they are medically stable.

ANEURYSMAL SUBARACHNOID HEMORRHAGE

Aneurysmal subarachnoid hemorrhage (SAH) occurs as a result of the rupture of a saccular (or berry) aneurysm related to a defect of the media or intima of the blood vessel wall. There are approximately 30,000 cases of aneurysmal SAH annually in the United States. SAH is a serious event with the potential for high mortality and morbidity. Approximately 10% of patients will die rapidly after a SAH, half succumb within 1 month, and only one third of patients are functional survivors. Three major factors that determine eventual outcome are the severity of the initial hemorrhage, the potential for rebleeding from the aneurysm, and the onset of cerebral vasospasm. Early diagnosis is imperative, yet one out of four patients is initially misdiagnosed and presents late, often following a second hemorrhage.

Following aneurysmal rupture, the extravasation of blood into the subarachnoid space evokes the classic presenting symptom of the abrupt onset of severe headache. Commonly associated signs and symptoms are vomiting, a transient loss of consciousness, photophobia, meningismus, and the onset of neurologic dysfunction. The clinician must be aware that more subtle presentations of aneurysmal hemorrhage occur. A relatively minor but persistent headache localized to the neck region in the absence of a chronic headache history should prompt careful consideration, as a third to one half of patients with SAH have had a recent acute and unusual headache caused by minute amounts of blood leaking from the aneurysm.

In the absence of an intracranial hematoma, the patient's level of consciousness is the most important indicator of prognosis. Patients with milder presenting symptoms such as a headache with nuchal rigidity, confusion, drowsiness, and mild focal neurologic signs generally have a favorable prognosis. Few patients who present in a coma or a moribund condition survive.

In addition to meningismus and altered consciousness, the location of the hemorrhage determines the occurrence of focal neurologic findings. A large aneurysm may also cause symptoms by progressive enlargement and its resultant mass effect; classically, a third-nerve palsy should alert the clinician to the potential presence of an aneurysm.

If the patient's history and clinical examination raise any suspicion of SAH, CT of the head, with or without contrast, should be obtained immediately. In about 90% of cases scanned within 24 hours of onset of the hemorrhage, CT will demonstrate the presence of blood in the subarachnoid space. Analysis of the distribution and density of blood may indicate the source of hemorrhage, and aneurysms greater than 1 cm in diameter may be highlighted by intravascular contrast. Further information regarding ventricular size and the presence of cerebral edema or infarction is acquired with imaging. The sensitivity of CT in SAH detection decreases by 10% per day after the ictus. When the CT results are equivocal or negative, direct CSF examination is mandatory. For immediate information following the lumbar puncture, prior to formal laboratory analysis, a vial of CSF can be spun down in the centrifuge. Traumatic hemorrhagic CSF can be distinguished from SAH in that the first tends to clear as the CSF is extracted; this difference can be noted by clearing fluid in subsequent tubes. If the supernatant is xanthochromic when compared with tap water, a diagnosis of SAH is confirmed. Although not available in all settings, spectrophotometry is more sensitive than visual inspection in detecting xanthochromia. A high opening CSF pressure and frank blood in the CSF are not always demonstrated. Laboratory analysis may reveal increased numbers of both red and white blood cells as well as an elevated CSF protein.

Angiography is obtained soon after the patient's admission to the hospital, to pinpoint the location of an aneurysm, rule out the possibility of other aneurysms or arteriovenous malformations, and define the anatomy in preparation for neurosurgical intervention. Although conventional catheter angiography remains the gold standard, MR angiography and CT angiography are rapidly increasing their role in the emergency department evaluation of these patients. The latter is easily obtained with spiral CT equipment, now available in many radiology departments.

Patients must be cared for in a critical care setting. Monitorings of central venous pressure, systemic arterial pressure, and intracranial pressure are instituted as necessary.

The fundamental objectives of preoperative management are to allow the brain to recover from the insult of the hemorrhage while minimizing the risks of rebleeding or cerebral ischemia. Experienced nursing care and observation are essential. If the patient is awake, he should be kept as calm and comfortable as possible with the use of analgesics (acetaminophen, codeine, demerol), sedation (diazepam, phenobarbital), and antiemetics. Anticonvulsants (phenobarbital, phenytoin) are often used prophylactically as seizures elevate intracranial pressure, increasing the risk of rebleeding. An adequate bowel program and the prevention of gastric inflammation with the use of antacids and H_2-blocking agents are imperative. These measures decrease the risk of rebleeding, which occurs at a rate of 4% in the first 24 hours, then at 1% to 2% per day for the first month, and at 3% per year after the initial 3 months. Rebleeding is the main cause of in-hospital mortality in patients with aneurysmal SAH; the best way to avoid this complication is by securing the aneurysm, either by surgical clipping or by endovascular coiling in poor surgical candidates or those with surgically inaccessible aneurysms.

The use of epsilon-aminocaproic acid (Amicar) to prevent rebleeding has decreased: Although its antifibrinolytic action appears to decrease the risk of rebleeding, its use has been associated with an increased incidence of both vasospasm and hydrocephalus.

The timing of neurosurgical intervention is critical. Early surgery may be complicated by the presence of blood, cerebral edema, and a medically unstable patient, while later surgery allows the opportunity for the onset of rebleeding and vasospasm. In general, patients with mild neurologic deficits and no evidence of vasospasm are early surgical candidates, while patients with more significant deficits are operated on later following medical stabilization and treatment for vasospasm when indicated. More severely affected patients may be better candidates for coiling, a procedure in which tiny detachable coils are deposited in the aneurysm through a catheter to promote thrombosis of the sac.

Delayed neurologic deficits caused by cerebral ischemia due to vasospasm are seen in up to 30% of patients, most commonly between the fifth and ninth day after the initial hemorrhage. Serial monitoring with noninvasive transcranial Doppler ultrasonography is in use to detect preclinical onset of cerebral vasospasm and monitor cerebral perfusion. The calcium channel–blocking agent nimodipine has been approved for prevention of cerebral vasospasm associated with aneurysmal SAH. Hypervolemic, hypertensive, and hemodilutional therapy ("triple-H therapy") may be necessary for the treatment of vasospasm-induced cerebral ischemia, usually with intravenous fluids, albumin, and occasionally vasopressors. However, these measures and the fundamental need for cerebral perfusion may be at odds with the risks of aneurysmal rebleeding; as it is much easier to manage these patients once the aneurysm is secured, early surgical clipping or endovascular coiling is usually attempted. Transluminal angioplasty with infusion of papaverine is recommended for patients who do not respond to triple-H therapy. Direct clot removal and cisternal deposition of fibrinolytic agents are still under investigation.

Other common complications of SAH include seizures, hydrocephalus, and hyponatremia. Seizures result from the irritative effects of subarachnoid blood. They produce increased intracranial pressure and systemic blood pressure, and by this mechanism they induce rebleeding from nonsecured aneurysms. Short-term administration of antiepileptics, usually phenytoin, is recommended. Obstructive hydrocephalus from an intraventricular clot occluding the aqueduct occurs in about a quarter of patients and may require the placement of a ventricular drain. Communicating hydrocephalus is usually a late complication and is thought to be related to obstruction of arachnoid villi. Finally, hyponatremia is probably caused by excessive natriuresis and not to the syndrome of inappropriate antidiuretic hormone (SIADH). Therefore, fluid restriction should be avoided as it is detrimental; rather, isotonic—and in rare occasions hypertonic—fluids should be administered.

The hazards and intricacies of caring for patients with aneurysmal SAH are clear and emphasize the need for a highly experienced nursing, medical, and surgical staff.

Incidental unruptured aneurysms are found in 0.5% to 1% of catheter cerebral angiographies and 1% to

6% of autopsies; they are multiple in up to 30% of cases. Tobacco use, by decreasing alpha-1-antitrypsin levels, is the main environmental risk factor, and a variety of genetic conditions have been associated with their presence: polycystic kidney disease, Ehler-Danlos type IV, neurofibromatosis type I, and Marfan's disease. The risk of rupture is 0.05 to 0.5% per year for aneurysms smaller than 10 mm, 1% per year for those larger than 10 mm, and even higher for giant aneurysms (>25 mm). Small aneurysms (< 10mm) are not usually surgically clipped. Close relatives of patients with cerebral saccular aneurysms should be screened for their presence, particularly those associated with one of the previously mentioned genetic conditions.

STATUS EPILEPTICUS

Status epilepticus (SE) is defined as a seizure lasting for more than 30 minutes, or intermittent serial seizures lasting for more than 30 minutes without return of consciousness. Although the term *status epilepticus* is most commonly associated with generalized tonic–clonic convulsive SE, in fact, this definition applies to any seizure type. The seizures may be generalized or partial (focal), convulsive, or nonconvulsive. Accordingly, the clinical manifestations of SE are extremely variable and run the gamut from acute confusional states, psychiatric disturbances, episodes of aphasia, and focal sensorimotor deficits to tonic–clonic convulsions with loss of consciousness. A high index of suspicion is required to make a diagnosis of nonconvulsive SE and therefore an electroencephalogram (EEG) should routinely be a part of the workup of the acute onset of altered mental status.

While isolated case reports of neurologic impairment following nonconvulsive SE are present in the literature, significant morbidity and mortality are generally associated with generalized tonic–clonic convulsive SE. Various studies over the last 20 years have reported a mortality from SE ranging from 8% to 50%. With more than 50,000 cases of SE each year, its impact is significant. As improved recognition and experience in treatment have developed, the mortality rate is now generally accepted as 10%. Brain damage in generalized convulsive SE is a consequence of the excessive neuronal excitation (so-called excitotoxicity) as well as the systemic complications of prolonged convulsive activity. The overall incidence of morbidity and mortality from SE is related to the aforementioned two factors, as well as to the underlying acute insult that precipitated SE.

The systemic manifestations are the sequelae of airway compromise, ventilatory failure, and excessive motor activity. Hypoxemia, respiratory acidosis, metabolic acidosis, hyperthermia, and, less commonly, rhabdomyolysis and fracture/dislocations have occurred. Laboratory investigations commonly demonstrate a peripheral leucocytosis, an acidotic pH, and a mild cerebrospinal fluid (CSF) pleocytosis.

The medical approach to SE must always take into account the underlying etiology of the prolonged seizure activity. It is important to remember that although the majority of patients who present with SE do not have a history of epilepsy, up to a third do. Although treatment is initially directed at the control of the seizures, in certain instances aggressive medical or surgical intervention is necessary. The three most common precipitating factors for SE are withdrawal from anticonvulsive medications, alcohol withdrawal, and cerebrovascular disease, which are each responsible for approximately one fifth of the cases. Metabolic disorders such as hyponatremia, hyper- or hypoglycemia, hypocalcemia, hepatic failure, and renal failure account for 10% to 15% of the cases reported. Other recognized etiologic conditions are anoxia, hypotension, infectious disorders (meningitis, abscess, encephalitis), tumors, trauma, and drug overdosage.

The general principles that guide a plan to minimize the morbidity and mortality associated with SE are early diagnosis, early intervention, a standard protocol to follow, and the prompt identification and management of underlying medical and surgical conditions. The fundamental step of recognition and diagnosis is often the greatest stumbling block. Ambulance staff and emergency room nursing and medical personnel must be educated to recognize the protean manifestations of seizure activity. Documentation of the time of onset of seizure activity is essential. The slowing or cessation of overt epileptic activity can be misleading. The observation and documentation of a gradual return of consciousness over the ensuing minutes is of paramount importance. Delays in diagnosis can often be traced to faulty communication among the staff members in attendance. It is well recognized that the longer the generalized convulsive status continues, the more difficult it is to control and the greater the possibility of irreversible brain injury.

Morbidity and mortality from SE are related to the following conditions: CNS damage from the causative illness or acute insult that resulted in SE, the metabolic consequences of prolonged SE, and prolonged electrical activity. It is now recognized that continuous electrical activity for more than 60 minutes, even while correcting metabolic derangements induced by the SE, results in at least hippocampal damage, and probably in more widespread damage as well. The chain of events leading to this brain damage may be induced by lack of gamma-aminobutyric acid (GABA), increased glutamate-mediated excitotoxicity, and calcium-induced neuronal death. These excitotoxic effects are compounded by significant metabolic alterations: In the first half hour of SE, acidosis with increased serum lactate, hyperglycemia, and blood pressure elevations are noted. With more prolonged SE, blood pressure does not increase with motor activity and may even drop, respiratory compromise worsens, hyperpyrexia and rhabdomyolysis may ensue from prolonged muscle activity, and significant sodium and potassium alterations develop. Cardiac arrhythmias may occur from CNS dysregulation, electrolyte abnormalities, or even medications employed in the treatment of SE.

Following the diagnosis of SE, the immediate response must be a timely and organized treatment plan to achieve the following objectives: basic life support, termination, prevention and treatment of complications of SE, identification of the cause of SE, and prevention of its reoccurrence (Table 25-2). The first steps are taken to assess vital signs and evaluate oxygenation. An oral airway is inserted and nasotracheal suction is performed if necessary. The need for oxygen therapy is evaluated by both clinical examination and arterial blood gas determination. Intravenous access is the next priority, and establishing two separate IV lines will optimize the patient's management. A second access not only serves as a backup in the event of a dislodging of the first IV line, but it also will be useful for the delivery of glucose, medications, and fluids aside from the needs of anticonvulsant therapy. Simultaneously, sufficient venous blood is drawn for a complete blood count, and to evaluate electrolytes, glucose, calcium, magnesium, blood urea nitrogen, liver function tests, anticonvulsant drug levels, toxicology screen, and ethanol level. An IV bolus of 50 ml of 50% glucose and thiamine (1 mg/kg) is administered as soon as the IV access is established. Electrocardiographic (ECG) monitoring is instituted immediately, and vital signs are checked regularly throughout the treatment protocol. EEG monitoring should begin at the earliest possible opportunity.

Specific treatment to terminate seizure activity is initiated with the infusion of benzodiazepines, as they are rapidly active and effective in controlling about 80% of all seizures (this figure does not reflect efficacy in SE). Intravenous lorazepam should be administered at a rate of 2 mg/min (0.1 mg/kg) to a maximal dose of 5 mg. Alternatively, IV diazepam may be given at a rate of 2 mg/min, until seizures stop or to a total of 20 mg. When available, lorazepam is preferable to diazepam, as it has a significantly longer duration of action. Infusion of the benzodiazepine is immediately followed by IV phenytoin 20 mg/kg at a rate no faster than 50 mg/min. Phenytoin must be delivered in normal saline as it will precipitate in a glucose solution. ECG and frequent blood pressure monitoring are essential. If hypotension or bradycardia develops, the rate of administration can be decreased or the infusion can be held until the vital signs stabilize. IV phenytoin should never be delivered by an automatic infusion pump to an unattended patient. If seizures are not controlled, a repeat bolus of phenytoin at 10 mg/kg can be administered.

Phosphenytoin, a prodrug that is converted to phenytoin, is posed to replace parenteral phenytoin. By virtue of its solubility, it does not require the addition of propylene glycol as a vehicle, which is thought to cause most of the clinically significant hypotension, arrhythmias, and local injection reactions of intravenous phenytoin administration. Absence of these side effects allows for a faster rate of infusion of phosphenytoin, usually at 100–150 mg/min. Dosage is expressed in phosphenytoin sodium equivalents (PE), thus requiring a loading dose of 20 PE/kg at the previously mentioned rate of administration. Although SE should be treated by the intravenous delivery of medications, phosphenytoin offers the additional advantage of intramuscular injection in those patients without IV access; therapeutic plasma concentrations are reached within 30 minutes by this route.

If seizures persist, elective endotracheal intubation is recommended at this point (if not done prior to this) before starting the IV infusion of phenobarbital. Phenobarbital is administered at a rate of 50–100 mg/min until seizures stop or to a loading dose of 2 mg/kg. Phenobarbital is a potent anticonvulsant and in combination with phenytoin is effective in controlling SE in the majority of cases. Unfortunately, it is also associated with significant degrees of respiratory depression and sedation. Therefore, the use of phenobarbital increases the risk of complications for the patient. In addition, postictal assessment of the patient's cognitive status is hindered by the long half-life of this drug.

When treatment is delivered in a timely and organized manner, the aforementioned medications can be administered within 1 hour. In the majority of cases, SE will be treated successfully at this point. However, if the seizures continue, begin IV pentobarbital with a loading dose of 2–3 mg/kg initially and then a continuous infusion of a solution of 100 mg/500 ml. Titrate the infusion rate to depress the background EEG to isoelectric for 4 hours. After this time, the infusion rate is gradually decreased. If epileptiform discharges reappear on the EEG or clinical seizures reoccur, repeat this procedure. If epileptic activity is terminated, the pentobarbital may be tapered over 12 to 24 hours.

TABLE 25–2. Management of Generalized Status Epilepticus (SE)

OBJECTIVES	TIME FRAME	INTERVENTION
Basic life support	0–5 min	1. Recognition of SE 2. Assessment of vital signs and oxygenation 3. Insert oral airway and administer oxygen if necessary. 4. Establish two intravenous lines for clear venous access. 5. Draw venous blood. 6. Draw arterial blood for evaluation of CBC, electrolytes, glucose, calcium, magnesium, BUN, LFTs, anticonvulsant levels, toxicology screen, and ethanol level. 7. Begin ECG and EEG monitoring.
	6–9 min	Administer IV bolus of 50 ml of 50% glucose and thiamine 1 mg/kg.
Termination of SE	10–30 min	1. Infuse IV lorazepam at a rate of 2 mg/min (0.1 mg/kg) to a maximum dose of 5 mg or infuse IV diazepam at a rate of 2 mg/min until seizures stop or to a total of 20 mg. 2. *Immediately follow with the infusion of IV fosphenytoin 20 PE/kg at a rate of 100 to 150 PE/min. If seizures persist, infuse another bolus of 10 PE/kg at the same rate. Alternatively, use IV phenytoin at 20 mg/kg at no more than 50 mg/min, followed if needed by 10 mg/kg bolus at the same rate.* 3. Monitor blood pressure, ECG, and respirations.
	31–60 min	1. If seizures persist, perform elective endotracheal intubation 2. Infuse IV phenobarbitol at a rate of 50–100 mg/min until seizures stop or to a loading dose of 20 mg/kg.
	1 h	1. *If seizures persist, begin IV phenobarbitol with a loading dose of 3–5 mg/kg followed by a continous infusion of 100 mg/500 ml at 1–4 mg/kg/hr until an isoelectric EEG is obtained.* 2. Maintain an isoelectric EEG pattern for 4 h and then gradually taper the infusion rate over 12–24 hours. 3. Repeat the procedure if clinical seizure activity or electrical epileptiform activity is observed.
Prevention and treatment of complications of SE	Throughout	1. Monitor vital signs regularly. 2. Monitor patient's volume status. 3. Maintain airway and suction as necessary to prevent aspiration 4. Review laboratory information promptly and intervene without delay.
Identification of cause of SE	Throughout	1. Obtain history from relatives and friends. 2. Review patient's volume status. 3. Maintain airway and suction as necessary to prevent aspiration. 4. Lumbar puncture, when indicated, *after CT done.* 5. Initiate IV antibiotic coverage when any suspicion of meningitis exists.
Prevention of reoccurence of SE	Following cesation of seizure activity	1. Continue to closely monitor anticonvulsant levels. 2. Initiate daily therapy with appropriate anticonvulsant levels. 3. Educate patient and family to ensure compliance with medication regimen.

BUN = blood urea nitrogen; CBC = complete blood count; LFTs = liver function tests; ECG = electrocardiogram; EEG = electroencephalogram; IV = intravenous; PE = phosphenytoin sodium equivalents; CT = computed tomography

Careful attention to prevention and management of complications of SE is ongoing throughout the treatment protocol. Effective control of hypertension, hyperthermia, and acidosis is required, but effective treatment of SE will reverse these problems. Hypotension may be the direct consequence of prolonged SE, but the effects of anticonvulsant medication, volume depletion, the sequelae of multiple trauma, or coincident cardiovascular disease must be considered and treated appropriately. The potential risks of rhabdomyolysis, aspiration pneumonia, or traumatic injury at the onset or during seizure activity must be recognized.

Two additional medications need to be mentioned. Children with well-established seizure patterns may develop seizure clusters or acute repetitive seizures (ARS), usually in the setting of an intercurrent illness. ARS may progress to SE if untreated. Rectal diazepam gel is approved for use in the prehospital setting for ARS, as it reduces the median seizure frequency. The recommended dose is 0.5 mg/kg for ages 2 through 5, 0.3 mg/kg for ages 6 through 11, and 0.2 mg/kg for older children. Its main side effect is somnolence. Parents of children with a predisposition for ARS can be easily trained to apply the gel at home. The second medication is intravenous valproate. Its role is mainly restricted to the rapid loading of patients requiring this drug. Its use in SE is limited as therapeutic serum concentrations cannot be reached consistently.

The management of SE cannot be separated from the exigency of identifying the underlying cause. Obtaining historical information from relatives or friends accompanying the patient or review of old medical records may reveal a pattern of noncompliance with medication or a recurrent history of alcohol binging and withdrawal. Reports of the recent onset of neurologic deficits, or a history of systemic disease with elevated temperature, raise the index of suspicion in new areas and will guide evaluation. CT of the head is obtained, with and without contrast (if renal function and allergies permit), to exclude the possibilities of neoplasm, cerebrovascular infarction, intracerebral hemorrhage, and traumatic injury. Following CT, lumbar puncture is often indicated and evaluation of CSF often reveals a moderate pleocytosis (up to 150 white blood cells) and an increase in CSF protein (up to 100 mg/dl) caused by the persistent seizure activity. Nonetheless, if there is any suspicion of meningitis, antibiotic therapy should be promptly begun and appropriate cultures sent for evaluation.

Following the successful treatment of SE, careful attention to serum anticonvulsant levels and the initiation of a daily dosing schedule of either an effective single anticonvulsant medication or a combination of anticonvulsants will help to prevent a reoccurrence of seizure activity. In the coming years, the development of new anticonvulsant medications as well as the introduction of new classes of drugs that may prevent the toxic consequences of excessive neuronal activity hold promise for continuing to reduce the morbidity and mortality of SE.

ACUTE ALTERATION OF MENTAL STATUS

Acute alterations of mental status are the most common neurobehavioral disorders seen in general hospitals. Studies have demonstrated an incidence of between 5% and 15% in hospitalized patients on medical/surgical floors, 20% and 30% in surgical intensive care units (ICUs), and even higher on geriatric wards. The use of numerous vague and redundant terms to describe this disorder (e.g., organic brain syndrome, acute cerebral insufficiency, organic psychosis, toxic–metabolic encephalopathy, acute confusional state, and exogenous psychosis) reflects the difficulties encountered in conceptualizing and categorizing these problems.

The differential diagnosis of a patient with an unexplained acute alteration of mental status is extensive. The approach to the patient should take into account the three broad areas of structural lesions, toxic–metabolic causes, and psychiatric etiologies. Structural lesions often distinguish themselves with focal or asymmetrical findings on neurologic exam and a more abrupt onset than that seen in metabolic disorders. In addition, the level of consciousness is more likely to fluctuate with metabolic than structural disorders. Inconsistencies on repeated examinations and atypical, nonanatomic findings may raise the suspicion of an underlying psychiatric problem.

The most common causes of acute confusional states, often associated with alterations of consciousness, are acquired metabolic disturbances. The metabolic encephalopathies are a diverse group of neurologic disorders characterized by an alteration of mental status caused by the failure of organs other than the brain. Cerebral dysfunction may result from three basic mechanisms: deficiency of a necessary metabolic substrate (e.g., hypoglycemia); disruption of the internal environment of the brain (e.g., dehydration); or the presence of a toxin or accumulation of a metabolic waste product (e.g., drug intoxication or uremia). Although the brain is, in effect, an innocent bystander, the alteration of personality, behavior, cognitive function, or level of alertness may be the presenting feature that brings the patient to medical attention.

Metabolic encephalopathies are usually characterized by an evolution from the patient's baseline mental status through stages of inattentiveness, disturbed memory, confusion, lethargy, somnolence, obtundation, and coma. The early stages of these deficits will often go unrecognized because of the patient's concurrent loss of insight and judgment.

The disturbance of higher cortical functions is illustrated by a wide range of signs and symptoms; inattention and distractibility are universal symptoms. Disorientation, memory impairment, emotional lability, disturbance of the sleep–wake cycle, and either increased or decreased psychomotor activity may be observed. Reduced ability to maintain and shift attention, as well as disorganized thinking with fluctuations over the course of the day, are characteristic. Perceptual disturbances may result in illusions, delusions, or hallucinations, which are usually visual and often unpleasant.

The sum of these disturbances is often characterized by delirium, a clouding of consciousness with reduced ability to sustain attention to environmental stimuli. As a result, the patient is unable to respond to events with the usual clarity, coherence, or speed.

Hepatic encephalopathy and uremic encephalopathy are frequent causes of altered mental status in hospitalized patients. Disorders of glucose regulation, osmolarity/sodium homeostasis, and derangement of calcium, magnesium, and phosphorous levels are also frequent offenders. Hypoxic–ischemic encephalopathy is often identified as the causative factor following cardiorespiratory arrest, ventilatory failure, or hypotensive episodes. Endocrine encephalopathies seen in Cushing's syndrome, Addison's disease, and thyroid disease are less common and may be overlooked.

Drug intoxication and drug withdrawal are very common causative factors. Acute alterations of mental status are especially associated with drugs that have anticholinergic properties, including many antidepressants, neuroleptics, antihistamines, antiparkinsonian agents, and over-the-counter cold preparations. High-dose steroids, narcotics, and sedatives may be the offending agent. Abused street drugs associated with violent behavior include amphetamines, cocaine, hallucinogens, minor tranquilizers/sedatives, and, of course, alcohol. Alteration of consciousness in alcoholic patients is a common presentation in the emergency room, and it should not be dismissed simply as intoxication in the face of a history of alcohol abuse. A blood ethanol level of 80 to 100 mg/dl correlates with a change in mental status. Sharp declines in blood ethanol levels 12 to 24 hours after intake may result in a tremulous state followed by alcohol withdrawal seizures, which are usually brief with subsequent normal neurologic functions. Prolonged or focal seizures, prolonged postictal state, or a focally abnormal neurologic examination should initiate a search for other causes of seizures. Alcoholics are particularly prone to head injury, and a brain imaging study may reveal epidural or subdural hematomas, intraparenchymal hemorrhage, or traumatic subarachnoid hemorrhage. They are also at risk for CNS infection, which is diagnosed by CSF examination. Coexistent hepatic failure, hypoglycemia, hyponatremia, or drug ingestion should be detected by appropriate testing. Prolonged postictal states due to nonconvulsive SE is revealed by prompt EEG monitoring. The clinician should be particularly alert to the possibility of Wernicke's encephalopathy, which is the manifestation of thiamine deficiency. It is clinically characterized by alteration of mental status, oculomotor dysfunction (which may be so subtle that it is represented only by nystagmus), and ataxia. As these manifestations can be present in alcoholics without Wernicke's encephalopathy (acute intoxication, cerebellar atrophy), it is wise to administer thiamine 100 mg/day IV, particularly before glucose is administered. Other vitamins should be supplemented, as alcoholics may be nutritionally compromised. Benzodiazepines are the mainstay of alcoholic withdrawal and alcoholic seizure management. Although chlordiazepoxide, diazepam, and lorazepam are commonly used, oxazepam may be preferable in patients with liver insufficiency as its clearance is less dependent on hepatic metabolism than other benzodiazepines. Dehydration is commonly seen in alcoholic withdrawal, so IV fluids should be provided. Magnesium may be in the low-normal range, but body stores are frequently depleted and should be replaced, and other electrolytes should be monitored. Hyponatremia should be corrected slowly, as rapid correction may lead to central pontine myelinolysis.

Management of the patient with an acute alteration of mental status involves two stages: identification and treatment of the underlying cause, and symptomatic treatment. Significant hypoxia or hypoglycemia demand especially quick recognition and treatment because of the potential for irreversible brain injury. Historical information must be obtained about systemic illnesses, drug or alcohol use, recent trauma, exposure to toxins, the baseline mental status, and the time frame of the change in mental function.

Factors predisposing to acute confusional states are a history of dementia, mental retardation, or preceding brain injury; these patients may be able to compensate in normal situations but may be "tipped over" by additional stressors. Psychological stress or anxiety, unfamiliar surroundings with loss of daily routine, disruption of sleep–wake cycles, and sensory understimulation or overstimulation are other precipitating factors. Both the very old and the very young patient are at special risk. Polypharmacy, the simultaneous use of multiple pharmacologic agents, is an especially important contributory factor.

While the alteration in mental states may be the presenting feature that brings the patient to medical attention, evidence of the underlying disorder is usually present on physical examination. A thoughtful examination includes inspection for the stigmata of hepatic, renal, or endocrine disorders. Scrutiny of the states of hydration and nutrition provides important information. Alterations in the patient's vital signs may provide clues to a wide diversity of problems, ranging from sepsis to elevated intracranial pressure. Evidence of head trauma should be sought in the obtunded or comatose patient.

Examination of the patient's mental status should be performed in a reproducible manner to guide subsequent reevaluations of disease progression and efficacy of therapy. Description of level of consciousness is best limited to a few commonly recognized descriptive terms, such as *alert, lethargic* (easily arousable), *stuporous* (difficult to arouse), and *comatose* (little response to external stimulation). The arbitrary imposition of labels to a wide continuum of behavior demands precise documentation of the patient's performance on standardized tests of arousability, orientation, attention, and memory. The Folstein Mini-Mental Exam and Glasgow Coma Scale provide convenient quantitative parameters for more precise follow-up.

The neurologic exam includes tests of pupillary control and ocular motility, including the oculocephalic and oculovestibular reflexes, and evaluation of respiratory pattern and motor responses to stimulation. Demonstration of intact brainstem function makes a structural lesion of the brainstem, including an elevation of intracranial pressure, less likely. Hyperreflexia may be seen in association with metabolic encephalopathy, but other evidence of upper motor neuron dysfunction is usually not demonstrated until advanced stages of alterations of consciousness. Asterixis, generalized tremor, and spontaneous myoclonus are often observed. Toxic encephalopathies should especially be considered in patients with dysarthria, nystagmus, ataxia, tremor, and dilated pupils.

Laboratory evaluation should screen for metabolic abnormalities and toxins, and they should include at least a blood count, platelet count, prothrombin time (PT), PTT, chemistry profile (electrolytes, glucose, blood urea nitrogen, creatinine, calcium, magnesium, phosphorous), liver function tests, ammonia level, thyroid function tests, arterial blood gas, urinalysis, and drug and toxicology screen. Information gathered during the history and physical exam will provide guidance in choosing from the following additional studies: serum osmolality, plasma cortisol level, syphilis serology, erythrocyte sedimentation rate, antinuclear antibody (ANA), vitamin B_{12}, folate, human immunodeficiency virus, ceruloplasmin, serum copper, urinary copper, and urinary porphobilinogen.

Neuroimaging is required following an acute change in mental status to exclude a structural lesion resulting in increased intracranial pressure or focal abnormalities. Patients with fluent aphasias from dominant temporoparietal lesions, or with nondominant parietal injury, are commonly misdiagnosed as delirious or psychotic; these situations are avoided by appropriate brain imaging. Specific CSF abnormalities are rare in metabolic encephalopathies; however, lumbar puncture may be necessary to rule out meningitis or encephalitis when previous evaluations have failed to reveal the cause of the change in mental state or when there is clinical suspicion of a CNS infection. There should be a low threshold for initiating this procedure. Brain imaging is recommended before a lumbar puncture to detect conditions of increased intracranial pressure and shift, which would contraindicate it.

An EEG should be routinely obtained in patients with metabolic encephalopathy or altered mental status of uncertain etiology. The EEG recording provides an objective evaluation of the degree of CNS dysfunction. Disorganization of the normal electroencephalographic patterns and generalized slowing are the most commonly observed changes. Seizure activity, particularly subclinical SE, as well as focal abnormalities may be identified. Often, the major value of EEG is in the use of serial studies to quantitatively and objectively gauge the degree of cerebral dysfunction.

While it is clear that the term *altered mental status* represents an extensive ensemble of behavior and a spectrum of levels of consciousness, there is a subset of patients who are especially challenging. Patients with disorientation, emotional lability, delusions, hallucinations, paranoid ideation, or intoxication may be agitated, aggressive, violent, and resistant to medical evaluation and treatment. Although it is best to avoid the use of drugs in confused and agitated patients, the patient's behavior may be potentially dangerous, may cause the patient profound distress, and may interfere with the provision of nursing and medical care.

The alternatives of chemical or physical restraints are both fraught with flaws and hazards. Intervention should be individualized and directed at the specific problem (anxiety, depression, insomnia, disturbance of sleep–wake cycles, agitation, hallucinations, delusions, and assaultiveness). The most commonly used agents are benzodiazepines and neuroleptics. Neuroleptics may be an appropriate choice but should not be used in this setting for the long-term management of behavior.

For the patient with acute agitation with psychiatric features, haloperidol may be administered in a dosage of 5 mg intramuscularly (IM) every 4 to 8 hours to a maximum of 15–30 mg/day. Delirious patients rarely require more than 10 mg of haloperidol daily, and often 2–4 mg/day will suffice. The therapeutic end point should be a manageable reduction in misperceptions and agitation, not a completely clear sensorium. When the predominant feature is anxiety, benzodiazepines (e.g., diazepam, 5–10 mg IM) are often sufficient.

There are some cautions to keep in mind when using neuroleptics or sedatives for organic cerebral dysfunction, particularly when the underlying etiology is unclear. One should be certain that the patient's level of consciousness is not worsening prior to administration. Intoxication with alcohol, overdosage with sedative or anticholinergic drugs, structural lesions with elevated intracranial pressure, and both CNS and systemic infections should be excluded. In some situations, these behaviors are a critical guide to the progression of the underlying process, and the use of physical restraints is preferable.

While the diagnosis and treatment of the commonplace disorder of alteration of mental status may be challenging and difficult in patients with multiple system failure or irreversible brain injury, a significant proportion of these patients are found to have reversible processes. These encounters, when approached with proficiency, can be especially rewarding.

ACUTE INTRACRANIAL HYPERTENSION

The main components of volume in the skull are the brain (1,400 ml), blood (1,400 ml), and CSF (150 ml). The latter two drain into the lower-resistance dural sinuses; in normal individuals, venous pressure is the main determinant of intracranial pressure (ICP). However, any increase in the volume of one of these components without a corresponding decrease in the volume of the other two will result in raised ICP; as volume in the cranium cannot change, adding volume will result initially in compensatory measures consisting of decrease in intracranial blood volume and transfer of CSF into the lumbar cistern. Once brain compliance is exhausted, small increases in ICP will result in displacement of brain matter through the foramen magnum. Cerebral blood flow (CBF) is normally maintained over a wide range of cerebral perfusion pressures (CPPs); this is defined as the difference between mean arterial blood pressure (MAP) and ICP. A CPP greater than or equal to 70 mm Hg ensures adequate cerebral perfusion; ICP is normally 5 to 20 cm H_2O, or 3 to 15 mm Hg. Constant CBF is obtained with MAPs from 50 to 150 mm Hg, but these values may be higher in chronic hypertensives. At the low end of this curve, CPP will drop and cerebral hypoperfusion will ensue, whereas at the high end of the curve, cerebral hyperperfusion with cerebral edema will occur. In disease states, the curve will become linear, and the CPP will approximate the CBF because of the loss of vessel autoregulation. Elevation of ICP or decrease in MAP will result in cerebral hypoperfusion.

Intracranial pressure may increase gradually over an extended period of time or suddenly in a matter of minutes to acutely threaten life. The prompt recognition and treatment of acutely raised intracranial pressure is vital to preserve brainstem function, and it may be lifesaving.

The cranial vault is divided incompletely into compartments by thick, fibrous bands of dura mater. The tentorium cerebelli is clinically the most important of these structures. It separates the lower brainstem and cerebellum from the cerebral hemispheres and diencephalon, delineating the infratentorial and supratentorial spaces. The midbrain lies within an opening in the tentorium called the tentorial notch, and it is bound laterally by fascicles of the oculomotor nerve and the medial portion of the temporal lobes (the uncus). This anatomic location renders the midbrain especially vulnerable to compression under conditions of increased intracranial pressure.

An acute rise in intracompartmental pressure, such as occurs with hypertensive hemorrhage, may result in downward displacement and herniation of neural structures. The midbrain, placed centrally in the tentorial notch, may be compressed by surrounding elements, compromising vital brainstem functions such as respiration, maintenance of consciousness, and cardioregulation. Coma and death may ensue. There are two main types of herniation syndromes: uncal and central. It is important that these syndromes be recognized early and that treatment be urgently instituted before further progression to irreversible brainstem damage occurs. Some of the mass lesions that can lead to herniation are listed in Table 25-3.

Central herniation occurs when diffusely raised supratentorial pressure compresses central brainstem structures and produces a progressive impairment of consciousness, respiratory irregularities, abnormal motor responses (posturing), and symmetrical mid-position unreactive pupils. Uncal herniation, on the other hand, occurs as a unilateral supratentorial mass lesion displaces the medial temporal lobe toward the tentorial notch. Early on, the oculomotor nerve becomes compressed between the encroaching uncus and the edge of the tentorial opening, producing a larger and less reactive pupil on that side. Hemiparesis may occur ipsilateral to the herniating uncus because of the compression of the contralateral cerebral peduncle against the far edge of the tentorial notch as the midbrain is displaced laterally (Kernohan's notch syndrome). More commonly, though, the hemiparesis is contralateral to the herniating uncus. In either case, hemiparesis is not a good clinical sign for localizing the side of the herniation. A dilated pupil (oculomotor nerve palsy) is ipsilateral to the herniation 95% of the time, and it is a reliable clinical indicator.

Unlike the situation that occurs with mass lesions, raised ICP may be distributed equally among the intracranial compartments with little risk of herniation and brainstem compression. Some of the more common causes of diffuse intracranial hypertension are listed in Table 25-4.

Symptoms and signs of intracranial hypertension are variable and depend on both the etiology and the rapidity with which the pressure increase develops. Headache, for example, is more likely to be a prominent symptom in more acute problems. Vomiting and alteration of consciousness may be seen; papilledema may be present in subacute or chronic conditions. The abducens nerve, by virtue of its extensive intracranial course, is particularly susceptible to traction injury

TABLE 25-3. Mass Lesions Associated with Brain Herniation

Neoplasm
Subdural hematoma
Epidural hematoma
Intraparenchymal hemorrhage
Abscess
Infarction

TABLE 25-4. Causes of Diffuse Intracranial Hypertension with Less Risk of Herniation

Hypoxia
Meningitis
Encephalitis
Head trauma without subdural or epidural hematoma
Subarachnoid hemorrhage
Malignant hyperthermia
Cerebral vein thrombosis
Pseudotumor cerebri
Lead encephalopathy

when the intracranial pressure is raised. Sixth nerve palsies, therefore, are frequently seen, but they have little localizing value.

The primary goal in raised ICP management is to decrease ICP while maintaining an adequate CPP (70 mm Hg). Therefore, judicious manipulations of systemic MAP is warranted, as well as good measurements of ICP. Although estimations of ICP can be deduced from clinical signs, this is unreliable. The gold standard for ICP monitoring is by direct ventricular pressure measurement through a ventriculostomy. This method is quite precise and allows for therapeutic CSF drainage to reduce ICP, but it may produce parenchymal damage and, with prolonged insertion of ventricular catheters, has a high incidence of infectious ventriculitis (particularly after 5 days). Other methods are safer, with fewer infectious complications, but also less precise. They include subarachnoid bolts, epidural transducers, and intraparenchymal fiberoptic transducers. noninvasive methods with transcranial Doppler are promising but not yet reliable.

The evaluation of patients with suspected intracranial hypertension should begin with a brief history from available sources and a brief physical examination. Patients who are unresponsive and in danger of herniation should be intubated immediately, and emergency treatment should be begun before diagnostic procedures are undertaken. In such catastrophic situations, mechanical hyperventilation is the fastest way of reducing intracranial pressure. It is desirable to keep the $PaCO_2$ between 25 and 30 mm Hg. The decreased $PaCO_2$ causes cerebral vasoconstriction, thereby reducing cerebral blood volume and intracranial pressure. Excessive hypocarbia may cause deleterious vasoconstriction. It is important not to compress the jugular veins with the tape used to secure the endotracheal tube.

Osmotic agents such as mannitol are given to decrease the water content of the brain. The starting dose is 500 ml of 20% mannitol given IV over 20 to 30 minutes (approximately 1 mg/kg). An indwelling urinary catheter is always inserted. Serum electrolytes and osmolality are monitored closely, using the latter as a guide to further dosing. A mannitol dose of 100–250 mg (0.25 mg/kg) can be given every 4 hours as necessary to keep the serum osmolality at 300 to 320 milliosmoles (mOsm) per liter.

Corticosteroids are administered if considerable vasogenic edema is present. Vasogenic edema occurs in those conditions that involve a breakdown of the blood–brain barrier and is seen commonly with brain neoplasms. Steroids are generally not effective for the type of edema that accompanies cerebral infarction (cytotoxic edema) and thus are not indicated in large hemispheric strokes. Steroids do not begin to work for several hours, so they are usually given concurrently with hyperventilation and hyperosmolar agents in acute situations. Methylprednisolone (Solu-Medrol) 250 mg or dexamethasone (Decadron) 10 mg IV can be used immediately, followed by Decadron 4 mg IV every 6 hours.

In some instances of rapidly progressing intracranial hypertension, none of the aforementioned measures are helpful and emergency neurosurgery is the preferred treatment. This is certainly the case with cerebellar hemorrhages or rapidly expanding epidural or subdural hematomas, where surgical decompression and evacuation may be lifesaving. Ventricular drainage of CSF can also rapidly decrease ICP and is easily performed at the bedside. Craniotomy is being increasingly performed for ICP control. Hypothermia and pentobarbital coma are last-resort measures that hold promise in the management of these patients.

There are a number of other general therapeutic measures that should be undertaken. Intravenous or enteral fluids should always be isotonic. Hypotonic solutions such as 5% dextrose or half-normal (0.45) saline will aggravate cerebral edema. Serum osmolarity under 280 mOsm/l should be corrected, and mild hyperosmolarity greater than 300 mOsm/l is desired. The *composition* of fluids replenished is a greater determinant in cerebral edema than the *amount* of fluids. Blood pressure should be modified to maintain a CPP of 70 to 120 mm Hg (remember that CPP = MAP – ICP). When CPP is greater than 120 and elevated ICP greater than 20, short-acting antihypertensives such as labetalol should be employed. Nitroprusside may worsen cerebral edema by dilating the cerebral vasculature. In patients with raised ICP and CPP under 70 mm Hg, elevation of MAP is required to avoid

hypoxic–ischemic injury, which in turn may lead to worsening cerebral edema. Vasopressors are sometimes used in this situation. Sedation is often required in ventilated patients, particularly those that "buck" the ventilator; in these patients, raised intrathoracic pressure elevates ICP by increasing venous resistance to CSF outflow. Short-acting sedatives are preferred; propofol is gaining popularity in this setting because of its very short half-life, which allows rapid discontinuation and reliable serial neurologic examinations.

Only after the patient's clinical status has been stabilized should a further evaluation with a head CT scan proceed. Because of the risk of precipitating herniation, a lumbar puncture should not be performed in any patient suspected of having increased intracranial pressure until a mass lesion is ruled out by a CT scan. A lumbar puncture may have to be performed prior to obtaining a CT scan if the patient is suspected of having bacterial meningitis and focal findings are not seen on the neurologic examination. In this instance, any delay in the diagnosis and administration of appropriate antibiotics may seriously threaten a favorable outcome.

ACUTE SPINAL CORD COMPRESSION

Acute compression of the spinal cord often presents insidiously with mild sensory disturbance, weakness, or sphincter or sexual dysfunction, but it may progress rapidly to irreversible paralysis if not corrected. Spinal cord compression is a common complication of metastatic disease, affecting 5% to 10% of cancer victims, but it also occurs with other conditions (Table 25-5). The most frequent metastatic tumors causing spinal cord compression include multiple myeloma, lymphoma, and carcinomas of the prostate, lung, breast, kidney, and colon.

Pain is the earliest symptom in the vast majority of patients and may be localized to the involved spinal area (96%) or radiate in a dermatomal pattern (90%) if the dorsal spinal roots are also involved. Pain may

TABLE 25-5. Common Causes of Acute Spinal Cord Compression

Metastatic cancer
Herniated disk
Abscess
Hematoma

be intensified by actions that increase intrathoracic pressure and consequently CSF pressure, such as coughing, sneezing, or straining at stool. Percussion tenderness over the spine is often a valuable clinical sign aiding localization.

The development of weakness, sensory loss, or erectile or sphincter dysfunction may progress quickly, and treatment should be started at the first sign of myelopathy. Thoracic cord compression is the most frequent site of involvement (70%), as it is the narrowest area of the spinal canal. It is followed in frequency by the lumbosacral (20%) and cervical (10%) areas. Up to one fifth of patients have multiple sites of cord compression. A very high dose of corticosteroids, such as dexamethasone 100 mg IV, is given immediately to reduce the edema caused by the compressing lesion, and this often provides dramatic pain relief and return of some neurologic function. In metastatic epidural cord compression, dexamethasone is continued at 24 mg IV every 6 hours for 24 hours, and then tapered over the next 48 hours to 6 mg every 6 hours, until more definite treatment is completed. Lower doses may be as effective. Gastric prophylaxis should be provided concurrently. An indwelling bladder catheter should be inserted. Bladder and bowel function should be monitored, with stool softeners and laxatives given as needed.

Diagnostic procedures to delineate the etiology and area of involvement should then be pursued. Discerning the cause is usually not difficult in patients with known cancer or recent trauma, but on occasion, spinal cord compression may be the initial manifestation of malignancy. Plain x-rays of the spine are abnormal in 84% to 94% of cases and may show evidence of bony erosion from metastatic disease, particularly loss of vertebral pedicles; however, they are of little help in imaging the soft-tissue structures that are invading the epidural or subdural spaces and compressing the spinal cord. MRI is the procedure of choice for visualizing the extent of anatomic involvement and spinal cord compression. It is superior to myelography in most instances because of its noninvasiveness and better resolution of anatomic structures. Spinal CT and bone scans play an important role in the diagnostic evaluations of these patients.

Specific treatment directed at the underlying process can begin once the etiology and location are defined. In metastatic disease, radiation therapy is started immediately and is especially valuable for the more radiosensitive tumors such as multiple myeloma and lymphoma. Surgical decompression is the treatment of choice for disc disease, epidural abscess, and hematoma, and it is sometimes indicated for metastatic disease in situations in which a tissue diagnosis

is needed, spinal stabilization is necessary, or further radiotherapy is not warranted.

The prognosis for meaningful functional recovery depends in large part on the functional state of the patient at presentation. While 80% of patients who are able to walk when they come to medical attention remain ambulatory after treatment, only 30% to 40% of nonambulatory persons with antigravity leg function regain ambulation, and only 5% of people with no antigravity leg strength are able to walk after therapy.

A high index of suspicion is required to make the diagnosis of epidural abscess, and a history of recent bacteremia or IV drug abuse is often obtained. The patient may or may not appear septic at the time of presentation. If epidural abscess is suspected, high-dose IV antibiotics should be given immediately (after sending blood and other appropriate cultures for analysis), while awaiting radiologic procedures and surgical decompression.

PERIPHERAL NERVOUS SYSTEM

MYASTHENIC CRISIS

Myasthenia gravis is an autoimmune disorder mediated by the binding of antibody to the postsynaptic acetylcholine receptor of striated muscle. Neuromuscular transmission is impaired, resulting in weakness and fatigability of voluntary muscles. Classically, a diurnal variation in strength is noted, which is stronger in the morning and weaker at night. Diplopia or ptosis is the initial symptom in about half of the cases. Dysphagia, chewing difficulty, nasal speech, and regurgitation of fluids are the presenting features in one third of patients, reflecting the involvement of bulbar musculature. Proximal extremity weakness, without bulbar or ocular involvement, is the least common presentation and is easily misdiagnosed.

A myasthenic crisis occurs when muscle weakness interferes with vital functions such as breathing and swallowing. Emergency intervention is then required. The mortality rate remains approximately 5% to 6%, with cardiac complications and aspiration pneumonia being the leading causes of death. A crisis may be precipitated most commonly by infection, but emotional stress, hypokalemia, thyroid disease, or, rarely, certain drugs (Table 25-6) may trigger a crisis. However, in one third of patients, no precipitant is identified. A crisis may also be caused by overmedication with anticholinesterase agents, the so-called cholinergic crisis. A cholinergic crisis may be heralded by an increase in muscarinic symptoms such as abdominal colic and

TABLE 25-6. Drugs That May Exacerbate the Weakness of Myasthenia Gravis

Aminoglycoside antibiotics
Quinine
Cardiac antiarrhythmics (e.g., quinidine, procainamide, propranolol, lidocaine)
Polymyxin
Colistin

diarrhea, with more severe muscarinic signs such as vomiting, lacrimation, hypersalivation, and miosis indicating impending danger. The differentiation of myasthenic from cholinergic crisis may be more academic than practical, however, because when faced with a patient whose respiratory function is severely compromised, the emergency management is the same protection of the airway and maintenance of adequate ventilation. Medication adjustments and discussion of precipitating factors may be done after the patient is safe in the ICU and on a mechanical ventilator.

It is rare for a crisis to be the first manifestation of myasthenia gravis. It is our policy to hospitalize any known myasthenic patient who complains of shortness of breath or difficulty swallowing, preferably in an intensive care setting. Frequent monitoring of the vital capacity is important, with endotracheal intubation performed when the vital capacity is less than 800 to 1,000 ml, or less than 15 ml/kg, or if dysphagia is so severe that there is a serious risk of aspiration. Maximal inspiratory pressure and maximal expiratory pressure are more sensitive in detecting ventilatory weakness than vital capacity. A reduction of maximal inspiratory pressure to less than 30% of that predicted for age and weight should alert the physician to impending respiratory failure and the need for mechanical ventilation. Arterial blood gases are not good predictors as they may be normal up to the onset of respiratory failure. Oral anticholinesterase agents are stopped in all patients and are withheld for 48 hours even if cholinergic crisis is not suspected. This is justified because an increased response to these drugs may occur after this "drug holiday," and often less medication may be needed once resumed.

Treatment begins with a shorter-acting drug, neostigmine (Prostigmin), 0.5 mg IM or 15 mg per nasogastric tube every 2 to 3 hours using the vital capacity or muscle strength as a guide to dosage titration. Once the optimal dose of neostigmine is found, the switch to the longer-acting agent pyridostigmine (Mestinon) can be made. Approximately 4 times the neostigmine dose is required every 3 to 4 hours. Corticosteroids may also be helpful in ending myasthenic crisis, but they should be used cautiously in the presence of infection. It should be kept in mind that steroids can initially worsen weakness and result in respiratory failure, particularly in the first few days of their being instituted. For this reason corticosteroids must initially be administered in a hospital setting, particularly if a high-dose regimen is chosen. Since the employment of steroids is usually required for several weeks or more after the crisis situation has passed, a better approach is alternate-day steroid therapy to minimize long-term side effects. Prednisone 100 mg, or its equivalent, is given on alternate days, with a gradual taper beginning only after the patient's status is clearly stabilized, usually several weeks after the crisis is over. Some authors favor giving high-dose IV corticosteroids on a daily basis early in the course before switching to alternate-day prednisone therapy.

Intravenous immune globulins (IVIG) or plasmapheresis is useful adjunct therapy in myasthenic crisis. Plasmapheresis is directed at removing the acetylcholine receptor antibody that causes myasthenia gravis. The effects of plasmapheresis alone are only temporary and may not occur for several days. IVIG is administered at 400 mg/kg daily for 3 to 5 consecutive days; it acts by blocking the noxious antibodies, but its immune-modulating effects are quite complex. Plasma exchange and IVIG have similar effectiveness, but the ease of administration of the latter makes it the more commonly used modality. Although it is an expensive medication, costs are comparable with plasma exchange.

Complications include a hyperviscosity syndrome with the possibility of cardiac or cerebral ischemia, a usually mild aseptic meningitis, acute renal failure, or an allergic reaction. It is important to draw pertinent serologic titers before IVIG administration, as many of these will altered by the administration of pooled IVIG. In particular, quantitative immune globulins and a careful history of upper respiratory infections should be obtained as immune IgA–deficient individuals can develop adverse responses to repeat administration of IVIG after being sensitized to it.

Any infection may precipitate a crisis, and an infectious source should be sought and treated aggressively. Many myasthenic patients are iatrogenically immunosuppressed and are highly susceptible to infection. If an infection is suspected, empiric therapy with broad-spectrum antibiotics is started at once after cultures have been sent. The change to more specific drugs is made when the cultures' sensitivities are available. The aminoglycosides are known to interfere with neuromuscular transmission but may be used when necessary. Chest roentgenogram, blood, urine, and sputum cultures on all myasthenic patients presenting with exacerbation should be routinely checked. In addition, a diligent search for infections is required in elderly or steroid-treated patients who may not manifest the usual systemic signs of infection.

GUILLAIN-BARRÉ SYNDROME

Acute inflammatory polyradiculoneuropathy, commonly referred to as the Guillain-Barré syndrome (GBS), is a symmetrical, rapidly progressive, demyelinating polyneuropathy that in its most fulminant form may lead to sudden respiratory failure and autonomic instability. It therefore should be considered a neurologic emergency. The mortality rate remains at 3% to 5% despite modern intensive care management.

The classic presentation is a fairly symmetrical, ascending, flaccid paralysis that usually begins in the lower extremities (10% begin in the upper extremities) and progresses upward, with the maximum deficit attained by 4 weeks. In contrast to other more slowly progressive polyneuropathies in which a distal weakness predominates, the greatest weakness in GBS is typically in the proximal muscles. Areflexia is the rule and may precede weakness. Many patients complain of distal paresthesias initially, but formal testing rarely demonstrates a significant sensory loss. In fact, patients with early GBS have been discharged from emergency rooms undiagnosed because of sensory complaints without findings. Facial weakness is seen in about half the cases. Fever should not be present at the onset. A prior history of a recent (within 4 weeks) respiratory or gastrointestinal illness is obtained in about half of the patients. A previous inoculation, surgery, hematologic malignancy, and hepatitis B or mycoplasma infection have also been associated with the syndrome.

Cerebrospinal fluid analysis within the first week may be normal—the classic albuminocytologic dissociation (increased protein and up to 10 mononuclear cells) usually appears after the second week of illness.

Nerve conduction studies may be entirely normal early in the course if the proximal root segments are not studied. The F and H responses measuring the motor and sensory proximal segments, respectively, may be the only abnormality noted early on. Profound slowing of nerve conduction velocity may appear on routine studies after several weeks of illness. Those cases that show evidence of secondary axonal degeneration with denervation on an electromyogram (EMG) will generally have a more protracted recovery.

Guillain-Barré syndrome is a neurologic emergency because of the life-threatening complications of respiratory failure and cardiovascular collapse that some-

times occur within 24 hours of the onset of symptoms. The patient must, therefore, be closely watched in an ICU or an intermediate care unit until the plateau phase of maximal deficit is reached. The vital capacity should be checked every 4 to 6 hours; if it is less than 800 ml, endotracheal intubation should be performed. Artificial ventilation may be required in up to 23% of patients. Autonomic instability may be severe, with marked fluctuations in blood pressure, tachycardia, and malignant arrhythmias. Cardiac arrhythmias are probably the main cause of death in the acute period, hence the need for continuous cardiac monitoring. Hypotension is usually mild and can be controlled with IV fluids; vasopressor agents are rarely needed. Extreme caution should be taken when treating hypertension. Because of the marked lability in blood pressure, only short-acting, easily titratable drugs such as IV nitroprusside should be used. Sustained tachycardia can be treated with small doses of beta-blockers if necessary. Corticosteroids, previously widely used in the acute phase of GBS, are no longer advocated, and a randomized double-blind study actually showed significantly slower improvement and more instances of relapse in the steroid-treated group. However, a recent pilot study found promise in the combination of IVIG and methylprednisolone.

Plasmapheresis, if performed within 2 weeks of the onset of symptoms, can significantly shorten the time it takes to attain a functional recovery; however, it does not decrease the incidence of respiratory failure. It is contraindicated in patients with severe autonomic instability. Thus, plasmapheresis, while probably an important treatment modality to invoke early in the course of GBS for long-term goals, is not a valuable therapy for the prevention of its life-threatening complications. Studies comparing high-dose IVIG with plasma exchange indicated a beneficial effect from prompt institution of IVIG, comparable to that seen with plasmapheresis. IVIG has become the treatment of choice for GBS in many centers because of its ease of administration, safety profile, and comparable cost. In spite of concerns of early recurrences with IVIG treatment (compared with plasmapheresis), most centers use IVIG as initial treatment of GBS. Plasmapheresis is often used in patients who do not respond to IVIG; it is recommended to wait 2 weeks before changing to the alternative modality, as the effects of either may not be immediately apparent.

Several other entities can cause a rapidly progressive and occasionally fatal flaccid paralysis that can mimic GBS (Table 25-7), and these should be differentiated because of variations in acute management.

Acute intermittent porphyria can cause a rapidly ascending flaccid paralysis with respiratory and

TABLE 25-7. Disorders That Can Mimic Guillain–Barré Syndrome

Acute intermittent porphyria
Diphtheria neuropathy
Botulism
Tick-bite paralysis
Poliomyelitis
Arsenic intoxication

autonomic involvement, but severe abdominal pain is usually the initial symptom, and seizures and psychosis often occur. Urine porphobilinogen and delta-aminolevulinic acid are elevated. Unlike in GBS, the CSF protein is usually normal. Attacks of acute intermittent porphyria may be precipitated by certain drugs such as barbiturates, phenytoin, some of the benzodiazepines, and sulfonamides. Treatment of acute attacks is aimed at the suppression of porphyrin synthesis with a high carbohydrate intake, as well as supportive management of the accompanying complications.

Diphtheric neuropathy occurs 1 to 2 months after the characteristic pharyngitis. The onset of weakness usually follows pronounced cranial nerve involvement by several weeks, and it may be associated with myocarditis. Unfortunately, by the time neurologic symptoms appear, specific therapy with antitoxin is ineffective and the mainstays of treatment are respiratory support and good nursing care.

The first neurologic symptoms of botulism are usually ocular, with blurred vision and diplopia. Intoxication usually presents with gastrointestinal symptoms. Unlike in GBS, the pupillary reflexes are lost and the CSF is normal. Sensation remains intact. The diagnosis is supported by nerve conduction studies with reduced amplitude of compound muscle action potentials and an incremental response following rapid repetitive nerve stimulation. Specific treatment with trivalent botulinum antitoxin is recommended. Nasogastric suctioning and enemas may help remove toxin from the gastrointestinal tract early in the illness. In wound botulism, surgical debridement and penicillin are the essentials of treatment. In food-borne botulism, the role of antibiotics is controversial because of the concern that rapid bacterial destruction might increase the release of toxin.

Tick-bite paralysis is caused by a natural endotoxin that interferes with the release of acetylcholine at the neuromuscular junction. It can present as a rapidly ascending paralysis with respiratory and bulbar involvement. A dramatic improvement occurs after the removal of the offending tick.

Poliomyelitis can produce a flaccid paralysis with respiratory involvement and can thus mimic GBS. However, the weakness of poliomyelitis is characteristically asymmetrical, and the disease usually presents as a febrile illness with gastrointestinal symptoms, myalgias, meningismus, and a CSF pleocytosis. Arsenical neuropathy can present as rapidly developing weakness and areflexia, with CSF and nerve conduction studies indistinguishable from those of GBS. However, the neuropathy is usually accompanied by gastrointestinal, hepatic, and hematologic manifestations of arsenic poisoning. The patient with arsenical neuropathy often complains of burning dysesthesia, a feature not common in GBS.

NEUROLEPTIC MALIGNANT SYNDROME

Neuroleptic malignant syndrome (NMS) is a potentially lethal complication associated with the use of agents that block the action of dopamine in the CNS. Although NMS is not exclusively associated with neuroleptic drugs, this syndrome continues to bear a name that reflects the initial circumstances in which it was recognized. Phenothiazines, butyrophenones, and thioxanthenes continue to be the classes of drugs most commonly implicated (Table 25-8). In general, a drug's potential for inducing NMS parallels its antidopaminergic potency. Accordingly, haloperidol, chlorpromazine, and fluphenazine have been identified as the most frequent offenders. Less commonly, NMS has also occurred with the use of a dopamine-

TABLE 25-8. Causes of Neuroleptic Malignant Syndrome

Dopamine-blocking agents
  Haloperidol (Haldol)
  Chlorpromazine (Thorazine)
  Fluphenazine (Prolixin)
  Clozapine (Clozaril)
  Thioridazine (Mellaril)
  Thiothixene (Navene)
  Trifluoperazine (Stelazine)
  Metaclopramide (Reglan)
Dopamine-depleting agents
  Tetrabenazine
Abrupt discontinuation of antiparkinsonian dopaminergic
  medications
Lithium

depleting agent such as tetrabenazine, and following the abrupt discontinuation of antiparkinsonian dopaminergic medication.

Because of a scarcity of reliable epidemiologic data, the incidence of NMS is not clearly established. Retrospective studies have documented the incidence of NMS among all patients exposed to neuroleptic drugs to be between 0.5% and 1%. NMS has been reported in all age groups and in both sexes. It is related neither to the duration of exposure to neuroleptics nor to toxic overdoses of neuroleptics; however, numerous predisposing factors in affected patients have been identified. NMS is associated with the initiation of neuroleptic medications at high dosages, the rapid upward titration of dose, as well as the use of long-acting depot neuroleptic preparations. Metabolic factors such as dehydration, physical exhaustion, and acute agitation with excessive sympathetic discharge have also been implicated.

The four cardinal features of NMS are hyperthermia, muscle rigidity, altered mental status and instability of the autonomic nervous system. An interruption of dopaminergic pathways is believed to be the primary etiology. A blockade of dopaminergic receptors in the striatum is thought to cause tonic contraction of skeletal muscles, which generates heat, and a similar blockade in the hypothalamus may disrupt thermoregulatory function. It is proposed that an analogous disruption of dopaminergic function in the mesocorticolimbic system may underlie the alteration of mental status and a blockade of dopamine receptors in the spinal cord may be responsible for the dysautonomia. It has also been postulated that reduction in serum iron levels may affect dopamine receptor sensitivity, making these patients more vulnerable to develop NMS.

Hyperthermia is present in all cases of NMS; however, the height of the temperature elevation is variable. Body temperature above 38°C (100.4°F) was noted in 92% of NMS patients, and higher temperatures, above 40°C (104°F), were recorded in 40%. Muscular rigidity, commonly described as "lead pipe" rigidity, is generalized in distribution and may be severe enough to compromise chest wall compliance, causing hypoventilation and the need for ventilatory support. Dysphagia may occur as a result of the rigidity of the pharyngeal musculature, placing the patient at risk for aspiration. Other commonly reported motor abnormalities include akinesia, bradykinesia, and involuntary movements, such as tremor and dystonia.

Mental status changes, often described as fluctuating states of consciousness, occur in 75% of affected patients. Progression through stages of agitation to alert mutism, stupor, and coma may be observed. Autonomic dysfunction is universal. Frequently reported manifestations are tachycardia, diaphoresis, blood pressure instability, urinary incontinence, cardiac dysrhythmias, and pallor or flushing of the skin. Infrequent findings include Babinski sign, hyperreflexia, seizures, opisthotonos, oculogyric crisis, chorea, and trismus. The clinical features of NMS typically develop over a 24- to 72-hour period and continue for approximately 5 to 10 days even when the offending agents are discontinued. Symptoms persist 2 to 3 times longer when depot preparations of neuroleptics were the etiologic agents.

Laboratory investigations can be instrumental in making the diagnosis of NMS and in recognizing metabolic alterations that mandate diligent monitoring and treatment. Two laboratory abnormalities that are consistently found are elevation of the blood creatinine phosphokinase (CPK) level and a polymorphonuclear leukocytosis. Myonecrosis due to intense sustained muscle contractions underlies the rise in CPK, which can vary widely from slightly elevated, to the hundreds of thousands. White blood cell determinations between 10,000 and 30,000 cells/mm^3 are found in the majority of cases. Electrolyte levels may reveal dehydration, and elevations of muscle enzymes are commonly seen. Lumbar puncture, when performed, demonstrates either normal CSF parameters or nonspecific changes. CT of the head is typically negative and EEG traces are either normal or consistent with a nonspecific encephalopathy.

The recognition of NMS can be troublesome. It is a clinical diagnosis. Commonly, the differential diagnoses of CNS infection (meningitis, encephalitis, postinfectious encephalomyelitis), malignant hyperthermia, acute lethal catatonia, and anticholinergic toxicity must carefully be ruled out. Other disorders with similar presentations include thyrotoxicosis, heat stroke, tetanus, and drug-induced parkinsonism. Most important, when the suspicion of NMS is raised, treatment should be initiated without delay. Management of NMS begins with the immediate withdrawal of neuroleptic medications as well as any other dopamine antagonists in use. In the acute setting, IV fluids may be required for volume repletion, metabolic abnormalities may require correction, and ice packs and cooling blankets may be indicated for hyperthermia. The two most commonly used agents for treatment of NMS are dantrolene sodium and bromocriptine. Dantrolene sodium is a muscle relaxant, and bromocriptine is a centrally acting dopamine agonist. These two medications used alone or in combination promote a reduction of body temperature and serum CPK by lessening skeletal muscle rigidity. Both dantrolene and bromocriptine have been shown to significantly shorten the time of clinical response to therapy as compared with supportive care.

If the syndrome is caused by orally administered neuroleptics, treatment with dantrolene and/or bromocriptine should be continued for at least 10 days, as reoccurrence may develop with early withdrawal from therapy. When depot neuroleptics were used, treatment may be required for 2 to 3 weeks. During this period, supportive care is maintained, with careful monitoring of nutrition, fluid balance, and metabolic parameters. Approximately 40% of patients with NMS suffer from medical complications. Respiratory complications, including ventilatory failure, aspiration pneumonia, pulmonary edema, and pulmonary embolism, are the sequelae of diminished chest wall compliance and prolonged immobility. Cardiovascular complications such as phlebitis, dysrhythmias, myocardial infarction, and cardiovascular collapse may be seen. There is a significant risk of renal failure as a result of the combined effects of volume depletion and myoglobinuria due to rhabdomyolysis.

Mortality may result from the cumulative effects of medical complications. Morbidity and mortality from NMS have decreased over the years: reports document a mortality rate of 25% before 1984 and 11.6% since 1984. The improvement in prognosis is attributed more to early recognition and treatment of the syndrome than to the use of any specific therapeutic agent.

As many patients who recover from NMS continue to require the use of dopamine-blocking agents, the question of the safety of reintroducing neuroleptics is relevant. Experience has shown that neuroleptic agents can be reintroduced safely in the majority of cases. Studies have demonstrated that a reoccurrence of NMS can best be avoided by waiting a sufficient amount of time so that a given episode of NMS has completely resolved, reintroducing low doses of low-potency neuroleptics, and ensuring that the patient is well hydrated and metabolically stable.

The diagnosis of NMS should come to mind when encountering any individual receiving neuroleptics who develops unexplained fever associated with muscle rigidity. Although there are numerous alternate diagnoses, the life-threatening potential of NMS demands that treatment should not be delayed if there is significant clinical suspicion.

QUESTIONS AND DISCUSSION

1. A 21-year-old woman is seen in the emergency room complaining of a feeling of tingling in her feet and hands for 1 day. She has no other neurologic complaints. She denies shortness of breath, exposure to drugs or toxins, or a recent viral illness. An examination reveals diffuse hyporeflexia with absent ankle jerks. Very careful sensory testing is normal despite the patient's complaints. The best course of action would be:

A. Discharge the patient with the diagnosis of "functional disorder" because of a paucity of objective findings.
B. Admit her to the hospital for close observation, watching carefully for signs of developing weakness or respiratory difficulty.
C. Perform a lumbar puncture in the emergency room, suspecting early Guillain-Barré syndrome (GBS), with plans to discharge the patient if the results are normal.

The answer is (B). Paresthesias without objective sensory findings occur commonly and early in GBS, often before clinical weakness develops. The key features in this case are the sensory complaints in the presence of diffuse hyporeflexia. The typically high CSF protein concentration without pleocytosis may not occur until after a few weeks of illness.

The next day, she complains of difficulty in walking and on examination shows a pulse of 120, diffuse areflexia, and bilateral proximal lower extremity weakness. The best management at this time would be:

A. Admit her to an ICU for cardiac monitoring, frequent vital capacities (with intubation if less than 800 ml), and lumbar puncture.
B. Observe her in a general medical ward with daily vital capacities and steroids.
C. Admit her to an ICU for cardiac monitoring, with monitoring of the vital capacity only if respiratory problems occur.
D. Admit her to an ICU for vital capacity and cardiac monitoring, and give high-dose steroids.

The answer is (A). With weakness now developing, it is clear that the patient has GBS. She should be monitored in an ICU setting and she should be watched closely for the development of cardiac arrhythmias and respiratory compromise. Vital capacities should be checked every 4 to 6 hours, with intubation done if less than 800 ml. Steroids have not been shown to be effective in GBS.

2. A 30-year-old man is brought to the emergency room after suddenly developing a severe generalized headache ("like being struck by lightning") while he was moving furniture. The headache was not associated with nausea or vomiting, photophobia, neck stiffness, or other neurologic complaints. There is no previous history of headaches and no family history. An examination reveals a young man in moderate distress. Temperature is 99°F, blood pressure 140/90, pulse 96. The general physical examination and neurologic examination are unremarkable. Choose the best plan of management:

A. Intramuscular meperidine, then discharge the patient with a prescription for ergotamine and a follow-up appointment in the neurology clinic
B. Narcotic analgesics and observation overnight in the emergency room, with plans for discharge if symptoms are improved
C. Immediate CT brain scan
D. Immediate lumbar puncture

The answer is (C). The sudden onset of a severe headache, especially if it occurs in a patient of this age during exertion, should bring to mind the possibility of aneurysmal subarachnoid hemorrhage. Meningismus or other physical findings may be absent with early sentinel leaks. The diagnostic procedure of choice is a CT brain scan followed by a lumbar puncture if no evidence of subarachnoid blood is seen on the CT.

A CT scan is done and is read as normal. What should be the next step?

A. Discharge the patient with a follow-up in neurology clinic.
B. Perform a lumbar puncture.

The answer is (B).

A lumbar puncture is performed and the results are as follows: opening pressure 260 mm of CSF, xanthochromic supernatant, 10 WBCs (100% monos), 200 RBCs, glucose 70 mg/dl, protein 50 mg/dl. What is the best course of action?

A. Admit the patient, send for cultures, and begin broad-spectrum antibiotics for presumed bacterial meningitis.

B. Admit the patient to a quiet, closely monitored bed; give sedatives, analgesics, stool softeners, and prophylactic anticonvulsants.
C. Discharge the patient, since the red cells are most likely due to a traumatic tap and the CSF profile is otherwise normal.

The answer is (B). The increased opening pressure, red cells, and xanthochromic fluid are consistent with a subarachnoid hemorrhage. A traumatic tap may have increased red cells but xanthochromia would not be present unless the specimen was left standing for several hours before centrifugation.

3. Generalized status epilepticus should be:

A. Diagnosed in the following situation: A patient has a series of seizures within a 2-hour period. Between fits, he is able to state that he recently quit a 2-quarts-per-day vodka habit
B. Diagnosed in the following situation: A patient has had continuous jerking movements of one limb for 6 hours but no loss of consciousness
C. Treated aggressively with immediate intubation and neuromuscular blockade to prevent rhabdomyolsis from intense muscular contractions
D. Treated with a fast-acting benzodiazepine followed immediately by a loading dose of a long-acting anticonvulsant such as phenytoin

The answer is (D). Generalized status epilepticus, by definition, involves a loss of consciousness as part of the ictus, without a regaining of consciousness between episodes. Neuromuscular blockade will abolish the motor activity but will have no effect on the underlying persistent epileptiform activity. Following preservation of an airway, blood sampling, and the establishment of intravenous access, first-line therapy is aimed at abolishing the epileptiform discharges with anticonvulsants.

4. Spinal cord compression should be considered in all of the following situations except:

A. Sudden onset of right arm and leg weakness, accompanied by sensory loss
B. Gradual onset of paraparesis associated with a loss of bowel and bladder function
C. Subacute proximal leg weakness associated with a beltlike sensation across the chest that increases with lifting heavy objects
D. Back pain associated with paraparesis

The answer is (A). In this case, the hemineurologic deficit is most likely secondary to a contralateral hemispheric infarct.

5. All of the following statements are true regarding the management of acute intracranial hypertension *except:*

A. Reduction of $PaCO_2$ is the quickest way of reducing intracranial pressure.
B. Corticosteroids are especially helpful in reducing the edema associated with infarction.
C. Emergency surgery is the preferred treatment for cerebellar hemorrhages.
D. Osmotic agents are helpful in reducing intracranial hypertension from any cause.

The answer is (B). Steroids are useful when considerable tumor edema (vasogenic edema) is present, but they are not particularly effective on the type of edema associated with cellular damage (cytoxic edema) such as occurs with infarction.

6. All of the following statements concerning the treatment of myasthenic crisis are false *except:*

A. Aminoglycoside antibiotics are contraindicated.
B. It is not necessary to differentiate a myasthenic from a cholinergic crisis because the emergency management is the same.
C. Anticholinesterase drugs are withdrawn for 48 hours only if a cholinergic crisis is suspected, then restarted at twice the previous dose.
D. Plasmapheresis is an important treatment modality because its effects are always immediate.
E. Although vital-capacity monitoring is important prior to intubation, it is not helpful in assessing a patient's progress after he has been placed on a mechanical ventilator.

The answer is (B). Emergency management of a crisis is the same regardless of etiology—the maintenance of adequate ventilation and the withdrawal of anticholinesterase medications. These drugs are then restarted after 48 to 72 hours at smaller doses. Aminoglycoside antibiotics may be used if necessary. Plasmapheresis may be helpful, but its effects are often delayed for several days. Vital-capacity monitoring may be a useful tool in assessing the adequacy of therapy in the crisis situation.

7. A 58-year-old hypertensive man is brought by ambulance to the emergency room at 10 PM with a witnessed 2-hour history of abrupt onset of inability to speak and right-sided weakness while at the dinner table. On examination, blood pressure was 180/100 mm Hg with a regular heart rate at 80 per minute; he was awake, unable to speak or follow verbal commands, and had complete paralysis of the right lower face and right arm, and moderate weakness of the right leg. An emergency brain CT is normal. What are the appropriate therapeutic measures?

A. Admit him to the regular floor for a search for the cause of the stroke; have the neurologist see the patient the next morning.
B. Start intravenous heparin.
C. Administer rt-PA 0.9 mg/kg, 10% as a bolus, the rest over 1 hour. Repeat brain CT 24 hours later, prior to anticoagulant or antiplatelet therapy.
D. Immediately intubate and hyperventilate.
E. Start a nitroprusside drip to lower systolic BP to 120–130 mm Hg.

The answer is (C). This patient appears to have suffered a left middle cerebral artery stroke. The abruptness of onset and the significant cortical involvement (as manifested by aphasia and the differential involvement of face and arm weakness greater than leg weakness) argues for an embolic event. Patients with significant neurologic deficits presenting within 3 hours of onset in the presence of a normal brain CT should receive thrombolytic therapy. Anticoagulation should be held until a follow-up brain CT excludes significant hemorrhagic transformation of the infarction. It is important not to lower the blood pressure, to ensure adequate perfusion to the ischemic penumbra. Management of acute ischemic stroke should be emergent; an experienced neurologist should evaluate the patient immediately and manage him in a stroke unit or ICU.

SUGGESTED READING

Adams HP: Trial of Org 10172 in acute stroke treatment: Preliminary results. 6th European Stroke Conference. Amsterdam, The Netherlands, May 28–31, 1997

Broderick JP, Brott TG, Tomsick T et al: Ultraearly evaluation of intracerebral hemorrhage. J Neurosurg 72:195, 1990

Byrne TN: Spinal cord compression from epidural metastases. N Engl J Med 327: 614, 1992

Charness ME, Simon RP, Greenberg DA. Ethanol and the nervous sytem. N Engl J Med 321:442, 1989

Chinese Acute Stroke Trial Collaborative Group: CAST: A randomised placebo-controlled trial of early aspirin use in 20,000 patients with acute ischaemic stroke. Lancet 349:1641, 1997

DeLorenzo RJ: Status epilepticus: Concepts in diagnosis and treatment. Semin Neurol 10:396, 1990

Devinsky O, Leppik I, Willmore LJ et al: Safety of intravenous valproate. Ann Neurol 38:670, 1995

Dickey W: The neuroleptic malignant syndrome. Prog Neurobiol 36:425, 1991

The Dutch Guillain-Barré Study Group. Treatment of Guillain-Barré syndrome with high-dose immune globulins combined with methylprednisolone: A pilot study. Ann Neurol 35:749, 1994

Factor SA, Singer C: Neuroleptic malignant syndrome. In: Weiner WJ (ed): Emergent and Urgent Neurology. Philadelphia, JB Lippincott, 1992

Gajdos P, Cherret S, Clair B et al: (Myasthenia Gravis Clinical Study Group): Clinical trial of plasma exchange and high-dose intravenous immunoglobulins in myasthenia gravis. Ann Neurol 41:789, 1997

Giroud M, Gras D, Escousse A et al: Use of injectable valproic acid in status epilepticus: A pilot study. Drug Invest 5:154, 1993

Grant R, Papadopoulos SM, Sandler HM et al: Metastatic epidural spinal cord compression: Current concepts and treatment. J Neurooncol 19:79, 1994

Hankey GJ, Hon C: Surgery for primary intracerebral hemorrhage: Is it safe and effective? A systematic review of case series and randomised trials. Stroke 28:2126, 1997

International Stroke Trial Collaborative Group: The International Stroke Trial (IST): A randomised trial of aspirin, subcutaneous heparin, both, or neither among 19435 patients with ischaemic stroke. Lancet 349:1569, 1997

International Study of Unruptured Intracranial Aneurysms Investigators: Unruptured intracranial aneurysms: risk of rupture and risks of surgical intervention. N Engl J Med 339:1725, 1998

Kazui S, Naritomi H, Yamamoto H et al: Enlargement of spontaneous intracerebral hemorrhage: Incidence and time course. Stroke 27:1783, 1996

King WA, Martin NA: Critical care of patients with subarachnoid hemorrhage. Neurosurg Clin North Am 5:767, 1994

Leppik IE: Status epilepticus. In: Wyllie E (ed): The Treatment of Epilepsy: Principles and Practice. Philadelphia, Lea and Febiger, 1993

Mayer SA, Dennis LJ: Management of increased intracranial pressure. Neurologist 4:2, 1998

The National Institute of Neurological Disorders and Stroke rt-PA Stroke Study Group: Tissue plasminogen activator for acute ischemic stroke. N Engl J Med 333: 1581, 1995

Plum F, Posner JB: Diagnosis of Stupor and Coma. Philadelphia, FA Davis, 1980

Ramsey RE, DeToledo J: Intravenous administration of fosphenytoin: Options for the management of seizures. Neurology. 46(s1):517, 1996

Reid RL, Quigley ME, Yen SS: Pituitary apoplexy. Arch Neurol 42:712, 1985

Ropper AH: The Guillain-Barré syndrome. N Engl J Med 326:1130, 1992

Runge JW, Allen FH: Emergency treatment of status epilepticus. Neurology 46(s1): 520, 1996

Schievink WI: Intracerebral aneurysms. N Engl Med J 336:28, 1997

Taylor CE, Selman WR, Ratcheson RA: Brain attack: The emergent management of hypertensive hemorrhage. Neurosurg Clin North Am 8:237, 1997

Thomas CE, Mayer SA, Gungor Y et al: Myasthenic crisis: Clinical features, mortality, complications, and risk factors for prolonged intubation. Neurology 48:1253, 1997

Van der Meche FG, Schmitz PI, and the Dutch Guillain-Barré Study Group: A randomized trial comparing intravenous immune globulin and plasma exchange in Guillain-Barré syndrome. N Engl J Med 326: 1123, 1992

Neurology for the Non-Neurologist, Fourth Edition, edited by William J. Weiner and Christopher G. Goetz. Lippincott Williams & Wilkins, Philadelphia © 1999.

C H A P T E R   2 6

Neurologic Complications of Human Immunodeficiency Virus Infection

Joseph R. Berger

Peter Portegies

In the spring of 1981, the Centers for Disease Control (CDC) in Atlanta reported on the occurrences of uncommon opportunistic infections (*Pneumocystis carinii* pneumonia) and malignancies (Kaposi's sarcoma) among previously healthy young homosexual men in New York and California. This newly recognized immunodeficiency state was referred to as the acquired immunodeficiency syndrome (AIDS). Shortly afterward, neurologic consequences of this illness were reported.

Within 3 years of its clinical description, a retrovirus, initially called lymphadenopathy-associated virus (LAV), human T-cell lymphotropic virus type III (HTLV-III), or AIDS-associated retrovirus (ARV), was convincingly demonstrated to be the etiologic agent. In 1986, this retrovirus was designated as human immunodeficiency virus (HIV). This virus is now referred to as HIV-1, since a second type was isolated from West African patients with AIDS.

HUMAN IMMUNODEFICIENCY VIRUS TYPE 1

The human immunodeficiency virus type 1 (HIV-1) is a member of a unique family of RNA viruses characterized by the presence of RNA-dependent DNA polymerase (reverse transcriptase), an enzyme enabling these RNA viruses to produce a DNA copy of this genome, which can then be incorporated into the host genome. Other characteristics of this family of viruses are their large size, the ability to produce cytopathic changes in infected cells, and the long incubation times before the development of clinical illness (typically, immunologic or neurologic disease). All known lentiviruses are capable of causing neurologic disease. In addition to the neurologic diseases that occur as a direct consequence of HIV-1 infection, a large number of neurologic disorders occur as a result of the accompanying immunosuppression.

SPECTRUM OF NEUROLOGIC DISEASES

Neurologic involvement occurs in at least 70% of patients who meet the CDC's clinical criteria for AIDS, and it is the presenting manifestation in 10% of HIV-infected patients. At autopsy, 80% to 90% are found to have neuropathologic abnormalities.

Each part of the neuraxis may be involved. Some of these neurologic complications occur in the early and clinically "latent" phases of the infection, while others are associated with advanced HIV-1 infection (Table 26-1). Therefore, from a clinical point of view (namely, differential diagnosis), it is useful to keep in mind the correlation between the neurologic complications and the level of immune compromise, generally reflected in the absolute CD4 T-lymphocyte cell count. With the advent of measures of HIV viral load, CD4 counts are not as commonly obtained; however, they are more reflective of the effect of the virus on immune function than the former. It is important to appreciate that very often, different neurologic complications may occur in one patient. Patients may manifest symptoms and signs from several neurologic disorders that have occurred concomitantly or, alternatively, various neurologic disorders may occur sequentially in the same patient. Additionally, the physician must never lose sight of the possibility that a given neurologic disorder in the HIV-infected individual is the result of a more common disorder, unrelated to the underlying viral illness. The most important neurologic complications in patients with AIDS reported in the literature are given in Table 26-2.

In this chapter, the description of the neurologic disorders accompanying HIV-1 infection will be classified according to their manifestations. The most common etiologies for each of these manifestations will be discussed. Some overlap between the categories occurs. The classification will include meningitis, global encephalopathy, focal neurologic disturbances of central origin, myelopathy, peripheral neuropathy, and myopathy.

MENINGITIS

Meningitis is a frequent occurrence in the patient with HIV-1 infection. Cerebrospinal fluid (CSF) studies are required for a precise identification of the etiology. In the asymptomatic stage of HIV-1 infection, HIV-1 itself is perhaps the most common cause of meningitis in the infected patient. The most important meningeal infection in AIDS patients is caused by *Cryptococcus neoformans*. Other common etiologies of meningitis include tuberculosis, syphilis, and lymphoma (Table 26-3).

HIV-1 MENINGITIS

An aseptic meningitis may occur at the time of seroconversion and in later stages of HIV-1 infection

TABLE 26-1. Neurologic Complications of HIV-1 Infection

EARLY

Acute syndromes associated with initial infection
Multiple sclerosis–like illness
Aseptic meningitis
Demyelinating neuropathies

LATE

AIDS dementia complex
Vacuolar myelopathy
Peripheral neuropathy
Myopathies
Cerebrovascular complications
Seizures
Opportunistic infections and neoplasms
    Cerebral toxoplasmosis
    Cryptococcal meningitis
    Progressive multifocal leukoencephalopathy
    Cytomegalovirus infections
    Syphilis
    Primary central nervous system lymphoma
    Meningitis lymphomatosis

TABLE 26-2. Incidence of Neurologic Complications in AIDS

Cerebral toxoplasmosis	10–20%
Cryptococcal meningitis	2–10%
Progressive multifocal leukoencephalopathy	2–5%
Cytomegalovirus polyradiculomyelopathy	2%?
Cytomegalovirus encephalitis	<1%?
Primary central nervous system lymphoma	2–13%
Meningitis lymphomatosis	0.5–3%
Aseptic meningitis	<5%?
AIDS dementia complex[a]	5–33%
Vacuolar myelopathy	20–30%[b]
Polyneuropathy	10–35%
Myopathy	<10%?

[a] Incidence of AIDS dementia complex has declined after introduction of zidovudine.
[b] Autopsy statistic, less frequently recognized on clinical grounds.

TABLE 26-3. Meningitides in HIV-1 Infection

HIV-1 meningitis
Cryptococcal meningitis
Tuberculous meningitis
Syphilitic meningitis
Listeria meningitis
Meningitis lymphomatosis (non-Hodgkin's lymphoma)

while the patient is systemically well. This aseptic meningitis has an acute and a chronic form. Patients present with headache, fever, and meningeal signs. Cranial neuropathies, especially of cranial nerves V, VII, and VIII, and long-tract signs have been noted. The CSF shows a mild mononuclear pleocytosis (< 200 cells/mm), with slightly elevated protein levels. The meningitis is presumed to result from direct HIV-1 infection of the meninges, because HIV-1 can, with the appropriate virologic procedures, be isolated from the CSF. Most cases have a self-limited monophasic course, but the syndrome tends to recur.

It is important to appreciate that a mild mononuclear pleocytosis (usually < 100 cells/mm), with or without an elevated protein, is common and well known in HIV-1–infected individuals, even in the absence of neurologic symptoms. It has become increasingly clear that these "background" CSF abnormalities may be confusing in establishing a diagnosis of neurosyphilis, aseptic meningitis, or the inflammatory neuropathies. CSF abnormalities observed with HIV-1 infection should be interpreted cautiously.

CRYPTOCOCCAL MENINGITIS

Cryptococcal meningitis is the most common mycotic infection involving the nervous system in patients with HIV-infection. The fungus *C. neoformans* has a worldwide distribution, is commonly encountered in the feces of pigeons, and is associated with disease in both immunocompetent and immunosuppressed patients. Meningitis results from hematogenous dissemination after a frequently asymptomatic pulmonary infection. The prevalence of this life-threatening opportunistic infection among AIDS patients is 2% to 10%.

Clinically, the disease manifests as subacute or chronic meningitis with headache, altered mentation, and fever. Headache may become severe, with nausea and vomiting. Neck stiffness is frequently absent. Papilledema (occasionally with visual loss) and sixth cranial nerve palsy may be present.

The diagnosis is based on CSF analysis: variable mononuclear pleocytosis, with mildly elevated pro-

tein and low glucose level. However, these CSF parameters may all be normal in patients with AIDS. The CSF opening pressure is usually increased. The fungus can often be easily recognized in India-ink preparation. Cryptococcal polysaccharide capsular antigen is nearly always positive in the CSF and serum, as are fungal cultures of CSF. Brain computed tomography (CT) scan is usually normal or shows nonspecific abnormalities; occasionally, mass lesions (e.g., cryptococcoma) may be present.

Standard therapy with amphotericin B given intravenously (> 0.3 mg/kg/day) with or without oral flucytosine (150 mg/kg/day) is effective in about 60% of cases. The oral triazole fluconazole (400 mg/day) is as effective as the more toxic regimen of intravenous (IV) amphotericin. However, amphotericin does appear to be superior in patients who are severely ill. Because relapses are so common in AIDS patients, maintenance treatment (after 6 to 8 weeks of induction) is recommended. Fluconazole (100–200 mg/day) is highly effective in preventing relapses.

TUBERCULOUS MENINGITIS

Mycobacterium tuberculosis and *Mycobacterium avium-intracellulare* (MAI) occur frequently in AIDS and are often extrapulmonary in nature. Involvement of the central nervous system (CNS) is almost always due to *M. tuberculosis*, although atypical mycobacterial infection of the CNS in AIDS has been reported.

Meningitis and mass lesions (tuberculous brain abscess, tuberculomas) due to *M. tuberculosis* have been described. When a mass lesion is suspected, brain biopsy is necessary to confirm the diagnosis. The response of AIDS patients to the standard therapy for *M. tuberculosis* (including isoniazid, rifampin, pyrazinamide, and streptomycin) is generally gratifying. The use of corticosteroids is controversial.

SYPHILITIC MENINGITIS

A retrospective (chart review) study estimated that neurosyphilis, strictly defined by the presence of reactive CSF VDRL, was present in approximately 1.5% of HIV-1–infected hospitalized patients. Diagnosing neurosyphilis can be quite problematic. First, in 40% to 60% of HIV-1 infected patients, the CSF may show a pleocytosis, elevated protein, an elevated immunoglobulin G synthesis rate, and oligoclonal bands, making it impossible to use these CSF findings as an indicator of active neurosyphilis. Second, the signs and symptoms of the clinical syndromes caused by HIV-1 infection (meningitis, strokes, myelopathy, dementia) can also occur in neurosyphilis. Third, the CSF serologic tests for neurosyphilis [VDRL and fluorescent treponemal antibody absorption (FTA-ABS)] may be negative in HIV-1–infected individuals with *Treponema pallidum* in the CSF.

Several diagnostic schemata have been used to establish the diagnosis; however, all have relied on indirect evidence of the presence of *T. pallidum,* because the organism is fastidious and requires the rather cumbersome use of animal inoculation for strict verification of its presence. The frequent presence of CSF abnormalities in the HIV-1 infection results in a loss of the specificity of these criteria. Although it is the most specific test for neurosyphilis, the CSF VDRL, as well as other nontreponemal tests, may be insensitive to the diagnosis of neurosyphilis. One suggested approach to the diagnosis of neurosyphilis is as follows: (1) a reactive CSF VDRL in the absence of gross blood contamination of CSF; or (2) a reactive CSF FTA-ABS in the absence of blood contamination occurring in association with a CSF pleocytosis (>5 cells/mm), increased protein (>50 mg%), an increased IgG index (>6), or oligoclonal bands in the absence of HIV infection or identifiable neurologic illness; or (3) a reactive CSF FTA-ABS in association with a neurologic illness compatible with neurosyphilis, unexplained by other disease, and responding to penicillin therapy; or (4) *T. pallidum* isolated from the CSF by animal inoculation.

T. pallidum in the CNS may be more aggressive in HIV-1–infected individuals, and the complications may be atypical. In addition to meningovascular syphilis, a polyradiculopathy has also been described. Patients who present with meningovascular syphilis after adequate treatment for primary syphilis, and with neurologic relapse after adequate treatment for secondary syphilis, have been described.

Unsuspected neurosyphilis is relatively common in HIV-1–infected individuals, and neurosyphilis should always be considered in the differential diagnosis of neurologic disease in HIV-infected persons. CSF examination should be performed in all HIV-1–seropositive persons with neurologic complaints and a history of syphilis or serologic evidence of syphilis, regardless of prior treatment. If neurosyphilis is suspected, patients should be treated for at least 10 days with aqueous penicillin G, 2 to 4 million units IV every 4 hours (12 to 24 million units each day).

LISTERIA MENINGITIS

Listeria is a gram-positive, rod-shaped, aerobic bacterium that is widespread in nature. Although infec-

tion with *Listeria monocytogenes* (usually meningitis, sometimes brain abscess) has been reported in HIV-1–infected individuals and patients with AIDS, the incidence remains low. Diagnosis of *Listeria* meningitis and treatment with high-dose IV penicillin or ampicillin are the same in AIDS patients and in immunocompetent individuals.

LYMPHOMATOUS MENINGITIS

Twelve percent to 33% of AIDS patients with systemic non-Hodgkin's lymphoma (usually high-grade B-cell neoplasms) have leptomeningeal infiltration with a positive CSF cytologic examination at diagnosis. Because of this high incidence, all AIDS patients with systemic lymphoma should have CSF examination as part of their staging evaluation.

Leptomeningeal lymphoma causes headache, encephalopathy, cranial nerve palsies, radicular pain, cauda equina syndrome, or hydrocephalus. An otherwise unexplained cranial polyneuropathy in a patient with AIDS is not infrequently the result of lymphomatous (usually large cell lymphoma) infiltration. A differential diagnostic list of the potential etiologies of cranial neuropathy in AIDS is presented in Table 26-4. Cytologic examination is the single most useful test for leptomeningeal lymphoma, but even after repeated high-volume taps, the cytologic analysis may remain persistently negative. Sometimes subarachnoid nodules or thickened roots can be seen on myelography or by contrast magnetic resonance.

Intrathecal chemotherapy with methotrexate (or cytosine arabinoside) is the primary treatment. An

---

TABLE 26-4. Etiologies of Cranial Nerve Palsies with HIV-1 Infection

Infectious meningitis
  Fungal (*Cryptococcus*)
  Bacterial (*M. tuberculosis, L. monocytogenes, T. pallidum*)
  Viral (HIV-1)
Neoplastic meningitis
  Meningitis lymphomatosa
Compression from mass lesion
  Infectious (toxoplasmosis)
  Neoplastic (central nervous system lymphoma)
Vasculitis
Inflammatory
  Guillain–Barré syndrome
  Chronic inflammatory polyradiculoneuropathy
Miscellaneous
  Malignant otitis externa

Ommaya reservoir should be inserted. Radiotherapy can be added to the symptomatic region. Corticosteroids may temporarily relieve symptoms.

ENCEPHALOPATHY

Both an alteration in cognitive abilities and a decline in level of consciousness may occur in HIV-1 infection. The former, a direct consequence of HIV-1 infection (AIDS dementia complex, HIV-1 encephalopathy, or HIV-associated cognitive/motor disorder), is usually insidious in nature. The latter is often associated with focal neurologic abnormalities and typically results from mass lesions of the brain, usually opportunistic infections or lymphoma. The evaluation of a global encephalopathy complicating HIV-1 infection requires a thorough physical and neurologic examination; laboratory studies that assess renal, liver, and thyroid function, electrolytes, syphilis serologies, vitamin B_{12} and folate levels; magnetic resonance imaging (MRI) of the brain, preferably with gadolinium (alternatively, CT may be employed but should be performed as a double-dose, delayed scan); and CSF analysis for routine studies (opening pressure, cell count and differential, protein, glucose), as well as detailed microbiologic studies, including VDRL, and cytology. A differential diagnosis list is given in Table 26-5.

HIV DEMENTIA

One of the most important neurologic syndromes in patients with AIDS is HIV dementia, otherwise referred to as AIDS dementia complex (ADC), HIV-1 encephalopathy, or HIV-associated cognitive/motor deficit. This dementia is characterized by disturbances in cognition, motor performance, and behavior. Patients complain of decreased concentration, forgetfulness, and slowing of thoughts. Tasks take more time to complete and have to be well planned in

advance. Patients become apathetic and lose interest in their environment. As a consequence, they may become socially withdrawn, which is often mistaken for depression. Motor symptoms include clumsiness, tremor, poor balance, unsteadiness of gait, and slowing of rapid alternating movements. Organic psychosis may develop in some patients. Cortical symptoms such as aphasia, alexia, and agraphia are lacking. The Mini-Mental State examination is often normal, though responses are delayed. Saccadic and pursuit eye movements are often slowed and inaccurate. Fine finger movements are slowed, snout response is common, and deep tendon reflexes are brisk. With time, increasing psychomotor slowing may progress to severe dementia with akinetic mutism, paraparesis, and incontinence. The clinical and neuropsychological abnormalities in ADC are compatible with what has been called a subcortical dementia.

The epidemiology and course of ADC have not yet been precisely defined and have been influenced by the introduction of zidovudine. The incidence of ADC has declined since the introduction of zidovudine. However, recent prevalence studies suggest that one third of patients with AIDS eventually develop a mild or severe form of ADC. In patients who develop ADC, there is no protracted decline in neuropsychological performance, but rather a precipitous change first affecting psychomotor speed. This further strengthens existing data suggesting that asymptomatic patients do not have gradually increasing neuropsychological dysfunction. It suggests an acute or a subacute rather than a cumulative process affecting the brain over a long period of time as the cause of ADC.

Diagnostic studies are important to exclude treatable infections and tumors. CT scan and MRI show cortical atrophy, enlargement of ventricles, or both in most patients. MRI may reveal patchy or diffuse increased signal intensity on T2-weighted images, usually in the periventricular white matter and centrum semiovale, without mass effect. However, these neuroradiologic abnormalities may occur in patients who are not demented. CSF analysis may reveal a mononuclear pleocytosis and increased protein level. HIV-1 antibodies may be found, and HIV-1 itself may be cultured from approximately 30% of patients with ADC. HIV-1 p24 core protein in CSF, which is independent of HIV-1 antigen in serum, is detectable in 50% of patients with ADC. In addition to these CSF markers, several immunologic markers support a diagnosis of ADC when other causes have been excluded. These include beta-2-microglobulin, neopterin, and quinolinic acid. Beta-2-microglobulin and neopterin

TABLE 26-5. **Encephalopathies (Diffuse Brain Disease) in HIV-1 Infection**

AIDS dementia complex (= HIV-1 encephalopathy)
Metabolic encephalopathies
Diffuse encephalitis
  Acute HIV-1 encephalitis
  Cytomegalovirus encephalitis
  Herpes simplex virus encephalitis
  Toxoplasmosis (diffuse form)

are markers of immune activation; quinolinic acid is a metabolic product of macrophage activation.

The gross pathology of HIV-1 encephalopathy is characterized by brain atrophy with sulcal widening, ventricular dilatation, and meningeal fibrosis. Histologically, the most common feature of this illness is white matter pallor, chiefly of the periventricular and central white matter. However, multinucleate giant cells, typically located in perivascular spaces, are the pathologic hallmark of this illness. Astrocytosis and perivascular mononuclear inflammation are commonly observed.

Zidovudine has been well substantiated as an effective treatment for ADC in both adults and children. Zidovudine crosses the blood–brain barrier, and treatment has been found to be associated with decreasing HIV-1 antigen levels in serum and CSF. However, anecdotal data suggest that highly active antiretroviral therapy (HAART) may substantially improve the manifestations of ADC. It has also been suggested that HAART has reduced the overall frequency of the disorder. Other therapies under development are directed at the potential mechanisms by which HIV may result in neuronal injury, including the use of N-methyl-d-aspartate antagonists.

CYTOMEGALOVIRUS ENCEPHALITIS

The clinical features of cytomegalovirus (CMV) encephalitis in AIDS are not uniform. Neurologic symptoms may include meningeal signs, disorientation, short-term memory deficits, apathy, dementia, coma, seizures, or brainstem involvement. CSF examination is often normal. Rarely, CMV can be isolated from the CSF. CT scan may reveal subependymal enhancement compatible with ventriculitis. Often the identification of CMV is based on typical intranuclear inclusions or identification of CMV antigen by immunocytochemistry, or both, at postmortem neuropathologic examination. The relative importance of CMV infection in many cases is unclear, and CMV often coexists with other infectious agents. Effective therapeutic regimens include the use of ganciclovir and foscarnet.

FOCAL NEUROLOGIC DISTURBANCES OF CENTRAL ORIGIN

Focal neurologic disturbances, such as hemianopsia, hemiparesis, and hemianesthesia, occurring with HIV-1 infection may result from a variety of lesions affecting the cerebrum. These lesions can be broadly classified in their order of frequency as opportunistic infections, tumors, and cerebrovascular disease. The most common opportunistic infections are toxoplasmosis and progressive multifocal leukoencephalopathy (PML) (Table 26-6). With rare exception, brain tumors occurring with AIDS are primary CNS lymphomas, although other primary CNS tumors and metastatic tumors have been reported. In the HIV-1–infected patient with focal neurologic signs, either a cranial MRI with gadolinium or a double-dose, delayed brain CT is mandated. The former is more sensitive, but brain CT scan is more specific, particularly with respect to toxoplasmosis. Therefore, these studies often prove to be complementary.

CEREBRAL TOXOPLASMOSIS

Infection with the intracellular protozoan *Toxoplasma gondii* has a worldwide distribution, is most often subclinical, and results in seropositivity and chronic, latent infection in immunocompetent individuals. However, it may present with lymphadenopathy or mononucleosis-like illness in otherwise healthy adults.

TABLE 26-6. Histopathology of Focal Brain Lesions in AIDS

1986[1] BEFORE EMPIRIC TOXO-THERAPY		1991[2] AFTER EMPIRIC TOXO-THERAPY (n = 50)	
Toxoplasmosis	50–70%	Toxoplasmosis	14
Lymphoma	10–25%	Lymphoma	14
Progressive multifocal leukoencephalopathy	10–22%	Progressive multifocal leukoencephalopathy	14
Nondiagnostic	10%	Nondiagnostic	4
Candida abscess	3%	HIV encephalopathy	3
Cryptococcoma	2%	Cryptococcoma	1
Kaposi sarcoma	2%	Atypical mycobacteria	1
Tuberculoma	1%	Stroke	1
Herpes simplex	1%	Metastasis	2

[1] De La Paz R., Enzmann D: Neuroradiology of acquired immunodeficiency syndrome. In: Rosenblum ML, Levy RM, Bredsen DE (eds): AIDS and the Nervous System, pp 121–154. New York, Raven Press, 1988.
[2] Levy RM, Russel E, Yungbluth M, et al.: Abstract WB 27, Seventh International Conference on AIDS, Florence, 1991.

Intracranial mass lesions or diffuse meningoencephalitis sporadically occurs. *Toxoplasma* cysts remain present in all tissues during latent infection. The seroprevalence in adults varies geographically and depends on certain risk factors (e.g., eating habits).

Cerebral toxoplasmosis is the leading cause of focal brain disease in AIDS patients and has a prevalence of 3% to 40%, depending on the seroprevalence of the population studied. Cerebral toxoplasmosis is the presenting opportunistic infection in at least 5% of the AIDS patient population. Clinically, patients present with constitutional symptoms, headache, and fever, followed by focal neurologic abnormalities, including focal seizures, aphasia, hemiparesis, and homonymous hemianopsia, depending on the localization of the lesions. This combination of focal abnormalities and signs of a global encephalopathy is very suggestive of cerebral toxoplasmosis.

Brain imaging is very important in establishing the diagnosis. A CT scan normally reveals multiple hypodense areas, usually with mass effect, and contrast enhancement (ring pattern or irregular nodules). MRI is more sensitive in detecting lesions. Serology is rarely diagnostic at the time CNS toxoplasmosis develops: IgM antibodies are rarely demonstrable and a fourfold rise of preexisting low IgG antibody titer or a high IgG antibody titer (higher than 1:512 in the Sabin–Feldman dye test), consistent with recrudescent infection, is usually absent. Likewise, antibody tests in CSF are rarely diagnostic and may even be negative in many patients. Even negative serology tests in CNS toxoplasmosis have been described.

In AIDS patients with suspected cerebral toxoplasmosis, based on clinical findings and CT scan abnormalities, empirical treatment is justifiable, reserving brain biopsy for atypical or refractory cases. The most effective therapy is a combination of pyrimethamine (50 mg/day) and sulfadiazine (6–8 g/day). Oral folinic acid is given to prevent hematologic side effects. Corticosteroids may be used for lesions associated with edema and mass effect. A considerable number of patients develop a rash due to the sulfadiazine. In these cases, clindamycin may represent an alternative therapy. Secondary prophylaxis is mandated because of the high rate of recurrence. For this maintenance treatment, the pyrimethamine–sulfa combination is effective.

PROGRESSIVE MULTIFOCAL LEUKOENCEPHALOPATHY

Progressive multifocal leukoencephalopathy is a demyelinating disease of the CNS that results from infection of oligodendrocytes with JC virus, a papovavirus first described in 1958 by Aström, Mancall, and Richardson in patients with lymphoma and leukemia. With rare exception, PML occurs in the clinical setting of cellular immunosuppression. Until the AIDS epidemic, the most common underlying illnesses were lymphoproliferative diseases, but since 1981, increasing numbers of individuals with PML have been recognized. Approximately 4% to 5% of all HIV-1–infected patients will develop PML, and in as many as 25% of HIV-1–infected individuals with PML this neurologic disease will be the presenting manifestation of AIDS.

The presentation of the AIDS patient with PML does not appear to be substantially different from that of patients with PML complicating other immunosuppressive conditions. The onset is insidious, with symptoms and signs suggesting multifocal disease. Hemiparesis is the most common presenting symptom. Headache and seizures are rare, and signs of elevated intracranial pressure are characteristically absent. The diagnosis is strongly supported but not confirmed on the basis of radiographic imaging. CT of the brain reveals hypodense lesions of the affected white matter that generally do not enhance with contrast administration and exhibit no mass effect. Cranial MRI shows a hyperintense lesion on T2-weighted images in the affected regions. As with the CT scan, contrast enhancement is an exception. The lesions are not confined to a vascular territory and are less diffusely distributed than MRI abnormalities in AIDS dementia complex. CSF specimens are nondiagnostic. Polymerase chain reaction for JC virus genome in the CSF of affected patients is positive in only about 30%. For the present, diagnostic certainty depends on the demonstration of typical histopathologic abnormalities at brain biopsy and detecting the virus. The histopathologic changes include demyelination, oligodendrocytes with large intranuclear inclusions, and large bizarre astrocytes with hyperchromatic nuclei. The JC virus can be demonstrated by using electron microscopy or by employing immunofluorescence or immunohistochemistry.

Occasionally, prolonged survival and spontaneous partial recovery in AIDS-associated PML have been described. The prognosis in these patients is generally poor, with a mean survival of 4 months. An effective treatment for PML in patients with AIDS has not been identified. The administration of cytosine arabinoside [cytarabine (ara-C)] either intrathecally or intravenously has demonstrated no value above placebo. Other therapies directed to the JC virus are under development.

PRIMARY CNS LYMPHOMA

Primary central nervous system lymphoma (PCNSL) is a non-Hodgkin lymphoma that arises within and is confined to the nervous system. The incidence of PCNSL has increased rapidly over the past 10 years. Of HIV-1–infected patients, 0.6% will present with PCNSL, and 2% to 13% can be expected to develop it. PCNSL is the second most frequent CNS mass lesion in adults with AIDS, and it is the most frequent in children with AIDS.

Clinically, most of the patients present with lethargy, confusion, memory loss, and personality change. The remaining patients present with hemiparesis, dysphasia, seizures, and cranial nerve deficits. CT appearance of PCNSL in AIDS patients is generally described as a mass, or multiple masses, exhibiting diffuse or ring enhancement with a predilection for the corpus callosum, basal ganglia, and periventricular areas, but toxoplasmosis may also appear as solitary or multiple, ring- or nodular-enhancing masses. It is therefore generally accepted that PCNSL is indistinguishable from toxoplasmosis. In the majority of patients with PCNSL, multiple lesions can be seen on MR or CT. However, among solitary MRI lesions, there is a predominance of lymphoma.

Cerebrospinal fluid examination is often not possible because of the mass effect of the tumor. However, up to 25% of patients with PCNSL have a positive cytology, and this can eliminate the need for a diagnostic biopsy. At autopsy, 100% of patients have leptomeningeal seeding. Histologic confirmation remains essential, and this should preferably be done by stereotactic biopsy. Corticosteroid administration can produce shrinkage of the tumor seen on CT or MRI scan because of the lysis of tumor cells, but this necrosis in the tumor makes it more difficult to establish the diagnosis. So, when PCNSL is a diagnostic consideration, corticosteroids should be withheld. Histologically, the majority of PCNSLs are large cell and large cell immunoblastic tumors of B-cell origin.

Radiotherapy is the treatment of choice. Patients with PCNSL may respond both clinically and radiologically to whole-brain radiotherapy (4,000 Gy). If possible, a boost of 1,500 cGy to the tumor bed can be added. With radiotherapy, median survival can be prolonged by 4 to 5 months. Leptomeningeal lymphoma should be treated with intrathecal chemotherapy: methotrexate or ara-C, using an Ommaya reservoir. Systemic chemotherapy may be of value.

CEREBROVASCULAR COMPLICATIONS

Some patients with AIDS suffer transient ischemic attacks or strokes. Sometimes, these cerebrovascular complications occur as the result of an underlying opportunistic infection or lymphoma, or occasionally they are secondary to marantic endocarditis. A unique CNS vasculitis may be observed in HIV-infected persons. In many cases, no underlying condition for the stroke is identified. Anticardiolipin antibodies may play an ancillary role in the pathogenesis of stroke in AIDS, as they are frequently found in HIV-infected patients. Treatment is no different from that which is used in the non-HIV-infected patient.

MYELOPATHY

Spinal cord disease is observed frequently in HIV-1 infection. In most instances, the disorder is ascribed solely to HIV-1 infection, a condition referred to as HIV-1–related vacuolar myelopathy. The diagnosis of this disorder, like that of HIV-1 encephalopathy, is one of exclusion. A number of other myelopathies may also occur with HIV-1 infection, including infectious myelopathies (CMV, herpes simplex type 2, herpes zoster, HTLV-I, mycobacteria, *T. pallidum*, and epidural abscesses), vascular myelopathies, epidural and intramedullary tumors, and a demyelinating myelopathy (Table 26-7). Diagnostically, the single most useful study is an MRI of the involved area of the spinal cord to exclude the possibility of a mass lesion. The CSF needs to be examined for treatable pathogens, including syphilis and the herpes viruses.

HIV-1–RELATED VACUOLAR MYELOPATHY

A vacuolar myelopathy has been reported in 20% to 25% of AIDS cases. The syndrome is often associated with AIDS dementia complex, but it may occur in isolation. Clinically, the syndrome is characterized by a slowly progressive spastic paraparesis, lower-extremity hyperreflexia (except when diminished as a result of concomitant peripheral neuropathy), gait ataxia, and impaired sensation with vibratory and position

---

TABLE 26-7. Myelopathies in HIV-1 Infection

HIV-1–associated vacuolar myelopathy
Cytomegalovirus polyradiculomyelopathy
Varicella-zoster virus radiculomyelopathy
HTLV-I–associated myelopathy
Lymphoma (epidural or intradural)
Vascular insults
Vitamin B_{12} deficiency

sense being disproportionately affected. A discrete sensory level is distinctly unusual. Sometimes urinary incontinence develops. No treatment has been unequivocally demonstrated to be of value in HIV-related vacuolar myelopathy. Zidovudine seems to have little efficacy, although controlled clinical trials are lacking.

Pathologic changes are most prominent in the thoracic cord and closely mimic the pathology of subacute combined degeneration of the spinal cord. There is degeneration of the posterior and lateral columns of the spinal cord. The vacuolation appears to result from swelling within the layers of the myelin sheaths. Microglial nodules and multinucleate giant cells can be detected in the affected spinal cord.

The role of HIV-1 in the pathogenesis of this myelopathy remains unclear. The virus has been demonstrated by *in situ* hybridization and immunohistochemical staining in mononuclear and multinucleated macrophages in the areas of vacuolar myelopathy. However, the myelopathy is probably not the result of productive HIV-1 infection, and a disturbance in vitamin B_{12} metabolism has been suggested. A trial of high-dose methionine in this condition is currently underway.

PERIPHERAL NEUROPATHIES

Several peripheral neuropathies are associated with HIV-1 infection. These include distal symmetrical polyneuropathy or HIV-1–associated predominantly sensory polyneuropathy, the inflammatory demyelinating polyneuropathies, mononeuropathy multiplex, autonomic neuropathy, CMV polyradiculomyelopathy, and the toxic polyneuropathies [associated with dideoxyinosine (ddI) and dideoxycytidine (ddC)] (Table 26-8). Some of them, like the inflammatory-demyelinating polyneuropathies, occur early in HIV-1 infection, and some of them, like the distal symmetrical polyneuropathy and CMV polyradiculomyelopathy, occur late. The neuromuscular complications of HIV-1 infection are considered common. Several studies suggest that even subclinical neuromuscular involvement occurs frequently. At least one third of patients with AIDS will develop symptoms of neuropathy.

INFLAMMATORY DEMYELINATING POLYNEUROPATHIES

A demyelinating polyneuropathy may occur acutely or chronically in HIV-infected individuals. These demyelinating neuropathies tend to occur early in the course of HIV infection. The HIV-1–associated

TABLE 26-8. Neuromuscular Complications of HIV-1 Infection

Neuropathies
   Distal symmetrical polyneuropathy
   Inflammatory demyelinating polyneuropathy (acute and chronic)
   Mononeuropathy multiplex
   Autonomic polyneuropathy
   Toxic neuropathies
   Cytomegalovirus polyradiculomyelopathy
Myopathies
   HIV-1–associated polymyositis
   Zidovudine-associated myopathy
   HIV wasting syndrome

acute inflammatory demyelinating polyradiculoneuropathy (HIV-1–associated Guillain–Barré syndrome) is similar to Guillain–Barré syndrome in patients not infected with HIV-1. Patients present with progressive weakness, areflexia, and minor sensory signs. However, CSF examination may reveal a mild mononuclear pleocytosis (and an elevated protein) in HIV-infected patients. The same CSF abnormalities may be found in the HIV-1–associated chronic inflammatory demyelinating polyneuropathy (HIV-1–associated CIDP). Electrophysiologic studies indicate features of primary demyelination and axonal loss. The pathogenesis of the inflammatory demyelinating polyneuropathies may be autoimmune. The clinical course of the neuropathies in HIV-infected individuals is variable, but most patients improve. Plasmapheresis has been suggested as the treatment of choice, but steroids may be effective as well. Some recover spontaneously.

DISTAL SYMMETRICAL POLYNEUROPATHY

Distal symmetrical polyneuropathy, or HIV-1–associated predominantly sensory polyneuropathy (HPSP), is the most common polyneuropathy in HIV-infection. This polyneuropathy has been diagnosed in up to 35% of patients with AIDS. The most frequent symptoms are paresthesias, numbness, pain, and dysesthesias affecting the feet. Ankle reflexes are decreased or absent, there is a decreased sensation to pain and vibration in the feet and legs, and weakness is usually mild. The hands are less often involved. In a small proportion of patients, pain is the most prominent feature. Most investigators believe that this painful distal sensory neuropathy is a subgroup of the HPSP. There is some epidemiologic evidence suggesting a relationship with CMV. Electrophysiologic studies demonstrate a polyneuropathy with features of both axonal degeneration and demyelin-ation, but pathologically the abnormalities found are predominantly axonal and the demyelination is largely secondary. HIV has been isolated from periph-eral nerves, but the pathogenesis remains unknown. Possible mechanisms include direct viral infection or a cell-mediated immune attack on components of peripheral nerve. Treatment is limited to providing symptomatic relief with tricyclic antidepressants, anti-convulsants, analgesics, or topical capsacin. Antiretro-viral therapy seems to have little efficacy, although clinical trials are lacking. The administration of re-combinant nerve growth factor appears to have effi-cacy in decreasing the degree of discomfort and may eventually be proven to speed nerve recovery.

MONONEUROPATHY MULTIPLEX

Mononeuropathy multiplex is characterized by sen-sory and motor deficits in the distributions of multi-ple spinal, cranial, or peripheral nerves. CSF reveals both pleocytosis and elevated protein level. Electro-physiologic studies suggest axonal neuropathy. Nerve biopsies have revealed necrotizing arteritis in some instances.

AUTONOMIC NEUROPATHY

Late in HIV-1 infection, a small number of patients develop an autonomic neuropathy that is clinically sig-nificant. Patients present with postural hypotension, bowel and bladder dysfunction, impotence, sweating abnormalities, presyncope, and sudden arrhythmias with the risk of death. Numerous factors may contrib-ute to these symptoms, but often the symptoms are due to small-fiber peripheral neuropathy. Extensive autonomic testing reveals both parasympathetic and sympathetic dysfunction in 50% of patients. Treatment is purely symptomatic, with the use of agents such as fludrocortisone for stabilization of blood pressure.

TOXIC POLYNEUROPATHIES

A painful peripheral neuropathy has been associated with the use of the dideoxynucleoside analogs ddI and ddC. The syndrome is characterized by burning pain and tingling in the feet and legs, starting 8 to 27 weeks after initiating ddI treatment. These neur-opathic symptoms have generally not been associated with significant abnormalities in nerve conduction studies. Some patients have reported marked im-provement in symptoms within 1 to 2 weeks of dis-continuing ddI. The neuropathy appears to be related to the total cumulative dose of ddI. The ddC neurop-athy is clinically similar to ddI neuropathy: It is also dose related, and significant recovery occurs in most patients. The findings in these ddI and ddC neurop-athies are consistent with a distal axonopathy primar-ily affecting sensory fibers.

CYTOMEGALOVIRUS POLYRADICULOMYELOPATHY

Cytomegalovirus polyradiculomyelopathy, or poly-radiculitis, has been increasingly recognized in pa-tients with AIDS. Patients present with lower-extremity and sacral paresthesias or pain, followed by a rapidly progressive flaccid paraparesis, with areflexia and sphincter disturbances. Sensory disturbances are usu-ally mild. The CSF reveals a pleocytosis with predom-inance of polymorphonuclear leukocytes. CMV has been detected in the CSF by several techniques, in-cluding culture, immunohistochemistry, *in situ* hy-bridization, and the detection of cytomegalic cells by cytologic examination. Myelographic examination may show thickened adherent lumbar nerve roots.

At autopsy, spinal roots have revealed extensive multifocal necrosis, acute inflammatory infiltrates, and vasculitis. Typical CMV inclusions are seen within endoneurial inflammatory cells, Schwann cells, and endothelial cells. Treatment with ganciclovir (DHPG), started early in the course of the disease, may stop pro-gression or even cause some improvement. The gan-ciclovir regimen recommended is 5 mg/kg IV every 12 hours for 2 to 3 weeks, followed by maintenance therapy, 5 mg/kg per day, 5 days per week.

MYOPATHIES

Several myopathies have been described in HIV-1—infected individuals. The most important are HIV-1—associated polymyositis and zidovudine-associated myopathy. Progressive proximal muscle weakness—often associated with myalgia, elevated serum creati-nine kinase (CK), myopathic EMG abnormalities, inflammatory infiltrates, and mitochondrial abnor-malities (by electron microscopy) in muscle biopsy—may be present in both types, and no features clearly discriminate between them.

HIV-1—associated polymyositis (or some authors prefer HIV-associated myopathy) has been described in all stages of HIV-1 infection. Patients present sub-acutely with progressive proximal weakness and myalgia, most prominent in the thighs. The weakness involves the legs and neck flexors more than the arms. CK elevation is mild or moderate. Patients usually have myopathic EMG abnormalities, and 50% may have nerve conduction abnormalities indicating an accompanying peripheral neuropathy. Pathologic findings include noninflammatory myofiber degeneration, myofiber necrosis with inflammatory infiltrates, nemaline rod bodies, cytoplasmic bodies, and mitochondrial abnormalities. The pathogenesis is unknown. A T-cell–mediated and major histocompatibility class I (MHC-I)-restricted cytotoxic process may be the underlying mechanism. HIV-1–associated polymyositis may respond to corticosteroids.

A zidovudine-associated myopathy occurs in a minority of patients who have been treated with zidovudine for at least 9 to 12 months. Muscle tenderness and weakness are preceded by CK elevation. In this myopathy, mitochondrial dysfunction, resulting from drug-induced inhibition of mitochondrial DNA polymerase, has been suggested as the direct cause of the myopathy. The cumulative dose of zidovudine might be important. Pathologically ragged-red fibers, indicative of abnormal mitochondria, coexist with inflammatory changes. Zidovudine-associated myopathy usually (but not always) responds to zidovudine withdrawal.

SUMMARY

In the diagnostic approach to a neurologic problem in an HIV-1–infected individual, it is critical to appreciate the following:

1. The degree of advancement of HIV-1 infection (or the level of immune compromise): Some neurologic complications occur early in HIV-1 infection, others occur late.
2. The anatomic site of involvement: Focal brain lesion or nonfocal disorder? CNS disease or neuromuscular complication?
3. Is there a single disease, or are multiple levels of the neuraxis involved simultaneously?
4. The prevalences of the neurologic complications: Some complications are common, others are rare.

Computed tomography or MRI scanning and CSF examination are the most important tools in confirming a presumed diagnosis and excluding others. Usually, lumbar puncture (if not contraindicated) follows CT or MRI scanning. Electrophysiologic studies may be helpful in neuromuscular complications.

Brain biopsy, muscle biopsy, neuropsychological examination, and electroencephalography may give additional and sometimes essential information in specific problems.

QUESTIONS AND DISCUSSION

1. A patient with AIDS presents with fever and very severe headache. Neurologic examination reveals no abnormalities (not even neck stiffness). Give a differential diagnosis and diagnostic approach.

Answer: Physicians should remember that the presence of headache alone in the HIV-infected person seldom indicates a serious underlying pathology. However, in a patient with AIDS (usually severely immunosuppressed) who presents with new-onset, severe headache with fever in the absence of focal neurologic abnormalities, cryptococcal meningitis is the most likely diagnosis. This meningitis often results in very severe headaches, as a result of raised intracranial pressure, without focal abnormalities, and in two thirds of patients without meningeal signs. When there is any doubt about focal abnormalities, CT or MRI should precede lumbar puncture. Other causes for meningitis include HIV-1, *M. tuberculosis, L. monocytogenes, T. pallidum,* and lymphomatous meningitis. HIV-1 (aseptic) meningitis usually occurs early in HIV-1 infection and the others occur less frequently than cryptococcal meningitis. CSF analysis will almost always provide the conclusive answer.

2. A patient with AIDS presents with apathy, slowness, and forgetfulness. He has no headache or fever. Can we conclude that the diagnosis is AIDS dementia complex?

Answer: No, we cannot. The diagnosis of AIDS dementia complex is one of exclusion. Clinically, this patient presents with frontal lobe dysfunction, so CT or MR should be performed. Frontal lobe toxoplasmosis, PML, and PCNSL have to be excluded. Chronic meningitis (syphilis, *M. tuberculosis, Listeria*) must also be excluded by CSF examination. If CT or MRI and CSF are negative, further support for the diagnosis of AIDS dementia complex can be obtained by neuropsychological examination, which may show abnormalities compatible with "subcortical dementia" and may help to exclude depression. CT or MRI and CSF examination may give additional support for a diagnosis of AIDS dementia complex. CT or MRI may show atrophy and diffuse white matter abnormalities; CSF analysis may reveal HIV-1 p24 antigen, and increased levels of beta-2-microglobulin, neopterin, and quinolinic acid. The diagnosis of AIDS dementia complex can be extremely difficult to make. Sometimes, longer follow-up is necessary to make a definite conclusion.

3. An HIV-infected patient presents with headache, fever, aphasia, and a slight right-sided hemiparesis. The day before, he had a seizure. His illness developed in 1 week. What is the most likely diagnosis?

Answer: The most likely diagnosis in an HIV-infected individual who presents with focal abnormalities is cerebral toxoplasmosis. This is the leading cause of cerebral mass lesions in patients with HIV infection. A CT or MRI scan was performed, which showed multiple ring-enhancing lesions with surrounding edema, compatible with cerebral toxoplasmosis. Because of its high incidence and the fact that toxoplasmosis is easily treatable, empiric treatment is usually justifiable. When the lesion is radiographically observed to be single and the toxoplasmosis serology is negative, the likelihood of its being toxoplasmosis is low and the physician should proceed to brain biopsy. The presence of a lesion that enhances in thallium single photon emission computed tomography is suggestive of PCNSL. A positive polymerase chain reaction for Epstein–Barr virus in the CSF is felt by many investigators to be diagnostic of PCNSL. If antitoxoplasmosis therapy is employed, most patients react favorably, both clinically and radiologically, within 5 days and almost invariably within 2 weeks. Among the differential diagnoses of focal abnormalities in AIDS are PCNSL (the second most common brain mass lesion in AIDS) and PML. PCNSL is clinically and radiologically indistinguishable from toxoplasmosis and has to be confirmed by brain biopsy. PML presents with a more protracted course and is radiologically different (white matter lesions, usually without contrast enhancement or mass effect). AIDS patients with focal lesions, without a favorable response to empiric antitoxoplasmosis treatment, require a brain biopsy to make a definite diagnosis.

4. A patient with AIDS presents with slowly progressive gait disturbances. On neurologic examination, he has a spastic paraparesis and a sensory ataxia. Give a differential diagnosis.

Answer: A slowly progressive spastic paraparesis with a sensory ataxia is usually caused by a myelopathy. There are several etiologic possibilities in a patient with AIDS. Medullary compression (e.g., an epidural tuberculous abscess or lymphoma) has to be excluded by MRI. CSF examination should exclude infectious agents, of which the most important are CMV, varicella-zoster virus, HTLV-I, and *T. pallidum*. Vitamin B_{12} deficiency should be ruled out. If the MRI and CSF are negative for the previously mentioned causes, the most likely diagnosis is HIV-1–related vacuolar myelopathy. This is a slowly progressive myelopathy that is related to HIV-infection and is often associated with AIDS dementia complex but may occur without dementia. Its pathogenesis is poorly understood, and zidovudine has no clear efficacy. The diagnosis is one of exclusion.

5. An AIDS patient with CMV retinitis presents with subacute low back pain and radicular pain in the left leg. Do you think this patient has a herniated lumbar disk?

Answer: HIV infection does not protect against herniated disks. But be careful! A very aggressive polyradiculomyelopathy caused by CMV has been described in patients with AIDS, and this syndrome may well present as if it were a herniated disk. In this syndrome, in days to weeks after the initial lumbago and radicular pain, a rapidly progressive flaccid paraparesis with sphincter disturbances may develop. The CSF reveals a pleocytosis with predominance of polymorphonuclear leukocytes. CMV may be cultured from the CSF, or CMV may be detected by immunohistochemistry or *in situ* hybridization. Treatment with ganciclovir, started early, may stop progression or even cause some improvement. In every AIDS patient with radicular pain in the legs who develops a paresis, a lumbar puncture should be done; when the previously mentioned CSF abnormalities are found, ganciclovir should be started while awaiting CSF culture.

SUGGESTED READING

Berger JR, Levy RM: AIDS and the Nervous System, 2nd Edition. Philadelphia, Lippincott-Raven, 1998

Gendelman HE, Lipton SA, Epstein L et al: The Neurology of AIDS. New York, Chapman & Hall, 1998

Harrison MJG, McArthur JC: AIDS and Neurology. New York, Churchill Livingstone, 1995

Price RW, Brew BJ, Sidtis J et al: The brain in AIDS: Central nervous system HIV-1 infection and AIDS dementia complex. Science 239:586, 1988

Rudge P (ed): Bailliere's Clinical Neurology Series: Neurological Aspects of Human Retroviruses. London, Bailliere Tindall, 1992

Simpson DM, Berger JR: Neurologic manifestations of HIV infection. Med Clin North Am 80:1363, 1996

Neurology for the Non-Neurologist, Fourth Edition, edited by William J. Weiner and Christopher G. Goetz. Lippincott Williams & Wilkins, Philadelphia © 1999.

C H A P T E R   2 7

Neurologic Disorders in Pregnancy

Kathleen M. Shannon

The majority of women who become pregnant do so at times in their lives of relative health and physical fitness. Fortunately, concomitant diseases are relatively rare in this population. However, the childbearing years overlap periods of increased risk for neurologic disorders such as migraine headache, vascular malformations, multiple sclerosis, and myasthenia gravis. Pregnancy enhances susceptibility to some conditions, such as venous and arterial thrombosis, or it may be the setting for conditions such as eclampsia, which do not occur in the nongravid state. An understanding of the physiologic changes of pregnancy and how they are likely to influence neurologic diseases forms the foundation on which decisions about diagnostic and therapeutic interventions are made.

The focus of this chapter is on the evaluation and treatment of neurologic disorders that are commonly encountered during pregnancy. For those conditions that commonly occur in the nongravid population as well, the reader is referred elsewhere in the text for more comprehensive discussion of the disease entities.

TERATOLOGY

Teratologic concerns weigh heavily on the minds of pregnant patients and their physicians. The result is a reluctance to perform neurodiagnostic tests, particularly where ionizing radiation is employed. There

is also a popular perception that the risk of malformation consequent to drug ingestion may be as high as 25%, even with drugs not known to be teratogenic. This perception commonly leads to noncompliance with prescribed medications.

Malformations are detected in 2% to 3% of live births; less than 5% are thought to result from exposure to teratogens. The effects of a teratogen depend on the dose reaching the fetus, the duration of exposure, the gestational age of the fetus at the time of the exposure, and simultaneous exposure to other agents. Two major classes of teratogens are of concern to the treating physician: ionizing radiation and drugs.

The effects of radiation on the developing fetus depend on the dose and duration of radiation absorbed by the conceptus and the stage of development at which exposure occurs. With the exception of myelography and fluoroscopy, fewer than 0.1% of neuroradiographic examinations properly performed with abdominal shielding expose the fetus to levels of radiation greater than 1 rad, a level that is not felt to pose significant risk to the fetus. In general, if a radiographic study is indicated for the diagnosis or management of a pregnant woman, the benefits far outweigh the risks to the fetus.

The risks of magnetic resonance imaging (MRI) to the fetus are not known. However, limited studies have not shown teratogenic potential, and it is believed to be safe for use during pregnancy.

Reports of drug teratogenicity are most often based on animal studies, anecdotal reports, or case control studies. Unfortunately, few drugs are known to be entirely without risk in pregnancy, and few are known to be teratogenic. For the majority of compounds, the actual risks to the fetus are unknown.

Because organogenesis occurs mainly during the first trimester, drugs should be avoided whenever possible during this time. Throughout pregnancy, prudent assessment of risk-to-benefit ratios is encouraged.

PERIPHERAL NERVOUS SYSTEM AND MUSCLE DISORDERS IN PREGNANCY

BACK PAIN AND DISC DISEASE

Back pain is almost universal during pregnancy and relates to changes in posture and relaxation of spinal joints and ligaments. The pain is usually localized to the back and buttock, or it radiates into the thighs. The cumulative incidence of back pain rises with the duration of pregnancy. Musculoskeletal back pain is treated with bed rest, analgesia, heat, and massage.

Disc disease in pregnancy is rare. When it occurs, the complaint is usually of unilateral low back pain radiating through the buttock into the foot. L5 and S1 radiculopathies are most common. Treatment should be conservative—with the same recommendations as for back pain. Steroid injections may benefit some who are refractory to conservative management. Surgery should be used only in refractory cases or when there is objective evidence by electromyography or examination of nerve compromise.

PLEXUS DISORDERS, POLYNEUROPATHIES, AND MONONEUROPATHIES

Pregnancy-associated brachial plexus neuropathy may be familial or sporadic. The clinical syndrome consists of pain followed by weakness of the shoulder and arm. Neurologic exam points to a plexus lesion rather than root or nerve lesion. Recovery usually begins 4 to 8 weeks after onset, irrespective of the time of onset relative to the pregnancy. Recovery is complete in 60% at 1 year and nearly 100% at 3 years. The syndrome may recur during subsequent pregnancies. Treatment is supportive.

Lesions of the lumbosacral plexus or nerves exiting the plexus most commonly are related to traumatic or forceps-manipulated delivery. Most are self-limited, although complete recovery may take many months.

Pregnancy-associated polyneuropathies can result from nutritional deficiencies and resemble those seen in the nonpregnant malnourished.

Acute idiopathic demyelinating polyneuropathy (AIDP, Guillain–Barré syndrome) occurs in women of childbearing age, but pregnancy does not seem to confer added risk of this disorder. AIDP presents as rapidly ascending motor neuropathy with autonomic dysfunction. The presentation and course do not differ from that in the nonpregnant population. AIDP does not adversely affect pregnancy outcome. Depending on the functional status of the patient at term, it may be necessary to assist delivery with forceps or vacuum extraction. Plasmapheresis has been shown to lessen the duration of severe symptoms in AIDP and is permissible during pregnancy. Special attention should be given to avoiding extreme fluid shifts during pheresis.

Chronic idiopathic demyelinating polyneuropathy (CIDP) shares an inflammatory etiology with AIDP. Patients have a chronic motor and large sensory fiber neuropathy with a remitting and relapsing course. CIDP may begin or relapse during pregnancy. For unknown reasons, the relapse rate is increased during pregnancy. Treatment with plasmapheresis, as described for AIDP, may be helpful. Alternative strategies include chronic corticosteroids and human immune globulin administration.

Mononeuropathies in pregnancy result from hormonal and fluid changes as well as disruptions in body mechanics secondary to the gravid uterus. Bell's palsy is an acute, idiopathic unilateral weakness of muscles innervated by the facial nerve. Retroauricular pain is commonly associated. The etiology is obscure, but viral infection, nerve edema, and hormonal influences have been implicated. Most cases occur in the third trimester. The prognosis for complete recovery is good, but some patients with very severe involvement may have residual paralysis. Treatment remains controversial. Prednisone, 40–60 mg daily for 10 days, has been said to improve long-term outcome.

Carpal tunnel syndrome, presenting as nocturnal pain and burning in the first three digits of the hand, is the most common peripheral neuropathy of pregnancy. The symptoms relate to compression of the median nerve as it traverses the carpal canal. Symptomatic treatment with splinting of the wrist at night and analgesics as needed is adequate for most patients. Because aspirin has been associated with fetal malformations and with complications during labor and delivery, acetaminophen is the preferred analgesic in pregnancy. Persistent carpal tunnel symptoms may require treatment with steroid injection into the tunnel. An occasional patient may need surgical release of the compressed nerve. Usually, symptoms resolve in the postpartum period. Meralgia paresthetica is seen in conditions that place undue pressure on the lateral femoral cutaneous nerve as it passes the inguinal ligament. As in the nonpregnant population, weight gain is largely responsible. Typically, patients notice symptoms beginning in the third trimester. Pain and burning affect the middle third of the lateral thigh. Treatment consists of weight loss if possible, avoidance of binding garments or belts, acetaminophen, and in some instances local injections of analgesics or transcutaneous nerve stimulation. Most patients recover after the pregnancy.

DISORDERS OF THE NEUROMUSCULAR JUNCTION OR MUSCLE

Myasthenia gravis (MG) is a disease of women of childbearing age and older men. MG is a disorder of neuromuscular junction transmission that manifests as fatigable weakness in skeletal muscle. MG rarely presents during pregnancy, but in patients with known MG, worsening can be expected in a third. One third of patients with MG improve, and one third remain stable during pregnancy. Although malignant thymoma is no more common during pregnancy than in the general MG population, pregnancy has been associated with an increased risk of widespread metastases. MG is not associated with a poorer outcome of pregnancy. Management of the MG patient who desires to become pregnant should include stabilization of the medication regimen. Corticosteroids may be continued during pregnancy, but immunosuppressants should be discontinued in favor of nonteratogenic therapies. Should thymectomy be indicated, it is best to perform this prior to pregnancy. When pregnancy occurs in the course of therapy, the risks and benefits of continuing the preexistent management plan should be weighed. There is little to be gained by discontinuing immunosuppressants once the patient has passed the phase of organogenesis, but such patients may be offered ultrasound imaging studies to assess malformations. It is permissible to initiate corticosteroids during pregnancy. Thymectomy may be undertaken if indicated, but the patient should be prepared for this with a course of plasmapheresis, which may also be needed for disease exacerbations occurring during pregnancy. Anticholinesterase agents such as pyridostigmine may be used during pregnancy. They may be particularly helpful and may be given parenterally during labor and parturition. It may be necessary to assist delivery with low forceps and vacuum extraction. It is wise to remember that patients on long-term corticosteroids may have adrenal suppression with a blunted response to stress, so they may require supplemental corticosteroids for delivery.

Special attention must be focused on the infant of the myasthenic mother following delivery. Up to 20% of these infants have transient neonatal myasthenia due to transfer of maternal anti–acetylcholine-receptor antibody. Such infants are floppy, with poor suck and cry, and ventilatory insufficiency. They should receive ventilatory assistance as indicated and may require tube feeding. Anticholinesterases may be required in some instances. The disease is self-limited and resolves as antibody titers fall, usually within 30 days of birth.

The course of muscular dystrophies is not altered by pregnancy. Muscular dystrophies do not adversely affect pregnancy outcome, but labor and delivery may be hindered by weakness and fatigability. It may be necessary to assist in the second stage of labor with forceps or vacuum extraction.

Polymyositis is an inflammatory disease involving proximal muscles. Tenderness and proximal muscle weakness, sometimes with rash (dermatomyositis), are accompanied by striking increases in creatinine phosphokinase and erythrocyte sedimentation rate. Other autoimmune diseases may be associated. Treatment is usually with corticosteroids or immunosuppressants. Adverse fetal outcome has been reported in half of pregnancies in polymyositis/dermatomyositis patients. Treatment of the pregnant woman with polymyositis/dermatomyositis stresses avoidance of teratogenic immunosuppressants, attention to steroid replacement peripartum, and support of the second stage of labor, as indicated.

CENTRAL NERVOUS SYSTEM DISORDERS IN PREGNANCY

HEADACHE

Headache is the most common neurologic symptom in pregnancy, and rarely does its presence reflect serious underlying pathology. Headaches that present during pregnancy and are severe or atypical, persistently unilateral, or associated with focal findings or papilledema, are indications for diagnostic evaluation. The most common headache encountered in the gravid patient is the tension or muscle-contraction headache. Such headaches are dull and persistent with band- or viselike pain lasting days to years. They are commonly associated with tension or spasm in the muscles of the scalp and neck, and they may respond in part to nonpharmacologic measures such as relaxation training, massage, and heat. When headaches are disabling, they may be treated with acetaminophen or codeine, which have been found to be safe analgesics in pregnancy. Migraine headaches are severe, throbbing, often unilateral headaches that may be preceded by a visual or sensory aura. They are often associated with nausea and vomiting. Migraine headache affects 5% to 10% of the general population, and a higher percentage of women in the childbearing years. Fifty percent to 74% of women with migraine experience some decrease in the frequency of severity of migraine during pregnancy. However, some are worsened, and migraine may first present during pregnancy, usually during the first trimester. Infrequent migraine headaches, like tension headaches, are treated with analgesics. Ergot preparations, which are the mainstay of abortive migraine therapy outside pregnancy, are not recommended during pregnancy because of their propensity to cause uterine contraction. When disabling headaches occur more frequently than once weekly and adequate control is not achieved with analgesics alone, prophylactic therapy may be indicated. Propranolol 80–320 mg daily is the treatment of choice for migraine prophylaxis, but this drug may be associated with fetal growth retardation, prematurity, respiratory depression, hypoglycemia, and hyperbilirubinemia. Relatively low doses of antidepressants, such as amitriptyline 25 mg, may also be helpful.

EPILEPSY

One in every 200 pregnancies occurs in an epileptic woman. Management issues include the effects of pregnancy on seizure frequency and anticonvulsant pharmacokinetics, the effects of epilepsy on pregnancy and fetal development, and the effects of anticonvulsants on fetal development.

Seizure frequency is increased in 5% to 46%, decreased in 19% to 44% and unchanged in 35% to 55% of patients. Patients whose epilepsy has been poorly controlled prior to pregnancy are more likely to be poorly controlled during pregnancy. Increased seizure frequency is most likely to occur during the first two trimesters, and it is often related to changes in serum drug levels (as a result of altered

pharmacokinetics or noncompliance) or to sleep deprivation.

Total concentrations of all anticonvulsants decrease during pregnancy. This reflects changes in dose, body weight, and plasma protein binding (see Table 27-1). Decreased levels are apparent during the first trimester, but become more pronounced throughout pregnancy and may be associated with exacerbation of seizures. Changes in protein binding make total drug levels unreliable in monitoring of epileptic patients, as free levels may remain unchanged or may increase. The clinician should use the patient's clinical condition, frequency of seizures, and drug levels to monitor epileptic drug therapy. Whenever possible, free anticonvulsant levels should be used to monitor drug levels.

In prospective studies of epileptic women, complications of pregnancy, including preeclampsia, hemorrhage, placental abruption, and preterm labor, occurred 1.5 to 3 times as frequently as in controls. Stillbirth, prematurity, intrauterine growth retardation, and cesarean section occurred with increased frequency in the pregnancies of patients with seizure disorders, and these were associated with increased neonatal morbidity. There has been no association found between anti-epileptic drug therapy and these complications. Although severe and prolonged convulsions may cause fetal heart decelerations, obvious

TABLE 27-1. Factors Affecting Drug Pharmacokinetics during Pregnancy

Absorption
  Slowed gastric emptying
  Increased mucus production
  Decreased acid secretion
Distribution
  Increased intravascular volume
  Increased extravascular volume
  Increased tissue volume
  Changes in plasma protein binding
    Decreased plasma protein concentration
    Decreased binding capacity of albumin
    Increased concentration of endogenous inhibitors
      of protein binding
Liver metabolism
  Induction of microsomal enzymes by circulating
    steroid hormones
  Centrilobular bile stasis
Renal excretion
  Increased renal plasma flow
  Increased glomerular filtration rate

neonatal sequelae of convulsions are rare, even in the case of status epilepticus.

The risk of major congenital malformations in children of epileptic mothers is twice that in the general population. These defects consist mainly of congenital heart malformations, facial clefts, and neural tube defects. Although the risk of major malformation is increased in nontreated epileptics compared to control patients, it is higher still in epileptics receiving anticonvulsant drugs. With the exception of the association between valproic acid and neural tube defects, there is no specific association with a particular drug and resulting malformation. Neural tube defects, ranging from spina bifida to complete failure of fusion of the neuraxis, may be seen in 1% to 2% of children of epileptic mothers treated with valproic acid during the first trimester.

Controlled studies have shown an excess of minor malformations in offspring of epileptic women. The anomalies, which are seen in up to 11% of infants exposed *in utero* to anticonvulsants, include epicanthal folds, hypertelorism, small nose with anteverted nares, and low nasal bridge, long philtrum, abnormal ears, low hairline, nail hypoplasia, distal phalangeal hypoplasia, and increased dermal arches. Similar anomalies have been shown to occur in children of epileptic women who have not been exposed to anticonvulsant drugs, which suggests that some of them may be genetically linked to epilepsy. Proposed mechanisms of anticonvulsant teratogenicity include folate deficiency induced by the agents themselves, and the effects of toxic intermediate metabolites.

Up to 10% of infants exposed to anticonvulsants *in utero* will develop hemorrhagic complications related to deficiency of vitamin K–dependent coagulation factors. Bleeding is usually within the first 24 hours of life and can be prevented in most instances by treating the mother for the last 4 weeks of pregnancy with vitamin K (20 mg orally daily) and by administering parenteral vitamin K to the infant immediately after delivery. Fresh frozen plasma can be used for acute hemorrhage if needed.

Patients in the childbearing years should be encouraged to inform the physician when they begin trying to have children. They should be counseled about the risks of anomalies in their offspring as well as the importance to fetal outcome of careful seizure control during pregnancy. It should be stressed that the likelihood they will have a normal infant is 90%. Vitamin replacement should begin before pregnancy. When possible, seizures should be managed with monotherapy and should be monitored closely to establish the level at which optimal control is achieved. Valproic acid and trimethadione should be avoided in patients likely to have children. With the exception of these two agents, the evidence that one anticonvulsant is less teratogenic than the others is not strong enough to justify removing a patient from a drug regimen under which her seizures are well controlled.

When epileptic patients present after they have become pregnant, there is little to be gained from changing the anticonvulsant regimen, as malformations may have already occurred. Patients who have been exposed to valproic acid during the first trimester should be offered ultrasound and amniocentesis with quantitation of alpha-fetoprotein levels at the 20th week of gestation to detect neural tube defects.

The previously well patient who has noneclamptic seizure during pregnancy should have its cause investigated. Most represent coincidental onset of idiopathic epilepsy, but an underlying structural lesion should be excluded. The choice of anticonvulsant should be dictated by the seizure type. Most physicians elect not to initiate anticonvulsants for a single uncomplicated seizure. When anticonvulsants are indicated, monotherapy is desirable; the dose should be optimized to the lowest dose that maintains seizure control.

Pregnant women taking anticonvulsants should have serum levels (preferably free drug levels) monitored on a monthly basis, and the dosage of medications should be adjusted to maintain levels in the range of those that controlled seizures before the pregnancy. Free drug levels more accurately reflect concentrations of active drug, and they are useful when seizures prove difficult to manage despite therapeutic serum drug levels.

CEREBROVASCULAR DISEASE

The differential diagnosis of stroke in pregnancy is listed in Table 27-2.

ISCHEMIC CEREBROVASCULAR DISEASE

Sixty percent to 80% of ischemic cerebrovascular events in pregnancy result from arterial occlusion. Most occur during the second and third trimesters and the first postpartum week, and they are related to cervical or cranial arterial disease or to cardiac disease with cardiogenic cerebral embolization. Patients with preexisting hypertension, diabetes mellitus, cigarette smoking, and familial hyperlipidemia are at particular

Table 27-2. Differential Diagnosis of Stroke during Pregnancy

Hemorrhagic
  Subarachnoid hemorrhage
    Aneurysm
    Arteriovenous malformation
  Intracerebral hematoma
    Hypertension
    Eclampsia
    Clotting disorder
Ischemic—arterial
  Embolism
    Cardiac disease
      Valve disease
      Arrhythmia
      Cardiomyopathy of pregnancy
    Systemic venous thromboembolism
      Patent foramen ovale
  Thrombosis
    Cervical arterial disease
      Atherosclerosis
      Takayasu's pulseless disease
      Fibromuscular dysplasia
      Carotid artery dissection
    Cranial arterial disease
      Arteritis
      Hypertension
    Hypercoagulable state
Ischemic—venous
  Infectious
  Aseptic
    Idiopathic
    Associated with coagulopathy

risk for atherosclerotic disease of the cervical and intracranial arteries. Cranial arterial disease may also result from infectious or noninfectious vasculitis or from longstanding hypertension. Coagulopathy may be related to changes in coagulation factors during pregnancy, to underlying sickle cell anemia, or to thrombotic thrombocytopenic purpura. Cardiogenic cerebral emboli originate on infected or damaged cardiac valves or from the cardiac chambers in the presence of hypokinetic wall segments or arrhythmias. Rarely, a patent foramen ovale will be the route for cerebral emboli originating in the systemic venous circulation, or for fat or amniotic fluid emboli.

The evaluation and treatment of arterial occlusion in the pregnant patient differ little from those in the general population. Computed tomography, MRI, and arteriography, if indicated, can be performed without significant risk to the fetus. When diagnostic evaluation indicates infarction due to carotid artery disease, a symptomatic, surgically accessible, highly stenosed artery can be approached surgically at a center with acceptably low morbidity and mortality rates. Conservative treatment with daily low-dose aspirin therapy may be advised as initial therapy for patients with surgically accessible lesions, as well as for those with nonsurgical lesions. The only clear indication for systemic anticoagulation is the prevention of recurrent emboli of cardiac origin.

Venous infarction in pregnancy and the puerperium may arise from infectious or noninfectious causes, although the incidence of the former is quite small in the antibiotic age. Most venous infarctions occur in the 2nd to 5th weeks after delivery. Typically, infarction is heralded by severe headache, nausea, and vomiting. Weakness of one or both legs may be accompanied by proximal arm weakness. Focal deficits are commonly progressive and may be accompanied by focal or generalized seizures and increased intracranial pressure. Consciousness is often impaired. Mortality during the acute phase approaches 25%, but the prognosis is good for patients who survive, and recovery is often complete. Diagnosis is based on clinical features, characteristic CT or MRI findings, or angiographic studies. Treatment is conservative and includes hospitalization, hydration, and antibiotic and anticonvulsant therapy when indicated. The role of anticoagulation is controversial, but a trial may be indicated for patients who are showing progressive deterioration, early in the course, without evidence of hemorrhage on imaging studies or lumbar puncture.

It should be noted that heparin does not cross the placenta, so it is not teratogenic. However, heparin exposure has been associated with an increased risk of prematurity or stillbirth, and also with osteopenia and pathologic fracture in the mother. However, it is the anticoagulant of choice prior to the 13th week of pregnancy. Although it is not without risk in the second and third trimesters, warfarin is a superior anticoagulant and is the drug of choice during the time between the 13th and 36th weeks of gestation. After the 36th week, heparin should again be used to minimize the risk of peripartum hemorrhage.

HEMORRHAGIC CEREBROVASCULAR DISEASE

An underlying arteriovenous malformation or aneurysm can be found in 93% of pregnant patients presenting with subarachnoid hemorrhage, and aggressive and immediate diagnostic evaluation of the pregnant woman presenting with subarachnoid hemorrhage is indicated.

Arteriovenous malformations tend to occur in younger primiparous women; the bleed tends to occur during the second trimester, with rebleed during labor, delivery, and subsequent pregnancies (see Table 27-3). It is recommended that the patient with arteriovenous malformations be delivered by elective cesarean section, and that the risks of future pregnancy be explained to her. Surgical intervention during pregnancy is avoided when possible.

Aneurysms tend to present in older multiparous women, usually during the last trimester, and the risk of rebleeding is greatest in the first 2 weeks after the initial bleed. Early surgical intervention is recommended. The risk of rebleeding is low during labor and delivery, and vaginal delivery may be allowed. It is recommended that forceps assistance be used in the second stage of labor.

ECLAMPSIA

Although maternal mortality from all causes has declined, preeclampsia and eclampsia continue to account for about 5% of maternal deaths. Eclampsia may have up to 20% maternal mortality and 53% infant mortality. It is largely a disease of nulliparous gravid women. When it occurs in multiparous women, it is usually associated with multiple gestation, chronic hypertension, diabetes, or renal failure. Hypertension (systolic ≥ 140 mm Hg, or increase of ≥30 mm Hg; diastolic ≥ 90 mm Hg, or increase of ≥15 mm Hg), usually occurring after the 20th week of pregnancy, is accompanied by proteinuria and edema. Other symptoms include headache, visual disturbance, epigastric pain, hyperreflexia, and consumptive coagulopathy. Eclampsia is differentiated from preeclampsia by the occurrence of central nervous system signs, usually seizure or coma. Other neurologic manifestations include lethargy, obtundation, flashing lights, cortical blindness, visual hallucinations, and other focal signs.

Gross neuropathologic features of eclampsia include patchy areas of infarction and petechial hemorrhage. Some patients have large hemorrhages in the cortical white matter, deep gray-matter structures, or brainstem. There is microscopic evidence of endothelial cell damage, vasospasm, and medial necrosis.

The pathogenesis of preeclampsia/eclampsia remains unknown. Putative causal factors include immunologic, placental or maternal endocrine or genetic factors, and alterations in prostaglandin metabolism.

The treatment of eclampsia remains controversial and targets multiple signs. First used in 1900 and widely accepted after 1925, magnesium sulfate has been considered the treatment of choice for preeclampsia and eclampsia by the obstetric community. Recently, a number of controlled studies have suggested that magnesium sulfate reduces the incidence of primary seizures in preeclamptic/eclamptic women and reduces the recurrence of seizures in women who have seized prior to its institution. However, there remains little evidence that maternal and neonatal morbidity are significantly reduced by this therapy. Although magnesium has been shown to have antiepileptic properties in experimental models of epilepsy, penetration into the central nervous system is poor and there is little evidence of anticonvulsant activity in humans.

Clearly, the mainstay of treatment in preeclampsia/eclampsia is control of hypertension. Adequate prenatal care must stress blood pressure surveillance, and action should be taken if the diastolic blood pressure exceeds 75 mm Hg in the second trimester and 85 mm Hg in the third trimester. Conservative measures, such as bed rest, should be supplemented with antihypertensive medications when the former fail. Methyldopa has an established safety record in pregnancy, as has hydralazine. Although less well studied, beta-adrenergic blocking agents and calcium-channel blockers are also believed to be safe enough in pregnancy to justify their use as antihypertensives. Acute hypertensive crisis accompanied by other clinical features of preeclampsia or eclampsia should be treated by bed rest, oral or parenteral antihypertensives, and close monitoring of parameters of fetal well-being.

TABLE 27-3. **Subarachnoid Hemorrhage in Pregnancy**

	AVM	ANEURYSM
Decade of presentation	3rd	4th
Presentation trimester	1–2	2–3
Time of rebleeding risk	Intrapartum	Postpartum
Surgery when gravid?	Not recommended	Recommended
Allow labor?	Not recommended	Postoperative

AVM = arteriovenous malformation.

Recent data suggest that an intensive program of monitoring both the patient and the fetus, coupled with bed rest and antihypertensive therapy, can be safely conducted in the home. Such a management strategy, either in the home or the hospital, has been shown to increase gestational age at delivery and decrease perinatal mortality. For severe hypertension when oral medications have failed, hydralazine and diazoxide have established roles, but the risk of cyanide toxicity in the neonate dictates against the use of sodium nitroprusside.

Whether or not magnesium sulfate has been used, seizures and status epilepticus should be treated aggressively with standard anticonvulsants. The deleterious effects of convulsions on the fetus far outweigh the central nervous system depression attributed to anticonvulsant drugs. Patients who have had magnesium sulfate therapy are at greater risk of respiratory depression, and they should be monitored more closely during treatment with benzodiazepines or barbiturates. Following the acute eclamptic period, it is recommended that anticonvulsants be continued through the 30th postpartum day to prevent seizure recurrence.

SUMMARY COMMENTS

Although as many as 45% of pregnant women are exposed to one or more medications during pregnancy, the majority enjoy uncomplicated pregnancies and are delivered of normal, healthy infants. The physician must function as diagnostician, medication prescriber, and counselor to pregnant women. A coherent approach to care during pregnancy is founded on comprehension of the effects of pregnancy on acute and chronic disease states, working knowledge of pharmacologic and teratologic principles, and sensitivity to the concerns of the mother about the outcome of pregnancy.

QUESTIONS AND DISCUSSION

1. A 40-year-old multiparous woman presents during the 32nd week of pregnancy with acute onset of severe headache, neck stiffness, and obtundation. What is the most likely diagnosis?

A. Ischemic brainstem stroke
B. Eclampsia
C. Subarachnoid hemorrhage due to cerebral aneurysm

D. Subarachnoid hemorrhage due to arteriovenous malformation

The answer is (C). The symptoms typify subarachnoid hemorrhage, and the usual etiology in a patient of this age and duration of gestation is aneurysm. An emergency CT scan should be performed to confirm this diagnosis.

2. The management of the well-controlled epileptic in her third trimester of pregnancy includes all but which one of the following:

A. If she is taking phenytoin, a change should be made to phenobarbital to minimize the risk of fetal malformation.
B. The dose of anticonvulsant should be determined by assessing the clinical control of seizures, by noting the presence of side effects, and by following drug levels.
C. Anticonvulsant levels should be checked approximately once monthly.
D. She should be given vitamin K supplementation to avoid hemorrhagic complications in the newborn.

The answer is (A). Although it has been believed for some time that phenobarbital is less teratogenic than other anticonvulsants, this is not supported by clinical studies. Patients who are well controlled on phenytoin should be maintained on this agent.

3. A 22-year-old primiparous woman in the 28th week of gestation has a blood pressure of 140/95, peripheral edema, and proteinuria. What is the most responsible course of management?

A. She should be sent home with magnesium supplements.
B. She should be admitted to the hospital and started immediately on parenteral magnesium sulfate.
C. She should be started on an intensive inpatient or home program of bed rest, maternal and fetal monitoring, and antihypertensive therapy if needed.
D. She should be admitted to the hospital and started on phenobarbital, 30 mg three times a day.

The answer is (C). The patient has pre-eclampsia. Recent studies have shown that pre-eclampsia can be managed in the outpatient setting with intensive bed rest, antihypertensive therapy if needed, and close monitoring of the fetus. If there is any significant risk of noncompliance with such a rigorous regimen, hospitalization may be required.

4. A 27-year-old woman in the 30th week of pregnancy complains of 4 days of back pain that radiates into her thighs. Her neurologic examination is normal. What should be your approach?

A. An electromyogram (EMG) should be ordered to evaluate for acute radiculopathy.

B. A computed tomography (CT) scan should be ordered to evaluate for acute radiculopathy.

C. Bed rest and analgesics should be prescribed.

D. A neurosurgical evaluation for chymopapain injection should be scheduled.

The answer is (C). Back pain is frequent in pregnancy, and it usually responds to conservative management. EMG is unlikely to be diagnostic of radiculopathy with this duration of symptoms. The CT scan may be abnormal, but interpretation is difficult in nonspecific back pain.

SUGGESTED READING

Astedt B: Antenatal drugs affecting vitamin K status of the fetus and the newborn. Semin Thromb Hemost 21:364, 1995

Buehler BA, Rao V, Finnell RH: Biochemical and molecular teratology of fetal hydantoin syndrome. Neurol Clin 12:741, 1994

Chien PF, Khan KS, Arnott N: Magnesium sulphate in the treatment of eclampsia and pre-eclampsia: An overview of the evidence from randomised trials [see comments]. Br J Obstet Gynaecol 103:1085, 1996

Donaldson JO: Neurology of Pregnancy. London, WB Saunders, 1989

Gleicher N (ed): Principles of Medical Therapy in Pregnancy. New York, Plenum, 1985

Hiilesmaa VK: Pregnancy and birth in women with epilepsy. Neurology 42(Suppl 5):8, 1992

Morrell MJ: The new antiepileptic drugs and women: Efficacy, reproductive health, pregnancy, and fetal outcome. Epilepsia 37(Suppl 6):S34, 1996

Sibai BM, Frangieh AY: Management of severe pre-eclampsia. Curr Opin Obstet Gynecol 8:110, 1996

Stanley FJ, Bower C: Teratogenic drugs in pregnancy. Med J Aust 145:596, 1986

Wiebers DO: Ischemic cerebrovascular complications of pregnancy. Arch Neurol 42:110, 1985

Neurology for the Non-Neurologist, Fourth Edition, edited by William J. Weiner and Christopher G. Goetz. Lippincott Williams & Wilkins, Philadelphia © 1999.

C H A P T E R 2 8

Principles of Neurorehabilitation

David S. Kushner

The World Health Organization has described disablement in terms of disease, impairment, disability, and handicap. In this conceptual model, disease is an underlying condition or pathologic process that results in an impairment. Impairment is an abnormality in physical or psychological capacity. Disability is the limitation an impairment places on an individual's ability to perform necessary routine daily functional activities. Handicap is the social disadvantage that results from disabilities that prevent an individual from fulfilling his/her expected role in society. Handicap is influenced in a society by physical barriers, social and cultural factors, and the attitudes of those involved.

A host of neurologic conditions exist that can result in static or progressive impairments. Neurologic disorders can occur at any point in an individual's lifetime and may be developmental, hereditary, infectious, autoimmune, metabolic, degenerative, vascular, neoplastic, or traumatic. Pathology may involve any part of the nervous system, from the central nervous system (including the brain or spinal cord) to the peripheral nervous system and the muscle (resulting in impairments such as disorders of strength, endurance, balance, coordination, mobility, cognition, perception, communication, swallowing, and sensation). The same neurologic impairments can vary in intensity between individuals depending on the pathologic cause or the region of the nervous sys-

tem affected. Similarly, the prognosis may differ with similar impairments but with different pathologic processes at work. For example, hemiparesis resulting directly from an area of brain infarction would be less likely to resolve than would hemiparesis resulting from demyelination or edema involving the same region of the brain.

Disabilities that may result from neurologic impairments can involve any of the routine daily functions of an individual from ordinary self care tasks, including grooming, toileting, bathing, dressing, and feeding, to the more complex tasks of independent living, including financial management, shopping, home making, and the ability to use a telephone or drive a car. Pathology at different sites of the nervous system can result in similar functional disability manifestations between individuals. For example, disorders affecting balance, coordination, cognition, or strength all may separately result in the inability of an individual to walk or to effectively perform routine self-care activities. In neurorehabilitation, functional disabilities are the focus of medical, restorative, adaptive, environmental, and social interventions.

Neurorehabilitation encompasses medical, physical, social, educational, and vocational interventions that can be provided in a variety of institutional and community settings. Professionals include specialized physicians, nurses, therapists, psychologists, social workers, dietitians, and orthotists. Goals include the prevention of secondary complications, treatment to reduce neurologic impairments, compensatory strategies for residual disabilities, patient/caretaker education, and maintenance of function. Anyone with neurologic impairments can benefit from neurorehabilitation, but the setting, approach, and limitations of treatment will vary with the type and extent of the disabilities. The objective is to match patient needs with capabilities of available programs. This chapter will focus on principles of neurorehabilitation, including a broad overview of the role of ongoing patient assessment, acute-care intervention, the determination of rehabilitation need and an appropriate setting, the rehabilitation management plan, and issues pertaining to community transition and neurorehabilitation outcomes. In addition, case presentations will be given in the Questions and Discussion section, to explore potential benefits and limitations of neurorehabilitation in a variety of neurologic conditions.

ROLE OF ASSESSMENT IN NEUROREHABILITATION

Ongoing and thorough patient assessment is a crucial aspect of the neurorehabilitation process. The goals of assessment change over the clinical course of rehabilitation from the acute hospitalization, to the transfer to a rehabilitation facility/program, to the transition back to the community. Initial concerns often include patient survival, level of consciousness, and response to acute treatments. Later concerns focus on specific neurologic impairments and a patient's functional abilities. Patient evaluation throughout the neurorehabilitation process involves clinical examinations and well-validated standardized measures performed by various members of the interdisciplinary team of rehabilitation specialists. This team is often composed of the physician (neurologist/physiatrist), nurses, a social worker, and therapists (including physical, occupational, speech, and recreational/vocational), and a psychologist.

The non-neurologist primary care physician should obtain a neurorehabilitation consultation for evaluation of all patients admitted to the hospital with acute neurologic impairments resulting in functional deficits. In addition, patients having chronic medical or neurologic conditions with functional deficits that may be related to deconditioning weakness, reduced joint mobility, or progression of the condition may also benefit from rehabilitation. In principle, a neuro-

rehabilitation evaluation should be obtained for all hospitalized or ambulatory clinic patients having functional decline in any routine daily functions including mobility, transfers, ambulation, or the ability to dress, bathe, feed, groom, speak, or carry out previously routine duties such as vocational or homemaking responsibilities.

The objectives of neurorehabilitation assessment during the acute hospital admission include documentation of the diagnosis, the impairments, and the disabilities, as well as identification of treatment needs. Subsequent reevaluation focuses on response to acute-care treatments and any changes in neurologic or medical status. Once patients are medically stable, the evaluation is geared toward identifying those who will benefit from further rehabilitation intervention and determining the appropriate rehabilitation setting. Recommendation may be made for referral to an interdisciplinary rehabilitation program, in an inpatient or an outpatient facility, or for selected individual rehabilitation services in an ambulatory care setting.

Upon admission to a neurorehabilitation program, assessment is performed to help develop a rehabilitation management plan with realistic goals and to document a baseline level of function for monitoring progress. Periodic weekly or biweekly reassessment during the rehabilitation program allows patient progress to be monitored, treatment regimens to be adjusted when necessary to maximize patient potential, and facilitation of discharge planning. Objectives of assessment after discharge include the evaluation of patient adaptation to the home environment and community setting, the determination of the need for further rehabilitation services, and the assessment of caregiver burden and needs.

Standardized assessment instruments in neurorehabilitation complement the neurologic examination in evaluating functional recovery. Standardized measurement scales facilitate reliable documentation of severity of functional disabilities, help to increase consistency of treatment decisions, facilitate communication between therapists, and provide a reliable basis for monitoring progress. Scales exist to measure many areas of neurologic function, such as consciousness, cognition, perception, communication, strength, mobility, balance, coordination, somatosensation, and affective function. For example, the Rancho Los Amigos Cognitive Scale is often used to document levels of cognitive recovery following a traumatic brain injury, and the Functional Independence Measure Scale is often used to assess levels of independence in areas of basic daily function. In addition, many other scales exist to help measure and quantify specific functional impairments and disabilities. Limitations of various standardized measurement scales are often counterbalanced by use of other scales and the neurologic examination.

Another important aspect of patient assessment in neurorehabilitation is the clarification of the complex relationship that exists between disease, impairment, and disability in any individual patient. Specific neurologic impairments may play a role in multiple functional disabilities. For example, a patient's inability to adequately self-feed, dress, or propel a wheelchair could separately result from impairments in strength, endurance, cognition, comprehension, perception, sensation, coordination, balance, lack of motivation, or the presence of pain or fatigue. Furthermore, individual impairments may have multiple possible etiologies. For example, fatigue may directly result from a neurologic disease process, or it may indirectly result from depression, sedative side-effects of various medications, or a lack of adequate sleep. Similarly, a patient's inability to effectively concentrate and attend to therapies may result from impairments of cognition or perception resulting directly from neurologic disease, or indirectly resulting from depression, the side-effects of medications, or the distraction of pain. Thus, the role of assessment in neurorehabilitation includes clarification of etiologies contributing to a patient's disabilities so that appropriate therapeutic interventions may be undertaken at any point during the rehabilitation process. In addition, certain treatments may be contraindicated or recovery may be limited by comorbid chronic conditions such as cardiovascular disease, chronic pulmonary disease, cancer, musculoskeletal disorders, or psychiatric conditions. Evaluation and treatment of poorly controlled comorbid medical conditions will also improve neurorehabilitation outcomes.

NEUROREHABILITATION DURING ACUTE CARE

Neurorehabilitation intervention should begin following an acute hospitalization once a neurologic diagnosis has been established and life-threatening problems are controlled. Highest priorities are the prevention of secondary complications, maintenance of general health functions, early mobilization, and resumption of self-care activities. Immediate neurorehabilitation concerns include the maintenance of homeostasis and the prevention of complications that could result from the particular neurologic condition. Maintenance of homeostasis is a priority in all neurologic patients in the acute-care hospital setting. Routine continuous monitoring of basic health functions can help to prevent further disability. Included in any rehabilitation program are efforts to ensure regulation and adequacy of nutrition/hydration, bladder/bowel function, and sleep. In addition, measures are commonly undertaken to prevent deep vein thrombosis, pulmonary embolism, skin ulcerations, orthostasis, development of joint contractures, and pneumonia, which all may result from impaired mobility. In those patients with disorders of swallowing or cognition, efforts are also undertaken to prevent malnutrition and dehydration. The prevention of recurrent stroke is a concern in those individuals having acute cerebrovascular disorders. Autonomic dysreflexia is of concern in individuals having spinal cord injury or disorders. Autonomic dysfunction including cardiovascular dysfunction is of concern in patients with the acute Guillain-Barré syndrome (acute demyelinating polyneuropathies). In addition, efforts to prevent falls and accidental fractures or joint dislocations are undertaken in all patients who may be at risk.

MAINTENANCE OF HOMEOSTASIS

Dehydration and malnutrition may be consequences of neurologic disorders resulting in dysphagia, inability to self-feed, confusion, or inability to communicate hunger or thirst. Reduction of risk may include monitoring daily intake of liquids and calories, weekly determinations of body weight, and supervision with meals. A formal dysphagia assessment may be indicated in certain patients (see Management of Dysphagia and Aspiration).

Bladder dysfunction is another possible consequence of neurologic disease. Dysfunction may result from neurologic conditions causing bladder hypertonicity, bladder hypotonicity, and areflexia or hyperactivity of the internal or external sphincters. Often, a urologic consultation and urodynamic testing is necessary. Treatment may involve a program of bladder training that may include intermittent bladder catheterization, certain medications, and toileting at regular intervals. Use of indwelling Foley catheters is avoided with the exceptions of urinary retention that cannot otherwise be controlled, patients with extensive skin ulcerations, or if incontinence interferes with fluid and electrolyte-balance monitoring.

Bowel dysfunction, and particularly constipation or fecal impaction, may occur in neurologic disease as a result of immobility, inadequate nutrition (food or fluid), cognitive impairment, neurogenic bowel, and even depression or anxiety. Treatment measures include the assurance of adequate intake of fluids and fiber, establishment of a regular toileting schedule, and judicious use of stool softeners or laxatives.

Insomnia may occur as a direct result of a neurologic disorder, or it may result indirectly from comorbidities including depression, agitation, anxiety, the side effects of medications, muscle spasms, pain, inability to move in bed, urinary frequency or incontinence, or interruptions related to the hospital environment. Inadequate sleep can result in daytime drowsiness and inability to fully benefit from rehabilitation therapies. Goals of management include determination and treatment of a specific etiology if one exists, alteration of the environment if necessary to reduce disturbances of sleep, adjustment of type, timing, and dose of offending medications, and if all else fails, limited judicious use of hypnotic medications.

PREVENTION OF DEEP VEIN THROMBOSIS

Acute prolonged immobility, and particularly the paralysis of one or both legs, places an individual at risk for deep vein thrombosis (DVT) and pulmonary embolism. Randomized trials have shown effective risk reduction with use of subcutaneous low-dose heparin or low-molecular-weight heparin products. In addition, warfarin, intermittent pneumatic compression, early mobilization, and elastic stockings have been shown to be effective. Management of DVT risk in neurorehabilitation often includes early mobilization, elastic stockings, and, in the absence of contraindications, mini-dose subcutaneous heparin.

PREVENTION OF SKIN BREAKDOWN

Risk factors for skin breakdown include impaired cognition, poor mobility, incontinence, spasticity, and obesity. Steps to maintain skin integrity in those at risk include systemic daily inspection, gentle routine skin cleansing, protection from moisture, maintenance of hydration and nutrition, efforts to improve patient mobility, frequent turning and repositioning of immobile patients, and avoidance of skin pressure or friction. Prior to discharge from the acute-care hospital setting, patients or caretakers should be educated on skin care issues.

PREVENTION OF JOINT CONTRACTURES

A patient's potential for functional recovery may be limited by the restriction of movement or pain that results from joint contractures. The joints of spastic paretic limbs are most at risk for contractures. Simple prolonged disuse of an extremity can also result in contractures. For example, a comatose individual with spastic hemiparesis is at risk for bilateral plantar flexion contractures, with one plantar flexion contracture related to spasticity and the other related to simple disuse. Spasticity often develops in individuals having so-called upper motor neuron lesions that result from disorders involving the brain or spinal cord. Spasticity may involve one extremity (monoparesis) to all four extremities (quadriparesis), depending on the underlying pathologic process. Routine prevention of contractures often include antispastic limb positioning, frequent range-of-motion exercises with passive or active stretching, and splinting or bracing where necessary. Other treatment options to further limit the effects of spasticity or reduce early contractures may include medications, progressive casting, surgical correction (i.e., tendon-release procedures), motor point blocks, botulinum toxin injections, or an intrathecal baclofen pump. Antispasticity medications exist with various sites of action, ranging from effects at the central nervous system to effects at the muscle. Patients with early contractures in a monoparesis or hemiparesis pattern may benefit from botulinum toxin injections of involved muscles. Patients with spastic quadriparesis may benefit from placement of an intrathecal baclofen pump. In general, botulinum toxin or intrathecal baclofen may be indicated if reduction of spasticity/early contractures will improve functional independence, hygiene, or comfort, or will decrease risk of skin breakdown.

PREVENTION OF PNEUMONIA

Pneumonia is a common complication of neurologic illness. Risk factors include depressed cognition, swallowing disorders, and impaired mobility. Risk-reduction programs include efforts toward early mobilization as well as prevention of aspiration through modification of diet, alteration of means of nutrition intake if necessary, and proper positioning during feedings. Prolonged bed rest can result in poor aeration of the lungs, atelectasis, and a greater likelihood for development of pneumonia. Early patient mobilization can minimize this risk.

MANAGEMENT OF DYSPHAGIA AND ASPIRATION

Dysphagia occurs in certain neurologic conditions and may lead to aspiration pneumonia. Swallowing dysfunction can occur as a result of impaired cognition or from incoordination or weakness of the muscles of deglutition. Thus, swallowing is assessed prior to oral feedings in those patients who may be at risk (patients having strokes, brain injuries, neuromuscular diseases, etc.). Signs of possible dysphagia include dysarthria, confusion, frequent coughing, choking on fluids, nasal regurgitation, and pneumonia. Currently, the gold standard of diagnosis is a modified barium swallow study, which can help clarify the phase of swallowing that may be impaired. Goals of dysphagia management include the prevention of aspiration, dehydration, and malnutrition; and the restoration of the ability to chew and swallow safely. Treatment includes oral motor exercises, compensatory feeding strategies, modification of food textures, or alternative methods of feeding such as nasogastric tubes or percutaneous endoscopic gastrostomy tubes.

PREVENTION OF FALLS, FRACTURES, AND DISLOCATIONS

A goal of neurorehabilitation intervention includes ensuring patient safety by preventing falls. The risk of falls is increased in patients having sensorimotor deficits, confusion, or difficulty with communication. Methods to prevent falls vary with the type and severity of the disabilities. A risk-reduction program may include supervision of high-risk patients, toileting at regular intervals, supervision of transfers and ambulation, adapted nurse-call systems, and patient/family education. The use of restraints is avoided whenever possible, as restraints may lead to other injuries or cause greater agitation in those already restless.

Another concern is prevention of shoulder dislocations in patients with paretic upper extremities. There is a tendency for subluxation to occur at the shoulder joint capsule as a result of the gravitational pull from the weight of a paretic arm. Preventive measures include maintenance of normal scapulohumeral positioning through physical measures, use of lap trays on wheelchairs, use of pull-sheets during bed positioning, and avoidance of excessive range-of-motion exercises. Caution must be taken with lap trays, as improper use can lead to nerve injuries or wrist flexion contractures; furthermore, sling arm supports may promote upper extremity flexion contractures if used improperly. The differential diagnosis for shoulder pain in those with paretic upper extremities also includes rotator cuff tears, adhesive capsulitis, bicipital tendonitis, reflex sympathetic dystrophy, arthritis, and previous injuries.

PREVENTION IN SPECIFIC NEUROLOGIC DISORDERS

Patients who have had an ischemic stroke are at substantial risk for a recurrent stroke. Often, the acute care team will determine the need for carotid endarterectomy, or anticoagulation with warfarin, ticlopidine, or aspirin. Neurorehabilitation can help with patient/family education regarding potential modifiable risk factors including hypertension, diabetes mellitus, cigarette smoking, alcohol consumption, drug abuse, obesity, high serum cholesterol, coronary artery disease, left ventricular hypertrophy, and atrial fibrillation.

Spinal cord injuries and disorders can result in a potential for autonomic dysreflexia. This is more likely with high-level cord pathology. Autonomic dysreflexia manifests as precipitous drops or elevations in blood pressure or pulse, often accompanied by a pounding headache, hyperventilation, and flushing or sweating above the level of the lesion. The cause is usually a noxious stimulus involving a numb portion of the body detectable only to the autonomic nervous system. Possible causes may include a full bladder, a fecal impaction, tight-fitting clothing or shoes, a skin irritation, a DVT, or an infection. Prevention includes a routine bowel and bladder program, daily skin inspection, and careful dressing. Treatment of acute autonomic dysreflexia includes blood pressure stabilization as well as determination and correction of the etiology.

Autonomic dysfunction may also occur in the setting of acute demyelinating polyneuropathy (Guillain-Barré syndrome). Autonomic symptoms including sinus tachycardia, bradycardia, facial flushing, hypotension, or hypertension, and profuse diaphoresis or even anhydrosis can occur. In addition, urinary retention may also occur in some patients. The autonomic dysfunction associated with acute demyelinating polyneuropathies often remit after a few weeks. Treatment is supportive and expectant.

EARLY MOBILIZATION AND RETURN TO SELF-CARE

Another goal of acute neurorehabilitation intervention is early patient mobilization and the encouragement of self-care activities. Early mobilization helps to prevent DVT, skin breakdowns, pneumonia, joint contractures, and constipation; it promotes early ambulation, better orthostatic tolerance, and performance of basic activities of daily living. Early participation in self-care activities can help to increase strength, endurance, awareness, communication, problem solving, and social activity. Mobilization and the encouragement of self-care is beneficial as soon as a patient's medical and neurologic condition is stabilized, and, if possible, within 1 to 2 days of admission to the hospital. Early mobilization is delayed or approached with caution in patients with coma, obtundation, evolving neurologic signs, intracranial hemorrhage, DVT, or persistent orthostasis.

Mobilization may be passive or active at first, depending on a patient's condition. It will variably progress from ability to move in bed, to sitting in bed, to sitting up, to transferring, to operating a wheelchair, to standing and bearing weight, and eventually to walking. Basic self-care activities, including feeding, grooming, toileting, bathing, and dressing, are encouraged as soon as possible. Training in compensatory strategies and use of adaptive devices are offered to any patient having persistent disability with any aspect of mobility or self-care.

DISCHARGE FROM ACUTE CARE

Ideally, acute-care discharge planning should begin shortly after admission. Objectives of rehabilitation involvement in the discharge process include the determination of need for further rehabilitation services, helping to select the best discharge environment, educating the patient and caretakers regarding pertinent issues, and ensuring continuity of care. Patients or caretakers should be instructed on the effects and prognosis of the neurologic condition, the prevention of potential complications, and the need and rationale for further treatments. The patient and family are included in the discharge decision-making process whenever possible.

DETERMINATION OF REHABILITATION NEED AND SETTING

A patient's medical condition and the extent of functional disabilities are the most important determinants of need for neurorehabilitation services and the choice of an appropriate rehabilitation setting. The neurologic condition, medical comorbidities, ability to tolerate physical activity, and ability to learn are all important considerations. Rehabilitation services can be provided in a variety of programs and settings following discharge from acute care. Neurorehabilitation

may continue in an inpatient rehabilitation hospital or the rehabilitation unit of an acute-care hospital, in a nursing home, in the patient's home, or in an outpatient facility. Determination of an appropriate program is based on patient needs and capabilities.

REHABILITATION PROGRAM CRITERIA

Referrals for neurorehabilitation programs are usually made on patients in an acute-care hospital setting, but patients with chronic stable impairments and disabilities may also be referred from ambulatory care settings. The rehabilitation specialist physician will often be consulted to help facilitate the evaluation and transfer process. Determination of the most appropriate rehabilitation setting is based on strict criteria.

Threshold criteria for admission to any active rehabilitation program include medical stability, one or more persistent disabilities, the ability to learn, and the endurance to sit supported at least 1 hour per day. More debilitated patients may benefit from rehabilitation services at home or in a supported living setting. Candidates for intense interdisciplinary inpatient rehabilitation require total to moderate assistance in either mobility or self-care function and are able to tolerate at least 3 hours of active daily therapy. Candidates for outpatient rehabilitation programs include patients with limited mild functional deficits who are otherwise able to live independently and those requiring supervision to minimal assistance with mobility or self-care. Patients having complex medical problems are candidates for inpatient programs having 24-hour medical supervision.

In general, the inability to learn that results from a fixed static lesion is a contraindication to active neurorehabilitation. However, some patients may have cognitive deficits that are temporary and that have the potential to clear over time as a lesion resolves (e.g., some cases of brain swelling, multiple sclerosis, or traumatic brain injury). In such cases, a trial admission to an active rehabilitation program is warranted. Also, some patients who are unable to learn may still benefit from a course of passive rehabilitation, such as those with severe spasticity who may have recently received botulinum toxin injections or an intrathecal baclofen pump. In cases such as those, vigorous passive range-of-motion exercises may further help to reduce early contractures to allow better hygiene, to help decrease pain and discomfort, and to prevent skin breakdown. In addition, families and caretakers of such patients can benefit from education regarding pertinent care issues, including a program of passive range-of-motion exercises as well as other preventive care.

PROGRAMS AND SETTINGS

Freestanding rehabilitation hospitals and rehabilitation units in acute-care hospitals usually offer intense comprehensive programs staffed by a full range of rehabilitation professionals. A physician certified in neurorehabilitation or psychiatry is available at all times for patient management issues. General practitioners and specialist medical consultants are generally available as needed. Weekly interdisciplinary team care plan conferences are held and attended by the physician, nurse, and therapists to establish goals, to develop a plan to achieve goals, to assess patient progress, to identify barriers to progress, and to facilitate revision of goals and the management plan when necessary. These programs are active and require greater physical and cognitive effort from patients than would be necessary in other rehabilitation settings.

Rehabilitation programs also exist at nursing facilities, which also may be hospital based or freestanding. Staff, rehabilitation services, and physician coverage vary between facilities. Usually supportive care and low-level rehabilitation services (so-called subacute rehabilitation programs) are offered. Programs may provide 1 hour of selected rehabilitation services 5 days a week, or comprehensive therapies that may include physical, occupational, speech, psychology, and recreational therapies several hours per day. Interdisciplinary team care plan conferences are usually held every 2 weeks. These programs can accommodate patients who have the potential to later become suitable candidates for further rehabilitation at an inpatient hospital, at home, or in an outpatient rehabilitation program.

Outpatient rehabilitation facilities may also be hospital based or freestanding and can provide selected rehabilitation therapies or comprehensive programs. Services and intensity vary with patient needs from 1 hour to several hours of therapy per day, from 1 to 5 days per week. Team care plan conferences are often held monthly to review patient progress. These programs allow a patient to reintegrate into home life while providing necessary therapies, rehabilitation equipment, social contact, and peer support.

Home rehabilitation programs vary in capabilities from comprehensive services to selected rehabilitation therapies. These programs are designed for patients who are medically stable. Advantages include that skills will be learned and applied at home where they are most necessary and some patients may function better in a familiar environment. Disadvantages include absence of peer support (fellow patients), limited availability of specialized rehabilitation equipment, and increased burden on caregivers.

REHABILITATION MANAGEMENT PLAN

Upon admission to a neurorehabilitation program, a patient management plan is formulated by the rehabilitation physician and the therapy team. The rehabilitation management plan includes a clear description of a patient's impairments, disabilities, and strengths; explicit short- and long-term functional goals; and specification of treatment strategies to achieve goals and to prevent secondary complications. The objective is to devise short- and long-term goals that are realistic in terms of patient potential. Overly ambitious goals can set a patient up for failure, and overly modest goals can limit a patient's potential for recovery. A rehabilitation management care plan is reevaluated on a regular basis based on patient progress, and it may be adjusted as needed to suit patient needs. Typically, in an intense multidisciplinary inpatient program, the management plan and patient progress are reviewed on a weekly basis; in less intense rehabilitation programs, the care plan is reviewed monthly.

MANAGEMENT OF IMPAIRED MOBILITY

Disabilities involving mobility may result from impairment that can include muscle weakness, abnormal muscle tone, loss of joint range of motion, delayed response time, abnormal muscle synergy patterns, abnormal muscle contraction sequencing (motor apraxia), abnormal coordination or balance, lack of endurance, pain, and sensory impairments (especially proprioception). Prior to treatment, the specific cause of motor dysfunction and impaired mobility must be determined. Options for treatment may include a program of remediation/facilitation, compensation, or task-specific motor retraining. Some degree of volitional movement is required in an affected limb for remediation/facilitation to be effective. This approach includes traditional exercises, resistive training, and forced sensory stimulation modalities to improve limb strength and function. In the compensation approach, the goal is to improve a patient's level of functional independence in performing self-care activities by teaching compensatory strategies that involves the unaffected limbs. The compensation approach can result in learned nonuse of an impaired limb and therefore is reserved for patients with a poor prognosis for recovery of sensorimotor function, or those whose motor recovery has plateaued. A program of task-specific motor retraining involves some components of both remediation/facilitation and compensation as well as employing environmental cues to assist in enhancement of performance of specific tasks. This approach may be helpful for patients having motor apraxias. The effectiveness of these functional approaches may be enhanced by treatment of specific causes of impaired mobility such as spasticity, contractures, or chronic pain, and use of orthotic devices, braces, and adaptive equipment when necessary. Adjunct modalities that may also aid in functional recovery include biofeedback, functional electrical stimulation, and various computerized retraining devices. In summary, patients with some voluntary motor control are encouraged to use an affected limb in functional tasks. Patients unable to use an affected limb are taught compensatory strategies. Adaptive devices are used if more natural methods are not available or cannot be learned, and orthotic devices/braces are indicated if joint or limb stabilization will help improve function or ambulation.

MANAGEMENT OF IMPAIRED COGNITION

Limitations in cognition or perception are important in planning and conducting rehabilitation efforts, in preparation for functional safety upon discharge, and in predicting a patient's ability to resume vocational activities. Cognitive deficits may involve difficulties of concentration, attention, orientation, memory, perception, and executive function. Causes may include specific brain lesions and environmental or nonenvironmental distractors. Nonenvironmental distractors may include chronic pain, vertigo, lack of motivation, diplopia, visual loss, hearing loss, fatigue, impulsiveness, the side effects of medications, the effect of emotional disturbances (e.g., depression, anxiety, or agitation), or intermittent seizures such as nonconvulsive seizures or brief absence or psychomotor seizures. Environmental distractors can include aspects of the hospital routine that may prevent adequate sleep at night such as late medications or busy/noisy therapy areas. Prior to treatment, specific etiologies are identified and a relevant management plan is devised. A cognitive remediation program often includes the efforts of an occupational therapist, a speech therapist, and a psychologist. Treatments emphasize cognitive retraining, substitution of intact abilities, and compensatory strategies. Irreversible cognitive deficits

that absolutely preclude learning are a contraindication to active neurorehabilitation (see previous section, Rehabilitation Program Criteria).

MANAGEMENT OF COMMUNICATION DISORDERS

Impairments of speech and language may include aphasias, disorders of pragmatics (right hemisphere communication disorders), and difficulties related to dysarthria. Management varies with etiology and often involves the services of a speech therapist and a psychologist. Treatment of aphasia targets problems of comprehension or expression. Specific goals variably include improving ability to speak, comprehend, read, or write; developing strategies to compensate for persistent problems; addressing associated adjustment issues; and teaching caregivers to communicate with the patient. Goals of treatment for right-hemisphere language disorders (i.e., right-hemispheric strokes with left hemineglect) include increasing the awareness of deficits, reinstating the pragmatics of communication, and providing appropriate compensatory strategies. Treatment goals for dysarthria include improving intelligibility of speech through special exercises, and compensatory strategies such as manipulation of respiration, phonation, resonation, articulation, and prosody.

MANAGEMENT OF EMOTIONAL DYSFUNCTION

Emotional disturbances such as depression, anxiety, apathy, mania, agitation, delusions, hallucinations, personality changes, and obsessive/compulsive behavior may occur in association with certain neurologic conditions. The etiology of emotional dysfunction complicating a neurologic condition may be multifactorial. Possible causes include organic brain damage, exacerbation of a preexisting psychiatric condition or personality disorder, the side effects of medications, acute medical conditions (e.g., electrolyte disturbances, hypothyroidism, or hyperthyroidism), chronic pain, environmental factors (e.g., interruption of sleep), or a reaction to functional loss. Emotional dysfunction can adversely affect participation in active rehabilitation and long-term outcomes. Effective treatment depends on an accurate diagnosis of etiology. A psychiatry consultation may be indicated. Management may include psychotherapy, a brief course of a psychoactive medication, a program of maladaptive behavior modification, and addressing specific etiologies. A behavior-modification program will involve the interdisciplinary team in redirecting and discouraging socially inappropriate behaviors while encouraging appropriate conduct.

MANAGEMENT OF CHRONIC PAIN

The physiologic and psychological causes and effects of chronic pain are quite complex. Pain occurs in many forms and may involve any portion of the body. The stimulus for pain may arise at the level of the peripheral nerves, the autonomic nervous system, or the central nervous system. Etiologies may include static or progressive disorders involving soft tissues, joints, bones, the viscera (internal organs), the peripheral nerves or nerve roots, and the central nervous system. Pain could result from pathology related to the postoperative state, trauma, burns, and a host of other conditions including degenerative, inflammatory, infectious, metabolic, or neoplastic disorders. Environmental factors may interact with internal factors to result in pain. For example, individuals having muscle spasticity, contractures, or decubitus skin ulcers often experience pain when being moved or repositioned. Also, the perception of pain may be modified by certain psychological factors, which can contribute to the onset, severity, exacerbation, and maintenance of chronic pain. It is known that chronic anxiety or depression can adversely influence the subjective experience of pain, and similarly chronic pain can result in the onset of chronic anxiety or depression. The pattern of behavior resulting from chronic pain may include irritability, anger, dysphoric moods, loss of self-confidence or self-esteem, poor treatment compliance, and deterioration of important social relationships (possibly including the doctor–patient relationship). The subjective experience of chronic pain may also adversely affect cognitive functioning and overall functional recovery outcomes. Concentration, attention, mental alertness, and capacity to perform complex neuropsychological tasks may be reduced by the direct distraction of pain, or indirectly impaired by associated fatigue, sleep deprivation, depression, anxiety, poor motivation, or the effects of analgesics. In addition, physical capacity, including mobility and the ability to perform self-care activities, may be diminished by chronic pain.

The treatment of chronic pain involves the identification and correction of causal factors whenever possible. A course of opioid or nonopioid analgesic, anxiolytic, or antidepressant medications may be useful. Long-term use of narcotic or anxiolytic medications should be avoided with few exceptions (e.g., cancer pain). Often, a psychological evaluation and course of psychotherapy may be beneficial for adjust-

ment issues and associated affective dysfunction. If there are prominent signs of affective dysfunction, a psychiatry consultation may be necessary. Pain and other somatic complaints rooted in emotional dysfunction may be refractive to traditional treatments but responsive to psychopharmacologic intervention. Physical modalities that may be helpful in a pain management program include thermotherapy (hot packs, ultrasound, analgesic creams), cryotherapy (cold packs), transcutaneous electrical nerve stimulation, massage, progressive joint mobilization, acupressure or acupuncture, biofeedback, relaxation exercises, and movement education regarding proper body mechanics. Consultation with an anesthesia/pain specialist for local anesthesia, regional blocks, epidural analgesics, or sympathetic nerve blocks may be helpful to break a cycle of pain. Refractive cases may require a surgical consultation. For example, orthopedic surgeons may be able to replace painful degenerative joints. Neurosurgeons may be able to correct or ablate sources of chronic neuropathic pain. Finally, compensation issues should also be considered in certain cases as a possible source of chronic pain.

DISCHARGE PLANNING

Discharge planning is an integral part of a rehabilitation management plan and involves the interdisciplinary team, the patient, and the family or caregivers. Objectives include the education of the patient or caregivers and the determination of the best living environment if other than home, family or caregiver capabilities, home accessibility, special equipment needs, disability entitlements, the ability to return to work or to school, driving issues including handicap parking needs, need for further rehabilitation therapies such as vocational rehabilitation, and necessary community services including appropriate medical follow-up. Discharge occurs when reasonable treatment goals have been achieved. Reasonable treatment goals can include the progression from one level of functional dependence to a more independent level that is realistic for that patient. For example, discharge may be indicated when a patient who initially required total assistance in certain mobility or self-care activities progresses to a level of moderate or minimal assistance or supervision. In general, inpatients are discharged from intense comprehensive rehabilitation programs when they progress to a level of minimal assistance in mobility, which may include proficiency in wheelchair operation or progression to ambulation with the physical assistance of another person with use of an assistive device, and ability to assist caregivers with transfers.

Discharge from an outpatient program often occurs when a level of supervision to independence is reached in mobility and self-care activities. Absence of patient progress in mobility or self-care function on two successive care plan evaluations suggests a functional plateau and a need to reconsider the treatment regimen or the rehabilitation setting. Interdisciplinary care plan conferences are held weekly in intense comprehensive inpatient programs, and bimonthly to monthly in outpatient or subacute rehabilitation programs. These meetings are held to allow interdisciplinary team members the chance to update one another on patient progress and potential problems. The care plan meetings facilitate the formulation of individualized rehabilitation management plans, modifications of existing plans, and the discharge planning process.

A crucial aspect of the discharge planning process is the determination of the best living environment and family caregiver capabilities. Therapeutic weekend day passes are often encouraged during a comprehensive inpatient rehabilitation program to allow a patient and caregivers the opportunity to test their abilities at home and in the community. Thus, problem areas of community transition may be identified, allowing therapists to focus special attention prior to discharge. In addition, some programs allow therapists to perform home consultations to determine potential safety hazards and special home equipment needs (e.g., wheelchair ramps, grab bars), to help patients and caregivers rehearse the daily routine, and to assess accessibility of community facilities that may still be used by the patient following discharge. Whether a patient is discharged to home or to an alternative living facility depends in part on patient/caregiver preferences and a realistic assessment of patient/caregiver capabilities. For example, an elderly, chronically ill spouse may not be able to care for the patient unless full-time help is available at home. Also, patients who previously lived independently may no longer be able to do so. In addition, some patients may require temporary placement in a transitional living program in preparation for more independent living. In other cases, the availability of home health-care services including a home health aide and a visiting nurse may allow a patient to be discharged to the home setting.

Another important objective of the discharge planning process is patient or caregiver education and training regarding pertinent care issues and community transition. This includes prevention of complications, necessary techniques such as safe car transfers, home exercises, proper use of necessary adaptive equipment or braces, routine care needs such as bladder catheterization or the use of alternative feeding devices, instruction on medication administration or potential side effects, information regarding specific precautions such as driving or the use of machinery, information regarding sexual issues, information regarding available community services that may include vocational or recreational programs and support groups, and instructions regarding discharge follow-up and continued therapy needs. The importance of continuity of care is emphasized. Usually, the team case manager will assist the patient and caregivers in arranging for necessary community services such as home health care and outpatient therapies. In addition, arrangements are made for important medical follow-up that often includes the primary medical physician, the neurorehabilitation specialist, and all other treating specialist physicians. Prior to discharge, a patient's functional baseline is documented to help monitor subsequent progress and maintenance of function. Also, disability entitlements are addressed, such as handicap parking needs, certification of disabilities, and clarification of a patient's ability to return to work or school. If necessary, arrangements are also made for special educational or vocational programs. Whenever possible, adaptive equipment or strategies are offered to allow individuals the ability to return to work or school.

NEUROREHABILITATION FOLLOW-UP AND COMMUNITY TRANSITION

Gaps in medical follow-up increase risks for institutionalization of patients having certain disabilities. Therefore, routine medical follow-up is encouraged following discharge from a neurorehabilitation program. The frequency of recommended follow-up varies with patient needs. Responsibility for coordination of outpatient medical care, rehabilitation services, and determination of further rehabilitation needs rests with the primary care physician, who may be the previous treating family physician, internist, pediatrician, or rehabilitation specialist. Goals of follow-up include assessment of a patient's health status, safety at home and in the community, and maintenance of function. In addition, if applicable, the follow-up physician should assess adequacy of family or caregiver interventions. Areas of concern include medical, physical, cognitive, emotional, and social function. Problems may develop once an individual begins to attempt resumption of previous community activities and social relationships. This is when the full impact of disabilities resulting from a neurologic condition may become apparent to the patient or the family. Changes in traditional family roles may also have profound consequences on the patient or the family members. Support groups and psychotherapy may be useful in certain situations. Also, the ability of a family member or caretaker to provide effective care for a patient with severe disabilities must be constantly reevaluated. Even committed caregivers may reach a point of desperation when providing continuous support without relief. Another concern is a patient's ability to maintain functional levels previously achieved during a rehabilitation program. Loss of function may occur secondary to exacerbation of medical comorbid conditions or the neurologic disorder, or from lack of stimulation, lack of self-confidence, physical barriers to activity, or inadvertent suppression of initiation by over-protective caregivers.

The need for continued or additional rehabilitation services also must be considered. Further outpatient rehabilitation needs vary with a patient's progress in an existing program and the extent of remaining disabilities. Goals of further rehabilitation services may include encouragement of recreational activities and the return to work or school. Specific rehabilitation programs exist to assess the capacity to perform certain activities such as the ability to drive or to return to work-related physical activities. Work-capacity assessments are available. In addition, handicap driving programs exist to assess driving safety as well as to teach adaptive strategies. The ability to drive is influenced by an individual's impairments, including visual/spatial and cognitive function. Adaptive driving instruction programs are available for appropriate patients. Another follow-up concern includes sexual function issues. Adaptive strategies, devices, and counselling can enhance sexual function in patients with disabilities and can even allow sexual reproduction for patients with spinal cord injuries. In summary, in an attempt to maximize quality of life and functional independence, neurorehabilitation outpatient follow-up concerns include medical, physical, cognitive, emotional, and social aspects of patient function during the transition back into the community.

NEUROREHABILITATION OUTCOMES

The effectiveness of a medical treatment may be measured in terms of biologic or functional changes in an individual, and cost efficiency. The biologic effectiveness of a medical treatment can be assessed in terms of changes in an impairment rating such as the degree of sensory loss, spasticity, or weakness. The functional effectiveness of a medical treatment may be measured by changes in disability or handicap scores. The cost efficiency of a medical treatment may be measured in terms of relative monetary savings or losses to the payer in relation to the outcome, which may include length of hospital stay or an individual's ability to return to work, school, or independent living. Variables that may complicate the assessment of a specific medical treatment outcome on an individual may include age, sex, social factors such as prior education, coexistent chronic medical or psychological problems, the effects of other treatments, and patient compliance. Numerous prior and ongoing outcome studies exist regarding the effectiveness of neurorehabilitation in terms of various neurologic impairments, disabilities, handicaps, and cost efficiency. The goal of these studies has been to determine the most effective and cost-efficient neurorehabilitation approaches for a host of specific neurologic impairments or disorders, while considering possible individual variables. Already, a number of specific neurorehabilitation interventions have been shown to be effective for a variety of impairments (e.g., various speech therapy language exercises for certain aphasias or dysphasias, and various occupational therapy/physical therapy interventions for certain problems of mobility). In addition, the multidisciplinary rehabilitation team approach has been shown to be effective in a variety of neurologic disorders such as stroke and traumatic brain or spinal cord injury. National collaborative rehabilitation outcome studies should continue to provide useful data for determination of model systems of care for a host of neurologic conditions and disorders.

QUESTIONS AND DISCUSSION

1. A 51-year-old woman with a history of multiple substance abuse developed difficulty swallowing. Two days later, she developed an acute onset of paraplegia and was admitted for an evaluation. She was diagnosed with an extensive retropharyngeal abscess with compression of the cervical spinal cord. She underwent surgical drainage of the abscess and was started on broad-spectrum intravenous antibiotics. One month later, she presents for neurorehabilitation with incomplete quadriplegia with four-fifths strength in the both arms and two-fifths strength at both legs. A low cervical sensory level is present, below which there is partial pin prick and light touch sensation to the toes. An

indwelling Foley catheter is in place and there is a small area of superficial skin breakdown at the sacrum involving only the epidermis.

The indwelling Foley catheter should be removed.

A. True
B. False

The answer is (A). This is a middle-aged woman presenting for neurorehabilitation with incomplete quadriplegia secondary to a compressive cervical myelopathy and having an area of superficial skin breakdown at her sacrum. The indwelling Foley catheter should be removed on admission and a program of bladder training should be started. Initially, bladder catheterizations should be performed at least every 6 hours, and postvoid residuals should be monitored closely. Bladder catheterization frequency may be tapered as postvoid residuals diminish. A urology consultation may be helpful in determining medications that may hasten recovery of bladder function. Superficial skin breakdown is not a contraindication to removal of the Foley catheter. However, if the area of skin ulceration penetrated through the dermis into the soft tissue or muscle, then Foley catheter removal might be contraindicated. Moisture from urine incontinence can contribute to further skin ulceration.

Short-term rehabilitation goals should include:

A. Patient/family education
B. Prevention of secondary complications
C. Compensatory strategies and strengthening
D. All of the above

The answer is (D). Short-term neurorehabilitation goals in this patient would include patient/family education, prevention of secondary complications, strengthening of deconditioned muscles and provision of compensatory strategies to overcome functional disabilities. Long-term prognosis for recovery of ambulation in this patient is fair, as there is already some movement and sensation present in both legs.

2. A previously healthy 49-year-old man developed progressive weakness that started in his legs following a flulike illness. A workup included a lumbar puncture, which demonstrated an elevated protein, and an electromyographic nerve conduction study that showed nerve demyelination with axonal involvement. He was diagnosed with Guillain-Barré syndrome and underwent a course of plasmapheresis. On admission for neurorehabilitation 2 months later, he presents with flaccid quadriplegia, with the ability to shrug his shoulders. Proprioception is intact down to the ankles but is absent at the toes. Reflexes are absent. Bulbar muscles are not involved.

Secondary complications here may include:

A. Dysautonomia
B. Pneumonia
C. Contractures
D. Skin breakdown
E. All of the above

At admission, ambulation should be set as a long-term neurorehabilitation goal in this patient.

A. True
B. False

The answer to the first part is (E), and the answer to the second part is (B). This is a middle-aged man who presents for neurorehabilitation with complete flaccid quadriplegia following an episode of acute demyelinating polyneuropathy with axonal involvement. He is at risk for complications of immobility including pneumonia, contractures, DVT, and skin breakdown. In addition, he is at risk for orthostasis and dysautonomia. The latter is a rare complication of Guillain-Barré syndrome that occurs most often during the acute illness rather than the convalescence. Ambulation would be an unrealistic long-term rehabilitation goal at the time of his admission, as he is presenting as a flaccid quadriplegic. However, many patients with acute demyelinating polyneuropathies present for rehabilitation with flaccid quadriplegia 1 to 2 months after onset of their illness and later recover the ability to ambulate. Therefore, ambulation would not be an impossibility in this patient. Short-term rehabilitation goals here would include patient education, prevention of secondary complications, and gradual mobilization with passive range-of-motion exercises to help strengthen deconditioned muscles and prevent development of contractures. Motor recovery may be delayed in this patient, as his polyneuropathy involves both demyelination and axonal nerve damage. Motor recovery occurs more rapidly in those individuals having only demyelination.

3. A 70-year-old woman underwent a coronary artery bypass graft and suffered a left hemispheric stroke 3 days later. Her hospital stay was complicated by pneumonia. Three weeks later, she is transferred for neurorehabilitation with a nasogastric feeding tube in place, expressive aphasia, a flaccid right arm, and two-fifths strength present in the right leg. She is able to follow simple commands. Mood and affect are flat to tearful.

The nasogastric feeding tube should be removed and a trial pureed diet with thickened liquids should be started:

A. True
B. False

Short-term rehabilitation goals in this patient should include:

A. Compensatory strategies
B. Bracing and splinting to enhance function and prevent contractures
C. Patient/family education
D. All of the above

The answer to the first part is (B), and the answer to the second part is (D). This is an elderly woman presenting for neurorehabilitation 3 weeks after the onset of a left hemispheric stroke. There is a nasogastric feeding tube in place that should not be removed until a swallowing study is performed to evaluate for aspiration. Previous history of pneumonia is suggestive of aspiration. A modified barium swallow study can be performed to document safety in all phases of swallowing with various food textures. Compensatory swallowing strategies are available for certain types of dysphagia, but a temporary alternative means of feeding may be necessary in patients at high risk for aspiration. Short-term rehabilitation goals in this patient should include compensatory strategies to overcome functional disabilities, bracing and splinting to enhance function and prevent contractures, prevention of secondary complications, and patient/family education. Gradual recovery of some functional abilities is likely in this patient. Prognosis for functional recovery is best in those having ability to comprehend and learn. Rehabilitation is still possible, though more difficult, in patients with receptive aphasias or hemineglect.

4. A 14-year-old boy was involved in a motor vehicle accident. He remained comatose for 5 days following admission. He was found to have a left ankle fracture and diffuse axonal brain injury. Three weeks later, on transfer for neurorehabilitation, he is restless and agitated with poor concentration and attention. He is nonverbal but attempts to follow some simple commands. There is diminished movement on the left side. A nasogastric feeding tube is in place and the left ankle is casted.

This patient is at risk for:

A. Falls
B. Inadvertent removal of a medical device
C. Elopement from the rehabilitation facility

Initial measures to ensure safety should include:

A. Redirection
B. Vail bed
C. Medications
D. One-to-one supervision
E. Restraints

The answers to the first part are (A) and (B). The answers to the second part are (A) and (D). This is a young man presenting for neurorehabilitation with a severe traumatic brain injury. He is confused, restless, and agitated, which places him at risk for falls and inadvertent removal of the nasogastric tube. Elopement from the facility is less likely as he is hemiparetic and confused. Initial measures to ensure safety would include one to one supervision. Redirection alone is unlikely to be successful, as he is confused with poor attention and concentration. A vail bed or restraints would most likely result in further agitation. Medications may be effective if one-to-one supervision fails to ensure safety and to redirect impulsive or aggressive behavior.

Cognitive improvement is expected in this patient:

A. True
B. False

The answer is (A). Cognitive improvement is expected. Cognitive function is most likely to improve in patients having traumatic brain injuries where coma lasted 13 days or less. These individuals will generally have selective impairments on neuropsychological testing at 1 year following injury. Those individuals having coma lasting 2 weeks to 29 days are more likely to have impairments in all areas of cognitive function at 1 year following trauma. More than half of those individuals having coma lasting more than 29 days will remain severely impaired in all areas of cognitive function 1 year following injury.

SUGGESTED READING

Delisa JA (ed): Rehabilitation Medicine. Principles and Practice. Philadelphia, JB Lippincott, 1993

Dikmen S, Machamer JE: Neurobehavioral outcomes and their determinants. J Head Trauma Rehabil 10:74, 1995

Dobkin BH: Impairments, disabilities and bases for neurological rehabilitation after stroke. J Stroke Cerebrovasc Dis 6:221, 1997

Gordon J: Assumptions underlying physical therapy intervention: Theoretical and historical perspectives. In: Carr J, Shepherd RB, Gordon J et al (eds): Movement Science Foundations for Physical Therapy in Rehabiliation. Rockville, MD, Aspen, 1987

Granger CV, Hamilton BB: UDS report: The uniform data system for medical rehabilitation report on the first admissions for 1990. Am J Phys Med Rehabil 71:108, 1992

Gresham GE, Duncan PW, Stason WB et al: Post-stroke rehabilitation: Clinical practice guideline. Rockville, MD, US Department of Health and Human Services (Agency for Healthcare Policy and Research), 1995

Hamilton BB, Laughlin JA, Granger CV, Kayton RM: Interater agreement of the seven level functional independence measures (FIM). Arch Phys Med Rehabil 72:790, 1991

Rothberg JS: The rehabilitation team: Future direction. Arch Phys Med Rehabil 62:407, 1981

Sivak M, Hill CS, Henson DL et al: Improved driving performance following perceptual training in persons with brain damage. Arch Phys Med Rehabil 65:163, 1984

Soderback I: The effectiveness of training intellectual functions in adults with acquired brain damage: An evaluation of occupational therapy methods. Scand J Rehabil Med 20:47, 1988

Umphred DA (ed): Neurological Rehabilitation. St. Louis, CV Mosby, 1990

Wade DT: Measurement in neurological rehabilitation. Oxford, Oxford University Press, 1992

Neurology for the Non-Neurologist, Fourth Edition,
edited by William J. Weiner and
Christopher G. Goetz. Lippincott
Williams & Wilkins, Philadelphia © 1999.

C H A P T E R   2 9

Medical–Legal Issues in the Care of the Patient with Neurologic Illness

Lois Margaret Nora
Robert E. Nora

In recent years, legal aspects of medical practice have assumed greater visibility and importance. This has been particularly apparent in the care of patients with neurologic disease. Although increased attention to medical–legal aspects of patient care are not welcomed by all, it is unlikely that the emphasis will diminish. Knowledge of, and comfort with, legal aspects of medical practice can contribute to optimal medical care.

Medical practice is affected by laws from three major sources: case, statutory, and administrative law. *Case law* (also called common law) is developed in the judicial system through the resolution of various criminal and civil matters. An important role of the courts is to interpret the various statutes passed by different legislative bodies. State and federal courts exist in parallel, and appellate review is available in both systems.

Many physicians are most concerned with this aspect of the legal system because of the recent increase in malpractice lawsuits. Malpractice cases are civil actions. Most malpractice cases allege that the physician was negligent in the care of the plaintiff. To win a lawsuit alleging negligence, the plaintiff must demonstrate by a preponderance of the evi-

dence (1) that the physician had a duty of care to the patient; (2) that the physician breached that duty; and (3) that the breach proximately caused injury to the plaintiff. Expert testimony must be used in most medical malpractice cases to establish what the physician's duty was and whether or not it was breached. In addition to proving his case, the plaintiff must also successfully counter any defenses brought by the physician.

It is important to be aware of the other sources of law that affect medical practice. *Statutory law* is developed by local, state, or federal legislative bodies and applies to persons within the jurisdictions of those legislatures. Federal and state laws on medical malpractice, abortion, living wills, and termination of treatment are examples of statutory laws. Variation in laws among different jurisdictions is common. The court system frequently is involved in interpreting statutes and in resolving conflicts that arise between different jurisdictions.

A third source of rules that may affect health care is *administrative law*. Some government agencies are empowered to make and enforce rules related to their specific activities; these rules constitute administrative law. The Internal Revenue Service, for example, has broad authority to make and enforce rules about the collection of taxes. Government agencies whose rulings impact medical practice include the Food and Drug Administration (FDA), state and federal drug enforcement agencies, and the Occupational Health and Safety Administration (OSHA), among others.

This chapter addresses three specific areas where medical and legal matters interface in the care of patients with neurologic illness. First, informed consent, a legal doctrine that affirms patient self-determination, is presented. The discussion then turns toward the aspects of brain death in clinical practice. The chapter concludes with a discussion of the common problem of licensing drivers with a seizure disorder.

INFORMED CONSENT

Informed consent has been recognized as a legal requirement for nearly a century.[1] Informed consent doctrine supports individual autonomy and states that patients have the right to understand proposed interventions (diagnostic and therapeutic, including medication) and to voluntarily consent to or reject those interventions. Unfortunate instances demonstrate that, even in recent years, medical and scientific practitioners have not always conformed to these expectations.[2,3]

Several assurances are necessary for informed consent. First, the patient must be competent. Second, the patient must be provided with understandable and adequate information about a proposed intervention. Third, the patient's consent must be given voluntarily.

A patient must be competent to give informed consent. In order to be competent to give informed consent, the patient must be *both* legally and clinically competent. Adults are presumed to be legally competent unless they have been legally declared incompetent. In general, minors are not considered legally competent. However, there are exceptions. A minor who has been legally emancipated is considered legally competent to make medical decisions. Also, some minors are legally competent to provide consent for certain interventions but not for others. For example, in some states, adolescents are legally competent to make reproductive health decisions, despite lacking legal competence to make other medical care decisions. When a person is legally incompetent, the appointed guardian should be approached to obtain consent.

Legal competence, by itself, is not enough. A person must also be clinically competent. Clinical competence implies that the patient can understand information, formulate a decision, and communicate his/her decision. Assistive devices (e.g., hearing aids, communication boards) can be helpful in maintaining a patient's clinical competence. Clinical competence is a medical decision. In some situations, not uncommonly in the setting of neurologic illness, a person may be legally competent but not clinically competent. Dementia, encephalopathy, and other conditions may render the patient incapable of providing informed consent for a variable period of time.

In the event of clinical incompetence, medical treatment can proceed in an emergency situation. Attempts should be made to contact members of the patient's family to obtain approval for the intervention, although their consent is not legally necessary if the treatment is a medical necessity.

In situations when consent from an incompetent person is not possible, two legal tests have been used to determine whether or not an intervention should proceed. These tests are *substituted judgment* and *best interest*. The substituted judgment test reviews the patient's prior actions, comments, and beliefs in an effort to determine what decision the patient would have made. The best interest approach looks at all the facts of the case and attempts to identify the action that would be in the best interest of the incompetent patient.

A judgment of legal and/or clinical incompetence for certain medical decision making should not preclude the patient's ability to participate in other decisions. Every attempt should be made to allow continued decision making by the patient (e.g., even as basic as what to eat for dinner).

The second requirement for informed consent is that adequate information be provided to the patient in an understandable fashion. Although other health-care personnel may be involved in obtaining consent, the physician remains responsible for ensuring adequate information provision as well as the other aspects of informed consent. Information provided to the patient should include the nature and purpose of the proposed intervention, its risks and anticipated benefits, alternatives to the proposed interventions, prognosis without the intervention, and prognosis with alternative interventions. The patient should be told of his rights to refuse and to withdraw a consent at any time.

The adequacy of information provided to a patient can be an issue in malpractice suits. Two different legal standards of information disclosure are recognized: the *professional standard* and the *material risk standard*. The professional standard requires the physician to give the patient information that other physicians of the same specialty, in the same community, would give to patients considering the same intervention. Expert testimony is necessary to delineate what this information consists of. This is the older of the two standards and is currently the choice of most courts.

The material risk standard requires the physician to provide any information that a reasonable person in the patient's position would want disclosed or would use in making a consent decision. Advocates of this standard identify its emphasis on the patient's need for information. Opponents point to its retrospective application as a major disadvantage.

The most appropriate approach is probably a hybrid. Physicians should communicate those risks that occur with great enough frequency or that are so severe, even if infrequent, that a usual patient would wish to know of them. For example, patients should be advised of the possibility of hirsutism and gingival hyperplasia with phenytoin use, and they should be given information about spinal headaches prior to lumbar puncture. In addition, if a physician is aware of a particular characteristic of a patient that would make a potential side effect more important to that patient, this side effect should be communicated, even if not generally discussed. For example, potential teratogenic effects of medications should be discussed with female patients who may become pregnant.

A third requirement of informed consent is that the patient must give consent voluntarily. Coercion invalidates consent. A physician should provide patients with advice and guidance regarding proposed therapies, but this must be done in a noncoercive way. No explicit or implicit threat of loss of medical or nursing care should be linked to a decision.

Consent discussion should be documented in the patient record. A patient-signed consent is not required for valid consent, but it can provide evidence of decision making by the patient. Prepared consent forms can be helpful, but the value of these documents should not be overestimated. Courts are suspicious of complicated documents that appear to be written to protect the physician rather than inform the patient.

Care must be taken that interventions remain within the scope of the consent given by the patient. Consent is given for a particular procedure and other procedures that are within the scope of that procedure or that can be reasonably expected. Consent is usually given to a particular individual and those working with that individual. The physician should not overextend the consent to procedures that are not logically associated with the consent or to personnel not reasonably anticipated by the patient.

In certain circumstances, an intervention can proceed without informed consent. Some exceptions to informed consent exist. In emergency situations, when there is significant, immediate risk to the patient, necessary therapy can proceed. A competent patient may waive his right to informed consent: the patient decides to "let the doctor decide." Although courts recognize patient waiver of informed consent, physicians should take care that waiver decisions are documented carefully, and they may wish to have the patient put the waiver in writing.

Therapeutic privilege is another exception to informed consent. This exception is used when the physician determines that an informed consent discussion will prove so detrimental to the patient's health that it should not be done. For example, some physicians have used this exception to justify not disclosing the risk of tardive dyskinesia when neuroleptic medications are prescribed to certain patients who, they fear, will refuse a potentially beneficial medication because of a severe, but unlikely, side effect.

Physicians must be extremely cautious in their use of therapeutic privilege. Courts may not be sympathetic to physicians' defending their use of therapeutic privilege when confronted by an uninformed patient who has suffered severe side effects. If a physician feels the use of therapeutic privilege is absolutely necessary, involving the patient's family in the decision may be beneficial. In addition, complete disclosure to the patient at the earliest opportunity is also advisable. The physician should keep contemporaneous clear documentation of reasons for the decision.

The right of a patient to give informed consent carries with it an obvious recognition of the patient's right of informed refusal. Patients have a legal right to refuse interventions, even if the refusal will result in the patient's death. Education and persuasion of the patient are the tools usually available to the physician confronted by a refusal. Physicians must inform patients of potential problems related to refusing a potential intervention, and this should also be documented.

Informed refusal is not an absolute right. Certain exceptions to the patient's right to refuse an intervention have been recognized, and judicial intervention is possible in certain situations. Courts will not permit informed refusal to be used as a means to commit suicide and may override a patient's refusal if deemed necessary for the protection of innocent third parties. The court may modify a patient's refusal in order to protect the standards of the medical profession or of an institution.

Legal proceedings against physicians for failure to obtain informed consent may take two forms. A physician may be sued for battery, an intentional unconsented-to touching of an individual (the patient) by another (the physician). As an intentional tort, punitive damages (monetary damages meant to punish the physician, not just recompense the patient) may be available if a physician is found liable. Except in extreme cases when no consent was obtained or when misrepresentation or fraud was used to obtain the consent, it is unlikely that battery will be alleged. The fact that malpractice insurance coverage is usually not available for intentional torts may also limit the use of a battery action by plaintiffs.

More commonly, failure to obtain informed consent will lead to a negligence suit. To win, the plaintiff must demonstrate by a preponderance of the evidence that (1) the injury sustained was a known risk of the therapy, (2) the physician failed to meet the applicable standard of care regarding information about the risk that caused the injury, and (3) the patient would not have consented to the therapy if the information had been provided. If these things are proved, the plaintiff can succeed, even if the sustained injury was a known complication of the intervention and did not result through any fault of the physician.

In summary, physicians remain responsible for informed consent even when others are involved in obtaining it. Information given to patients should be adequate and understandable. Patients must be legally and clinically competent, and assent to interventions must be given voluntarily. Written documentation may help provide evidence of patient decision making, although written documentation is neither required nor guaranteed to relieve the physician of liability.

In the case of legal incompetence, guardians should be approached for consent. When a patient is legally competent but clinically incompetent, medical care can proceed in an emergency situation. Intervention by the courts may be necessary in determining nonemergency care for incompetent patients.

In the case of informed refusal, care must be taken to inform the patient of risks of refusal. Although informed refusal is allowed, even when misguided or life threatening, courts do recognize exceptions to the doctrine. Excellent medical and nursing care should continue regardless of a patient's individual treatment decisions.

BRAIN DEATH

Death was traditionally defined clinically by the lack of cardiac and pulmonary functioning. In recent years, medical and technological advances make artificial ventilation and continued cardiac rhythm possible even when death of the brain has occurred. As a result, it is necessary to recognize that irreversible and total brain death is an additional means of demonstrating death of the patient.

The concept that irreversible coma was equivalent to death was first articulated by the Harvard criteria in 1968.[4] A National Institutes of Health Collaborative Study in 1977 studied brain death further, and in 1981 the President's Commission for the Study of Ethical Problems in Medicine and Biomedical and Behavioral Research published a treatise on the issue.[5, 6] In 1980, the United States Uniform Determination of Death Act codified brain death as a legally acceptable definition of death, and states were encouraged to adopt this law.[7] These studies and opinions have contributed to a gradual acceptance in the United States of brain death as a medical and legal criterion for death. Practice parameters and diagnosis guidelines for brain death have been developed in recent years.[8,9]

The laws of most states currently define death as either the irreversible cessation of circulation and pulmonary functioning *or* the irreversible cessation of complete brain functioning. This does not imply that there are two types of death. Instead, two mechanisms for determining death in a given patient are delineated.

There are two critical aspects in the determination of brain death: (1) the total cessation of functioning of the total brain (including the brainstem) and (2) the irreversibility of the condition. Potential legal difficulties related to brain death can be avoided by a rigorous medical approach to establishing the condition. In addition, careful and considerate communication with the patient's family members contributes to optimal medical care and the avoidance of legal problems.

The diagnosis of brain death should be made by one familiar with the process. This will usually be a neurologist, neurosurgeon, or critical care specialist. Any physician with a real or perceived conflict of interest in the diagnosis (e.g., member of a transplant team) should not be involved in making the diagnosis.

A diagnosis of brain death is established in three interrelated steps. First, an etiology should be established, and certain conditions that can mimic brain death, but are reversible, must be excluded. The second step is the clinical evaluation of the patient. Third, laboratory tests provide confirmation of the diagnosis and prognosis. Careful attention to these three steps will ensure that complete cessation of brain functioning and its irreversibility are established. Physicians should also be aware of any specific institutional requirements for establishing brain death. For example, some institutions require certain tests or a formal checklist approach.

Certain prerequisites are necessary for a diagnosis of brain death. The brain death criteria to be discussed have been established for adults; these criteria should not be used in children under 5 years of age. Specific consultation with experts in pediatric neurology and critical care should be obtained when diagnosing brain death in a young child.

The reason for the patient's condition must be known. In general, brain death should not be diagnosed without a clear etiology. The most common causes of brain death are head trauma, intracerebral hemorrhage, and anoxia following a cardiopulmonary arrest. A careful history, a careful examination, and various laboratory tests (e.g., computed tomographic scanning) may be helpful in determining the etiology.

Medical conditions that can mimic brain death must be ruled out prior to making a diagnosis of brain death. These include hypothermia, metabolic dysfunction, and drug intoxication. In the setting of hypothermia, the temperature must be corrected prior to a diagnosis. Barbiturate and anesthetic agents are the most frequently implicated drugs in this setting, but tricyclic antidepressants and other medications have also been reported. In the setting of drug intoxication, endocrine derangement, or metabolic dysfunction, brain death can be established only after correction of the problem or with demonstration of lack of cerebral circulation.

The second component of the brain death evaluation is the clinical examination. The clinical examination establishes the total absence of brain (cerebral and brainstem) functioning and helps rule out those conditions that may mimic brain death. The patient must be in deep coma unresponsive to any external stimuli, including pain. Any form of purposeful response, seizure activity, or decerebrate or decorticate posturing is inconsistent with the diagnosis of brain death.

All activities, including reflexes, mediated by the cortex and the brainstem must be absent. Pupils are usually dilated but may be midpoint. The light reflex must be absent. Other brainstem reflexes, including doll's eye, calorics, corneal, gag, swallow, and cough, must be absent.

The brainstem controls respiration, and the evaluation of brain death should include formal apnea testing to rule out the ability of the brainstem to maintain respiration. Following extended ventilation with 90% to 100% oxygen, the patient is discontinued from the respirator. Arterial blood gases are drawn, and an endotracheal catheter with 100% oxygen running at 6 liters is placed. If the patient has had no spontaneous respiratory efforts after 5 minutes, blood gases are redrawn and the patient placed once again on the ventilator. If a $PaCO_2$ of 60 is not obtained, testing should continue with gradual prolongation of the off-ventilator period until this level is reached. If no spontaneous respiratory attempts are made with a $PaCO_2$ of 60, it can be said with confidence that the patient has no spontaneous respiration.

Although brainstem reflexes are completely absent with brain death, certain spinal-mediated reflexes can be preserved. The presence of these reflexes does not preclude the diagnosis, and it is important that members of the health-care team and the patient's family are aware that such movements do not constitute purposeful activity. Confirmatory tests are mandatory when specific components of clinical testing cannot be reliably evaluated.

The third aspect of a brain death evaluation is laboratory testing. These tests can help rule out conditions that can mimic brain death, confirm the neurologic examination, and establish the irreversibility of the condition.

The electroencephalogram (EEG) has been an important part of brain death evaluation for many years. Care must be taken to obtain a technically acceptable EEG when evaluating a patient for brain death; this can be difficult in the intensive care setting. The presence of cortical activity on an EEG is inconsistent with a diagnosis of brain death. Extended electrocerebral silence (ECS), although consistent with brain death, is not pathognomonic for the process. ECS can be seen in certain reversible conditions, including drug overdose.

Evoked potentials can also be helpful in making the diagnosis of brain death. Evoked potentials may be less likely than other EEG activity to be affected in certain metabolic conditions. The presence of cortical and brainstem evoked responses rules out brain death. The absence of evoked potentials is confirmatory, but not absolute, evidence.

The complete cessation of blood flow to the nor-mothermic adult brain for 10 minutes or more is incompatible with life. Blood flow studies that demon-strate no intracranial circulation for 10 minutes or more provide compelling and conclusive evidence of irreversible brain death. Cerebral blood flow studies, by way of angiography or radionuclide imaging, can be very helpful in the diagnosis of brain death.

It is critically important that adequate time be allowed for complete evaluation and serial observa-tions of the patient during the determination of brain death. Repeat clinical examination 6 hours after the first is recommended. The time necessary to reach the diagnosis will vary depending on the etiol-ogy of the patient's condition, the clinical expertise of the examiner, and the use of various diagnostic tests. Generally, the patient should be observed for at least 12 hours. In some instances, this time period may be shortened, but confirmatory diagnostic test-ing is critically important in these shorter time peri-ods. Pressure for organ harvesting and other con-cerns should not prevent the careful and complete process necessary to reach the diagnosis.

Some legal difficulties related to brain death have resulted from poor communication with the patient's family members. Probably the most frequent error in the clinical setting, as well as in literature about brain death, is the suggestion that the brain-dead patient is somehow still alive. This is usually done by referring to the brain as dead but the body as alive. For exam-ple, a family member is told the "patient is dead [because of brain death], but we are keeping the body alive [because of desire for organ donor possi-bilities]." This is confusing information for the fam-ily, made more so by the chest movements created by the ventilator and the cardiac rhythm bleeping on a monitor. The situation is further complicated if activ-ities around the patient elicit some form of spinal reflex response.

It is extremely important to communicate that brain death is one way that death is diagnosed and that brain death *is death*. Families must be helped to understand that their loved one is dead. Continued pharmaco-logic and technological supports should be described in terms of perfusing organs (particularly when the specific organs are being considered for donation) rather than keeping the body alive. Pharmacologic and technological support should be discontinued as soon as feasible following the diagnosis of brain death; allowing families their good-byes prior to discontinua-tion of machinery may be appropriate, but extended technological support of dead bodies is not.

Although organ harvesting is possible in the ab-sence of family consent (e.g., when there is a valid donor card), physicians will usually not do so without family consent. From a risk-management perspective, this is appropriate. When there is a possibility of organ donation, it should be discussed with the fam-ily early in the care of the patient by persons un-involved in diagnostic and treatment decisions about the patient. Many organ procurement programs have personnel specially trained to perform these tasks. In no event should undue pressure be exerted on fam-ily members to consent to organ harvesting. One institution was successfully sued for refusing to dis-continue organ support systems and release the body of a brain-dead teenager to his family while physi-cians persisted in encouraging the family to consent to organ harvesting.[10]

Somatic death inevitably follows brain death within several days. When there are no organ harvesting con-siderations, there may be fewer pressures to declare the patient brain dead and discontinue treatment. This may be a particularly tempting course of action when there is family dissension about terminating organ support systems. Nonetheless, this course of action must be balanced against the ethics of using lim-ited resources (including nursing and medical support staff) to support a corpse.

EPILEPSY AND LICENSING OF DRIVERS

The issue of motor vehicle driving and seizures is complex. Driving a car is an important life activity for most adults, and limitations may have important occupational and social impacts. Most persons with controlled seizure disorders can drive safely and with-out incident. However, some seizures pose a risk of injury and death to a patient who is driving when they occur, and there is a risk to others. Persons who have uncontrolled seizures of this type should not drive. The laws about epilepsy and driver-licensing vary among the states, and the treating physician should be aware of the requirements in his/her own locale.[11]

Several areas of legal interest occur in the man-agement of the patient with seizures who wishes to drive. First, what should the physician tell the seizure patient about driving? How should this be docu-mented? Second, what are the state Department of Motor Vehicle (DOMV) requirements and proce-dures for licensing people with seizures? How does the physician participate in the patient's obtaining a license? Finally, when a person with an active seizure disorder drives against medical advice, how does the physician balance his duty to maintain patient confidences with his duty to warn the state about behavior that places the patient and others in danger?

Physicians should inform patients with seizures of any recommended life-style, recreational, or occupational limitations related to the seizure disorder. To abstain from driving is a common recommendation following a seizure, particularly those that involve an alteration in consciousness or loss of motor control. Most states have a mandatory seizure-free interval, and physicians must be aware of their own state's regulations regarding licensing. In states with a mandatory seizure-free period, requirements vary from 3 months to 2 years. Restricted licenses are available in many states and may represent a way that persons can drive despite not meeting the statutory seizure-free interval. Examples are licenses that allow emergency driving only, or that allow driving to and from work only, or that limit driving to daylight hours.

Some states do not have a mandatory seizure-free interval prior to licensure; instead, decisions are based on individualized determinations. In such states, important data considered in each decision include the length of time since the last seizure, seizure type, precipitants, and other factors reasonably expected to affect the applicant's ability to control a motor vehicle. The DOMV in these states frequently solicits the recommendation of the treating physician.

The physician should make a medical judgment about necessary driving limitations, incorporating state requirements into his recommendations. If a restricted license or some other exception to the state rules appears appropriate, the physician can work with the patient and the state agency. Recommendations about driving restrictions, as well as other occupational and recreational limits, should be carefully documented in the patient's chart. One effective method of documentation is to have the patient record his understanding of what he has been advised in the chart. This process encourages discussion between the physician and patient and provides clear evidence of patient involvement.

The physician may find that direct interaction with the state's DOMV or similar agency is necessary. In several states, physicians are required to report patients with seizure disorders to the DOMV or another state agency. Mandatory reporting is, however, not common and is considered by many authorities unwise for many reasons. It infantilizes the patient, diminishes patient responsibility, and interposes a third party in the patient–physician relationship. Nonetheless, in these states, physicians can be penalized by the state, and they can potentially be held liable to third parties who are injured as a result of a seizure if this reporting activity is not accomplished. Although the physician is immunized from suit for providing such information to the state, the patient should still be told that the information will be transmitted.

In general, no information about a patient's medical condition should be released without the express consent of the patient. Many states require that the physician fill out periodic reports on persons with seizures who drive. Physicians must fill out these forms honestly and are usually immunized from suit for doing so. Nonetheless, it is wise to inform patients that the information is being sent. Office staff should be aware that complying with a state DOMV request does not mean that other requests (e.g., from the patient's employer) should be complied with.

Physicians should be aware of the drivers licensing procedures in their state. Typically, applicants for initial or renewal licensure complete forms developed by the DOMV. These forms may ask generally or specifically about seizure disorders. When a seizure disorder is identified, DOMV personnel may act on available information or may ask for more.

Once adequate information is available, DOMV personnel may grant the license, refuse it, or refer the question to a medical advisory panel, a group of experts who advise the state on the correct procedures as well as individual cases. If DOMV personnel refuse a license, a patient may be able to appeal to the medical advisory panel that reviews cases, and it may contact the physician for additional information. Based on its recommendation, the applicant may subsequently be granted or denied licensure. In some settings, negative decisions by the panel may be appealed through the court system.

Perhaps the most difficult problem that a physician can face occurs when a patient with poorly controlled seizures persists in driving despite medical advice. What is a physician to do in such instances? In states with mandatory reporting, the physician is not only able to report such behavior but may be required to do so. In some states, statutory immunities have been granted to physicians who warn of the risky behavior of a patient to third parties. In other states, there is no clear law on the subject. A model drivers licensing statute developed by the Epilepsy Foundation of America in conjunction with physician experts proposes that physicians be immunized for reporting, in good faith, patients with seizures who drive despite loss of consciousness or loss of bodily control.[12] Also, a health professional was found liable for not notifying

474 NEUROLOGY FOR THE NON-NEUROLOGIST

the identified potential victim of a patient who threatened her.[13] Although the law is not settled, it is unlikely that a court would find a physician liable for breaching confidentiality if he notified the state when a patient refused to comply with medical advice and continued driving despite ongoing seizures that made such behavior unsafe.

Additional information on the status of state and federal laws in this changing area can be obtained from the Epilepsy Foundation of America by phone at 1-800-EFA-1000, or on their Web site, www.efa.org.

QUESTIONS AND DISCUSSION

1. For informed consent to be valid:

A. It must be given voluntarily.
B. It must be given after information is supplied to the patient in an understandable fashion.
C. The patient must be competent.
D. It must be accompanied by a witnessed form.

Answers (A) and (C) are correct. (B) is correct unless the patient has waived the information provision or unless the physician has used the therapeutic privilege exception (which should be used only cautiously). (D) is incorrect: Although informed consent should be documented, a specific form and witnessing is not absolutely necessary. Informed-consent forms may be useful in demonstrating consent, but they are not foolproof and if not "user friendly" can actually do more harm than good.

2. An adult patient is competent to provide consent unless he has been judged incompetent in legal proceedings. True or false?

The statement is false. A patient must be both clinically and legally competent to provide informed consent. An adult patient is presumed to be legally competent unless he has been found incompetent in judicial proceedings. Clinical competence is a medical decision. A patient may be clinically incompetent even though legally competent.

3. A 50-year-old man is found collapsed on a city street by paramedics who initiate cardiopulmonary resuscitation and take him to the hospital. One hour later, he is in the emergency room on a ventilator, totally unresponsive to all stimuli, and without brainstem reflexes. He has a completed donor card. The most appropriate action at this time is:

A. To pronounce brain death and call the transplant team to come in and recover the organs
B. To call the family to see if they agree with the organ donation
C. To observe the patient in the emergency department for 2 more hours to ensure that there is no change in the exam
D. To transfer the patient to an intensive care setting for further evaluation and workup

The answer is (D). The diagnosis of irreversible and total brain death has not been established. There is no clear etiology for this patient's clinical condition; there is no indication that conditions that can produce this clinical picture, but that might be reversible (e.g., drug overdose), have been ruled out. It is unlikely that a complete exam to establish brain death in this setting, including anoxia testing, has been performed. This patient should receive additional evaluation prior to being declared dead.

Although the family's consent for organ retrieval is not absolutely necessary in the presence of a valid organ donor card, most physicians wish to obtain consent of next of kin prior to organ retrieval.

4. In a state with mandatory reporting of persons with seizure disorders, the physician has a duty to inform the patient's family and employer of the diagnosis. True or false?

The statement is false. Mandatory reporting requirements apply only to the specific state agency mentioned in the statute. Disclosure to any other person or institution is precluded by the physician's duty to maintain patient confidences.

5. Actions to be taken when a patient with uncontrolled seizures continues to operate a motor vehicle include the following:

A. Educate the patient about the risks to himself and others.
B. Carefully document discussions with the patient about driving, and have the patient document his understanding of the discussion in the record as well.
C. In states with mandatory reporting, conform with the requirements of the applicable statute.
D. In cases in which patient education has been ineffective and the patient continues to place himself and others at risk by driving despite poor control of seizures, inform the patient of the need to report to the state Department of Motor Vehicles, and do so.

The answer is all of the above. Patient education is an important aspect of handling driving restrictions because of uncontrolled seizures. When a patient with uncontrolled seizures persists in driving despite warnings of the risk to self and others, the physician should inform the patient of the need to report to the state. Some states provide immunity for the physician who reports in these instances. Although not all states provide immunities, it is unlikely that a suit for breach of confidentiality would be successful. In some states, a physician may be found liable for failing to report dangerous behavior on the part of a patient.

SUGGESTED READING

1. *Schloendorff v. Society of New York Hospitals*, 211 N.Y. 125, 105 N.E. 2d 92 (1914)

2. Brandt AM: Racism and research: The case of the Tuskegee Syphilis Study. Hastings Cent Rep 8:21, 1978

3. *Hyman v. Jewish Chronic Disease Hospital*, 251 N.Y. 2d 818 (1964), 206 N.E. 2d 338 (1965)

4. A definition of irreversible coma: Report of the Ad Hoc Committee of the Harvard Medical School to examine the definition of brain death. JAMA 205:337, 1968

5. National Institutes of Health: A collaborative study: An appraisal of the criteria of cerebral death. A summary statement. JAMA 237:982, 1977

6. President's Commission for the Study of Ethical Problems in Medicine and Biomedical and Behavioral Research: Defining Death. A Report on the Medical, Legal and Ethical Issues in the Determination of Death. 1981

7. 12 Uniform Laws annotated 237 Cum. Sups. 1983

8. Quality Standards Subcommittee of the American Academy of Neurology: Practice parameters for determining brain death in adults. Neurology 45:1012, 1995

9. Widkicks EFM: Determining brain death in adults. Neurology 45:1003, 1995

10. *Strachan v. John F. Kennedy Memorial Hospital*, 583 A. 2d 346 (N.J. 1988)

11. Krumholz A: Driving and epilepsy: A historical perspective and review of current regulations. Epilepsia 35:668, 1994

12. American Academy of Neurology, American Epilepsy Society, and Epilepsy Foundation of America: Consensus statements, sample statutory provisions, and model regulations regarding driver licensing and epilepsy. Epilepsia 35:606, 1994

13. *Tarasoff v. Board of Regents of the University of California*, 17 Cal. 3d 425, 551 P. 2d 334 (1976)

Page numbers followed by f indicate figures; those followed by t indicate tables.